CANCER PREVENTION – FROM MECHANISMS TO TRANSLATIONAL BENEFITS

Edited by **Alexandros G. Georgakilas**

Cancer Prevention – From Mechanisms to Translational Benefits
Edited by Alexandros G. Georgakilas

Published by InTech
Janeza Trdine 9, 51000 Rijeka, Croatia

Publishing Process Manager Dejan Grgur

Technical Editor Teodora Smiljanic

Cover Designer InTech Design Team

Additional hard copies can be obtained from orders@intechopen.com

Cancer Prevention – From Mechanisms to Translational Benefits,
Edited by Alexandros G. Georgakilas
p. cm.
ISBN 978-953-51-0547-3

For EU product safety concerns:
IN TECH d.o.o., Prolaz Marije Krucifikse Kozulić 3, 51000 Rijeka, Croatia,
info@intechopen.com or visit our website at intechopen.com.

Meet the editor

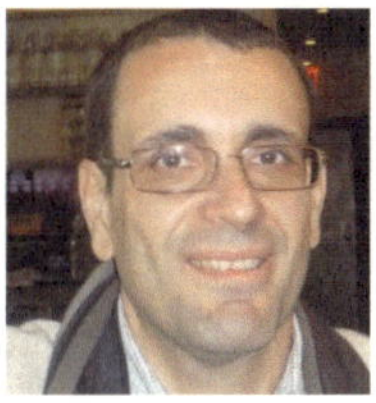

Dr Alexandros G. Georgakilas is an Associate Professor of Biology at East Carolina University (ECU) in Greenville, NC. He is responsible for the DNA Damage and Repair laboratory at ECU, USA, and has trained several graduate (1 PhD and 8 MSc) and undergraduate students. His work has been funded by various sources like East Carolina University, NC Biotechnology Center and International Cancer Control (UICC), which is the largest cancer fighting organization of its kind with more than 400 member organizations across 120 countries. He holds several editorial positions in scientific journals and his research work has been published in more than 50 peer-reviewed high profile journals like Cancer Research, Journal of Cell Biology and Proceedings of National Academy of Sciences USA, and has more than 900 citations. Ultimately, he hopes to translate his work of basic research into clinical applications using DNA damage clusters as cancer or radiation biomarkers for oxidative stress.

Contents

Preface

There is growing evidence on the importance of studies focusing on mechanisms and strategies leading to cancer prevention. The plethora of approaches include regulation of oxidative stress using antioxidant therapies, carefully balanced diets and living habits, epidemiological evidence and molecular approaches on the role of key biological molecules such as antioxidant enzymes, vitamins, proteins and naturally occurring free radical scavengers as well as controversial results and clinical applications. These are some of the topics that this book highlights. Furthermore, it provides comprehensive reviews of the state-of-the-art techniques and advances of cancer prevention research of different areas and how all this knowledge can be translated into therapeutic benefits as well as controversies. The primary target audience for the book includes PhD students, researchers, biologists, medical doctors and professionals who are interested in mechanistic studies on cancer prevention, clinical approaches and associated topics.

In section 1, top experts discuss a diverse set of carcinogenesis mechanisms with emphasis in oxidative stress, DNA damage and inflammation. Specifically, Dr Li Yang and colleagues discuss the targeting of tumor microenvironments and cancer prevention. Dr Du's chapter concentrates on the role of inflammatory reactive oxygen species (ROS) in Fanconi anemia hematopoiesis and leukemogenesis. Dr Eddy Yang and colleagues concentrate on the interplay between inflammation, DNA damage and cancer exploring the positive roles of vitamin D, retinoid and antioxidants. Dr Cofre's chapter focuses on Kaiso protein and prognosis of cancer discussing especially the role of immunohistochemistry in the current epigenetic paradigm. Finally, for this section, Drs. Showalter and Czerniecki 'dissect' very successfully the targeting of molecular pathways for prevention of high-risk breast cancer.

In section 2, chapters focus on the contribution of specific dietary and lifestyle patterns to cancer as well as in prevention. Dr Novaković and colleagues discuss how nutrition, physical activity, tobacco and alcohol use may contribute to carcinogenesis and the necessary lifestyle changes to prevent the appearance of a malignancy. Dr Kotzev's chapter concentrates on the prevention of colorectal cancer and especially the various risk and protective factors for colorectal polyps and cancer. Dr. Wada's work focuses on the preventive effects of food components and commonly used supplements in colorectal cancer as well as controversies. Dr Kaliora's and Dr Kountouri's chapter discusses the exciting chemopreventive activity of Mediterranean medicinal plants while Dr De Souza's comprehensive review chapter explores critically the dietary manipulation for therapeutic effect in prostate cancer. Dr Barone's work discusses extensively the roles of phytoestrogens as nutritional modulators in colon cancer prevention. On the same note, Dr Akpinar-Bayizit and colleagues concentrate on the unique therapeutic potential of pomegranate and its products for prevention of cancer. Last but not least, Dr Sanghvi and colleagues focus on the prevention of cervical cancer in women living with HIV in the developing word.

The last section of this book, section 3, targets strategies for effective prevention and translational benefits i.e. from the bench to the clinic. The chapter by Dr Kreps on strategic communication for cancer prevention and control, and especially the ways for reaching and influencing vulnerable audiences opens the discussion in this section. Dr Lichtveld and colleagues concentrate on the advantageous creation of a sustainable cancer workforce through focusing on disparities and cultural competence. Dr Morré and Dr Morré shed light on the opportunities for cancer prevention based simply on early and reliable detection. The comprehensive review by Dr Phillips and Dr Crawford critically presents the changing landscape of prostate cancer chemoprevention with all current strategies and future directions. In a more clinical direction, Dr Craina and colleagues concentrate on the current advances in the field of therapeutic strategies in endometrial cancer. Finally, our concluding chapter for this book, by Dr Roca-Pardiñas and colleagues targets the significance of reducing false positives in CAD mammographic schemes for detecting breast microcalcificacions, a type of radiologic signs of irregular shape.

Dr. Alexandros Georgakilas,
PhD, Associate Professor,
Head of DNA Damage and Repair Laboratory,
Biology Department,
Howell Science Complex,
East Carolina University,
Greenville NC,
USA

Section 1

Mechanisms of Carcinogenesis, Role of Oxidative Stress, Inflammation and DNA Damage

Targeting Tumor Microenvironments for Cancer Prevention and Therapy

Li V. Yang[1,2,3], Reid D. Castellone[1] and Lixue Dong[1]
[1]*Department of Internal Medicine, Division of Hematology/Oncology,*
[2]*Department of Anatomy and Cell Biology, Brody School of Medicine,*
East Carolina University, Greenville, North Carolina,
[3]*UNC Lineberger Comprehensive Cancer Center, Chapel Hill,*
North Carolina,
U.S.A.

1. Introduction

Solid tumors comprise not only cancer cells but also host stromal cells, such as vascular cells, inflammatory/immune cells, and cancer-associated fibroblasts. The crosstalk between cancer cells and stromal cells plays an important role in tumor growth, metastasis, and response to antitumor therapy (Hanahan and Weinberg, 2011; Joyce and Pollard, 2009; Petrulio et al., 2006). Cancer cells with oncogenic mutations are central to tumor formation. Endothelial cells in tumors form new blood vessels (angiogenesis) which bring oxygen and nutrients to the growing tumor (Ferrara and Kerbel, 2005), and also regulate leukocyte infiltration and tumor cell metastasis (Chouaib et al., 2010). Inflammatory cells have both tumor-promoting and tumor-preventing effects (Grivennikov et al., 2010; Hanahan and Weinberg, 2011). Fibroblasts are the most abundant cells in the tumor stroma and have been demonstrated to have tumor-promoting activities (Bhowmick et al., 2004). Moreover, cancer cells within tumors are heterogeneous and composed of distinct subpopulations with different states of tumorigenicity. One subpopulation of cells that has recently been extensively studied is the cancer initiating cell or cancer stem cell (CSC) (Cho and Clarke, 2008), which exhibits high capacity of generating new tumors.

The microenvironment in solid tumors is very distinct from that in normal tissues. Due to deregulated cancer cell metabolism, highly heterogeneous vasculature and defective blood perfusion, the tumor microenvironment is characterized by hypoxia and acidosis (Cairns et al., 2006; Gatenby et al., 2006; Gatenby and Gillies, 2004). The uncontrolled proliferation of tumor cells results in a growing mass that rapidly consumes oxygen, glucose and nutrients (Gatenby and Gillies, 2004). When an oxygen diffusion limit is reached, some regions of a tumor become hypoxic. Cancer cells rely heavily upon glycolysis ('Warburg effect') to generate ATP and metabolic intermediates for biosynthesis (Gatenby and Gillies, 2004; Vander Heiden et al., 2009). There is much evidence to link the connection between the adaptation to hypoxia and the development of an aggressive tumor phenotype in both experimental and clinical settings (Chang et al., 2011; Gatenby and Gillies, 2004). In addition to hypoxia, the existence of acidosis is a defining hallmark of the tumor microenvironment.

This condition arises mainly due to an increase in the production of lactic acid by glycolysis along with other proton sources (Gatenby and Gillies, 2004; Helmlinger et al., 2002; Yamagata et al., 1998). Acidosis is a selection force for cancer cell somatic evolution, modulates cancer cell invasion and metastasis, and affects the efficacy of some chemotherapeutic drugs (Cairns et al., 2006; Gatenby et al., 2006; Gatenby and Gillies, 2004).

Here we will describe cellular heterogeneity, hypoxia, and acidosis in the tumor microenvironment, and discuss some recent progresses in targeting tumor angiogenesis, inflammation, hypoxia and acidosis-related pathways for cancer prevention and therapy.

2. Tumor microenvironments and cancer progression

2.1 Complex cellular components in solid tumors

Tumor is an aberrantly proliferating tissue that contains cancerous cells and host stromal cells such as vascular cells, inflammatory cells, and fibroblasts. These cells are crucial for cancer initiation, progression and metastasis and have been exploited as targets for cancer therapy and prevention (Ferrara and Kerbel, 2005; Fukumura and Jain, 2007; Hanahan and Weinberg, 2011).

2.1.1 Vascular cells

Tumor blood vessels, like normal vessels, are composed of endothelial cells, pericytes/smooth muscle cells and basement membrane. However, all of these components are morphologically and/or functionally different from the normal counterparts (Baluk et al., 2005).

Tumor-associated endothelial cells (TECs) are the major player in the formation of tumor vasculature through sprouting from pre-existing blood vessels (a process called 'angiogenesis'). During blood vessel formation, endothelial cells proliferate, migrate and form the inner layer of a lumen, followed by basement membrane formation and pericyte attachment. Angiogenesis is stimulated by excessive pro-angiogenic factors secreted by tumor cells or stromal cells in an oxygen-depleted microenvironment. Moreover, bone marrow-derived endothelial progenitor cells recruited to tumor stroma can contribute to blood vessel construction by incorporating into vessels (Lyden et al., 2001). New blood vessel formation is critical for tumor development and progression, as it delivers nutrients and oxygen to growing tumor and removes metabolic wastes. In addition, vascular endothelial cells form a barrier between circulating blood cells, tumor cells and the extracellular matrix (ECM), thus playing a central role in regulating the trafficking of leukocytes and tumor cells (Chouaib et al., 2010). In this regard, endothelial cells are critical for boosting a host immune defense against cancer cells and for controlling tumor metastasis. However, the 'gate-keeping' function of endothelial cells in tumors is heavily compromised. TECs are not tightly associated with each other, resulting in wider inter-endothelial junctions that cause plasma leakage and hemorrhage (Hashizume et al., 2000). Consequently, tumor vasculature is often leaky and less efficient in blood perfusion, leading to high interstitial fluid pressure, hypoxia and acidic extracellular pH that significantly affect the delivery and efficacy of chemotherapeutic drugs. The leaky blood vessels also facilitate the intravastion of tumor cells and promote tumor metastasis.

TECs are different from endothelial cells in normal tissues at several aspects. It has been reported that human hepatocellular carcinoma-derived endothelial cells, when compared to the ones from adjacent normal liver tissue, show increased apoptosis resistance, enhanced angiogenic activity and acquire more resistance to the combination of angiogenesis inhibitor with chemotherapeutic drugs (Xiong et al., 2009). Studies have also revealed distinct gene expression profiles of TECs and identified cell-surface markers distinguishing tumor versus normal endothelial cells (Seaman et al., 2007).

In blood vessels, pericytes are smooth muscle cell-like cells that cover the vascular tube. They are intimately associated with endothelial cells and embedded within the vascular basement membrane, and play an important role in the maintenance of blood vessel integrity. Pericytes in tumors are different from normal ones: in tumors, pericytes are often less abundant and more loosely attached to the endothelial layer (Abramsson et al., 2002; Morikawa et al., 2002). The abnormality in pericytes weakens the vessel wall and increases vessel leakiness. Pericytes express several markers, though none is pericyte-exclusive, including α-smooth muscle actin (αSMA), platelet-derived growth factor receptor-β (PDGFR-β) and NG2 (Gerhardt and Betsholtz, 2003; McDonald and Choyke, 2003). PDGF-B signaling is important for pericyte recruitment and attachment to endothelial cells during vascular development (Abramsson et al., 2002; Abramsson et al., 2003).

2.1.2 Inflammatory/immune cells

Tumors are often infiltrated by inflammatory cells, such as macrophages, neutrophils, lymphocytes, mast cells, and myeloid progenitors. This phenomenon was initially observed by Rudolf Virchow more than a century ago and thought as an immunological response attempting to eliminate cancer cells. Whereas immune cells play a role in recognizing and eradicating early cancer cells (Kim et al., 2007), mounting evidence has also shown that inflammatory cells within tumors can enhance tumor initiation and progression by helping cancer cells acquire hallmark capabilities (Grivennikov et al., 2010; Hanahan and Weinberg, 2011). Inflammation is considered as an 'enabling characteristic' of tumor biology (Hanahan and Weinberg, 2011).

Pathological studies show that the abundance of certain types of infiltrating inflammatory cells, such as macrophages, neutrophils and mast cells, is correlated with poor prognosis of cancer patients (Murdoch et al., 2008). Tumor associated macrophages (TAMs), along with mast cells, neutrophils and other immune cells, produce cytokines (e.g. TNFα and IL-1), chemokines (e.g. CCL2 and CXCL12), angiogenic factors (e.g. VEGF, PDGF, FGF and IL-8), and matrix-degrading enzymes (e.g. MMPs, cathepsin proteases and heparanase) (Grivennikov et al., 2010; Karnoub and Weinberg, 2006). Some inflammatory cells, particularly neutrophils, also generate reactive oxygen and nitrogen species. These bioactive factors promote cancer cell proliferation, invasion and resistance to apoptosis through, for instance, the interleukin-JAK/STAT pathway (Ara and Declerck, 2010), and induce new blood vessel formation in the tumor. Extracelluar matrix-degrading enzymes promote cancer cell invasion and metastasis, whereas accumulation of reactive oxygen and nitrogen species can cause DNA mutagenesis, suppress DNA repair enzymes, increase genomic instability, and aggravate cancer progression.

While the tumor-promoting effects of infiltrating inflammatory cells have been well documented, certain types of immune cells, particularly cytotoxic T cells and natural killer cells, exhibit anti-tumor activities. The high numbers of these cells within a tumor predict a favorable prognosis (de Visser, 2008; Fridman et al., 2011). Immune surveillance is considered as an important mechanism to inhibit carcinogenesis and maintain tumor dormancy (Kim et al., 2007). Evading immune destruction by downregulating tumor antigens, suppressing immune cell function and other means is an emerging hallmark of cancer cells and plays important roles in cancer progression and metastasis (Hanahan and Weinberg, 2011). With regard to cancer therapy, blockade of CTLA-4 (cytotoxic T lymphocyte-associated antigen 4), a negative regulator of T cells, by the monoclonal antibody, ipilimumab, improved overall survival in patients with metastatic melanoma treated in combination with dacarbazine (Robert et al., 2011a). Moreover, expansion of tumor-infiltrating lymphocytes *ex vivo* and adoptive T-cell transfer immunotherapy led to regression of metastatic melanoma and durable responses in patients (Dudley et al., 2002; Rosenberg et al., 2011).

2.1.3 Fibroblasts

Fibroblasts account for the majority of stromal cells within solid tumors and are the principal source of ECM constituents (Chang et al., 2002). Fibroblasts in tumors are termed as cancer-associated fibroblasts (CAFs).

Tumors have been described as wounds that do not heal (Dvorak, 1986). Indeed, it has been observed that tumor-associated fibroblasts are biologically similar to the ones involved in wound healing or fibrosis (Ryan et al., 1973; Schor et al., 1988). Fibroblasts involved in these processes produce more ECM proteins and proliferate faster than the normal counterparts from healthy tissues (Castor et al., 1979; Muller and Rodemann, 1991). Fibroblasts with these properties are referred as "activated fibroblasts" or "myofibroblasts", due to their characteristic expression of α-smooth muscle actin (α-SMA) (Gabbiani, 2003; Ronnov-Jessen et al., 1996). Fibroblasts can be activated by various stimuli, such as transforming growth factor-β (TGFβ), epidermal growth factor (EGF), platelet-derived growth factor (PDGF) and fibroblast growth factor 2 (FGF2) (Zeisberg et al., 2000).

CAFs play an important role in promoting tumor initiation and progression by stimulating angiogenesis and tumor cell growth and invasion (Shimoda et al., 2010). The existence of a large number of CAFs in tumors is often associated with poor prognosis (Maeshima et al., 2002; Surowiak et al., 2006). CAFs produce growth factors, cytokines, chemokines and ECM proteases to stimulate angiogenesis and cancer cell proliferation and invasion. For example, CAFs secrete elevated levels of stromal cell-derived factor 1 (SDF-1; also called CXCL12) that facilitates angiogenesis by recruiting endothelial progenitor cells into the tumor (Orimo et al., 2005). SDF-1 can also interact with the CXCR4 receptor expressed on the surface of cancer cells, thus stimulating tumor cell growth and promoting tumor progression *in vivo* (Orimo and Weinberg, 2006). TGFβ, another factor produced by CAFs, is a critical mediator of the epithelial-to-mesenchymal transition (EMT); therefore, CAFs might contribute to EMT in nearby cancer cells and promote their invasiveness (Shimoda et al., 2010). Moreover, CAFs facilitate cancer cells to invade ECM and metastasize by releasing ECM-degrading proteases, such as matrix metalloproteinases (MMPs) (Boire et al., 2005; Sternlicht et al., 1999).

CAFs can maintain the myofibroblastic properties even after several passages *in vitro* without further signaling from carcinoma cells. How do CAFs acquire and maintain their activated phenotype? There are some controversial results with regard to the presence of somatic genetic alterations in CAFs. It has been reported that stroma microdissected from various human cancers exhibited some genetic alterations, such as chromosomal loss of heterozygosity (LOH) and somatic mutations (Currie et al., 2007; Kurose et al., 2002; Moinfar et al., 2000; Paterson et al., 2003; Tuhkanen et al., 2004; Wernert et al., 2001). Other reports also demonstrated that in the process of tumor development, fibroblasts that have lost p53 activity were clonally selected, leading to a highly proliferative stroma (Hill et al., 2005; Kiaris et al., 2005). In contrast, several genome-wide genetic analyses, including CGH and SNP arrays, were not able to detect any genetic alterations in the myofibroblasts isolated from various human cancers (Qiu et al., 2008; Walter et al., 2008). Other studies have suggested that epigenetic modifications within the genome of CAFs, such as DNA methylation, might be the reason (Hu et al., 2005; Jiang et al., 2008). Further studies are required to clarify these issues.

2.1.4 Cancer stem/initiating cells

Although cancer can originate from a single transformed cell, not all the cancer cells within a tumor are identical; in other words, cancer cells become heterogeneous during the somatic evolution process, reflected by distinct tumor regions with different histopathological characteristics and various degrees of tumor hallmark capacities. Moreover, mounting evidence indicates that tumor cells are also heterogeneous with regard to the capability to generate new tumors (Cho and Clarke, 2008; Lobo et al., 2007). Multiple studies showed that distinct subpopulations of cancer cells could be sorted from primary tumor samples based on their cell-surface antigen profiles. When different subpopulations of cells were injected into immune-deficient mice, only a subset of cells was able to propagate tumor growth, whereas other cells were unable to induce tumor regeneration (Lobo et al., 2007). This population of cancer cells has also been demonstrated to have the ability of self-renewal and differentiation, two hallmark characteristics of stem cells (Clarke et al., 2006). In addition, these cells also expresses some markers of normal stem cells (Al-Hajj et al., 2003); hence, these cells are termed as 'cancer stem cells' (CSCs; also referred as cancer initiating cells or tumorigenic cancer cells).

CSCs were initially identified in leukemia (Bonnet and Dick, 1997; Lapidot et al., 1994) and later in solid tumors that include cancers of breast, brain, pancreas, head and neck, and colon (Al-Hajj et al., 2003; Dalerba et al., 2007; Li et al., 2007; O'Brien et al., 2007; Prince et al., 2007; Ricci-Vitiani et al., 2007; Singh et al., 2004). Studies of leukemia stem cells suggest that, CSCs may arise from normal stem cells that acquire oncogenic mutations and undergo transformation (Fialkow, 1990; Lapidot et al., 1994; Lobo et al., 2007), or progenitor cells that gain the ability to self-renew through oncogenic transformation (Cozzio et al., 2003; Krivtsov et al., 2006; So et al., 2004). However, recent observations suggest that CSCs may also be derived from non-CSCs via the EMT process (Mani et al., 2008; Morel et al., 2008; Singh and Settleman, 2010), which plays an important role in morphogenesis and in promoting tumor cell motility and invasiveness (Hugo et al., 2007; Thiery, 2003). This model indicates that whereas CSCs can differentiate into non-CSCs; non-CSCs may also be reprogrammed and converted to CSCs, suggesting the existence of a dynamic interconversion between CSCs and non-CSCs that is controlled by the tumor microenvironment (Gupta et al., 2009). Such plasticity of CSC state is absent in the conventional depiction of normal stem cells, and has changed the perception of CSCs biology.

With regard to the frequency of CSC representation in tumors, there are conflicting results and ongoing controversies. Initially, CSCs were described to exist only as small subpopulations within tumors (Bonnet and Dick, 1997; Lapidot et al., 1994); moreover, since normal stem cells are usually rare, it was assumed that CSCs should also be rare. However, recent studies on human melanoma suggested that as many as a quarter of the cancer cells could be CSCs (Kelly et al., 2007; Quintana et al., 2008). This disparity on the frequency of CSCs reported were partially attributed to the experimental xenograft conditions in which the ability of human tumor cells to seed and grow in a mouse tissue may vary (Quintana et al., 2008). The plasticity of CSCs state may also in part account for the differences of CSCs representation. The balance of the interconversion between CSCs and non-CSCs could be shifted in one direction or another in response to microenvironmental signals (Santisteban et al., 2009; Till et al., 1964). It is suggested that the proportion of CSCs may differ between tumor types, dependent on stromal microenvironment and somatic mutations within tumors as well as tumor progression stage (Gupta et al., 2009).

The existence of CSCs has attracted growing attention as CSCs may provide explanations for some puzzled clinical problems and imply novel cancer therapies (Clevers, 2011). CSCs have been shown to be more resistant to a variety of conventional radio/chemotherapies than non-CSCs (Chiu et al., 2010; Diehn et al., 2009; Li et al., 2008). Together with their ability to regenerate tumor and to colonize distant organs (Hermann et al., 2007), CSCs are proposed to be responsible for cancer recurrence following chemotherapy or radiation treatment, and for metastases that appear after surgical removal of a primary tumor. In addition, CSCs hypothesis implies that development of novel and more effective treatments that target the 'seeds' of the tumors might be a promising improvement of current therapy regimen. However, the plasticity of CSC phenotype implies that eliminating CSCs alone may not effectively cure tumors as they can be regenerated from non-CSCs, calling for dual targeting therapeutic regimens (Gupta et al., 2009). Moreover, there are controversies about the CSCs model and the experimental strategy employed to define the existence of CSCs. There are rising concerns about the xenograft assay, a typical experimental strategy in the CSC research, in which sorted cancer cells are xenotransplanted into immunodeficient mice. However, this method could induce cellular stress of the isolated cancer cells; moreover, the species barrier and the transplantation procedure within this approach could complicate the process of CSC identification (Clevers, 2011). It will be of importance to devise new strategies to detect functional presence of CSCs within a tumor.

2.2 Angiogenesis

The growth and progression of tumors rely on blood vessels to acquire oxygen and nutrients and to remove metabolic wastes (Papetti and Herman, 2002). During the early stage of tumor development, once the size of a tumor mass reaches the diffusion limit for oxygen and nutrients, it may stay in a dormancy state with a steady rate of cell proliferation and death (Fukumura and Jain, 2007). Some human tumors can remain dormant for a number of years. However, the steady state may be disturbed as oxygen-deprived tumor cells release angiogenic factors that trigger the 'angiogenic switch' and initiate new blood vessel formation from nearby existing ones (a process called angiogenesis) (Hanahan and

Folkman, 1996; Hanahan and Weinberg, 2000). Angiogenesis expands the tumor vascular network, enabling malignant cell proliferation and metastasis. Therefore, angiogenesis is a rate-limiting step in tumor development and progression.

Angiogenesis is controlled by a fine-tuned equilibrium between angiogenic and angiostatic factors (Baeriswyl and Christofori, 2009; Bergers and Benjamin, 2003; Carmeliet and Jain, 2000). Under normal physiological conditions, this balance is tightly regulated, so that the 'angiogenic switch' is 'on' only when needed and otherwise remains 'off'. Moreover, the newly formed vessels rapidly mature and become quiescent. By contrast, in tumors, the balance between positive and negative controls is disrupted due to an overproduction of pro-angiogenic factors. Consequently, new blood vessels are constantly produced in tumors. To date, more than two dozen pro-angiogenic factors and similar number of anti-angiogenic factors have been identified. Key pro-angiogenic molecules include vascular endothelial growth factor (VEGF), angiopoietin 1 (Ang1), platelet-derived growth factor (PDGF), placenta growth factor (PlGF), fibroblast growth factor 2 (FGF2), hepatocyte growth factor (HGF), among others (Adini et al., 2002; Papapetropoulos et al., 1999). Important angiogenic inhibitors include thrombospondin, angiostatin, endostatin, canstatin and tumstatin (Folkman, 2006; Kazerounian et al., 2008; Nyberg et al., 2005).

VEGF signaling pathway is the most prominent and best characterized pro-angiogenic pathway (Ferrara et al., 2003). The VEGF family includes VEGF-A, B, C, D, and PlGF (Ferrara, 2002; Hicklin and Ellis, 2005). VEGF-A (also called VEGF) is the major regulator of tumor angiogenesis. There are several isoforms of VEGF-A, with 121, 165, 189 and 206 amino acids, which are generated by alternative splicing (Houck et al., 1991; Tischer et al., 1991). VEGF-A mainly binds to VEGF receptor 2 (VEGFR-2) and triggers various downstream signaling pathways to up-regulate genes that stimulate endothelial cell proliferation, migration and survival and increase vascular permeability (Dvorak, 2002; Shibuya and Claesson-Welsh, 2006). VEGF is expressed at elevated levels in most types of human cancer. This can be caused by diverse genetic and epigenetic factors (Kerbel and Folkman, 2002; Kerbel, 2008). Hypoxia, a hallmark of tumor microenvironment, is an important inducer of VEGF through the hypoxia-inducible factor (HIF) 1α and 2α (Semenza, 2003). In addition, inflammatory cytokines, growth factors and chemokines can also induce VEGF expression. Other genetic causes include activation of oncogenes, such as mutant ras (Rak et al., 1995), or inactivation of tumor-suppressor genes, such as the von Hippel-Lindau (VHL) tumor suppressor (Patard et al., 2009).

In addition to VEGF, there are other important signaling pathways that regulate angiogenesis. Endothelial cell-associated delta-like ligand (Dll) 4-notch signaling pathway acts as negative feedback mechanism of VEGF signaling to prevent excessive tumor angiogenesis (Lobov et al., 2007; Ridgway et al., 2006). HGF/c-Met signaling can induce VEGF and VEGFR expression and also promote angiogenic proliferation and survival (You and McDonald, 2008). FGF2 signaling can stimulate angiogenesis independent of VEGF (Beenken and Mohammadi, 2009). PDGF-B signaling is important for the recruitment of pericytes to nascent blood vessels and stabilization/maturation of the vasculature (Lindahl et al., 1997). The angiopoietins (Ang-1, 2), interacting with the Tie2 receptor, act in cooperation with VEGF to promote angiogenesis and stabilize and mature new vasculature (Augustin et al., 2009). PlGF, signaling through VEGFR1, is another growth factor that induces endothelial cell proliferation, migration and survival (Fischer et al., 2007).

Moreover, endothelial progenitor cells can also be recruited and contribute to the formation of new blood vessels.

Due to the imbalanced expression of pro- and anti-angiogenic factors (Jain, 2005), tumor vasculature is often abnormal in architecture and function (Baluk et al., 2005; Fukumura and Jain, 2007). In contrast to the well-organized normal vascular tree, tumor blood vessels are highly variable in size, shape, and branching pattern. They are tortuous, dilated, irregularly shaped, and lack the normal hierarchy of arterioles, capillaries and venules. The structure of vessel wall is also defective, with large inter-endothelial junctions and loose perivascular cells attachment (McDonald and Choyke, 2003; Morikawa et al., 2002). Hence, tumor blood vessels are often leaky and hemorrhagic. Vascular permeability in tumor is generally higher than that in normal tissues, leading to increased interstitial fluid pressure. Also, blood flow in tumor vessels is irregular, slower, oscillating, and sometimes can even reverse the direction. Therefore, in spite of the production of excess blood vessels, the perfusion efficiency in tumor is still low. The aberrant tumor vasculature fails to meet the demand of growing tumor for nutrients and oxygen, as well as to adequately remove waste products. Chronically, the tumor microenvironment becomes hypoxic and acidic (Fukumura and Jain, 2007). As stated in more detail in the following sections, hypoxia and acidosis are selection forces for cancer cell somatic evolution and also significantly affect radiation sensitivity and chemotherapeutic efficacy.

As angiogenesis plays a critical role in tumor growth and progression, anti-angiogenesis therapy has been developed aiming to halt tumor growth by depriving cancer cells of the blood supply (Ferrara and Kerbel, 2005). Most of the angiogenesis inhibitors target the VEGF signaling pathway, including antibodies directly against VEGF and small molecules inhibiting its receptors. These anti-angiogenic agents have provided clinical benefits in patients with various types of cancers. Detailed discussion on anti-angiogenesis therapy is presented in the Section 3.1.

2.3 Hypoxia

The defective architecture and functionality of tumor blood vessels results in the occurrence of hypoxic regions in solid tumors (Fukumura and Jain, 2007; Gatenby and Gillies, 2004). Hypoxia is further exacerbated by the uncontrolled and rapid proliferation of tumor cells. These cancerous cells consume large amounts of oxygen and nutrients during their rapid divisions, further dictating the need for ample blood supply. As the oxygen diffusion limit is reached and the partial pressure of oxygen, pO_2, drops towards zero, cells must adapt and rely upon alternative means to acquire energy in this hypoxic microenvironment (Bertout et al., 2008; Cairns et al., 2006; Fukumura and Jain, 2007; Gatenby and Gillies, 2004, 2007). A common adaptation strategy is the dependence upon glycolytic metabolism, coined the 'Warburg Effect' (Gatenby and Gillies, 2004; Warburg, 1956). In cancer cells, a large portion of glucose is utilized through glycolysis, by which each glucose molecule is converted to two ATP and two lactic acid molecules. In contrast, normal cells obtain the majority of their ATP through oxidative phosphorylation, which results in the release of 36 ATP from one glucose molecule (Gatenby and Gillies, 2004; Vander Heiden et al., 2009). While less efficient in ATP production, glycolysis generates intermediate molecules as substrates for nucleotide, lipid and amino acid biosynthesis, which is crucial for rapidly dividing cancer cells (Vander Heiden et al., 2009). It is proposed that the acquisition of glycolytic metabolism offers a selective advantage for cancerous cells, allowing them to adopt a more malignant phenotype (Gatenby and Gillies, 2004; Vander Heiden et al., 2009).

In addition to the noted alteration in the mode of energy acquisition, hypoxia is also known to regulate gene expression of cells. To proliferate and thrive in a hypoxic environment, cancer cells must modulate numerous cellular pathways. For example, pathways that initiate the acquisition of a motile and invasive phenotype, such as the c-Met pathway (Eckerich et al., 2007), are activated to facilitate cancer cells to leave the primary, hypoxic tumor (Hanahan and Weinberg, 2011). It has been discovered that hypoxia-inducible factor 1 (HIF-1) is a master regulator of many of the pathways that allow cancer cells to thrive in a hypoxic environment (Bertout et al., 2008; Semenza, 2007a, b). HIF-1 is reported to control the transcription of many genes, including those needed for maintaining cell viability, vascularization, glucose uptake, and metabolic reprogramming. HIFs are known to regulate pro-angiogenic and pro-glycolytic pathways. In animal models, HIF-1 overexpression has been associated with invasion, tumor growth and increased vascularization. Furthermore, HIF-1α overexpression has been correlated with an increase in patient mortality (Rankin and Giaccia, 2008; Semenza, 2007a). HIF proteins have also recently been attributed to the survival and self-renewal of cancer stem cells (CSCs), which are involved in cancer cell propagation and the development of aggressive and metastatic phenotypes (Heddleston et al., 2010; Wang et al., 2011). The Notch and Oct4 pathways, responsible for maintaining the stem cell phenotype, have been reported to be under the regulatory control of HIF protein. Due to the immense involvement of HIF-1 in transcriptional regulation of genes that promote survival and progression of cancer cells in a hypoxic environment, it serves as a target of anti-cancer therapies (Semenza, 2007a; Tennant et al., 2010).

Another effect of hypoxia lies in the resistance of cancer cells to chemotherapy and radiation treatment (Cairns et al., 2006; Gatenby and Gillies, 2004). Oxygen is known to increase the effectiveness of radiation therapy as it is a potent radiosensitizer. In turn, hypoxia can invoke a resistance of cancer cells to radiation and some forms of chemotherapy (Cairns et al., 2006). This hypoxia-induced resistance can be attributed, among many factors, to an inability in chemotherapy and radiation to induce cell cycle arrest, DNA breaks, and apoptosis (Wilson and Hay, 2011). Furthermore, hypoxia can up-regulate the expression of genes known to cause resistance to chemotherapeutics, such as multidrug resistance gene (MDR1), and downregulate the expression of apoptosis regulating genes (Bertout et al., 2008).

2.4 Acidosis

As discussed above, cancer cells develop a modified form of energy metabolism in which glucose incorporated by the tumor is mainly converted into ATP and lactic acid through glycolysis even in the presence of oxygen (Gatenby and Gillies, 2004; Vander Heiden et al., 2009; Warburg, 1956). In addition, it is believed this switch to a glycolytic phenotype, although inefficient in ATP production, is overall beneficial for rapidly dividing cancer cells (Cairns et al., 2011; Vander Heiden et al., 2009). However, the glycolytic metabolism directly results in the development of acidic interstitial pH in the tumor microenvironment, another stress that cancer cells must evolve to evade.

Acidosis is another defining hallmark of the tumor microenvironment. Interstitial accumulation of hydrogen ions is due to the production of lactic acid from glycolysis and other proton sources from, such as, ATP hydrolysis and carbonic acid (Gatenby and Gillies, 2004; Helmlinger et al., 2002; Yamagata et al., 1998). Whereas the intracellular pH of cancer cells is kept neutral, an extracellular pH of 6.5-6.8 is often observed in the interstitial space of tumors (Griffiths et al., 2001). To maintain a relatively neutral intracellular pH, cancer cells utilize an array of acid-base transporters, such as sodium/hydrogen exchangers, vacuolar-type H^+-ATPases, and monocarboxylate transporters, to extrude the excess protons from cancer cells (Izumi et al., 2003; Webb et al., 2011).

Just as the ability for tumor cells to adapt to a hypoxic microenvironment offers a distinct evolutionary advantage towards an aggressive phenotype, so does the ability for cancer cells to survive in an acidic microenvironment. Upon exposure to the low extracellular pH found in and around solid tumors, many of the normal, non-cancerous cells in the surrounding tissue undergo cell death, often attributed to p53-dependent pathways. Cancer cells that have evolved to be immune to this notable acidosis are often left highly invasive and aggressive (Gatenby and Gillies, 2004). Acidosis is also known to contribute towards tumor cell invasion through the release of proteolytic enzymes that degrade extracellular matrix. Hypoxia and acidosis have been reported to increase the secretion and activity of matrix metalloproteinases (MMPs) and other matrix-degrading enzymes (Bourguignon et al., 2004; Johnson et al., 2000; Ridgway et al., 2005).

Acidosis also plays a role in the cytotoxic effectiveness of radiation and chemotherapy. Microenvironmental acidosis has been shown to invoke a resistance to radiation-induced apoptosis of cancer cells (Hunter et al., 2006). Acidic extracellular pH can also modulate the uptake of chemotherapeutic drugs, especially the weak acid and weak base drugs (Cairns et al., 2006; Gerweck et al., 2006). In the acidic tumor microenvironment, weak base drugs, such as doxorubicin, exist in a highly charged state. In turn, the uptake of these drugs across the plasma membrane is inhibited, thereby reducing the ability of the chemotherapeutic drugs to reach their cytotoxic target. In contrast, weak acid drugs, such as chlorambucil, exist in a non-charged state at acidic pH and, therefore, have increased cell permeability.

2.5 Somatic evolution and cancer cell metastasis

As normal cells are transformed to pre-malignant tumor cells and further towards malignant and metastatic tumors, the process of somatic evolution is actively used (Gatenby and Gillies, 2004). Cancer cells arise through gene mutations. Oncogenes with a dominant gain of function arise, while tumor suppressor genes become inactivated through a loss of function. As a result of somatic evolution, some of the traits that promote the cancerous phenotype include the evasion of apoptosis, limitless replicative potential, sustained angiogenesis, the ability for invasion and metastasis, and deregulated energy metabolism (Hanahan and Weinberg, 2011).

Carcinogenesis and Darwinian dynamics draw an analogy as new phenotypes are generated through heritable genetic changes and subsequent selection for the fittest by the environment (Gatenby and Gillies, 2004, 2008). It has been proposed that hypoxia and acidosis both apply extreme constraints and act as selection forces for progressive tumor cells. Cancer cells that have gained immunity to these conditions, such as through the Warburg effect and other adaptations, display a distinct advantage over neighboring normal cells. Cancer cells that are able to thrive in the harsh environment are highly aggressive with a resistant phenotype. Communication between tumor cells and the microenvironment is crucial for the cells to take advantage of the changes in the microenvironment and develop a malignant phenotype (Gatenby and Gillies, 2004; Lorusso and Ruegg, 2008).

There are many mechanisms by which cancer cell somatic evolution is driven by the microenvironmental selection forces. Primarily, various pathways crucial for cancer cell survival under the hypoxic and acidotic conditions are activated, such as those that promote a downregulation of apoptosis, a switch to glycolytic metabolism, and an upregulation of HIFs (Gatenby and Gillies, 2004; Heddleston et al., 2010; Vander Heiden et al., 2009; Wilson and Hay, 2011). Cancer cells resistant to acidosis and hypoxia often acquire p53 mutations. As p53 is important for apoptosis, cells that have a mutation in this gene exhibit an advantage as they are often immune to the cytotoxic microenvironment (Bertout et al., 2008). In addition, many tumor cells develop a very active sodium/hydrogen exchange system and other proton transport mechanisms, which facilitate the extrusion of excess protons (Izumi et al., 2003; Webb et al., 2011). The resulting cytoplasmic alkalinization is thought to be crucial for cell reproduction in the acidic environment. Therefore, the hallmarks of the tumor microenvironment, such as hypoxia and acidosis, actively function as selection forces to shape cancer cell phenotypes during the somatic evolution process (Gatenby and Gillies, 2004; Webb et al., 2011).

The ability to acquire a metastatic phenotype via somatic evolution is one of the most devastating properties of cancer cells, and is directly correlated with an increase in patient morbidity and mortality (Fidler, 2002; Steeg, 2006). Current cancer therapy approaches, such as surgery, radiation and chemotherapy, can be effective in controlling primary, localized tumor. However, these modes of treatment are severely limited in retarding the spread of cancer as they do little to impair metastasis. It is therefore evident that the development of novel means of combating tumor cell metastasis is crucial towards the eradication and control of this disease.

The general steps of tumor metastasis involve the initial acquisition of motility and invasiveness, intravasation, transit in the blood or lymph, extravasation and finally arrest and growth at a new site (Fidler, 2002; Sahai, 2007; Steeg, 2006). The tumor microenvironment plays a large role in the ability of cancer cells to acquire a metastatic phenotype. As previously touched upon, two of the defining characteristics of the tumor microenvironment, hypoxia and acidosis, both actively select for more invasive and metastatic phenotypes (Chang et al., 2011; Gatenby et al., 2006; Gatenby and Gillies, 2004). It is also reported that inflammatory cells, fibroblasts and other stromal cells in the tumor microenvironment can contribute to the progression of a tumor towards a more malignant, metastatic phenotype (Joyce and Pollard, 2009; Lorusso and Ruegg, 2008).

3. Tumor microenvironments as targets for cancer prevention and therapy

Cellular components and molecular pathways associated with tumor microenvironments have been exploited as targets for cancer prevention and therapy. In fact, combination therapy targeting both cancer cells and other related cells and pathways, such as vascular cells and immune cells, can lead to more effective cancer treatment (Cairns et al., 2006; Ferrara and Kerbel, 2005; Luo et al., 2009). Therapeutic approaches modulating angiogenesis, inflammation, and hypoxia and acidosis pathways will be discussed below.

3.1 Anti-angiogenesis cancer therapy

As described in the 'angiogenesis' session, tumors rely on angiogenesis to grow and disseminate. Therefore, it has been proposed that tumor growth can be inhibited by starving tumor cells through angiogenesis blockade (Folkman, 1971). Since VEGF is a major regulator of tumor angiogenesis, a number of agents targeting VEGF and its receptors have been developed and several have been approved by the Food and Drug Administration (FDA) for clinical applications. Among them, bevacizumab (Avastin, Genentech/Roche) is a humanized monoclonal antibody directly against VEGF (Ferrara et al., 2004; Presta et al., 1997), and sunitinib (Sutent, Pfizer) and sorafenib (Nexavar, Bayer) are small molecule inhibitors that target multiple receptor tyrosine kinases (RTK), including VEGF receptors and PDGF receptors (Faivre et al., 2007; Kupsch et al., 2005; O'Farrell et al., 2003).

Bevacizumab was approved by the FDA in 2004 on the basis of the survival benefit observed in a randomized phase III clinical trial, in which bevacizumab was administrated in combination with chemotherapy in patients with previously untreated metastatic colorectal cancer (Hurwitz et al., 2004). The clinical benefit of bevacizumab was also evaluated in other cancer types. The combination of bevacizumab with paclitaxel and carboplatin in patients with previously untreated nonsquamous non-small-cell lung cancer (NSCLC) improved primary endpoint of overall survival (OS) (Sandler et al., 2006). Moreover, the combined regimen of bevacizumab with 5-fluorouracil, leucovorin, and oxaliplatin (FOLFOX) were used to treat patients with previously treated metastatic colorectal cancers and prolonged progression-free survival (PFS) and OS (Giantonio et al., 2007). More recently, bevacizumab monotherapy was approved as a second-line therapy for glioblastoma multiforme (GBM) (Cohen et al., 2009). Some severe adverse effects of bevacizumab therapy, including gastrointestinal perforation and arterial thromboembolic complications, were observed in a small percentage of patients. Other side effects such as hypertension were also noticed (Eskens and Verweij, 2006; Verheul and Pinedo, 2007). Notably, in addition to the oncologic application, VEGF inhibitors are also used to treat the neovascular (wet) age-related macular degeneration (AMD), as VEGF has been demonstrated to be a mediator of ischemia-induced intraocular neovascularization (Chen et al., 1999; Ferrara et al., 2006; Gragoudas et al., 2004; Ng et al., 2006; Rosenfeld et al., 2006).

Sunitinib and sorafenib are RTK inhibitors that inhibit the tyrosine phosphorylation of VEGFRs, PDGFRs, c-kit, and Flt-3 (Fabian et al., 2005; Smith et al., 2004). Sunitinib has been reported to prolong the time to progression in imatinib-refractory gastrointestinal stromal tumors (Goodman et al., 2007). Sunitinib was also approved by FDA for the treatment of metastatic renal cell carcinoma (Motzer et al., 2009; Motzer et al., 2006). Sorafenib has been shown to increase PFS in patients with metastatic renal cell carcinoma (Escudier et al., 2007). In addition, sorafenib was approved for treating hepatocellular carcinomas (Lang, 2008; Llovet et al., 2008). Pazopanib, another RTKI, was approved for the treatment of metastatic renal cell carcinoma (Sternberg et al., 2010). Moreover, there are other anti-angiogenic agents under investigation that target other signaling molecules involved in angiogenesis, such as antibodies against angiopoietin-2 and PlGF which have been shown to delay tumor growth in preclinical models (Fischer et al., 2007; Oliner et al., 2004).

There were also some clinical trials with angiogenesis inhibitors that did not show significant clinical benefits. For instance, the combination of bevacizumab with gemcitabine didn't show improved PFS or OS in patients with chemotherapy-naïve advanced pancreatic cancer (Kindler et al., 2010). An earlier phase III trial of bevacizumab combined with gemcitabine and erlotinib for the same type of cancer increased PFS but didn't improve primary endpoint of OS either (Van Cutsem et al., 2009). PFS, although an indicator of the efficacy of drugs, is a poor surrogate for OS, as PFS benefits are not always translated into OS benefits (Wilkerson and Fojo, 2009). The controversies about whether to keep the FDA's approval of bevacizumab for metastatic breast cancer provide such an example. In 2008, bevacizumab was approved for treating breast cancer in combination with chemotherapy based on the results from the clinical trial E2100 (Miller et al., 2007). However, the study was only able to show an improved primary endpoint of PFS but not OS. Several subsequent clinical trials showed similar results (Miles et al., 2010; Robert et al., 2011b), which leads to recent recommended withdrawal of bevacizumab by FDA for metastatic breast cancer (Lenzer, 2011).

Another major problem is that, even in those successful trials, the VEGF pathway inhibitors can only generate transitory clinical responses in most patients, with increased survival typically measured in months (Kerbel, 2008). Almost inevitably, temporary tumor shrinkage or stasis was followed by tumor relapse and progression. The modest responses to the anti-angiogenic agents are partly due to the existence of resistance to the therapeutics (Bergers and Hanahan, 2008). Tumor cells and the stroma they reside in can adapt to the presence of angiogenesis inhibitors by acquiring means to evade angiogenesis blockade and sustain blood vessel and tumor growth. One important compensatory response is that, when the VEGF signaling pathway is inhibited, tumor may activate or up-regulate the expression of alternative pro-angiogenic factors, such as FGF2, PlGF, and PDGF pathways (Fernando et al., 2008); or in other cases, there are pre-existing redundant pro-angiogenic factors in the treated tumors (Bergers and Hanahan, 2008).

Furthermore, a growing list of studies indicates that anti-angiogenic therapies may even lead to increased tumor invasiveness and metastasis (Ebos et al., 2009; Paez-Ribes et al., 2009). Questions and concerns have been raised about the efficacy and safety of antiangiogenic agents in blocking different stages of tumor progression. Potential mechanisms of the increased metastasis may involve both tumor-dependent and host-mediated responses (Ebos and Kerbel, 2011), such as increased expression of pro-metastatic proteins (Pennacchietti et al., 2003; Rofstad and Halsor, 2002), induction of tumor cell EMT (Higgins et al., 2007), and pericyte dysfunction (Bergers et al., 2003), among others. Perhaps the most prevailing proposition is that inhibition of angiogenesis could elicit an elevated level of tumor hypoxia, which selects for cancer cell populations that are able to grow in low oxygen environments and promote tumor invasion and metastasis (Rapisarda and Melillo, 2009). Studies have demonstrated that hypoxia-induced mechanisms, such as the up-regulation of c-Met and interleukin 8 (Pennacchietti et al., 2003; Rofstad and Halsor, 2002; Steeg, 2003), can promote cancer cells to disseminate to distant locations (Kienast et al., 2010).

As a breakthrough in cancer treatment, anti-angiogenesis therapies have provided survival benefits in certain cancer types and represent an important complement to the traditional chemotherapy strategies. However, there are ongoing challenges, such as the lack of lasting benefits for the majority of patients and an emerging, though still controversial, possibility that increased tumor invasion and metastasis might in some instances be induced by anti-angiogenesis therapy. It will be of importance to understand the molecular basis of the treatment limitations and to formulate improved strategies to overcome them. For example, combining anti-angiogenic therapy with anti-hypoxia agents or anti-metastatic agents might help overcome the metastatic phenotype induced by increased tumor hypoxia.

3.2 Anti-inflammation in cancer chemoprevention and therapy

Numerous studies show that inflammation plays an important role in cancer initiation, progression and metastasis. As described in the Section 2, infiltrating inflammatory cells such as macrophages, mast cells and neutrophils produce reactive oxygen and nitrogen species, growth factors, cytokines, chemokines, proteases and other bioactive factors in the tumor microenvironment (de Visser et al., 2006; Grivennikov et al., 2010). These bioactive factors can induce DNA mutagenesis, inhibit DNA repair enzymes, stimulate cancer cell proliferation, degrade extracellular matrix, and promote cancer cell invasion and metastasis. On the other hand, certain types of infiltrating immune cells, such as cytotoxic T cells and natural killer cells, can inhibit tumor progression.

Chronic inflammation is closely associated with the development of some types of cancers. For instance, patients with inflammatory bowel disease or ulcerative colitis have an increased risk of developing colorectal cancer (Xie and Itzkowitz, 2008). Chronic *Helicobacter pylori* infection and ulcers are associated with gastric cancer and mucosa-associated lymphoid tissue lymphoma. Infection with hepatitis B virus increases the risk of developing liver cancer (Pages et al., 2010). Furthermore, epidemiological studies indicate that the use of aspirin and other nonsteroidal anti-inflammatory drugs is associated with a reduced cancer incidence. These widely documented observations provide the rationale to assess anti-inflammatory agents in cancer chemoprevention and therapy (Kashfi, 2009).

Nonsteroidal anti-inflammatory drugs (NSAIDs) have been extensively evaluated for cancer chemoprevention. Aspirin (acetylsalicylic acid), a prototype NSAID, inhibits the cyclooxygenase (COX) enzymes and suppress the production of prostaglandins and thromboxanes. Aspirin exhibits chemopreventive effects on colon cancer in several randomized trials. A recent study performed a 20-year follow-up of 5 randomized trials to investigate the long-term effects of aspirin (75-300 mg daily) on colorectal cancer incidence and mortality (Rothwell et al., 2010). 391 of 14,033 patients (2.8%) had colorectal cancer during a median 18.3-year follow-up. Compared to the control group, the incidence of colon cancer, but not rectal cancer, was lower in the aspirin group. Furthermore, the benefit of aspirin increased with the duration of treatment. Allocation to aspirin treatment for 5 years or longer reduced the risk of proximal colon cancer by ~ 70% and also decreased the risk of rectal cancer. Moreover, a meta-analysis of 3 randomized controlled trials showed that, in more than 2,000 patients with previously resected colorectal adenomas, the aspirin groups (dose range from 81 to 325 mg per day), in comparison to the placebo groups, had a lower rate of tumor recurrence (Gao et al., 2009). In addition to colorectal cancer, a recent study showed that daily aspirin treatment for 5 years or longer reduced the mortality from several common types of solid cancers (Rothwell et al., 2011). However, not all studies supported the protective role of aspirin in cancer prevention. In the Woman's Health Study, a low dose (100 mg) of aspirin every other day for an average 10 years of treatment did not reduce the risk of total, breast, colorectal, and other cancers (Cook et al., 2005). The major adverse effects of aspirin treatment are gastrointestinal bleeding and ulceration.

In addition to aspirin, COX-2 specific inhibitors have been tested as cancer chemopreventive agents. There are two COX genes in the cell: COX-1 is constitutively expressed in many tissues and COX-2 is induced upon inflammation and other stimuli (Botting, 2010). Earlier clinical studies showed that the COX-2 inhibitor, celecoxib (400 mg twice per day for 6 month), resulted in approximately 30% reduction in polyp number and size in familial adenomatous polyposis (FAP) patients (Steinbach et al., 2000). However, studies found that prolonged use of COX-2 inhibitors increased the risk of cardiovascular events in a dose-related manner (Baron et al., 2008; Solomon et al., 2005; Solomon et al., 2006). These findings led to the discontinuation of the clinical trials and the withdrawal of the drugs from the market. Clearly, drugs with improved safety profiles are required for the long-term use in cancer chemoprevention. In this respect, the "old" NSAID, aspirin, has been widely used to prevent cardiovascular diseases and, therefore, has a favorable cardiovascular profile.

Inflammatory chemokines and their receptors have also been exploited as targets for cancer therapy. Chemokines are a family of chemotactic cytokines that bind to cognate G protein-coupled receptors. Forty-seven chemokine members have been identified and are divided into 4 subfamilies: the CC subfamily, the CXC subfamily, the CX3C subfamily, and the XC subfamily. The chemokine receptors are comprised of the CCR subfamily, the CXCR subfamily, CX3CR1, and XCR1 (Lazennec and Richmond, 2010). In the tumor microenvironment, various chemokines are produced by cancer cells, inflammatory cells, fibroblasts, and endothelial cells. Chemokines can stimulate cancer cell growth and metastasis, recruit inflammatory cells, and promote tumor angiogenesis.

Stromal cell-derived factor-1 (SDF-1, also named CXCL12) and its receptor CXCR4 play important roles in the mobilization and homing of hematopoietic stem cells and the metastasis of cancer cells. AMD3100 (plerixafor), developed by Genzyme, is a small molecule that antagonizes the binding of CXCL12 to its receptor CXCR4, and was recently approved by FDA for stem cell mobilization in non-Hodgkin's lymphoma and multiple myeloma patients (Pusic and DiPersio, 2010). Clinical trials demonstrated that AMD3100 (plerixafor), together with G-CSF, significantly increased the mobilization of hematopoietic stem cells for autologous stem cell transplantation in patients with multiple myeloma and non-Hodgkin's lymphoma (DiPersio et al., 2009a; DiPersio et al., 2009b). AMD3100 (plerixafor) can also be used as a chemosensitizing agent. Studies showed that AMD3100 (plerixafor) impeded the interaction between leukemia cells and the bone marrow microenvironment, mobilized cancer cells into peripheral blood, and increased the sensitivity of multiple myeloma cells and acute myeloid leukemia cells to chemotherapeutic drugs (Azab et al., 2009; Nervi et al., 2009). Furthermore, CXCL12/CXCR4 inhibitors have therapeutic effects on other non-hematological cancers. In pre-clinical models, blockade of CXCR4 has been shown to inhibit the migration and metastasis of melanoma cells, oral squamous cell carcinoma cells, and gastric cancer cells (Kim et al., 2010; Uchida et al., 2011; Zhao et al., 2011). CXCR4 inhibitors could also chemosensitize and suppress the growth of pancreatic and ovarian cancer cells (Righi et al., 2011; Singh et al., 2010). Besides CXCL12/CXCR4, inhibitors for other chemokines/receptors, such as CCL2 and CCR4, are also undergoing clinical development for the treatment of leukemia and solid tumors (Lazennec and Richmond, 2010).

3.3 Molecular targeting of hypoxia pathways

As described in the Section 2, hypoxia inhibits the tumor killing effects of radiation and also regulates cancer cell apoptosis, invasiveness and metabolism (Cairns et al., 2006; Gatenby and Gillies, 2004). Hypoxia-inducible factors (HIFs) are master regulators of cell hypoxia responses and control the expression of numerous genes involved in angiogenesis, glycolytic metabolism, glucose transport, erythropoiesis, and other processes (Semenza, 2007b). Increased expression of HIFs is correlated with a worse prognosis in many types of cancers. Thus, HIFs have been proposed as a potential target for cancer therapy. Inhibitors of the HIF pathway have been developed and tested in preclinical models and/or clinical trials (Semenza, 2007a).

PX-478, a HIF-1α inhibitor, showed remarkable antitumor activity in human cancer xenograft models (Welsh et al., 2004), and also enhanced radiosensitivity of human pancreatic cancer xenografts (Schwartz et al., 2009). It has been shown that the degradation of HIF-1α can be induced through inhibiting the chaperone protein HSP90 (Isaacs et al., 2002). The HSP90 inhibitor, 17-AAG (Tanaspimycin), exhibited anti-tumor activities in multiple cancer cell models. A recent phase II clinical trial showed that 17-AAG (Tanaspimycin) plus trastuzumab had significant anti-cancer activity in $HER2^+$ breast cancer patients previously progressing on trastuzumab (Modi et al., 2011). It should, however, be noted that HIF-1α degradation is only one of the effects of HSP90 inhibitors as HSP90 is required for preventing the degradation of many other proteins.

As a response and adaptation to hypoxia in the tumor microenvironment, cancer cells rely substantially on glycolysis for ATP production. It was discovered by Otto Warburg decades ago that cancer cells preferentially utilize glycolytic metabolism even under aerobic conditions (known as 'Warburg effect') (Warburg, 1956). Since glycolysis only generates 2 ATP molecules per glucose, tumor cells evolve a compensatory mechanism by up-regulating the level of glucose transporters and significantly increasing glucose uptake.

Genes involved in glycolytic metabolism have been proposed as potential cancer therapeutic targets (Tennant et al., 2010). Studies demonstrate that HIFs directly activate the transcription of glucose transporters (e.g. GLUT1) and several key glycolytic enzymes (Semenza, 2007b). Some oncogenes and tumor suppressors, such as Myc, PI3K, p53 and PTEN, can also regulate the expression of genes important for glycolysis and cell metabolism (Dang et al., 2009; Tennant et al., 2010). A recent chemical screening identified a compound, STF-31, which could inhibit the glucose transporter 1 (GLUT1) and the Warburg effect, induce cell death of renal cell carcinoma and inhibit the growth of tumor xenografts (Chan et al., 2011). Agents have also been developed to target the enzymes in the glycolysis pathway. One such agent is the hexokinase inhibitor, 2-deoxyglucose, which has been shown to have anti-tumor activities in multiple cancer cell models (Loar et al., 2010; Zhang and Aft, 2009). Other potential anti-cancer targets in the glycolysis cascade includes pyruvate kinase, the tumor-specific pyruvate kinase M2 (PKM2) isoform, pyruvate dehydrogenase kinase 1 (PDK1), among others (Tennant et al., 2010; Vander Heiden et al., 2009). Inhibitors of these enzymes, such as TLN-232 and dichloroacetate (DCA), are being evaluated in clinical trials. A recent study showed that DCA had anti-tumor activities in glioblastoma patients (Michelakis et al., 2010).

Furthermore, major regulators of metabolic pathways, such as mTOR (mammalian target of rapamycin) and AMPK (AMP-activated protein kinase), have been employed as important targets for cancer therapy. In particular, the mTOR inhibitors, everolimus and temsirolimus, have been approved by FDA for the treatment of advanced renal cell carcinoma with clinical benefits in prolonging progression free survival and overall survival (Kwitkowski et al., 2010; Motzer et al., 2008). Moreover, epidemiological studies indicated that the cancer incidence is lower in diabetic patients treated with the AMPK agonist metformin (Bo et al., 2011). In a short-term prospective clinical trial, metformin treatment reduced colorectal aberrant crypt foci in non-diabetic patients (Hosono et al., 2010). These results indicate that metformin may be a useful agent for cancer prevention and therapy (Gonzalez-Angulo and Meric-Bernstam, 2010; Li, 2011).

In addition to targeting hypoxia-related molecular pathways, hypoxia itself can be utilized for cancer therapy. Bioreductive prodrugs, which are activated in hypoxic environments, have been evaluated as potential anti-cancer agents to selectively kill hypoxic tumor cells. For instance, apaziquone (EO9), a bioreductive prodrug, was used through instillation to treat bladder cancer and significantly reduced the rate of tumor recurrence in the clinical trials (Hendricksen et al., 2009; Jain et al., 2009).

Hypoxia as a hallmark of the tumor microenvironment has also been exploited to develop imaging approaches for cancer diagnosis. A family of nitroimidazole derivatives has been used as chemical tracers to detect hypoxia in tissues. A PET probe, ^{18}F-fluoromisonidazole (FMISO), has been applied to detect hypoxic regions in solid tumors and to assess the change of tumor hypoxia status in response to therapy such as anti-angiogenesis treatment (Szeto et al., 2009; Valable et al., 2011). In addition, the up-regulation of hypoxia-responsive glucose transporters in tumor cells has been utilized for [^{18}F] fluorodeoxyglucose positron emission tomography (FDG-PET). As the uptake of glucose is substantially increased in cancer cells, the radioactive [^{18}F] fluorodeoxyglucose tracer is preferentially accumulated in the tumor and can be detected by positron emission tomography (Buerkle and Weber, 2008). FDG-PET has been widely used in the clinic to detect tumors and metastases and assess the response of tumors to therapeutics.

3.4 Molecular targeting of acidosis-related pathways

In addition to hypoxia, extracellular acidosis is another major hallmark of the tumor microenvironment. To avoid the harmful accumulation of protons and decrease of intracellular pH (pHi), cancer cells must use the cellular transporter system to expel excess acids from the cells. Carbonic anhydrases (CA), monocarboxylate transporters (MCT), vacuolar-type H^+-ATPase proton pump (V-ATPase), and sodium/hydrogen exchangers (NHE) play important roles in cellular pH regulation (Izumi et al., 2003; Swietach et al., 2010; Webb et al., 2011). Furthermore, recent studies have shown that a family of proton-sensing G protein-coupled receptors regulates the behavior of tumor cells, immune cells, and blood vessels (Ludwig et al., 2003; Mogi et al., 2009; Yang et al., 2007). Targeting these pH regulators may be utilized to kill cancer cells or to augment the effects of other anti-cancer agents.

Carbonic anhydrase (CA) enzymes catalyze the reversible reaction between carbon dioxide and bicarbonate: $CO_2 + H_2O \leftrightarrow HCO_3^- + H^+$, and facilitate the transport of CO_2 and H^+ ions for pH regulation (Swietach et al., 2010). There are 15 CA isoforms, I to XV, in mammalian cells, located in the cytosol, mitochondrion, extracellular plasma membrane, or secreted. In particular, the isoform IX (CAIX) has been extensively studied in cancer biology (Swietach et al., 2010). The expression of CAIX is strongly induced by hypoxia and regulated by HIF-1.

CAIX has been used as an endogenous marker to delineate hypoxic regions in solid tumors and is a prognostic marker of aggressive cancers. Inhibition of CAIX has been shown to suppress tumor growth in xenograft models (Chiche et al., 2009). CAIX small molecule inhibitors and antibodies have been developed and evaluated as potential anti-cancer therapeutics. A CAIX monoclonal antibody exhibited anti-tumor activities in the mouse xenograft model of colorectal cancer (Zatovicova et al., 2010). Moreover, CAIX inhibitors were shown to increase the therapeutic effects of tumor radiation (Dubois et al., 2011).

Monocarboxylate transporters (MCT) facilitate the efflux of lactate and protons from cells. The up-regulation of MCTs has been observed in a variety of tumors such as breast, colorectal, ovarian, prostate, and central nervous system carcinomas, and associated with cancer progression and poor prognosis in some instances (Fang et al., 2006; Froberg et al., 2001; Pertega-Gomes et al., 2011; Pinheiro et al., 2010; Pinheiro et al., 2008). MCT1 and MCT4 were related to the invasiveness of human lung cancer cells and drug resistance of ovarian cancer cells (Chen et al., 2010; Izumi et al., 2011). Inhibition of MCT1 could retard the growth of cancer cells in culture and animal models (Fang et al., 2006; Sonveaux et al., 2008). MCTs may, therefore, represent potential targets for cancer treatment.

Vacuolar-type H^+-ATPases (V-ATPases) are multi-subunit, complex enzymes that transport protons from the cytoplasm to vacuolar lumens or to extracellular space (Izumi et al., 2003). These proton pumps are important for maintaining intracellular and extracellular pH homeostasis. V-ATPases overexpression has been detected in many types of tumors such as oral squamous cell cancer and melanoma (Nishisho et al., 2011; Perez-Sayans et al., 2010). Studies showed that V-ATPases increased cancer metastasis and drug resistance (Nishisho et al., 2011; You et al., 2009). Inhibition of V-ATPases by small molecule inhibitors or small interfering RNA suppressed tumor growth and metastasis, induced tumor cell apoptosis, and overcame chemoresistance in several cancer models (De Milito et al., 2007; Lu et al., 2005; Nishisho et al., 2011; You et al., 2009).

Sodium/hydrogen exchangers (NHE) regulate the pH homeostasis of cells by extruding intracellular H^+ in exchange of extracellular Na^+ at a 1:1 ratio. Nine NHE isoforms have been identified in mammalian cells (De Vito, 2006). NHEs were found to regulate cytoskeletal structures and tumor cell migration and invasion (Paradiso et al., 2004). Treatment with NHE1 inhibitors sensitized the paclitaxel-induced apoptosis of human breast cancer cells (Reshkin et al., 2003). Moreover, increased activity of NHE was observed in doxorubicin-resistant human colon cancer cells and the treatment with the NHE inhibitor 5-(N-ethyl-N-isopropyl)-amiloride (EIPA) sensitized the resistant cells to doxorubicin (Miraglia et al., 2005). Inhibition of NHEs has also been shown to reduce the proliferation and VEGF production of leukemia cells (He et al., 2007; Turturro et al., 2007).

Proton-sensing G protein-coupled receptors (GPCRs), including GPR4, TDAG8 (GPR65), OGR1 (GPR68), and G2A (GPR132), can be activated by acidic extracellular pH to transduce multiple downstream signaling pathways such as the G_s/cAMP, G_q/phospholipase C/Ca^{2+}, and G_{13}/Rho pathways (Ludwig et al., 2003; Murakami et al., 2004; Radu et al., 2005; Tobo et al., 2007; Wang et al., 2004; Yang et al., 2007). Different from the proton transporters, the proton-sensing GPCRs do not directly transport protons but, instead, perceive acidic extracellular pH to trigger signal transduction. Potential roles of the proton-sensing GPCRs in cancer biology have been emerging, with differential roles for each family member in a cell context-dependent manner. Activation of GPR4 by acidic pH has been shown to inhibit tumor cell migration, invasion and metastasis and suppress microvascular outgrowth (Castellone et al., 2011; Yang et al., 2007). Overexpression of OGR1 also inhibited the migration and metastasis of prostate cancer cells and the effects were attributed to the constitutive activity of the receptor but not pH sensing function (Singh et al., 2007). Overexpression of TDAG8, however, enhanced the development of lung cancer cells (Ihara et al., 2010). TDAG8, as well as GPR4, exhibited transforming activities when ectopically overexpressed in immortalized cell lines (Sin et al., 2004). Furthermore, the proton-sensing GPCRs have been shown to regulate immune cell function and inflammatory responses (Ichimonji et al., 2010; Mogi et al., 2009; Onozawa et al., 2011). These observations suggest that the proton-sensing GPCRs may represent novel targets for cancer treatment, inflammation inhibition, and chemoprevention.

Taken together, the acid-base transporters and proton-sensing receptors described above are important for cancer cells to sense and adapt to the acidic tumor microenvironment. Further research is warranted to validate these pH regulators as potential targets for cancer therapy and chemoprevention. Moreover, acidity itself in the tumor microenvironment can also be exploited for cancer detection and treatment. Recent studies showed that a technology using the pH low insertion peptide (pHLIP), a peptide that forms α-helix at acidic pH and inserts across cell membrane, could be applied to image prostate cancer xenografts in mice by positron emission tomography (Vavere et al., 2009). Acidity in the tumor microenvironment may also be utilized to design pro-drugs that are activated or become more potent at acidic pH to differentially kill cancer cells.

4. Concluding remarks

Cancer cells do not exist in isolation; instead, they closely interact with blood vessels, inflammatory cells, and fibroblasts in a unique tumor microenvironment characterized by hypoxia and acidosis. The interaction between cancer cells and the tumor microenvironment plays a pivotal role in cancer progression and somatic evolution, which follows very similar principles of Darwinian selection. It is increasingly recognized that in addition to killing cancer cells, targeting the components of the tumor microenvironment can help develop more effective approaches for cancer prevention and therapy. For instance, anti-angiogenesis therapy, combined with conventional chemotherapy, has shown significant clinical benefits in multiple cancer types (Ferrara and Kerbel, 2005; Kerbel, 2008). Furthermore, a number of agents targeting inflammation, cancer cell metabolism, and hypoxia and acidosis pathways have been developed and added to the arsenal for cancer treatment, detection, diagnosis, prognosis and chemoprevention.

While significant progress has been made to understand the tumor-microenvironment interaction, considerable knowledge gaps still remain. This aspect is exemplified by the lessons learned from anti-angiogenesis therapy. Whereas angiogenesis inhibitors have offered therapeutic benefits in cancer patients, some unexpected adverse effects deserve a close attention. In certain experimental settings, anti-angiogenesis therapy has been shown to promote tumor invasion and metastasis (De Bock et al., 2011; Ebos and Kerbel, 2011; Ebos et al., 2009). The underlying cause is largely attributed to the anti-angiogenesis therapy-induced hypoxia, which is known to stimulate cancer cell metastasis. These observations illustrate that cancer cells constantly evolve and adapt to the changing tumor microenvironment during therapeutic interventions and/or tumor development. In addition to hypoxia, other microenvironmental factors, such as acidosis and low nutrients, are also important selection forces that have a significant impact on cancer cell somatic evolution. The experience of anti-angiogenesis therapy once again underscores the fact that tumors comprise not just cancer cells and these cancer cells are continuously evolving. It is necessary to target multiple cell components and molecular pathways (both cancer cell-intrinsic and microenvironment-related) in order to devise more effective strategies for the treatment and prevention of cancer.

5. Acknowledgment

We thank Dr. Adam Asch for reading the manuscript. The research in the authors' laboratory has been supported by the American Heart Association, Brody Brothers Endowment Fund, Golfers against Cancer, and North Carolina Biotechnology Center (to L.V.Y). We apologize to these whose work could not be cited due to the space limitation of this manuscript.

6. References

Abramsson, A., Berlin, O., Papayan, H., Paulin, D., Shani, M., and Betsholtz, C. (2002). Analysis of mural cell recruitment to tumor vessels. Circulation *105*, 112-117.

Abramsson, A., Lindblom, P., and Betsholtz, C. (2003). Endothelial and nonendothelial sources of PDGF-B regulate pericyte recruitment and influence vascular pattern formation in tumors. J Clin Invest *112*, 1142-1151.

Adini, A., Kornaga, T., Firoozbakht, F., and Benjamin, L.E. (2002). Placental growth factor is a survival factor for tumor endothelial cells and macrophages. Cancer Res *62*, 2749-2752.

Al-Hajj, M., Wicha, M.S., Benito-Hernandez, A., Morrison, S.J., and Clarke, M.F. (2003). Prospective identification of tumorigenic breast cancer cells. Proc Natl Acad Sci U S A *100*, 3983-3988.

Ara, T., and Declerck, Y.A. (2010). Interleukin-6 in bone metastasis and cancer progression. Eur J Cancer *46*, 1223-1231.

Augustin, H.G., Koh, G.Y., Thurston, G., and Alitalo, K. (2009). Control of vascular morphogenesis and homeostasis through the angiopoietin-Tie system. Nat Rev Mol Cell Biol *10*, 165-177.

Azab, A.K., Runnels, J.M., Pitsillides, C., Moreau, A.S., Azab, F., Leleu, X., Jia, X., Wright, R., Ospina, B., Carlson, A.L., *et al.* (2009). CXCR4 inhibitor AMD3100 disrupts the interaction of multiple myeloma cells with the bone marrow microenvironment and enhances their sensitivity to therapy. Blood *113*, 4341-4351.

Baeriswyl, V., and Christofori, G. (2009). The angiogenic switch in carcinogenesis. Semin Cancer Biol *19*, 329-337.

Baluk, P., Hashizume, H., and McDonald, D.M. (2005). Cellular abnormalities of blood vessels as targets in cancer. Curr Opin Genet Dev *15*, 102-111.

Baron, J.A., Sandler, R.S., Bresalier, R.S., Lanas, A., Morton, D.G., Riddell, R., Iverson, E.R., and Demets, D.L. (2008). Cardiovascular events associated with rofecoxib: final analysis of the APPROVe trial. Lancet *372*, 1756-1764.

Beenken, A., and Mohammadi, M. (2009). The FGF family: biology, pathophysiology and therapy. Nat Rev Drug Discov *8*, 235-253.

Bergers, G., and Benjamin, L.E. (2003). Tumorigenesis and the angiogenic switch. Nat Rev Cancer *3*, 401-410.

Bergers, G., and Hanahan, D. (2008). Modes of resistance to anti-angiogenic therapy. Nat Rev Cancer *8*, 592-603.

Bergers, G., Song, S., Meyer-Morse, N., Bergsland, E., and Hanahan, D. (2003). Benefits of targeting both pericytes and endothelial cells in the tumor vasculature with kinase inhibitors. J Clin Invest *111*, 1287-1295.

Bertout, J.A., Patel, S.A., and Simon, M.C. (2008). The impact of O2 availability on human cancer. Nat Rev Cancer *8*, 967-975.

Bhowmick, N.A., Neilson, E.G., and Moses, H.L. (2004). Stromal fibroblasts in cancer initiation and progression. Nature *432*, 332-337.

Bo, S., Ciccone, G., Rosato, R., Villois, P., Appendino, G., Ghigo, E., and Grassi, G. (2011). Cancer mortality reduction and metformin. A retrospective cohort study in type 2 diabetic patients. Diabetes Obes Metab.

Boire, A., Covic, L., Agarwal, A., Jacques, S., Sherifi, S., and Kuliopulos, A. (2005). PAR1 is a matrix metalloprotease-1 receptor that promotes invasion and tumorigenesis of breast cancer cells. Cell *120*, 303-313.

Bonnet, D., and Dick, J.E. (1997). Human acute myeloid leukemia is organized as a hierarchy that originates from a primitive hematopoietic cell. Nat Med *3*, 730-737.

Botting, R.M. (2010). Vane's discovery of the mechanism of action of aspirin changed our understanding of its clinical pharmacology. Pharmacol Rep *62*, 518-525.

Bourguignon, L.Y., Singleton, P.A., Diedrich, F., Stern, R., and Gilad, E. (2004). CD44 interaction with Na+-H+ exchanger (NHE1) creates acidic microenvironments leading to hyaluronidase-2 and cathepsin B activation and breast tumor cell invasion. J Biol Chem *279*, 26991-27007.

Buerkle, A., and Weber, W.A. (2008). Imaging of tumor glucose utilization with positron emission tomography. Cancer Metastasis Rev *27*, 545-554.

Cairns, R., Papandreou, I., and Denko, N. (2006). Overcoming physiologic barriers to cancer treatment by molecularly targeting the tumor microenvironment. Mol Cancer Res *4*, 61-70.

Cairns, R.A., Harris, I.S., and Mak, T.W. (2011). Regulation of cancer cell metabolism. Nat Rev Cancer *11*, 85-95.

Carmeliet, P., and Jain, R.K. (2000). Angiogenesis in cancer and other diseases. Nature *407*, 249-257.

Castellone, R.D., Leffler, N.R., Dong, L., and Yang, L.V. (2011). Inhibition of tumor cell migration and metastasis by the proton-sensing GPR4 receptor. Cancer Lett *312*, 197-208

Castor, C.W., Wilson, S.M., Heiss, P.R., and Seidman, J.C. (1979). Activation of lung connective tissue cells in vitro. Am Rev Respir Dis *120*, 101-106.

Chan, D.A., Sutphin, P.D., Nguyen, P., Turcotte, S., Lai, E.W., Banh, A., Reynolds, G.E., Chi, J.T., Wu, J., Solow-Cordero, D.E., *et al.* (2011). Targeting GLUT1 and the Warburg Effect in Renal Cell Carcinoma by Chemical Synthetic Lethality. Sci Transl Med *3*, 94ra70.

Chang, H.Y., Chi, J.T., Dudoit, S., Bondre, C., van de Rijn, M., Botstein, D., and Brown, P.O. (2002). Diversity, topographic differentiation, and positional memory in human fibroblasts. Proc Natl Acad Sci U S A *99*, 12877-12882.

Chang, Q., Jurisica, I., Do, T., and Hedley, D.W. (2011). Hypoxia predicts aggressive growth and spontaneous metastasis formation from orthotopically grown primary xenografts of human pancreatic cancer. Cancer Res *71*, 3110-3120.

Chen, H., Wang, L., Beretov, J., Hao, J., Xiao, W., and Li, Y. (2010). Co-expression of CD147/EMMPRIN with monocarboxylate transporters and multiple drug resistance proteins is associated with epithelial ovarian cancer progression. Clin Exp Metastasis *27*, 557-569.

Chen, Y., Wiesmann, C., Fuh, G., Li, B., Christinger, H.W., McKay, P., de Vos, A.M., and Lowman, H.B. (1999). Selection and analysis of an optimized anti-VEGF antibody: crystal structure of an affinity-matured Fab in complex with antigen. J Mol Biol *293*, 865-881.

Chiche, J., Ilc, K., Laferriere, J., Trottier, E., Dayan, F., Mazure, N.M., Brahimi-Horn, M.C., and Pouyssegur, J. (2009). Hypoxia-inducible carbonic anhydrase IX and XII promote tumor cell growth by counteracting acidosis through the regulation of the intracellular pH. Cancer Res *69*, 358-368.

Chiu, P.P., Jiang, H., and Dick, J.E. (2010). Leukemia-initiating cells in human T-lymphoblastic leukemia exhibit glucocorticoid resistance. Blood *116*, 5268-5279.

Cho, R.W., and Clarke, M.F. (2008). Recent advances in cancer stem cells. Curr Opin Genet Dev *18*, 48-53.

Chouaib, S., Kieda, C., Benlalam, H., Noman, M.Z., Mami-Chouaib, F., and Ruegg, C. (2010). Endothelial cells as key determinants of the tumor microenvironment: interaction with tumor cells, extracellular matrix and immune killer cells. Crit Rev Immunol *30*, 529-545.

Clarke, M.F., Dick, J.E., Dirks, P.B., Eaves, C.J., Jamieson, C.H., Jones, D.L., Visvader, J., Weissman, I.L., and Wahl, G.M. (2006). Cancer stem cells--perspectives on current status and future directions: AACR Workshop on cancer stem cells. Cancer Res *66*, 9339-9344.

Clevers, H. (2011). The cancer stem cell: premises, promises and challenges. Nat Med *17*, 313-319.

Cohen, M.H., Shen, Y.L., Keegan, P., and Pazdur, R. (2009). FDA drug approval summary: bevacizumab (Avastin) as treatment of recurrent glioblastoma multiforme. Oncologist *14*, 1131-1138.

Cook, N.R., Lee, I.M., Gaziano, J.M., Gordon, D., Ridker, P.M., Manson, J.E., Hennekens, C.H., and Buring, J.E. (2005). Low-dose aspirin in the primary prevention of cancer: the Women's Health Study: a randomized controlled trial. JAMA *294*, 47-55.

Cozzio, A., Passegue, E., Ayton, P.M., Karsunky, H., Cleary, M.L., and Weissman, I.L. (2003). Similar MLL-associated leukemias arising from self-renewing stem cells and short-lived myeloid progenitors. Genes Dev *17*, 3029-3035.

Currie, G.P., Kennedy, A.M., Paterson, E., and Watt, S.J. (2007). A chronic pneumothorax and fitness to fly. Thorax *62*, 187-189.

Dalerba, P., Dylla, S.J., Park, I.K., Liu, R., Wang, X., Cho, R.W., Hoey, T., Gurney, A., Huang, E.H., Simeone, D.M., *et al.* (2007). Phenotypic characterization of human colorectal cancer stem cells. Proc Natl Acad Sci U S A *104*, 10158-10163.

Dang, C.V., Le, A., and Gao, P. (2009). MYC-induced cancer cell energy metabolism and therapeutic opportunities. Clin Cancer Res *15*, 6479-6483.

De Bock, K., Mazzone, M., and Carmeliet, P. (2011). Antiangiogenic therapy, hypoxia, and metastasis: risky liaisons, or not? Nat Rev Clin Oncol *8*, 393-404.

De Milito, A., Iessi, E., Logozzi, M., Lozupone, F., Spada, M., Marino, M.L., Federici, C., Perdicchio, M., Matarrese, P., Lugini, L., *et al.* (2007). Proton pump inhibitors induce apoptosis of human B-cell tumors through a caspase-independent mechanism involving reactive oxygen species. Cancer Res *67*, 5408-5417.

de Visser, K.E. (2008). Spontaneous immune responses to sporadic tumors: tumor-promoting, tumor-protective or both? Cancer Immunol Immunother *57*, 1531-1539.

de Visser, K.E., Eichten, A., and Coussens, L.M. (2006). Paradoxical roles of the immune system during cancer development. Nat Rev Cancer *6*, 24-37.

De Vito, P. (2006). The sodium/hydrogen exchanger: a possible mediator of immunity. Cell Immunol *240*, 69-85.

Diehn, M., Cho, R.W., Lobo, N.A., Kalisky, T., Dorie, M.J., Kulp, A.N., Qian, D., Lam, J.S., Ailles, L.E., Wong, M., *et al.* (2009). Association of reactive oxygen species levels and radioresistance in cancer stem cells. Nature *458*, 780-783.

DiPersio, J.F., Micallef, I.N., Stiff, P.J., Bolwell, B.J., Maziarz, R.T., Jacobsen, E., Nademanee, A., McCarty, J., Bridger, G., and Calandra, G. (2009a). Phase III prospective randomized double-blind placebo-controlled trial of plerixafor plus granulocyte colony-stimulating factor compared with placebo plus granulocyte colony-stimulating factor for autologous stem-cell mobilization and transplantation for patients with non-Hodgkin's lymphoma. J Clin Oncol *27*, 4767-4773.

DiPersio, J.F., Stadtmauer, E.A., Nademanee, A., Micallef, I.N., Stiff, P.J., Kaufman, J.L., Maziarz, R.T., Hosing, C., Fruehauf, S., Horwitz, M., *et al.* (2009b). Plerixafor and G-CSF versus placebo and G-CSF to mobilize hematopoietic stem cells for autologous stem cell transplantation in patients with multiple myeloma. Blood *113*, 5720-5726.

Dubois, L., Peeters, S., Lieuwes, N.G., Geusens, N., Thiry, A., Wigfield, S., Carta, F., McIntyre, A., Scozzafava, A., Dogne, J.M., *et al.* (2011). Specific inhibition of carbonic anhydrase IX activity enhances the in vivo therapeutic effect of tumor irradiation. Radiother Oncol *99*, 424-431.

Dudley, M.E., Wunderlich, J.R., Robbins, P.F., Yang, J.C., Hwu, P., Schwartzentruber, D.J., Topalian, S.L., Sherry, R., Restifo, N.P., Hubicki, A.M., *et al.* (2002). Cancer regression and autoimmunity in patients after clonal repopulation with antitumor lymphocytes. Science *298*, 850-854.

Dvorak, H.F. (1986). Tumors: wounds that do not heal. Similarities between tumor stroma generation and wound healing. N Engl J Med *315*, 1650-1659.

Dvorak, H.F. (2002). Vascular permeability factor/vascular endothelial growth factor: a critical cytokine in tumor angiogenesis and a potential target for diagnosis and therapy. J Clin Oncol *20*, 4368-4380.

Ebos, J.M., and Kerbel, R.S. (2011). Antiangiogenic therapy: impact on invasion, disease progression, and metastasis. Nat Rev Clin Oncol *8*, 210-221.

Ebos, J.M., Lee, C.R., Cruz-Munoz, W., Bjarnason, G.A., Christensen, J.G., and Kerbel, R.S. (2009). Accelerated metastasis after short-term treatment with a potent inhibitor of tumor angiogenesis. Cancer Cell *15*, 232-239.

Eckerich, C., Zapf, S., Fillbrandt, R., Loges, S., Westphal, M., and Lamszus, K. (2007). Hypoxia can induce c-Met expression in glioma cells and enhance SF/HGF-induced cell migration. Int J Cancer *121*, 276-283.

Escudier, B., Eisen, T., Stadler, W.M., Szczylik, C., Oudard, S., Siebels, M., Negrier, S., Chevreau, C., Solska, E., Desai, A.A., *et al.* (2007). Sorafenib in advanced clear-cell renal-cell carcinoma. N Engl J Med *356*, 125-134.

Eskens, F.A., and Verweij, J. (2006). The clinical toxicity profile of vascular endothelial growth factor (VEGF) and vascular endothelial growth factor receptor (VEGFR) targeting angiogenesis inhibitors; a review. Eur J Cancer *42*, 3127-3139.

Fabian, M.A., Biggs, W.H., 3rd, Treiber, D.K., Atteridge, C.E., Azimioara, M.D., Benedetti, M.G., Carter, T.A., Ciceri, P., Edeen, P.T., Floyd, M., *et al.* (2005). A small molecule-kinase interaction map for clinical kinase inhibitors. Nat Biotechnol *23*, 329-336.

Faivre, S., Demetri, G., Sargent, W., and Raymond, E. (2007). Molecular basis for sunitinib efficacy and future clinical development. Nat Rev Drug Discov *6*, 734-745.

Fang, J., Quinones, Q.J., Holman, T.L., Morowitz, M.J., Wang, Q., Zhao, H., Sivo, F., Maris, J.M., and Wahl, M.L. (2006). The H+-linked monocarboxylate transporter (MCT1/SLC16A1): a potential therapeutic target for high-risk neuroblastoma. Mol Pharmacol *70*, 2108-2115.

Fernando, N.T., Koch, M., Rothrock, C., Gollogly, L.K., D'Amore, P.A., Ryeom, S., and Yoon, S.S. (2008). Tumor escape from endogenous, extracellular matrix-associated angiogenesis inhibitors by up-regulation of multiple proangiogenic factors. Clin Cancer Res *14*, 1529-1539.

Ferrara, N. (2002). VEGF and the quest for tumour angiogenesis factors. Nat Rev Cancer *2*, 795-803.

Ferrara, N., Damico, L., Shams, N., Lowman, H., and Kim, R. (2006). Development of ranibizumab, an anti-vascular endothelial growth factor antigen binding fragment, as therapy for neovascular age-related macular degeneration. Retina *26*, 859-870.

Ferrara, N., Gerber, H.P., and LeCouter, J. (2003). The biology of VEGF and its receptors. Nat Med *9*, 669-676.

Ferrara, N., Hillan, K.J., Gerber, H.P., and Novotny, W. (2004). Discovery and development of bevacizumab, an anti-VEGF antibody for treating cancer. Nat Rev Drug Discov *3*, 391-400.

Ferrara, N., and Kerbel, R.S. (2005). Angiogenesis as a therapeutic target. Nature *438*, 967-974.

Fialkow, P.J. (1990). Stem cell origin of human myeloid blood cell neoplasms. Verh Dtsch Ges Pathol *74*, 43-47.

Fidler, I.J. (2002). Critical determinants of metastasis. Semin Cancer Biol *12*, 89-96.

Fischer, C., Jonckx, B., Mazzone, M., Zacchigna, S., Loges, S., Pattarini, L., Chorianopoulos, E., Liesenborghs, L., Koch, M., De Mol, M., *et al.* (2007). Anti-PlGF inhibits growth of VEGF(R)-inhibitor-resistant tumors without affecting healthy vessels. Cell *131*, 463-475.

Folkman, J. (1971). Tumor angiogenesis: therapeutic implications. N Engl J Med *285*, 1182-1186.

Folkman, J. (2006). Angiogenesis. Annu Rev Med *57*, 1-18.

Fridman, W.H., Galon, J., Pages, F., Tartour, E., Sautes-Fridman, C., and Kroemer, G. (2011). Prognostic and predictive impact of intra- and peritumoral immune infiltrates. Cancer Res *71*, 5601-5605.

Froberg, M.K., Gerhart, D.Z., Enerson, B.E., Manivel, C., Guzman-Paz, M., Seacotte, N., and Drewes, L.R. (2001). Expression of monocarboxylate transporter MCT1 in normal and neoplastic human CNS tissues. Neuroreport *12*, 761-765.

Fukumura, D., and Jain, R.K. (2007). Tumor microenvironment abnormalities: causes, consequences, and strategies to normalize. J Cell Biochem *101*, 937-949.

Gabbiani, G. (2003). The myofibroblast in wound healing and fibrocontractive diseases. J Pathol *200*, 500-503.

Gao, F., Liao, C., Liu, L., Tan, A., Cao, Y., and Mo, Z. (2009). The effect of aspirin in the recurrence of colorectal adenomas: a meta-analysis of randomized controlled trials. Colorectal Dis *11*, 893-901.

Gatenby, R.A., Gawlinski, E.T., Gmitro, A.F., Kaylor, B., and Gillies, R.J. (2006). Acid-mediated tumor invasion: a multidisciplinary study. Cancer Res *66*, 5216-5223.

Gatenby, R.A., and Gillies, R.J. (2004). Why do cancers have high aerobic glycolysis? Nat Rev Cancer *4*, 891-899.

Gatenby, R.A., and Gillies, R.J. (2007). Glycolysis in cancer: a potential target for therapy. Int J Biochem Cell Biol *39*, 1358-1366.

Gatenby, R.A., and Gillies, R.J. (2008). A microenvironmental model of carcinogenesis. Nat Rev Cancer *8*, 56-61.

Gerhardt, H., and Betsholtz, C. (2003). Endothelial-pericyte interactions in angiogenesis. Cell Tissue Res *314*, 15-23.

Gerweck, L.E., Vijayappa, S., and Kozin, S. (2006). Tumor pH controls the in vivo efficacy of weak acid and base chemotherapeutics. Mol Cancer Ther *5*, 1275-1279.

Giantonio, B.J., Catalano, P.J., Meropol, N.J., O'Dwyer, P.J., Mitchell, E.P., Alberts, S.R., Schwartz, M.A., and Benson, A.B., 3rd (2007). Bevacizumab in combination with oxaliplatin, fluorouracil, and leucovorin (FOLFOX4) for previously treated metastatic colorectal cancer: results from the Eastern Cooperative Oncology Group Study E3200. J Clin Oncol *25*, 1539-1544.

Gonzalez-Angulo, A.M., and Meric-Bernstam, F. (2010). Metformin: a therapeutic opportunity in breast cancer. Clin Cancer Res *16*, 1695-1700.

Goodman, V.L., Rock, E.P., Dagher, R., Ramchandani, R.P., Abraham, S., Gobburu, J.V., Booth, B.P., Verbois, S.L., Morse, D.E., Liang, C.Y., *et al.* (2007). Approval summary: sunitinib for the treatment of imatinib refractory or intolerant gastrointestinal stromal tumors and advanced renal cell carcinoma. Clin Cancer Res *13*, 1367-1373.

Gragoudas, E.S., Adamis, A.P., Cunningham, E.T., Jr., Feinsod, M., and Guyer, D.R. (2004). Pegaptanib for neovascular age-related macular degeneration. N Engl J Med *351*, 2805-2816.

Griffiths, J.R., McIntyre, D.J., Howe, F.A., and Stubbs, M. (2001). Why are cancers acidic? A carrier-mediated diffusion model for H+ transport in the interstitial fluid. Novartis Found Symp *240*, 46-62; discussion 62-47, 152-153.

Grivennikov, S.I., Greten, F.R., and Karin, M. (2010). Immunity, inflammation, and cancer. Cell *140*, 883-899.

Gupta, P.B., Chaffer, C.L., and Weinberg, R.A. (2009). Cancer stem cells: mirage or reality? Nat Med *15*, 1010-1012.

Hanahan, D., and Folkman, J. (1996). Patterns and emerging mechanisms of the angiogenic switch during tumorigenesis. Cell *86*, 353-364.

Hanahan, D., and Weinberg, R.A. (2000). The hallmarks of cancer. Cell *100*, 57-70.

Hanahan, D., and Weinberg, R.A. (2011). Hallmarks of cancer: the next generation. Cell *144*, 646-674.

Hashizume, H., Baluk, P., Morikawa, S., McLean, J.W., Thurston, G., Roberge, S., Jain, R.K., and McDonald, D.M. (2000). Openings between defective endothelial cells explain tumor vessel leakiness. Am J Pathol *156*, 1363-1380.

He, B., Deng, C., Zhang, M., Zou, D., and Xu, M. (2007). Reduction of intracellular pH inhibits the expression of VEGF in K562 cells after targeted inhibition of the Na+/H+ exchanger. Leuk Res *31*, 507-514.

Heddleston, J.M., Li, Z., Lathia, J.D., Bao, S., Hjelmeland, A.B., and Rich, J.N. (2010). Hypoxia inducible factors in cancer stem cells. Br J Cancer *102*, 789-795.

Helmlinger, G., Sckell, A., Dellian, M., Forbes, N.S., and Jain, R.K. (2002). Acid production in glycolysis-impaired tumors provides new insights into tumor metabolism. Clin Cancer Res *8*, 1284-1291.

Hendricksen, K., van der Heijden, A.G., Cornel, E.B., Vergunst, H., de Reijke, T.M., van Boven, E., Smits, G.A., Puri, R., Gruijs, S., and Witjes, J.A. (2009). Two-year follow-up of the phase II marker lesion study of intravesical apaziquone for patients with non-muscle invasive bladder cancer. World J Urol *27*, 337-342.

Hermann, P.C., Huber, S.L., Herrler, T., Aicher, A., Ellwart, J.W., Guba, M., Bruns, C.J., and Heeschen, C. (2007). Distinct populations of cancer stem cells determine tumor growth and metastatic activity in human pancreatic cancer. Cell Stem Cell *1*, 313-323.

Hicklin, D.J., and Ellis, L.M. (2005). Role of the vascular endothelial growth factor pathway in tumor growth and angiogenesis. J Clin Oncol *23*, 1011-1027.

Higgins, D.F., Kimura, K., Bernhardt, W.M., Shrimanker, N., Akai, Y., Hohenstein, B., Saito, Y., Johnson, R.S., Kretzler, M., Cohen, C.D., *et al.* (2007). Hypoxia promotes fibrogenesis in vivo via HIF-1 stimulation of epithelial-to-mesenchymal transition. J Clin Invest *117*, 3810-3820.

Hill, R., Song, Y., Cardiff, R.D., and Van Dyke, T. (2005). Selective evolution of stromal mesenchyme with p53 loss in response to epithelial tumorigenesis. Cell *123*, 1001-1011.

Hosono, K., Endo, H., Takahashi, H., Sugiyama, M., Sakai, E., Uchiyama, T., Suzuki, K., Iida, H., Sakamoto, Y., Yoneda, K., *et al.* (2010). Metformin suppresses colorectal aberrant crypt foci in a short-term clinical trial. Cancer Prev Res (Phila) *3*, 1077-1083.

Houck, K.A., Ferrara, N., Winer, J., Cachianes, G., Li, B., and Leung, D.W. (1991). The vascular endothelial growth factor family: identification of a fourth molecular species and characterization of alternative splicing of RNA. Mol Endocrinol *5*, 1806-1814.

Hu, M., Yao, J., Cai, L., Bachman, K.E., van den Brule, F., Velculescu, V., and Polyak, K. (2005). Distinct epigenetic changes in the stromal cells of breast cancers. Nat Genet *37*, 899-905.

Hugo, H., Ackland, M.L., Blick, T., Lawrence, M.G., Clements, J.A., Williams, E.D., and Thompson, E.W. (2007). Epithelial--mesenchymal and mesenchymal--epithelial transitions in carcinoma progression. J Cell Physiol *213*, 374-383.

Hunter, A., Hendrikse, A., Renan, M., and Abratt, R. (2006). Does the tumor microenvironment influence radiation-induced apoptosis? Apoptosis *11*, 1727-1735.

Hurwitz, H., Fehrenbacher, L., Novotny, W., Cartwright, T., Hainsworth, J., Heim, W., Berlin, J., Baron, A., Griffing, S., Holmgren, E., *et al.* (2004). Bevacizumab plus irinotecan, fluorouracil, and leucovorin for metastatic colorectal cancer. N Engl J Med *350*, 2335-2342.

Ichimonji, I., Tomura, H., Mogi, C., Sato, K., Aoki, H., Hisada, T., Dobashi, K., Ishizuka, T., Mori, M., and Okajima, F. (2010). Extracellular acidification stimulates IL-6 production and Ca(2+) mobilization through proton-sensing OGR1 receptors in human airway smooth muscle cells. Am J Physiol Lung Cell Mol Physiol *299*, L567-577.

Ihara, Y., Kihara, Y., Hamano, F., Yanagida, K., Morishita, Y., Kunita, A., Yamori, T., Fukayama, M., Aburatani, H., Shimizu, T., *et al.* (2010). The G protein-coupled receptor T-cell death-associated gene 8 (TDAG8) facilitates tumor development by serving as an extracellular pH sensor. Proc Natl Acad Sci U S A *107*, 17309-17314.

Isaacs, J.S., Jung, Y.J., Mimnaugh, E.G., Martinez, A., Cuttitta, F., and Neckers, L.M. (2002). Hsp90 regulates a von Hippel Lindau-independent hypoxia-inducible factor-1 alpha-degradative pathway. J Biol Chem *277*, 29936-29944.

Izumi, H., Takahashi, M., Uramoto, H., Nakayama, Y., Oyama, T., Wang, K.Y., Sasaguri, Y., Nishizawa, S., and Kohno, K. (2011). Monocarboxylate transporters 1 and 4 are involved in the invasion activity of human lung cancer cells. Cancer Sci *102*, 1007-1013.

Izumi, H., Torigoe, T., Ishiguchi, H., Uramoto, H., Yoshida, Y., Tanabe, M., Ise, T., Murakami, T., Yoshida, T., Nomoto, M., *et al.* (2003). Cellular pH regulators: potentially promising molecular targets for cancer chemotherapy. Cancer Treat Rev *29*, 541-549.

Jain, A., Phillips, R.M., Scally, A.J., Lenaz, G., Beer, M., and Puri, R. (2009). Response of multiple recurrent TaT1 bladder cancer to intravesical apaziquone (EO9): comparative analysis of tumor recurrence rates. Urology *73*, 1083-1086.

Jain, R.K. (2005). Normalization of tumor vasculature: an emerging concept in antiangiogenic therapy. Science *307*, 58-62.

Jiang, L., Gonda, T.A., Gamble, M.V., Salas, M., Seshan, V., Tu, S., Twaddell, W.S., Hegyi, P., Lazar, G., Steele, I., *et al.* (2008). Global hypomethylation of genomic DNA in cancer-associated myofibroblasts. Cancer Res *68*, 9900-9908.

Johnson, L.L., Pavlovsky, A.G., Johnson, A.R., Janowicz, J.A., Man, C.F., Ortwine, D.F., Purchase, C.F., 2nd, White, A.D., and Hupe, D.J. (2000). A rationalization of the acidic pH dependence for stromelysin-1 (Matrix metalloproteinase-3) catalysis and inhibition. J Biol Chem *275*, 11026-11033.

Joyce, J.A., and Pollard, J.W. (2009). Microenvironmental regulation of metastasis. Nat Rev Cancer *9*, 239-252.

Karnoub, A.E., and Weinberg, R.A. (2006). Chemokine networks and breast cancer metastasis. Breast Dis *26*, 75-85.

Kashfi, K. (2009). Anti-inflammatory agents as cancer therapeutics. Adv Pharmacol *57*, 31-89.

Kazerounian, S., Yee, K.O., and Lawler, J. (2008). Thrombospondins in cancer. Cell Mol Life Sci *65*, 700-712.

Kelly, P.N., Dakic, A., Adams, J.M., Nutt, S.L., and Strasser, A. (2007). Tumor growth need not be driven by rare cancer stem cells. Science *317*, 337.

Kerbel, R., and Folkman, J. (2002). Clinical translation of angiogenesis inhibitors. Nat Rev Cancer *2*, 727-739.

Kerbel, R.S. (2008). Tumor angiogenesis. N Engl J Med *358*, 2039-2049.

Kiaris, H., Chatzistamou, I., Trimis, G., Frangou-Plemmenou, M., Pafiti-Kondi, A., and Kalofoutis, A. (2005). Evidence for nonautonomous effect of p53 tumor suppressor in carcinogenesis. Cancer Res *65*, 1627-1630.

Kienast, Y., von Baumgarten, L., Fuhrmann, M., Klinkert, W.E., Goldbrunner, R., Herms, J., and Winkler, F. (2010). Real-time imaging reveals the single steps of brain metastasis formation. Nat Med *16*, 116-122.

Kim, M., Koh, Y.J., Kim, K.E., Koh, B.I., Nam, D.H., Alitalo, K., Kim, I., and Koh, G.Y. (2010). CXCR4 signaling regulates metastasis of chemoresistant melanoma cells by a lymphatic metastatic niche. Cancer Res *70*, 10411-10421.

Kim, R., Emi, M., and Tanabe, K. (2007). Cancer immunoediting from immune surveillance to immune escape. Immunology *121*, 1-14.

Kindler, H.L., Niedzwiecki, D., Hollis, D., Sutherland, S., Schrag, D., Hurwitz, H., Innocenti, F., Mulcahy, M.F., O'Reilly, E., Wozniak, T.F., *et al.* (2010). Gemcitabine plus bevacizumab compared with gemcitabine plus placebo in patients with advanced pancreatic cancer: phase III trial of the Cancer and Leukemia Group B (CALGB 80303). J Clin Oncol *28*, 3617-3622.

Krivtsov, A.V., Twomey, D., Feng, Z., Stubbs, M.C., Wang, Y., Faber, J., Levine, J.E., Wang, J., Hahn, W.C., Gilliland, D.G., *et al.* (2006). Transformation from committed progenitor to leukaemia stem cell initiated by MLL-AF9. Nature *442*, 818-822.

Kupsch, P., Henning, B.F., Passarge, K., Richly, H., Wiesemann, K., Hilger, R.A., Scheulen, M.E., Christensen, O., Brendel, E., Schwartz, B., *et al.* (2005). Results of a phase I trial of sorafenib (BAY 43-9006) in combination with oxaliplatin in patients with refractory solid tumors, including colorectal cancer. Clin Colorectal Cancer *5*, 188-196.

Kurose, K., Gilley, K., Matsumoto, S., Watson, P.H., Zhou, X.P., and Eng, C. (2002). Frequent somatic mutations in PTEN and TP53 are mutually exclusive in the stroma of breast carcinomas. Nat Genet *32*, 355-357.

Kwitkowski, V.E., Prowell, T.M., Ibrahim, A., Farrell, A.T., Justice, R., Mitchell, S.S., Sridhara, R., and Pazdur, R. (2010). FDA approval summary: temsirolimus as treatment for advanced renal cell carcinoma. Oncologist *15*, 428-435.

Lang, L. (2008). FDA approves sorafenib for patients with inoperable liver cancer. Gastroenterology *134*, 379.

Lapidot, T., Sirard, C., Vormoor, J., Murdoch, B., Hoang, T., Caceres-Cortes, J., Minden, M., Paterson, B., Caligiuri, M.A., and Dick, J.E. (1994). A cell initiating human acute myeloid leukaemia after transplantation into SCID mice. Nature *367*, 645-648.

Lazennec, G., and Richmond, A. (2010). Chemokines and chemokine receptors: new insights into cancer-related inflammation. Trends Mol Med *16*, 133-144.

Lenzer, J. (2011). FDA committee votes to withdraw bevacizumab for breast cancer. BMJ *343*, d4244.

Li, C., Heidt, D.G., Dalerba, P., Burant, C.F., Zhang, L., Adsay, V., Wicha, M., Clarke, M.F., and Simeone, D.M. (2007). Identification of pancreatic cancer stem cells. Cancer Res *67*, 1030-1037.

Li, D. (2011). Metformin as an Antitumor Agent in Cancer Prevention and Treatment. J Diabetes.

Li, X., Lewis, M.T., Huang, J., Gutierrez, C., Osborne, C.K., Wu, M.F., Hilsenbeck, S.G., Pavlick, A., Zhang, X., Chamness, G.C., *et al.* (2008). Intrinsic resistance of tumorigenic breast cancer cells to chemotherapy. J Natl Cancer Inst *100*, 672-679.

Lindahl, P., Johansson, B.R., Leveen, P., and Betsholtz, C. (1997). Pericyte loss and microaneurysm formation in PDGF-B-deficient mice. Science *277*, 242-245.

Llovet, J.M., Ricci, S., Mazzaferro, V., Hilgard, P., Gane, E., Blanc, J.F., de Oliveira, A.C., Santoro, A., Raoul, J.L., Forner, A., *et al.* (2008). Sorafenib in advanced hepatocellular carcinoma. N Engl J Med *359*, 378-390.

Loar, P., Wahl, H., Kshirsagar, M., Gossner, G., Griffith, K., and Liu, J.R. (2010). Inhibition of glycolysis enhances cisplatin-induced apoptosis in ovarian cancer cells. Am J Obstet Gynecol *202*, 371 e371-378.

Lobo, N.A., Shimono, Y., Qian, D., and Clarke, M.F. (2007). The biology of cancer stem cells. Annu Rev Cell Dev Biol *23*, 675-699.

Lobov, I.B., Renard, R.A., Papadopoulos, N., Gale, N.W., Thurston, G., Yancopoulos, G.D., and Wiegand, S.J. (2007). Delta-like ligand 4 (Dll4) is induced by VEGF as a negative regulator of angiogenic sprouting. Proc Natl Acad Sci U S A *104*, 3219-3224.

Lorusso, G., and Ruegg, C. (2008). The tumor microenvironment and its contribution to tumor evolution toward metastasis. Histochem Cell Biol *130*, 1091-1103.

Lu, X., Qin, W., Li, J., Tan, N., Pan, D., Zhang, H., Xie, L., Yao, G., Shu, H., Yao, M., *et al.* (2005). The growth and metastasis of human hepatocellular carcinoma xenografts are inhibited by small interfering RNA targeting to the subunit ATP6L of proton pump. Cancer Res *65*, 6843-6849.

Ludwig, M.G., Vanek, M., Guerini, D., Gasser, J.A., Jones, C.E., Junker, U., Hofstetter, H., Wolf, R.M., and Seuwen, K. (2003). Proton-sensing G-protein-coupled receptors. Nature *425*, 93-98.

Luo, J., Solimini, N.L., and Elledge, S.J. (2009). Principles of cancer therapy: oncogene and non-oncogene addiction. Cell *136*, 823-837.

Lyden, D., Hattori, K., Dias, S., Costa, C., Blaikie, P., Butros, L., Chadburn, A., Heissig, B., Marks, W., Witte, L., *et al.* (2001). Impaired recruitment of bone-marrow-derived endothelial and hematopoietic precursor cells blocks tumor angiogenesis and growth. Nat Med *7*, 1194-1201.

Maeshima, A.M., Niki, T., Maeshima, A., Yamada, T., Kondo, H., and Matsuno, Y. (2002). Modified scar grade: a prognostic indicator in small peripheral lung adenocarcinoma. Cancer *95*, 2546-2554.

Mani, S.A., Guo, W., Liao, M.J., Eaton, E.N., Ayyanan, A., Zhou, A.Y., Brooks, M., Reinhard, F., Zhang, C.C., Shipitsin, M., *et al.* (2008). The epithelial-mesenchymal transition generates cells with properties of stem cells. Cell *133*, 704-715.

McDonald, D.M., and Choyke, P.L. (2003). Imaging of angiogenesis: from microscope to clinic. Nat Med *9*, 713-725.

Michelakis, E.D., Sutendra, G., Dromparis, P., Webster, L., Haromy, A., Niven, E., Maguire, C., Gammer, T.L., Mackey, J.R., Fulton, D., *et al.* (2010). Metabolic modulation of glioblastoma with dichloroacetate. Sci Transl Med *2*, 31ra34.

Miles, D.W., Chan, A., Dirix, L.Y., Cortes, J., Pivot, X., Tomczak, P., Delozier, T., Sohn, J.H., Provencher, L., Puglisi, F., *et al.* (2010). Phase III study of bevacizumab plus docetaxel compared with placebo plus docetaxel for the first-line treatment of human epidermal growth factor receptor 2-negative metastatic breast cancer. J Clin Oncol *28*, 3239-3247.

Miller, K., Wang, M., Gralow, J., Dickler, M., Cobleigh, M., Perez, E.A., Shenkier, T., Cella, D., and Davidson, N.E. (2007). Paclitaxel plus bevacizumab versus paclitaxel alone for metastatic breast cancer. N Engl J Med *357*, 2666-2676.

Miraglia, E., Viarisio, D., Riganti, C., Costamagna, C., Ghigo, D., and Bosia, A. (2005). Na+/H+ exchanger activity is increased in doxorubicin-resistant human colon cancer cells and its modulation modifies the sensitivity of the cells to doxorubicin. Int J Cancer *115*, 924-929.

Modi, S., Stopeck, A., Linden, H., Solit, D., Chandarlapaty, S., Rosen, N., D'Andrea, G., Dickler, M., Moynahan, M.E., Sugarman, S., *et al.* (2011). HSP90 Inhibition Is Effective in Breast Cancer: A Phase II Trial of Tanespimycin (17-AAG) Plus Trastuzumab in Patients with HER2-Positive Metastatic Breast Cancer Progressing on Trastuzumab. Clin Cancer Res *17*, 5132-5139.

Mogi, C., Tobo, M., Tomura, H., Murata, N., He, X.D., Sato, K., Kimura, T., Ishizuka, T., Sasaki, T., Sato, T., *et al.* (2009). Involvement of proton-sensing TDAG8 in extracellular acidification-induced inhibition of proinflammatory cytokine production in peritoneal macrophages. J Immunol *182*, 3243-3251.

Moinfar, F., Man, Y.G., Arnould, L., Bratthauer, G.L., Ratschek, M., and Tavassoli, F.A. (2000). Concurrent and independent genetic alterations in the stromal and epithelial cells of mammary carcinoma: implications for tumorigenesis. Cancer Res *60*, 2562-2566.

Morel, A.P., Lievre, M., Thomas, C., Hinkal, G., Ansieau, S., and Puisieux, A. (2008). Generation of breast cancer stem cells through epithelial-mesenchymal transition. PLoS One *3*, e2888.

Morikawa, S., Baluk, P., Kaidoh, T., Haskell, A., Jain, R.K., and McDonald, D.M. (2002). Abnormalities in pericytes on blood vessels and endothelial sprouts in tumors. Am J Pathol *160*, 985-1000.

Motzer, R.J., Escudier, B., Oudard, S., Hutson, T.E., Porta, C., Bracarda, S., Grunwald, V., Thompson, J.A., Figlin, R.A., Hollaender, N., *et al.* (2008). Efficacy of everolimus in advanced renal cell carcinoma: a double-blind, randomised, placebo-controlled phase III trial. Lancet *372*, 449-456.

Motzer, R.J., Hutson, T.E., Tomczak, P., Michaelson, M.D., Bukowski, R.M., Oudard, S., Negrier, S., Szczylik, C., Pili, R., Bjarnason, G.A., *et al.* (2009). Overall survival and updated results for sunitinib compared with interferon alfa in patients with metastatic renal cell carcinoma. J Clin Oncol *27*, 3584-3590.

Motzer, R.J., Michaelson, M.D., Redman, B.G., Hudes, G.R., Wilding, G., Figlin, R.A., Ginsberg, M.S., Kim, S.T., Baum, C.M., DePrimo, S.E., *et al.* (2006). Activity of SU11248, a multitargeted inhibitor of vascular endothelial growth factor receptor and platelet-derived growth factor receptor, in patients with metastatic renal cell carcinoma. J Clin Oncol *24*, 16-24.

Muller, G.A., and Rodemann, H.P. (1991). Characterization of human renal fibroblasts in health and disease: I. Immunophenotyping of cultured tubular epithelial cells and fibroblasts derived from kidneys with histologically proven interstitial fibrosis. Am J Kidney Dis *17*, 680-683.

Murakami, N., Yokomizo, T., Okuno, T., and Shimizu, T. (2004). G2A is a proton-sensing G-protein-coupled receptor antagonized by lysophosphatidylcholine. J Biol Chem *279*, 42484-42491.

Murdoch, C., Muthana, M., Coffelt, S.B., and Lewis, C.E. (2008). The role of myeloid cells in the promotion of tumour angiogenesis. Nat Rev Cancer *8*, 618-631.

Nervi, B., Ramirez, P., Rettig, M.P., Uy, G.L., Holt, M.S., Ritchey, J.K., Prior, J.L., Piwnica-Worms, D., Bridger, G., Ley, T.J., *et al.* (2009). Chemosensitization of acute myeloid leukemia (AML) following mobilization by the CXCR4 antagonist AMD3100. Blood *113*, 6206-6214.

Ng, E.W., Shima, D.T., Calias, P., Cunningham, E.T., Jr., Guyer, D.R., and Adamis, A.P. (2006). Pegaptanib, a targeted anti-VEGF aptamer for ocular vascular disease. Nat Rev Drug Discov *5*, 123-132.

Nishisho, T., Hata, K., Nakanishi, M., Morita, Y., Sun-Wada, G.H., Wada, Y., Yasui, N., and Yoneda, T. (2011). The a3 isoform vacuolar type H-ATPase promotes distant metastasis in the mouse B16 melanoma cells. Mol Cancer Res *9*, 845-855.

Nyberg, P., Xie, L., and Kalluri, R. (2005). Endogenous inhibitors of angiogenesis. Cancer Res *65*, 3967-3979.

O'Brien, C.A., Pollett, A., Gallinger, S., and Dick, J.E. (2007). A human colon cancer cell capable of initiating tumour growth in immunodeficient mice. Nature *445*, 106-110.

O'Farrell, A.M., Abrams, T.J., Yuen, H.A., Ngai, T.J., Louie, S.G., Yee, K.W., Wong, L.M., Hong, W., Lee, L.B., Town, A., *et al.* (2003). SU11248 is a novel FLT3 tyrosine kinase inhibitor with potent activity in vitro and in vivo. Blood *101*, 3597-3605.

Oliner, J., Min, H., Leal, J., Yu, D., Rao, S., You, E., Tang, X., Kim, H., Meyer, S., Han, S.J., *et al.* (2004). Suppression of angiogenesis and tumor growth by selective inhibition of angiopoietin-2. Cancer Cell *6*, 507-516.

Onozawa, Y., Komai, T., and Oda, T. (2011). Activation of T cell death-associated gene 8 attenuates inflammation by negatively regulating the function of inflammatory cells. Eur J Pharmacol *654*, 315-319.

Orimo, A., Gupta, P.B., Sgroi, D.C., Arenzana-Seisdedos, F., Delaunay, T., Naeem, R., Carey, V.J., Richardson, A.L., and Weinberg, R.A. (2005). Stromal fibroblasts present in invasive human breast carcinomas promote tumor growth and angiogenesis through elevated SDF-1/CXCL12 secretion. Cell *121*, 335-348.

Orimo, A., and Weinberg, R.A. (2006). Stromal fibroblasts in cancer: a novel tumor-promoting cell type. Cell Cycle *5*, 1597-1601.

Paez-Ribes, M., Allen, E., Hudock, J., Takeda, T., Okuyama, H., Vinals, F., Inoue, M., Bergers, G., Hanahan, D., and Casanovas, O. (2009). Antiangiogenic therapy elicits malignant progression of tumors to increased local invasion and distant metastasis. Cancer Cell *15*, 220-231.

Pages, F., Galon, J., Dieu-Nosjean, M.C., Tartour, E., Sautes-Fridman, C., and Fridman, W.H. (2010). Immune infiltration in human tumors: a prognostic factor that should not be ignored. Oncogene *29*, 1093-1102.

Papapetropoulos, A., Garcia-Cardena, G., Dengler, T.J., Maisonpierre, P.C., Yancopoulos, G.D., and Sessa, W.C. (1999). Direct actions of angiopoietin-1 on human endothelium: evidence for network stabilization, cell survival, and interaction with other angiogenic growth factors. Lab Invest *79*, 213-223.

Papetti, M., and Herman, I.M. (2002). Mechanisms of normal and tumor-derived angiogenesis. Am J Physiol Cell Physiol *282*, C947-970.

Paradiso, A., Cardone, R.A., Bellizzi, A., Bagorda, A., Guerra, L., Tommasino, M., Casavola, V., and Reshkin, S.J. (2004). The Na+-H+ exchanger-1 induces cytoskeletal changes involving reciprocal RhoA and Rac1 signaling, resulting in motility and invasion in MDA-MB-435 cells. Breast Cancer Res *6*, R616-628.

Patard, J.J., Rioux-Leclercq, N., Masson, D., Zerrouki, S., Jouan, F., Collet, N., Dubourg, C., Lobel, B., Denis, M., and Fergelot, P. (2009). Absence of VHL gene alteration and high VEGF expression are associated with tumour aggressiveness and poor survival of renal-cell carcinoma. Br J Cancer *101*, 1417-1424.

Paterson, R.F., Ulbright, T.M., MacLennan, G.T., Zhang, S., Pan, C.X., Sweeney, C.J., Moore, C.R., Foster, R.S., Koch, M.O., Eble, J.N., *et al.* (2003). Molecular genetic alterations in the laser-capture-microdissected stroma adjacent to bladder carcinoma. Cancer *98*, 1830-1836.

Pennacchietti, S., Michieli, P., Galluzzo, M., Mazzone, M., Giordano, S., and Comoglio, P.M. (2003). Hypoxia promotes invasive growth by transcriptional activation of the met protooncogene. Cancer Cell *3*, 347-361.

Perez-Sayans, M., Reboiras-Lopez, M.D., Somoza-Martin, J.M., Barros-Angueira, F., Diz, P.G., Rey, J.M., and Garcia-Garcia, A. (2010). Measurement of ATP6V1C1 expression in brush cytology samples as a diagnostic and prognostic marker in oral squamous cell carcinoma. Cancer Biol Ther *9*, 1057-1064.

Pertega-Gomes, N., Vizcaino, J.R., Miranda-Goncalves, V., Pinheiro, C., Silva, J., Pereira, H., Monteiro, P., Henrique, R.M., Reis, R.M., Lopes, C., *et al.* (2011). Monocarboxylate transporter 4 (MCT4) and CD147 overexpression is associated with poor prognosis in prostate cancer. BMC Cancer *11*, 312.

Petrulio, C.A., Kim-Schulze, S., and Kaufman, H.L. (2006). The tumour microenvironment and implications for cancer immunotherapy. Expert Opin Biol Ther *6*, 671-684.

Pinheiro, C., Albergaria, A., Paredes, J., Sousa, B., Dufloth, R., Vieira, D., Schmitt, F., and Baltazar, F. (2010). Monocarboxylate transporter 1 is up-regulated in basal-like breast carcinoma. Histopathology *56*, 860-867.

Pinheiro, C., Longatto-Filho, A., Scapulatempo, C., Ferreira, L., Martins, S., Pellerin, L., Rodrigues, M., Alves, V.A., Schmitt, F., and Baltazar, F. (2008). Increased expression of monocarboxylate transporters 1, 2, and 4 in colorectal carcinomas. Virchows Arch *452*, 139-146.

Presta, L.G., Chen, H., O'Connor, S.J., Chisholm, V., Meng, Y.G., Krummen, L., Winkler, M., and Ferrara, N. (1997). Humanization of an anti-vascular endothelial growth factor monoclonal antibody for the therapy of solid tumors and other disorders. Cancer Res *57*, 4593-4599.

Prince, M.E., Sivanandan, R., Kaczorowski, A., Wolf, G.T., Kaplan, M.J., Dalerba, P., Weissman, I.L., Clarke, M.F., and Ailles, L.E. (2007). Identification of a subpopulation of cells with cancer stem cell properties in head and neck squamous cell carcinoma. Proc Natl Acad Sci U S A *104*, 973-978.

Pusic, I., and DiPersio, J.F. (2010). Update on clinical experience with AMD3100, an SDF-1/CXCL12-CXCR4 inhibitor, in mobilization of hematopoietic stem and progenitor cells. Curr Opin Hematol *17*, 319-326.

Qiu, W., Hu, M., Sridhar, A., Opeskin, K., Fox, S., Shipitsin, M., Trivett, M., Thompson, E.R., Ramakrishna, M., Gorringe, K.L., *et al.* (2008). No evidence of clonal somatic genetic alterations in cancer-associated fibroblasts from human breast and ovarian carcinomas. Nat Genet *40*, 650-655.

Quintana, E., Shackleton, M., Sabel, M.S., Fullen, D.R., Johnson, T.M., and Morrison, S.J. (2008). Efficient tumour formation by single human melanoma cells. Nature *456*, 593-598.

Radu, C.G., Nijagal, A., McLaughlin, J., Wang, L., and Witte, O.N. (2005). Differential proton sensitivity of related G protein-coupled receptors T cell death-associated gene 8 and G2A expressed in immune cells. Proc Natl Acad Sci U S A *102*, 1632-1637.

Rak, J., Mitsuhashi, Y., Bayko, L., Filmus, J., Shirasawa, S., Sasazuki, T., and Kerbel, R.S. (1995). Mutant ras oncogenes upregulate VEGF/VPF expression: implications for induction and inhibition of tumor angiogenesis. Cancer Res *55*, 4575-4580.

Rankin, E.B., and Giaccia, A.J. (2008). The role of hypoxia-inducible factors in tumorigenesis. Cell Death Differ *15*, 678-685.

Rapisarda, A., and Melillo, G. (2009). Role of the hypoxic tumor microenvironment in the resistance to anti-angiogenic therapies. Drug Resist Updat *12*, 74-80.

Reshkin, S.J., Bellizzi, A., Cardone, R.A., Tommasino, M., Casavola, V., and Paradiso, A. (2003). Paclitaxel induces apoptosis via protein kinase A- and p38 mitogen-activated protein-dependent inhibition of the Na+/H+ exchanger (NHE) NHE isoform 1 in human breast cancer cells. Clin Cancer Res *9*, 2366-2373.

Ricci-Vitiani, L., Lombardi, D.G., Pilozzi, E., Biffoni, M., Todaro, M., Peschle, C., and De Maria, R. (2007). Identification and expansion of human colon-cancer-initiating cells. Nature *445*, 111-115.

Ridgway, J., Zhang, G., Wu, Y., Stawicki, S., Liang, W.C., Chanthery, Y., Kowalski, J., Watts, R.J., Callahan, C., Kasman, I., *et al.* (2006). Inhibition of Dll4 signalling inhibits tumour growth by deregulating angiogenesis. Nature *444*, 1083-1087.

Ridgway, P.F., Ziprin, P., Alkhamesi, N., Paraskeva, P.A., Peck, D.H., and Darzi, A.W. (2005). Hypoxia augments gelatinase activity in a variety of adenocarcinomas in vitro. J Surg Res *124*, 180-186.

Righi, E., Kashiwagi, S., Yuan, J., Santosuosso, M., Leblanc, P., Ingraham, R., Forbes, B., Edelblute, B., Collette, B., Xing, D., *et al.* (2011). CXCL12/CXCR4 Blockade Induces Multimodal Antitumor Effects That Prolong Survival in an Immunocompetent Mouse Model of Ovarian Cancer. Cancer Res *71*, 5522-5534.

Robert, C., Thomas, L., Bondarenko, I., O'Day, S., M, D.J., Garbe, C., Lebbe, C., Baurain, J.F., Testori, A., Grob, J.J., *et al.* (2011a). Ipilimumab plus dacarbazine for previously untreated metastatic melanoma. N Engl J Med *364*, 2517-2526.

Robert, N.J., Dieras, V., Glaspy, J., Brufsky, A.M., Bondarenko, I., Lipatov, O.N., Perez, E.A., Yardley, D.A., Chan, S.Y., Zhou, X., *et al.* (2011b). RIBBON-1: randomized, double-blind, placebo-controlled, phase III trial of chemotherapy with or without bevacizumab for first-line treatment of human epidermal growth factor receptor 2-negative, locally recurrent or metastatic breast cancer. J Clin Oncol *29*, 1252-1260.

Rofstad, E.K., and Halsor, E.F. (2002). Hypoxia-associated spontaneous pulmonary metastasis in human melanoma xenografts: involvement of microvascular hot spots induced in hypoxic foci by interleukin 8. Br J Cancer *86*, 301-308.

Ronnov-Jessen, L., Petersen, O.W., and Bissell, M.J. (1996). Cellular changes involved in conversion of normal to malignant breast: importance of the stromal reaction. Physiol Rev *76*, 69-125.

Rosenberg, S.A., Yang, J.C., Sherry, R.M., Kammula, U.S., Hughes, M.S., Phan, G.Q., Citrin, D.E., Restifo, N.P., Robbins, P.F., Wunderlich, J.R., *et al.* (2011). Durable complete responses in heavily pretreated patients with metastatic melanoma using T-cell transfer immunotherapy. Clin Cancer Res *17*, 4550-4557.

Rosenfeld, P.J., Brown, D.M., Heier, J.S., Boyer, D.S., Kaiser, P.K., Chung, C.Y., and Kim, R.Y. (2006). Ranibizumab for neovascular age-related macular degeneration. N Engl J Med *355*, 1419-1431.

Rothwell, P.M., Fowkes, F.G., Belch, J.F., Ogawa, H., Warlow, C.P., and Meade, T.W. (2011). Effect of daily aspirin on long-term risk of death due to cancer: analysis of individual patient data from randomised trials. Lancet *377*, 31-41.

Rothwell, P.M., Wilson, M., Elwin, C.E., Norrving, B., Algra, A., Warlow, C.P., and Meade, T.W. (2010). Long-term effect of aspirin on colorectal cancer incidence and mortality: 20-year follow-up of five randomised trials. Lancet *376*, 1741-1750.

Ryan, G.B., Cliff, W.J., Gabbiani, G., Irle, C., Statkov, P.R., and Majno, G. (1973). Myofibroblasts in an avascular fibrous tissue. Lab Invest *29*, 197-206.

Sahai, E. (2007). Illuminating the metastatic process. Nat Rev Cancer *7*, 737-749.

Sandler, A., Gray, R., Perry, M.C., Brahmer, J., Schiller, J.H., Dowlati, A., Lilenbaum, R., and Johnson, D.H. (2006). Paclitaxel-carboplatin alone or with bevacizumab for non-small-cell lung cancer. N Engl J Med *355*, 2542-2550.

Santisteban, M., Reiman, J.M., Asiedu, M.K., Behrens, M.D., Nassar, A., Kalli, K.R., Haluska, P., Ingle, J.N., Hartmann, L.C., Manjili, M.H., *et al.* (2009). Immune-induced epithelial to mesenchymal transition in vivo generates breast cancer stem cells. Cancer Res *69*, 2887-2895.

Schor, S.L., Schor, A.M., Grey, A.M., and Rushton, G. (1988). Foetal and cancer patient fibroblasts produce an autocrine migration-stimulating factor not made by normal adult cells. J Cell Sci *90 (Pt 3)*, 391-399.

Schwartz, D.L., Powis, G., Thitai-Kumar, A., He, Y., Bankson, J., Williams, R., Lemos, R., Oh, J., Volgin, A., Soghomonyan, S., *et al.* (2009). The selective hypoxia inducible factor-1 inhibitor PX-478 provides in vivo radiosensitization through tumor stromal effects. Mol Cancer Ther *8*, 947-958.

Seaman, S., Stevens, J., Yang, M.Y., Logsdon, D., Graff-Cherry, C., and St Croix, B. (2007). Genes that distinguish physiological and pathological angiogenesis. Cancer Cell *11*, 539-554.

Semenza, G.L. (2003). Targeting HIF-1 for cancer therapy. Nat Rev Cancer *3*, 721-732.

Semenza, G.L. (2007a). Evaluation of HIF-1 inhibitors as anticancer agents. Drug Discov Today *12*, 853-859.

Semenza, G.L. (2007b). Hypoxia-inducible factor 1 (HIF-1) pathway. Sci STKE *2007*, cm8.

Shibuya, M., and Claesson-Welsh, L. (2006). Signal transduction by VEGF receptors in regulation of angiogenesis and lymphangiogenesis. Exp Cell Res *312*, 549-560.

Shimoda, M., Mellody, K.T., and Orimo, A. (2010). Carcinoma-associated fibroblasts are a rate-limiting determinant for tumour progression. Semin Cell Dev Biol *21*, 19-25.

Sin, W.C., Zhang, Y., Zhong, W., Adhikarakunnathu, S., Powers, S., Hoey, T., An, S., and Yang, J. (2004). G protein-coupled receptors GPR4 and TDAG8 are oncogenic and overexpressed in human cancers. Oncogene *23*, 6299-6303.

Singh, A., and Settleman, J. (2010). EMT, cancer stem cells and drug resistance: an emerging axis of evil in the war on cancer. Oncogene *29*, 4741-4751.

Singh, L.S., Berk, M., Oates, R., Zhao, Z., Tan, H., Jiang, Y., Zhou, A., Kirmani, K., Steinmetz, R., Lindner, D., *et al.* (2007). Ovarian cancer G protein-coupled receptor 1, a new metastasis suppressor gene in prostate cancer. J Natl Cancer Inst *99*, 1313-1327.

Singh, S., Srivastava, S.K., Bhardwaj, A., Owen, L.B., and Singh, A.P. (2010). CXCL12-CXCR4 signalling axis confers gemcitabine resistance to pancreatic cancer cells: a novel target for therapy. Br J Cancer *103*, 1671-1679.

Singh, S.K., Hawkins, C., Clarke, I.D., Squire, J.A., Bayani, J., Hide, T., Henkelman, R.M., Cusimano, M.D., and Dirks, P.B. (2004). Identification of human brain tumour initiating cells. Nature *432*, 396-401.

Smith, J.K., Mamoon, N.M., and Duhe, R.J. (2004). Emerging roles of targeted small molecule protein-tyrosine kinase inhibitors in cancer therapy. Oncol Res *14*, 175-225.

So, C.W., Karsunky, H., Wong, P., Weissman, I.L., and Cleary, M.L. (2004). Leukemic transformation of hematopoietic progenitors by MLL-GAS7 in the absence of Hoxa7 or Hoxa9. Blood *103*, 3192-3199.

Solomon, S.D., McMurray, J.J., Pfeffer, M.A., Wittes, J., Fowler, R., Finn, P., Anderson, W.F., Zauber, A., Hawk, E., and Bertagnolli, M. (2005). Cardiovascular risk associated with celecoxib in a clinical trial for colorectal adenoma prevention. N Engl J Med *352*, 1071-1080.

Solomon, S.D., Pfeffer, M.A., McMurray, J.J., Fowler, R., Finn, P., Levin, B., Eagle, C., Hawk, E., Lechuga, M., Zauber, A.G., *et al.* (2006). Effect of celecoxib on cardiovascular events and blood pressure in two trials for the prevention of colorectal adenomas. Circulation *114*, 1028-1035.

Sonveaux, P., Vegran, F., Schroeder, T., Wergin, M.C., Verrax, J., Rabbani, Z.N., De Saedeleer, C.J., Kennedy, K.M., Diepart, C., Jordan, B.F., *et al.* (2008). Targeting lactate-fueled respiration selectively kills hypoxic tumor cells in mice. J Clin Invest *118*, 3930-3942.

Steeg, P.S. (2003). Angiogenesis inhibitors: motivators of metastasis? Nat Med *9*, 822-823.

Steeg, P.S. (2006). Tumor metastasis: mechanistic insights and clinical challenges. Nat Med *12*, 895-904.

Steinbach, G., Lynch, P.M., Phillips, R.K., Wallace, M.H., Hawk, E., Gordon, G.B., Wakabayashi, N., Saunders, B., Shen, Y., Fujimura, T., *et al.* (2000). The effect of celecoxib, a cyclooxygenase-2 inhibitor, in familial adenomatous polyposis. N Engl J Med *342*, 1946-1952.

Sternberg, C.N., Davis, I.D., Mardiak, J., Szczylik, C., Lee, E., Wagstaff, J., Barrios, C.H., Salman, P., Gladkov, O.A., Kavina, A., *et al.* (2010). Pazopanib in locally advanced or metastatic renal cell carcinoma: results of a randomized phase III trial. J Clin Oncol *28*, 1061-1068.

Sternlicht, M.D., Lochter, A., Sympson, C.J., Huey, B., Rougier, J.P., Gray, J.W., Pinkel, D., Bissell, M.J., and Werb, Z. (1999). The stromal proteinase MMP3/stromelysin-1 promotes mammary carcinogenesis. Cell *98*, 137-146.

Surowiak, P., Suchocki, S., Gyorffy, B., Gansukh, T., Wojnar, A., Maciejczyk, A., Pudelko, M., and Zabel, M. (2006). Stromal myofibroblasts in breast cancer: relations between their occurrence, tumor grade and expression of some tumour markers. Folia Histochem Cytobiol *44*, 111-116.

Swietach, P., Hulikova, A., Vaughan-Jones, R.D., and Harris, A.L. (2010). New insights into the physiological role of carbonic anhydrase IX in tumour pH regulation. Oncogene *29*, 6509-6521.

Szeto, M.D., Chakraborty, G., Hadley, J., Rockne, R., Muzi, M., Alvord, E.C., Jr., Krohn, K.A., Spence, A.M., and Swanson, K.R. (2009). Quantitative metrics of net proliferation and invasion link biological aggressiveness assessed by MRI with hypoxia assessed by FMISO-PET in newly diagnosed glioblastomas. Cancer Res *69*, 4502-4509.

Tennant, D.A., Duran, R.V., and Gottlieb, E. (2010). Targeting metabolic transformation for cancer therapy. Nat Rev Cancer *10*, 267-277.

Thiery, J.P. (2003). Epithelial-mesenchymal transitions in development and pathologies. Curr Opin Cell Biol *15*, 740-746.

Till, J.E., McCulloch, E.A., and Siminovitch, L. (1964). A Stochastic Model of Stem Cell Proliferation, Based on the Growth of Spleen Colony-Forming Cells. Proc Natl Acad Sci U S A *51*, 29-36.

Tischer, E., Mitchell, R., Hartman, T., Silva, M., Gospodarowicz, D., Fiddes, J.C., and Abraham, J.A. (1991). The human gene for vascular endothelial growth factor. Multiple protein forms are encoded through alternative exon splicing. J Biol Chem *266*, 11947-11954.

Tobo, M., Tomura, H., Mogi, C., Wang, J.Q., Liu, J.P., Komachi, M., Damirin, A., Kimura, T., Murata, N., Kurose, H., *et al.* (2007). Previously postulated "ligand-independent" signaling of GPR4 is mediated through proton-sensing mechanisms. Cell Signal *19*, 1745-1753.

Tuhkanen, H., Anttila, M., Kosma, V.M., Yla-Herttuala, S., Heinonen, S., Kuronen, A., Juhola, M., Tammi, R., Tammi, M., and Mannermaa, A. (2004). Genetic alterations in the peritumoral stromal cells of malignant and borderline epithelial ovarian tumors as indicated by allelic imbalance on chromosome 3p. Int J Cancer *109*, 247-252.

Turturro, F., Lawson, M., Friday, E., and Welbourne, T. (2007). Targeting the Na(+)/H(+) exchanger: an old concept with new perspectives in the treatment of hematological malignancies. Leuk Res *31*, 1449-1450.

Uchida, D., Onoue, T., Kuribayashi, N., Tomizuka, Y., Tamatani, T., Nagai, H., and Miyamoto, Y. (2011). Blockade of CXCR4 in oral squamous cell carcinoma inhibits lymph node metastases. Eur J Cancer *47*, 452-459.

Valable, S., Petit, E., Roussel, S., Marteau, L., Toutain, J., Divoux, D., Sobrio, F., Delamare, J., Barre, L., and Bernaudin, M. (2011). Complementary information from magnetic resonance imaging and (18)F-fluoromisonidazole positron emission tomography in the assessment of the response to an antiangiogenic treatment in a rat brain tumor model. Nucl Med Biol *38*, 781-793.

Van Cutsem, E., Vervenne, W.L., Bennouna, J., Humblet, Y., Gill, S., Van Laethem, J.L., Verslype, C., Scheithauer, W., Shang, A., Cosaert, J., *et al.* (2009). Phase III trial of bevacizumab in combination with gemcitabine and erlotinib in patients with metastatic pancreatic cancer. J Clin Oncol *27*, 2231-2237.

Vander Heiden, M.G., Cantley, L.C., and Thompson, C.B. (2009). Understanding the Warburg effect: the metabolic requirements of cell proliferation. Science *324*, 1029-1033.

Vavere, A.L., Biddlecombe, G.B., Spees, W.M., Garbow, J.R., Wijesinghe, D., Andreev, O.A., Engelman, D.M., Reshetnyak, Y.K., and Lewis, J.S. (2009). A novel technology for the imaging of acidic prostate tumors by positron emission tomography. Cancer Res *69*, 4510-4516.

Verheul, H.M., and Pinedo, H.M. (2007). Possible molecular mechanisms involved in the toxicity of angiogenesis inhibition. Nat Rev Cancer *7*, 475-485.

Walter, K., Omura, N., Hong, S.M., Griffith, M., and Goggins, M. (2008). Pancreatic cancer associated fibroblasts display normal allelotypes. Cancer Biol Ther *7*, 882-888.

Wang, J.Q., Kon, J., Mogi, C., Tobo, M., Damirin, A., Sato, K., Komachi, M., Malchinkhuu, E., Murata, N., Kimura, T., *et al.* (2004). TDAG8 is a proton-sensing and psychosine-sensitive G-protein-coupled receptor. J Biol Chem *279*, 45626-45633.

Wang, Y., Liu, Y., Malek, S.N., and Zheng, P. (2011). Targeting HIF1alpha eliminates cancer stem cells in hematological malignancies. Cell Stem Cell *8*, 399-411.

Warburg, O. (1956). On the origin of cancer cells. Science *123*, 309-314.

Webb, B.A., Chimenti, M., Jacobson, M.P., and Barber, D.L. (2011). Dysregulated pH: a perfect storm for cancer progression. Nat Rev Cancer *11*, 671-677.

Welsh, S., Williams, R., Kirkpatrick, L., Paine-Murrieta, G., and Powis, G. (2004). Antitumor activity and pharmacodynamic properties of PX-478, an inhibitor of hypoxia-inducible factor-1alpha. Mol Cancer Ther *3*, 233-244.

Wernert, N., Locherbach, C., Wellmann, A., Behrens, P., and Hugel, A. (2001). Presence of genetic alterations in microdissected stroma of human colon and breast cancers. Anticancer Res *21*, 2259-2264.

Wilkerson, J., and Fojo, T. (2009). Progression-free survival is simply a measure of a drug's effect while administered and is not a surrogate for overall survival. Cancer J *15*, 379-385.

Wilson, W.R., and Hay, M.P. (2011). Targeting hypoxia in cancer therapy. Nat Rev Cancer *11*, 393-410.

Xie, J., and Itzkowitz, S.H. (2008). Cancer in inflammatory bowel disease. World J Gastroenterol *14*, 378-389.

Xiong, Y.Q., Sun, H.C., Zhang, W., Zhu, X.D., Zhuang, P.Y., Zhang, J.B., Wang, L., Wu, W.Z., Qin, L.X., and Tang, Z.Y. (2009). Human hepatocellular carcinoma tumor-derived endothelial cells manifest increased angiogenesis capability and drug resistance compared with normal endothelial cells. Clin Cancer Res *15*, 4838-4846.

Yamagata, M., Hasuda, K., Stamato, T., and Tannock, I.F. (1998). The contribution of lactic acid to acidification of tumours: studies of variant cells lacking lactate dehydrogenase. Br J Cancer *77*, 1726-1731.

Yang, L.V., Radu, C.G., Roy, M., Lee, S., McLaughlin, J., Teitell, M.A., Iruela-Arispe, M.L., and Witte, O.N. (2007). Vascular abnormalities in mice deficient for the G protein-coupled receptor GPR4 that functions as a pH sensor. Mol Cell Biol *27*, 1334-1347.

You, H., Jin, J., Shu, H., Yu, B., De Milito, A., Lozupone, F., Deng, Y., Tang, N., Yao, G., Fais, S., *et al.* (2009). Small interfering RNA targeting the subunit ATP6L of proton pump V-ATPase overcomes chemoresistance of breast cancer cells. Cancer Lett *280*, 110-119.

You, W.K., and McDonald, D.M. (2008). The hepatocyte growth factor/c-Met signaling pathway as a therapeutic target to inhibit angiogenesis. BMB Rep *41*, 833-839.

Zatovicova, M., Jelenska, L., Hulikova, A., Csaderova, L., Ditte, Z., Ditte, P., Goliasova, T., Pastorek, J., and Pastorekova, S. (2010). Carbonic anhydrase IX as an anticancer therapy target: preclinical evaluation of internalizing monoclonal antibody directed to catalytic domain. Curr Pharm Des *16*, 3255-3263.

Zeisberg, M., Strutz, F., and Muller, G.A. (2000). Role of fibroblast activation in inducing interstitial fibrosis. J Nephrol *13 Suppl 3*, S111-120.

Zhang, F., and Aft, R.L. (2009). Chemosensitizing and cytotoxic effects of 2-deoxy-D-glucose on breast cancer cells. J Cancer Res Ther *5 Suppl 1*, S41-43.

Zhao, B.C., Wang, Z.J., Mao, W.Z., Ma, H.C., Han, J.G., Zhao, B., and Xu, H.M. (2011). CXCR4/SDF-1 axis is involved in lymph node metastasis of gastric carcinoma. World J Gastroenterol *17*, 2389-2396.

2

Inflammatory ROS in Fanconi Anemia Hematopoiesis and Leukemogenesis

Wei Du
Division of Experimental Hematology and Cancer Biology, Cincinnati Children's Hospital Medical Center, Cincinnati, Ohio USA

1. Introduction

Fanconi anemia (FA) is a genetic disorder characterized by bone marrow failure (BMF), clonal proliferation of hematopoietic stem cells, and transformation to leukemia and other cancers (Ames *et al.*, 1995; Boglilo *et al.*, 2002; Cohen-Haguenauer *et al.*, 2006; Cumming *et al.*, 2001; Fagerlie *et al.*, 2001; Jonkers *et al.*, 2001; Suematsu *et al.*, 2003). Somatic cell fusion studies show FA is genetically heterogeneous. So far mutations in 15 genes have been identified in FA or FA-like patients (Cohen-Haguenauer *et al.*, 2006; Joenje *et al.*, 1987; Jonkers *et al.*, 2001; Lensch *et al.*, 1999; Stoepker *et al.*, 2011; Yamamoto *et al.*, 2011). The genes encoding the groups A (FANCA), B (FANCB), C (FANCC), D1 (FANCD1/BRCA2), D2 (FANCD2), E (FANCE), F (FANCF), G (FANCG), -I (FANCI/KIAA1794), J (FANCJ/ BRIP1), L (FANCL), M (FANCM), N (FANCN/PALB2), O/RAD51C and P/SLX4 proteins have been cloned (de Winter *et al.*, 1998, 2000a, 2000b; Howlett *et al.*, 2002; Joenje *et al.*, 2000; Letitus *et al.*, 2004; Levran *et al.*, 2005; Lo Ten Foe *et al.*, 1996; Meetei *et al.*, 2003, 2004, 2005; Meindl *et al.*, 2010; Reid *et al.*, 2006; Smogorzewska *et al.*, 2007; Somyajit *et al.*, 2010; Strathdee *et al.*, 1992; Timmers *et al.*, 2001; Xia *et al.*, 2006; Yamamoto *et al.*, 2011). The latter two genes are still thought of as tentative as they do not fall within a defined category biologically and the patients carrying these gene mutations are limited. The majority of mutations are found in *FANCA*, *FANCC* and *FANCC* genes in FA patients (Table 1). Recent studies on the biological function of these FA proteins have demonstrated that eight of the FA proteins (namely, FANCA, B, C, E, F, G, L, and M) form a nuclear multiprotein complex (Collins *et al.*, 2005; D'Andrea *et al.*, 2003; de Winter *et al.*, 2000; Meetei *et al.*, 2003; Smogorzewska *et al.*, 2007; Tischkowitz *et al.*, 2003; Walsh *et al.*, 1994), which functions as a nuclear E3 ubiquitin ligase that monoubiquitinates downstream FANCD2/FANCI dimer in response to DNA damage or DNA replication stress. This FANCD2/FANCI heterodimer then recruits other downstream FA proteins including FANCD1 (which is the breast cancer protein BRCA2), and the recently identified FANCJ, FANCN, FANCO and another breast cancer protein, BRCA1 (D'Andrea *et al.*, 2010), to nuclear loci containing damaged DNA and consequently influence important cellular processes such as DNA replication, cell-cycle control, and DNA damage repair. The core complex also interacts with the FAAP100 and FAPP24 proteins, which are also crucial components in the pathway (Ciccia *et al.*, 2007; Horejsi *et al.*, 2009; Collis *et al.*, 2008, Fig 1). FANCM and its interacting proteins, such as FAAP24 and MHF1, MHF2, also play a role in controlling the processing and stabilization of stalled replication forks (Schwab *et al.*, 2010; Luke-Glaser *et al.*, 2010; Singh *et al.*, 2010).

Subtype	FA Patients Estimated %	Chromosome Location	Protein Products (kd)	Function
A	60.9	16q24.3	163	FA core complex
B	2.0	Xp22.31	95 (FAAP95)	FA core complex
C	7.6	9q22.3	63	FA core complex
D1	5.0	13q12-13	380 (BRCA2)	RAD51 recruitment
D2	4.7	3p25.3	155,162	Involved in DNA damage repair
E	3.5	6p21-22	60	FA core complex
F	2.0	11p15	42	FA core complex
G	6.9	9p13	68 (XRCC9)	FA core complex
I	2.8	15q25-16	140 (FANCI/KIAA1794)	Required for maintenance of chromosomal stability
J	1.7	17q22-q24	140 (FANCJ/BACH1/BRIP1)	5'>3' DNA helicase/ATPase
L	0.4	2p16.1	43(FANCL/PHF9/POG)	FA core complex,FAAP43 ubiqutin ligase
M	0.3	14q21.3	250	FA core complex/ATPase/translocase
N	2.1	16p12.1	130 (FANCN/PALB2)	Regulation of BRCA2 location
O	Rare	17q25.1	42 (FANCO/RAD51C)	Involved in HRR of DSB
P	Rare	16p13.3	200 (FANCP/SLX4)	Protect genome stability
BRCA1	-	17q21	208	E3 ubiquitin ligase Required for FANCD2 targeting to DNA damage site
FAAP100	-	17q25.1	100	Required for D2 mono-Ub
FAAP24	-	19q13.11	24	Required for D2 mono-Ub
MHF1	-	1p36.22	16 (FAAP16)	Interact with FANCM
MHF2	-	17q25.3	10 (FAAP10)	Interact with FANCM

Table 1. Complementation groups and interaction proteins of Fanconi Anemia.

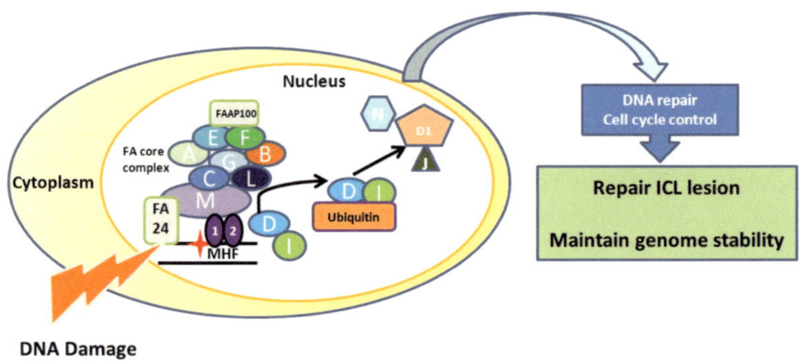

Fig. 1. Function of the FA pathway. Eight FA proteins form a nuclear core complex, which acts as ubiquitin ligase. FANCM interacts with FAAP24, FAAP100 as well as MHF1 and MFH2, resulting in complex chromatin loading and controlling the processing and stabilization of stalled forks, respectively. In response to DNA damage or replication stress, nuclear core complex monoubiquitinates two other FA proteins, FANCD2 and FANCI, which then recruit other downstream FA proteins FANCD1, FANCJ, and FANCN to damaged DNA and involved in DNA repair, cell-cycle control to repair ICL (interstrand crosslink) lesions and to maintain genome stability.

Many studies indicate that FA proteins might play specific roles in hematopoiesis by governing the responses of hematopoietic cells to both genotoxic and cytotoxic stresses. Loss of FA functions causes excessive apoptosis of HSC and progenitor cells (HSC/P) cells leading to BMF in the early stage of FA. As the disease progresses, apoptosis as well as genomic instability impose a selective pressure on FA HSC/P cells and promote the development of mutant clones, which could be transformed to leukemia (Cumming *et al.*, 1996, 2001; Fagerlie *et al.*, 2001; Haneline *et al.*, 1998, 1999, 2003; Koh *et al.*, 1999; Li X *et al.*, 2004; Li Y *et al.*, 1997; Maciejewski *et al.*, 1995; Nakata *et al.*, 2004; Pang *et al.*, 2001a, 2001b, 2002; Rathbun *et al.*, 1997, 2000; Si *et al.*, 2006; Walsh *et al.*, 1994; Wang *et al.*, 1998; Whitney *et al.*, 1996).

2. FA hematopoiesis

Hematological abnormalities are among the most important clinical features of FA. Children with FA often develop pancytopenia during the first few years of life. Complications of BM failure (BMF) are the major causes of morbidity and mortality of FA, and 80% of FA patients die from BMF (Bagby *et al.*, 2003; Buchwald *et al.*, 1998; Fagerlie *et al.*, 2001; Kutler *et al.*, 2003; Lensch *et al.*, 1999; Liu *et al.*, 2000). In addition, patients with FA have high risk of developing myelodysplasia (MDS) or acute myeloblastic leukemia (AML) (Bagby *et al.*, 2003; Buchwald *et al.*, 1998; D'Andrea *et al.*, 2003; Fagerlie *et al.*, 2001; Kennedy *et al.*, 2005; Tischkowitz *et al.*, 2003). During the BMF-MDS-AML progression, FA patients frequently develop clonal chromosomal abnormalities in the BM HSC/P cells. In fact, secondary occurred clonal cytogenetic abnormalities, such as 3q addition, 5q deletion and monosomy 7, are common in in children with FA who have evolved to MDS and AML and non-FA patients with MDS and AML after alkylating agents treatment (Freie *et al.*, 2004; Fridman *et al.*, 2003; Futaki *et al.*, 2002; Giaccia *et al.*, 1998; Lina-Fineman *et al.*, 1995; Rubin *et al.*, West *et al.*, 2000).

Excessive apoptosis and subsequent failure of the HSC compartment led to progressive BMF in FA patients have been documented from *in vitro* and *in vivo* studies. However, the molecular etiology of BMF and leukemia in FA remains to be elucidated. Compelling evidence suggest that altered expression of certain growth factors and cytokines, such as reduced expression of interleukin-6 (IL-6) and granulocyte-macrophage colony stimulating factor (GM-CSF) but increased secretion of mitotic inhibitor TNF-α in patient BM cells, may in part be responsible for hematopoietic disease progression in FA (de Cremoux *et al.*, 1996; Dufour *et al.*, 2003; Rosselli *et al.*, 1992; 1994; Schultz *et al.*, 1993; Stark *et al.*, 1993). It is conceivable that these alterations may change the BM microenvironment (for instance, leading to factor deprivation or constant exposure to mitogenic inhibitors) and cause deregulation of cellular homeostasis. It has also been shown that FA BM cells are hypersensitive to a variety of extracellular cytokines, including interferon-γ (IFN-γ) and tumor necrosis factor α (TNF-α) (Dufour *et al.*, 2003; Fagerlie *et al.*, 2001; Haneline *et al.*, 1998; Koh *et al.*, 1999; Li X *et al.*, 2004; Li Y *et al.*, 2004; Nakata *et al.*, 2004; Pang *et al.*, 2001a, 2001b, 2002; Rathbun *et al.*, 1997, 2000; Reid *et al.*, 2006; Rosselli *et al.*, 1992; Schultz *et al.*, 1993; Si *et al.*, 2006; Wang *et al.*, 1998; Whitney *et al.*, 1996), which may subsequently lead to cell apoptosis. Indeed, studies of FA patients have demonstrated that BM from FA patients has decreased number of colony-forming progenitors, as well as a reduction in colony size (Doneshbod–Skibba *et al.*, 1980; Gluckman *et al.*, 1989). These data demonstrate defective hematopoiesis in FA (Bagby *et al.*, 2003; Fagerlie *et al.*, 2001; Tischkowitz *et al.*, 2003).

In contrast to FA patients, mouse models deficient for several FA genes, including *Fanca, Fancc, Fancd2* and *Fancg*, do not show no spontaneous hematological defects or leukemia development (Cheng *et al.*, 2000; Whitney *et al.*, 1996; Wong & Buchwald, 2002; Yang *et al.*, 2001). Studies in the Fanca and Fancc mouse models show that while blood count and the number of committed BM progenitors are normal in FA mice as compared to WT mice; however, when subjected to sublethal dose of DNA cross-linking agent mitomycin C (MMC), which does not affect WT mouse cells, to the mutant mice experienced progressive decrease of all peripheral blood parameters, as well as early and committed progenitors, and eventually died within 8 weeks (Chen *et al.,* 1996; Whitney *et al.,* 1996). These results suggest that loss of FA genes in mouse models results in compromised defects in response to environmental insults (Chen *et al.,* 1996; Whitney *et al.,* 1996; Pang *et al.,* 2000; Rathbun *et al.,* 1997; Haneline *et al.,* 1998; Wong & Buchwald, 2002).

Similar to FA-C patients, BM cells from *Fancc-/-* mice show compromised colony growth capacity following IFN-γ, TNF-α and MIP-1α treatment (Haneline *et al.,* 1998). Literatures suggest that IFN-γ and TNF-α suppress colony growth forming ability of FA mouse BM cells by upregulating other cellular receptors, such as the fas receptor (CD95) (Young *et al.,* 1997). Increase in CD95 expression has been found in CD34+ cells from children with FA as well as the CD34+ fraction of hematopoietic progenitors in *Fancc-/-* mice, which is associated with increased apoptosis (Cumming *et al.,* 1996; Otsuki *et al.,* 1999). The hypersensitivity of *Fancc-/-* hematopoietic cells to IFN-γ and TNF-α is also mediated through activation of the RNA-dependent protein kinase (PKR) pathway, which is reported to initiate apoptosis in some instances, as an elevated level of activated PKR was found in *Fancc-/-* mouse embryonic fibroblasts (Pang *et al.,* 2001, 2002; Zhang *et al.,* 2004). Several groups independently showed compromised hematopoietic engraftment and reconstitution after BM transplantation of FA HSCs (Haneline *et al.,* 2003; Zhang *et al.,* 2007). Deregulation of apoptotic responses in hematopoietic cells may account at least in part for the nearly universal development of BM failure in children with inactivating FA mutations.

3. Inflammation and FA

Inflammation is a biological process orchestrated mainly by myeloid cells and accompanied by infection or phagocytosis (Balwill *et al.,* 2001). Increased oxidative stress in FA patients may be the result of an increased burden of endogenously produced oxidants as well as increased amounts of ROS generated by various inflammatory cytokines. Many studies indicate a correlation between elevated circulating pro-inflammatory cytokines and anemia in patients with leukemia-related BM diseases (Hakim *et al.,* 1993), but direct evidence for the mechanistic link between inflammation and BMF or leukemia is lacking.

There is evidence showing that patients with FA have abnormally high levels of TNF-α (Fagerlie *et al.,* 2001; Fiers *et al.,* 1999; Freie *et al.,* 2003), which is a major mediator of inflammation and ROS production (Liu *et al.,* 2003; Lohrum *et al.,* 1999). Inappropriate induction or activation of TNF-α signaling has been implicated in the pathogenesis of numerous common diseases such as arthritis, heart attacks, and cancer (Ekbom *et al.,* 1990; Jonsson *et al.,* 2005; Mantovani *et al.,* 2002; Marx *et al.,* 2004). It is conceivable that the presence of TNF-α and increased oxidative stress in FA BM may account for profound physiologic changes, including the development of BMF and progression to leukemia.

Similar to TNF-α, IL-1β and IL-6 are also well-known pro-inflammatory cytokines with a wide range of biological activities in immune regulation, hematopoiesis, inflammation and oncogenesis (Ibanez *et al.,* 2009). It has been demonstrated that IL-1β is overexpressed in FA-A patients (de Cremoux *et al.,* 1996). The elevated levels of IL-1*β* were completely reverted by complementation of functional FANCA into FA-A lymphocytes. In addition, the constitutive activation of the PI3K-Akt pathway in FA cells upregulates the expression of IL-1β through an NF-κB independent mechanism and this overproduction activates the proliferation of tumour cells (Ibanez *et al.,* 2009). IL-6 is the chief stimulator of the production of most acute phase proteins (Scheller *et al.,* 2011), whereas the other implicated cytokines influence subgroups of acute phase proteins. Recent studies demonstratethe presence of a defect in IL-6 production in FA patients (Coussens *et al.,* 2002; Cumming *et al.,* 1996), suggesting that this cytokine may partly be responsible for pancytopenia associated with BMF, the major clinical feature of FA, in FA patients. In addition, it has been reported that *Fancc-/-* HSC/P cells had altered growth and apoptosis responses to combinations of stimulatory cytokines, most dramatically in response to a combination of factors that included interleukin-3 (IL-3) and IL-6 (Aubé *et al.,* 2002).

4. FA oxidant hypersensitivity

Even in steady state, hematopoietic cells are exposed to various ROS, which are routinely generated during metabolic or inflammatory process. ROS induce a variety of responses in hematopoietic cells, including cellular proliferation and growth inhibition (Howlett *et al.,* 2002; Ichijo *et al.,* 1997). Like cells from other tissues, hematopoietic cells have developed several mechanisms to prevent the damage induced by oxidative stress. First, antioxidant enzymes, including superoxide dismutases (SODs), catalase, glutathione peroxidases and peroxiredoxins, can directly eliminate ROS. Secondly, other cellular enzymes can function to repair DNA damage induced by ROS in hematopoietic tissues. While FA murine models do not recapitulate some of the major FA clinical manifestations such as BM failure and leukemia, hematopoietic cells from FA knockout mice exhibit extreme oxidant sensitivity. Extensive studies have demonstrated FA oxidant hypersensitivity by using primary and immortalized cell cultures as well as *ex vivo* materials from patients (Bogliolo *et al.,* 2002; Cohen–Haguenauer *et al.,* 2006; Cumming *et al.,* 1996; Futaki *et al.,* 2002; Hadjur *et al.,* 2001; Kruyt *et al.,* 1998; Pagano *et al.,* 2005; Park *et al.,* 2004; Saadatzadeh *et al.,* 2004). It has also been shown that reoxygenation-generated oxidative stress, which is associated with significant DNA damage and inhibition of colony formation capacity (Ames *et al.,* 1993; Hammond *et al.,* 2003; Chen *et al.,* 2000), induced senescence of bone marrow progenitor cells from *Fancc-/-* mice compared to their counterparts. While these studies suggest a correlation between oxidative stress and FA disease progression, the mechanism by which oxidative stress influences the function of FA HSC/P cells has not been systematically studied. A number of hypotheses regarding the effect of oxidative stress in FA have been suggested, including the proposal that ROS could damage DNA and inability of FA HSC/P cells to repair such damage would result in exacerbated genomic instability leading to apoptosis and malignant transformation.

Three major FA core complex components, FANCA, FANCC, and FANCG (Bagby *et al.,* 2003; Kennedy *et al.,* 2000; Green *et al.,* 2009), were found to interact with a variety of cellular factors that primarily function in redox-related processes (Table 2), such as FANCC protein interacts with NADPH cytochrome P450 reductase and glutathione S-transferase P1-1 (Cumming *et al.,* 1996; Kruyt *et al.,* 1998), which are involved in either triggering or detoxifying reactive intermediates including ROS. It has also been demonstrated that *Fancc-/-* mice with deficiency in the anti-oxidative enzyme Cu/Zn superoxide dismutase demonstrated a defective hematopoiesis (Hadjur *et al.,* 2001). *Fancc-/-* cells exhibit hyperactivation of ASK1, a serine-threonine kinase that plays an important role in redox apoptotic signaling (Saadatzadeh *et al.,* 2004). Another FA protein, FANCG, interacts with cytochrome P450 2E1, which is associated with the production of reactive oxygen intermediates, and mitochondrial anti-oxidant enzyme peroxiredoxin-3 (Futaki *et al.,* 2002, Mukhopadhyay *et al.,* 2006), which suggested a possible role of FANCG in protection against oxidative DNA damage. Furthermore, FANCA and FANCG interact upon oxidative stress (Park *et al.,* 2004). These findings indicate a crucial role of FA proteins in oxidative stress signaling. We recently found that FANCD2 associated with FOXO3a, a master regulator in response to oxidative stress (Huang *et al.,* 2007; Li *et al.,* 2010; Tsai *et al.,* 2008). While these observations point to the involvement of FA proteins in oxidative stress response, the molecular pathways in which FA proteins function to modulate physiologic oxidative stress have not been defined.

FA proteins	*Redox-related factors*	*References*
FANCA	FANCG	Park *et al.*, 2004
FANCC	NADPH cytochrome P450 (RED)	Kruyt *et al.*, 1998
	Glutathine S-transferase P1-1 (GSTP1)	Cumming *et al.*, 2001
	Cu/Zn superoxide dismutase (SOD)	Hadjur *et al.*, 2001
	Apoptosis signal-regulating kinase 1 (ASK1)	Saadatzadeh *et al.*, 2004
FANCG	Cytochrome P450 2E1 (CYP2E1)	Futaki *et al.*, 2002
	Mitochondrail anti-oxidant enzyme peroxiredoxin-3	Mukhopadhyay *et al.*, 2006
FANCD2	Forkhead transcription factor FOXO3a	Li *et al.*, 2010

Table 2. Fanconi anemia proteins in redox signaling.

5. Oxidative stress response in FA hematopoietic cells: a FOXO3a connection

Forkhead transcription factors of the FOXO class O including FOXO1, FOXO3a, FOXO4 and FOXO6, are implicated in the regulation of diverse physiologic processes, including cell cycle arrest, apoptosis, DNA repair, stress resistance, and metabolism (Brunet *et al.,* 2004; Huang *et al.,* 2007). It has been established previously that members of the FOXO family are negatively regulated by PKB/c-Akt in response to insulin/IGF signaling, and are involved in regulating cell cycle progression and cell death (Geert *et al.,* 2002; Essers *et al.,* 2004). Among these FOXO proteins, FOXO3a functions as a master regulator of oxidative stress (Huang *et al.,* 2007; Tsai *et al.,* 2008). Several recent studies demonstrate that FOXO3a protects quiescent HSCs from oxidative stress (Tothova *et al.,* 2002, 2007; Miyamoto *et al.,* 2005). Some other studies also indicatethat Foxo3a is involved in inflammatory responses, such as inflammatory arthritis, intestinal inflammation, rheumatoid blood and synovial tissue, angiogenesis and postnatal neovascularization etc. (Turrel-Davin *et al.,* 2009; Potente *et al.,* 2005; Jonsson *et al.,* 2005; Walbert *et al.,* 2004).

While strong evidence indicates that FA cells, including hematopoietic cells from FA patients, are intolerant to oxidative stress (Cohen-Haguenauer *et al.,* 2006; Cumming *et al.,* 2001; Du *et al.,* 2008; Futaki *et al.,* 2002; Hadjur *et al.,* 2001; Kruyt *et al.,* 1998; Paganno *et al.,*

2005; Park *et al.*, 2004; Saadatzadeh *et al.*, 2004; Schindler *et al.*, 1988; Zhang *et al.*, 2005) and certain FA proteins interact with cellular factors involved in redox metabolism (Aggarwal *et al.*, 2003; Ames *et al.*, 1995; Bagby *et al.*, 2003), the molecular pathways in which FA proteins function to modulate physiologic oxidative stress have not been defined. Our recent identification of the FANCD2-FOXO3a complex (Li *et al.*, 2010) and preliminary characterization of impaired anti-oxidant defense in primary BM cells from FA patients opened new research opportunities to extend the functional study on the roles of FA proteins in the context of oxidative stress. We envision a model (Fig 2) in which the FA proteins regulate oxidative stress response through mechanisms involving functional interplay with the major oxidative stress-responsive transcription factor FOXO3a and protection of anti-oxidant genes from oxidative damage. Loss of these FA protein functions leads to elevated levels of ROS. As a consequence, FA HSC/P cells accumulate excessive DNA damage and increased genomic instability. However, further studies remains to be done in this context.

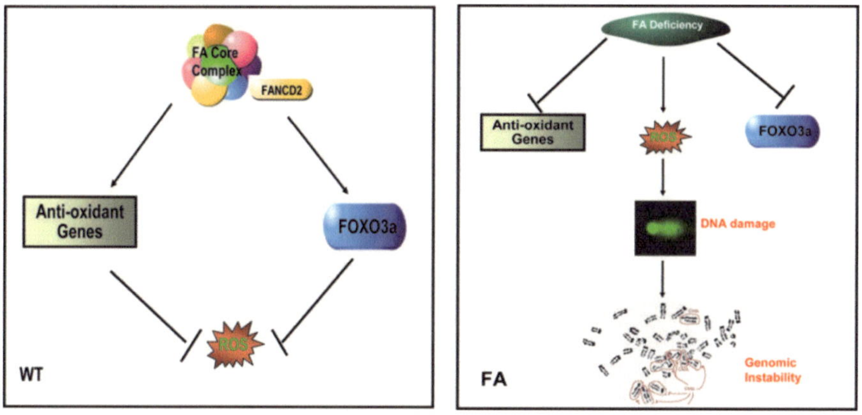

Fig. 2. A model for the role of FA proteins in oxidative stress signaling. In WT cells, the FA pathway helps keep cellular levels of ROS in check through functional interaction with the FOXO3a oxidative stress responsive pathway and safeguarding cellular anti-oxidant genes. In FA cells, both the FOXO3a pathway and the anti-oxidant defense are impaired due to loss of the FA protein functions. As a result, FA cells accumulate high levels of ROS, which damages DNA leading to genomic instability.

6. The FA syndrome links inflammatory ROS to leukemogenesis

Certain chronic inflammatory conditions have long been known to link to cancer. There is compelling evidence that chronic inflammation increases the risk of human cancers such as hepatocellular carcinoma, colon and bladder cancers, B cell lymphomas, and visceral malignancies (Kuper *et al.*, 2000; Mackay *et al.*, 2001; Martin *et al.*, 2011; Suematsu *et al.*, 2003; Umeda *et al.*, 2002; Ziech *et al.*, 2010), probably through the unbalanced machinery between DNA damage and repair (Fig. 3.).

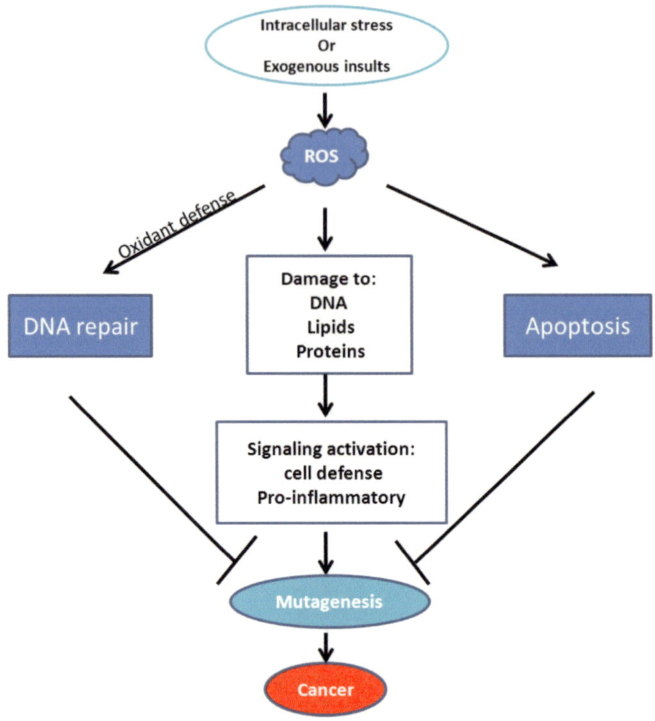

Fig. 3. Possible mechanisms for induction of oxidative stress and DNA damage and the roles in carcinogenesis. Intracellular stress or exogenous insults induces ROS production, which damages DNA, lipids and proteins. Over-produced ROS leads to cell death and activates cell defense machinery, including DNA repair and other cellular signaling pathways to maintain genome stability. Insufficient DNA repair or apoptosis causes mutagenesis, which results in cancer development.

Oxidative stress is considered as an important pathogenic factor in leukemia-prone bone marrow diseases like FA (Bogliolo *et al.,* 2002; Cohen–Haguenauer *et al.,* 2006; Cumming *et al.,* 1996; Futaki *et al.,* 2002; Hadjur *et al.,* 2001; Joenje *et al.,* 1987; Kruyt *et al.,* 1998; Mukhopadhyay *et al.,* 2006; Pagano *et al.,* 2005; Park *et al.,* 2004; Saadatzadeh *et al.,* 2004; Schindler *et al.,* 1988; Zhang *et al.,* 2005a, 2005b). The expression of inflammatory mediators, particularly the pro-inflammatory cytokines TNF-α, interleukin-1beta (IL-1β), and IL-6 in these patients is often associated with increased production of ROS either as a component of their immune response or as a consequence of increased metabolism (Macciò *et al.,* 1998; Mantovani *et al.,* 1997; Mantovani *et al.,* 2002; Tischkowitz *et al.,* 2004). Many studies have shown a correlation between elevated circulating pro-inflammatory cytokines and anemia in patients with leukemia-related BM diseases but direct evidence for the mechanistic link between inflammation and leukemia is lacking.

Normal hematopoiesis is maintained by dynamic interactions between HSCs and the bone marrow microenvironment, which is a complex system consisting of a variety of cell types, including stromal cells of nonhematopoietic, mesenchymal origin as well as hematopoietically derived stromal macrophages producing extracellular matrix components and hematopoietic growth factors (Bhatia *et al.,* 1995; Konopleva & Michael, 2007; Marina *et al.*, 2007). Alterations of pro-inflammatory cytokine expression such as reduced IL-6 and increased TNF-α, which are often found in FA patient cells, may account for BM microenvironment changes such as growth factor deprivation or constant exposure to mitogenic inhibitors. These alterations may subsequently cause deregulation of cellular homeostasis in FA (de Cremoux *et al.*, 1996; Dufour *et al.*, 2003; Rosselli *et al.*, 1992, 1994; Schultz *et al.*, 1993; Stark *et al.*, 1993) at least partially through upregulation of ROS production.

ROS induce a variety of responses in HSCs, including cellular proliferation and apoptosis (Nakamura *et al.*, 1997; Nakata *et al.*, 2004). ROS can also cause DNA damage and drive HSCs into cell division, which is essential for DNA repair processes (Wilson A *et al.*, 2008). There is strong evidence that HSCs are activated and thus functionally exhausted by oxidative stress. Mice with mutations in the ATM or FOXO genes, as well as various DNA repair genes exhibit premature exhaustion of HSCs due to accumulation of ROS or DNA damage, indicating that cellular balance between ROS and antioxidant defense as well as DNA repair is crucial for the maintenance of HSC self-renewal and hematopoietic function (Rossi *et al.*, 2007; Nijnik *et al.*, 2007).

The inflammatory cytokine TNF-α, which is overproduced in FA patients, has been considered as one important pathological factor involved in the abnormal hematopoiesis in FA. Extensive evidence demonstrated that excessive apoptosis of FA hematopoietic cells induced by TNF-α, may contribute to at least partially the pathophysiology of BM failure in FA. The c-JUN NH2-terminal kinase (JNK) and nuclear factor-kappa B (NF-κB) pathways are two well-established pathway involved in TNF-α-induced ROS production (Nakata *et al.*, 2004; Ma *et al.*, 2009; Ventura *et al.*, 2004). The JNK kinase can be activated by TNF-α-induced ROS. This activation then in turn leads to more ROS production, and sustained JNK activation in NF-κB-deficient cells was suggested to depend on ROS. It has been shown that TNF-α–induced ROS production at inflammatory sites causes DNA damage and therefore cause mutation and cancer (Aggarwal *et al.*, 2003; Kryston *et al.*, 2011; Martin *et al.*, 2011 Sedelnikova *et al.*, 2010; Suematsu *et al.*, 2003; Wajant *et al.*, 2003; Ziech *et al.*, 2010). One possible mechanism is through Oxidation of bases and generation of DNA strand interruptions. However, the accurate measurement of oxidative stress is a hallmark of disease diagnosis as well as treatment. Recently, HPLC associated with tandem mass spectrometry (MS/MS) or electrochemical detector (ECD) together with optimized DNA extraction conditions has been developed as a relevant analytical approach for measuring oxidatively base damage in cellular DNA (Cadet *et al.*, 2006, 2010). Our recent studies demonstrated the inflammatory ROS-mediated hematopoietic suppression and increased chromosomal aberrations in *Fancc-/-* mice, which is associated with impaired oxidative DNA-damage repair, implicating a role of FA pathway in maintaining genomic stability (Sejas *et al.*, 2007; Zhang *et al.*, 2007). Further studies indicated that TNF-α not only is a pro-apoptotic signal suppressing FA hematopoietic progenitor activity, but also promotes leukemic transformation of FA hematopoietic stem/progenitor cells (Li *et al.*, 2007). Therefore, FA disease progression to leukemia is governed not only by genetic changes intrinsic to the FA cells, but also by epigenetic and environmental factors and that TNF-α-mediated inflammation is one of the most important epigenetic and environmental factors contributing to FA leukemogenesis. Recent study indicate that FA hematopoietic cells are prone to clonal hematopoiesis and malignancy, which is associated with increased cytogenetic abnormalities and myeloid malignancies in *Fancc-/-* BM cells (Haneline *et al.*, 1998, 1999, 2003; Li X *et al.*, 2004; Si *et al.*, 2006). While the role of FA proteins in the regulation of TNF-α-induced ROS production remains to be elucidated, several hypotheses have been proposed, including that FA proteins protect chromosomal DNA from ROS attack or facilitate the repair of oxidative DNA damage, which in turn downstream ROS signaling. It is also possible that FA proteins can regulate the biosynthesis of ROS metabolic molecules, such as glutathione and the expression of antioxidant enzymes (such as glutathione Stransferases and catalase). However, there is no direct evidence for any of these assumptions so far. Another potential target is the redox-sensitive transcription factor NF-κB, a major player involved in transcription regulating during differentiation and inflammation (Dhar *et al.*, 2006). The activation of NF-κB is known to enhance inflammation and promote cancer (Coussens *et al.*, 2002; Fiers *et al.*, 1999; Macdougal *et al.*, 2002). In addition, chronic exposure of FA BM cells to proinflammatory cytokine TNF- α creates an environment selects for somatically mutated preleukemic stem cell clones which are apoptosis-resistant and acquire proliferative advantage (Li *et al.*, 2007). Patients with these TNF-α-resistant BM cells may advance to MDS and AML via a mechanism involving genomic instability, coupled with inflammation driven by high NF-κB transcriptional activity (Fig. 4).

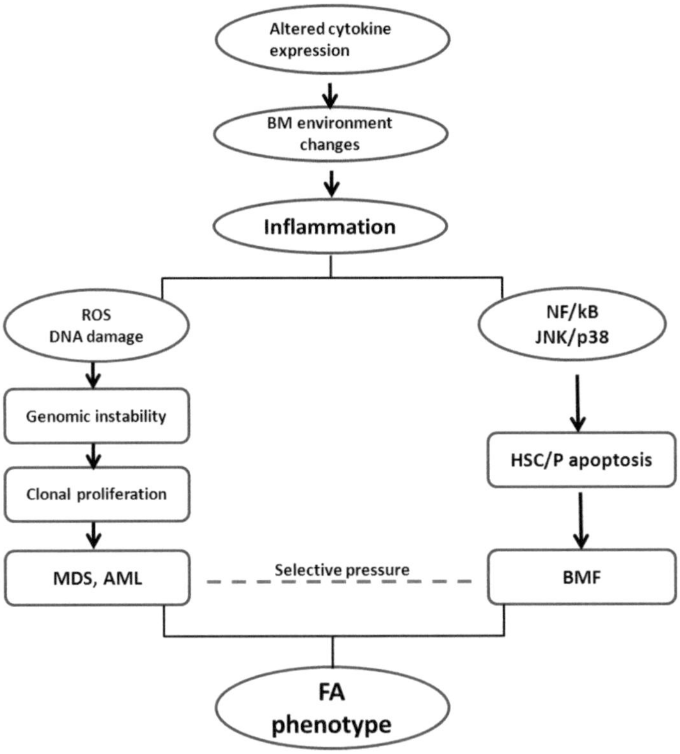

Fig. 4. The pro-inflammatory cytokines and their potential role in FA pathophysiology. Overproduced pro-inflammatory cytokines (TNF-α, IL-6, IL-1β etc.) plays roles in not only pro-apoptotic signal suppressing FA hematopoietic progenitor activity, but also promoting leukemic transformation of FA HSC/P cells, which lead to typical phenotype of FA patients.

7. Functional interaction between the FA proteins and other oxidative stress response pathways

Recent findings of a reduction of the HSC pool and a deficient repopulating capacity in Foxo3a knockout animals (Miyamoto *et al.*, 2007) indicate that FOXO3a plays essential regulatory roles in HSC maintenance through a mechanism of regulating ROS. This is consistent with our recent finding that FANCD2 forms complex with FOXO3a in response to oxidative stress (Li *et al.*, 2010). In addition, we observed several hematopoietic defects in FA mice deficient for Foxo3a (unpublished data). These results suggest that the FA proteins functionally interplay with other oxidative stress response pathways. Indeed, our preliminary results with primary BM cells from FA-A patients show that certain genes functioning in anti-oxidant defense and ROS metabolism fail to respond to oxidative stress (unpublished data). This suggests that one critical function of FA proteins under oxidative stress is to safeguard the expression of these anti-oxidant defense genes through DNA damage repair or gene promoter protection. While these observations indicate that the FA pathway functionally interacts with other cellular oxidative stress response pathways, the molecular mechanisms by which FA proteins function to modulate physiologic oxidative stress remain to be elucidated. Further investigation into the roles of FA proteins in oxidative DNA-damage response and repair, and the functional relationship between inflammatory ROS and genomic instability during FA leukemogenesis not only will advance our understanding of the function of FA proteins in hematopoiesis but also may suggest new targets for therapeutic prevention and treatment of BM failure and cancer progression of the disease.

8. Conclusion

Given other known genomic instability syndromes such as ataxia telangiectasia, Nijmegen breakage syndrome, xeroderma pigmentosum, and Werner syndrome rarely develop BM failure and leukemia, FA has been considered an excellent disease model for studying oxidative stress response in cancer development. Further investigation into the function of FA proteins in oxidative damage response and repair will help shed new light on the role of FA proteins in the maintenance of normal hematopoiesis under conditions of oxidative stress, and yield valuable information on whether targeting components of FA-related oxidative stress signaling pathways may be therapeutically useful in the prevention and treatment of FA BMF and leukemia. In addition, while FA is a rare disease, understanding functional interaction between FA proteins and other critical oxidative stress signaling pathways provides a unique opportunity to mechanistically comprehend and potentially intervene in these physiologically important processes.

9. References

Aggarwal, B.B. (2003) Signaling pathways of the TNF superfamily: a double-edged sword. *Nature Rev Immunol* 3: 745–756.

Ames, B.N., Gold, L.S., & Willett WC. (1995) The causes and prevention of cancer. *Proc Natl Acad Sci USA.* 92: 5258–5265.

Aubé, M., Lafrance, M., Charbonneau, C., Goulet, I. & Carreau, M. (2002) Hematopoietic stem cells from fancc(-/-) mice have lower growth and differentiation potential in response to growth factors. *Stem Cells.* 20(5): 438-447.

Bhatia, R., McGlave, P.B., Dewald, G.W., Blazar, B.R. & Verfaillie, C.M. (1995) Abnormal Function of the Bone Marrow Microenvironment in Chronic Myelogenous Leukemia: Role of Malignant Stromal Macrophages. *Blood* 85: 3636-3645

Bagby, G.C. Jr. (2003) Genetic basis of Fanconi anemia. *Curr Opin Hematol* 10: 68–76

Balkwill, F. & Mantovani, A. (2001) Inflammation and cancer: back to Virchow? *Lancet* 357: 539–545.

Bogliolo, M., Cabré, O., Callén, E., Castillo, V., Creus, A., Marcos, R., & Surrallés, J. (2002) The Fanconi anaemia genome stability and tumour suppressor network. *Mutagenesis* 17: 529–538.

Brunet, A., Sweeney, L.B., Sturgill, J.F., Chua, K.F., Greer, P.L., Lin, Y., Tran, H., Ross, S.E., Mostoslavsky, R., Cohen, H.Y., Hu, L.S., Cheng, H.L., Jedrychowski, M.P., Gygi, S.P., Sinclair, D.A., Alt, F.W. & Greenberg, M.E. (2004) Stress-dependent regulation of FOXO transcription factors by the SIRT1 deacetylase. *Science* 303: 2011-2015.

Buchwald, M. & Moustacchi, E. (1998) Is Fanconi anemia caused by a defect in the processing of DNA damage? *Mutat Res* 408: 75–90.

Cadet, J., Berger, M., Douki, T. & Ravanat, J. L. (2006) *Rev. Physiol. Biochem. Pharmacol.* 131: 1-87.

Cadet, J., Douki, T. & Ravanat, J.L. (2010) *Free Rad. Biol. Med.* 49: 9-21.

Chen, M., Tomkins, D.J., Auerbach, W., McKerlie, C., Youssoufian, H., Liu, L., Gan, O., Carreau, M., Auerbach, A., Groves, T., Guidos, C.J., Freedman, M.H., Cross, J., Percy, D.H., Dick, J.E., Joyner, A.L. & Buchwald, M. (1996) Inactivation of Fac in mice produces inducible chromosomal instability and reduced fertility reminiscent of Fanconi anaemia. *Nat. Genet.* 12, 448–451.

Chen, Q.M. (2000) Replicative senescence and oxidant-induced premature senescence. Beyond the control of cell cycle checkpoints. *Ann. N. Y. Acad. Sci.* 908, 111–125.

Cheng, N.C., van de Vrugt, H.J., van der Valk, M.A., Oostra, A.B., Krimpenfort, P., de Vries, Y., Joenje, H., Berns, A. & Arwert, F. (2000) Mice with a targeted disruption of the Fanconi anemia homolog Fanca. *Hum. Mol. Genet.* 9, 1805–1811

Ciccia, A., Ling, C., Coulthard, R., Yan, Z., Xue, Y., Meetei, A.R., Laghmani, el. H., Joenje, H., McDonald, N., de Winter, J.P., Wang, W. & West, S.C. (2007) Identification of FAAP24, a Fanconi anemia core complex protein that interacts with FANCM. *Mol Cell.* 25: 331–343.

Cohen-Haguenauer, O., Pult, B., Bauche, C., Daniel, M.I., Casalb, I., Levy, V., Dausset, J., Boiron, M., Auclair, C., Gluckman, E. & Marty, M. (2006) In vivo repopulation ability of genetically corrected bone marrow cells from Fanconi anemia patients. *Proc Natl Acad Sci USA* 103:2340–2345.

Collins, N. & Kupfer, G.M. (2005) Molecular pathogenesis of Fanconi anemia. *Int J Hemato* 82: 176–183.

Collis, S.J., Ciccia, A., Deans, A.J., Horejsi, Z., Martin, J.S., Maslen, S.L., Skehel, J.M., Elledge, S.J., West, S.C. & Boulton, S.J. (2008) FANCM FAAP24 function in ATR-mediated checkpoint signaling independently of the Fanconi anemia core complex. *Mol Cell.* 32:313–324.

Cumming, R.C., Liu, J.M., Youssoufian, H. & Buchwald, M. (1996) Suppression of apoptosis in hematopoietic factor-dependent progenitor cell lines by expression of the FAC gene. *Blood* 88: 4558–4567.

Cumming, R.C., Lightfoot, J., Beard, K., Youssoufian, H., O'Brien, P.J. & Buchwald, M. (2001) Fanconi anemia group C protein prevents prevents apoptosis in hematopoietic cells through redox regulation of GSTP1. *Nat Med* 7: 814–820.

Coussens, L.M. & Werb, Z. (2002) Inflammation and cancer. *Nature* 420: 860–867.

D'Andrea, A.D. & Grompe, M. (2003) The Fanconi anaemia/BRCA pathway. *Nat Rev Cancer* 3: 23–34.

D'Andrea, A.D. (2010) Susceptibility pathways in Fanconi's anemia and breast cancer. *N Engl J Med.* 362(20):1909-1919.

de Cremoux, P., Gluckman, E., Podgorniak, M.P., Menier, C., Thierry, D., Calvo, F. & Socie, G. (1996) Decreased IL-1 beta and TNF alpha secretion in long-term bone marrow culture supernatant from Fanconi's anaemia patients. *Eur J Haematol* 57: 202–207.

de Winter, J.P., Waisfisz, Q., Rooimans, M.A., van Berkel, C.G., Bosnoyan-Collins, L., Alon, N., Carreau, M., Bender, O., Demuth, I., Schindler, D., Pronk, J.C., Arwert, F., Hoehn, H., Digweed, M., Buchwald, M. & Joenje, H. (1998) The Fanconi anaemia group G gene FANCG is identical with XRCC9. *Nat Gene* 20: 281–283.

de Winter, J.P., Leveille, F., van Berkel, C.G., Rooimans, M.A., can Der, W.L., Steltenpool, J., Demuth, I., Morgan, N.V., Alon, N., Bosnoyan-Collins, L., Lightfoot, J., Leegwater, P.A., Waisfisz, Q., Komatsu, K., Arwert, F., Pronk, J.C., Mathew, C.G., Digweed, M., Buchwald, M. & Joenje, H. (2000) Isolation of a cDNA representing the Fanconi anemia complementation Group E gene. *Am Hum Gene* 67:1306–1308.

de Winter, J.P., Rooimans, M.A., van Der Weel, L., van Berkel, C.G., Alon, N., Bosnoyan-Collins, L., de Groot, J., Zhi, Y., Waisfisz, Q., Pronk, J.C., Arwert, F., Mathew, C.G., Scheper, R.J., Hoatlin, M.E., Buchwald, M. & Joenje. H. (2000) FANCF encodes a novel protein with homology to ROM. *Nat Gene* 24: 15–16.

Dhar SK, Lynn BC, Daosukho C, St Clair DK. Identification of nucleophosmin as an NF-kappaB co-activator for the induction of the human SOD2 gene. J Biol Chem. 2004 Jul 2;279(27):28209-28219.

Doneshbod-Skibba, G., Martin, J. & Shahidi, N. (1980) Myeloid and erythroid colony growth in non-anemic patients with Fanconi's anemia. *Br J Haematol* 44: 33–38.

Du, W., Adam, Z., Rani, R., Zhang, X. & Pang, Q. (2008) Oxidative stress in Fanconi anemia hematopoiesis and disease progression. *Antioxidants & Redox Signaling* 10:1909-1921.

Dufour, C., Corcione, A., Svahn, J., Haupt, R., Poggi, V., Beka'ssy, A.N., Scime, R., Pistorio, A. & Pistoia, V. (2003) TNF-alpha and IFNgamma are overexpressed in the bone marrow of Fanconi anemia patients and TNF-alpha suppresses erythropoiesis in vitro. *Blood* 102: 2053–2059.

Essers, M.A., Weijzen, S., de Vries-Smits, A.M., Saarloos, I., de Ruiter, N.D., Bos, J.L. & Burgering, B.M. (2004) FOXO transcription factor activation by oxidative stress mediated by the small GTPase Ral and JNK. *EMBO J.* 23(24):4802-1812.

Fagerlie, S.R., Diaz, J., Christianson, T.A., McCartan, K., Keeble, W., Faulkner, G.R. & Bagby, G.C. (2001) Functional correction of FA-C cells with FANCC suppresses the expression of interferon -inducible genes. *Blood* 97: 3017–3024.

Fagerlie, S., Lensch, M.W., Pang, Q. & Bagby, G.C. Jr. (2001) The Fanconi anemia group C gene product: signaling functions in hematopoietic cells. *Exp Hematol* 29: 1371–1381.

Fiers, W., Beyaert, R., Declercq, W. & Vandenabeele, P. (1999) More than one way to die: Apoptosis, necrosis and reactive oxygen damage. *Oncogene* 18: 7719–7730.

Freie, B., Li, X., Ciccone, S.L., Nawa, K., Cooper, S., Vogelweid, C., Schantz, L., Haneline, L.S., Orazi, A., Broxmeyer, H.E., Lee, S.H. & Clapp, D.W. (2003) Fanconi anemia type C and p53 cooperate in apoptosis and tumorigenesis. *Blood* 102: 4146–4152.

Freie, B.W., Ciccone, S.L., Li, X., Plett, P.A., Orschell, C.M., Srour, E.F., Hanenberg, H., Schindler, D., Lee, S.H. & Clapp, D.W. (2004) A role for the Fanconi anemia C protein in maintaining the DNA damage-induced G2 checkpoint. *J Biol Chem* 279: 50986–50993.

Fridman, J.S. & Lowe, S.W. (2003) Control of apoptosis by p53. *Oncogene* 22: 9030–9040.

Futaki, M., Igarashi, T., Watanabe, S., Kajigaya, S., Tatsuguchi, A., Wang, J. & Liu, J.M. (2002) The FANCG Fanconi anemia protein interacts with CYP2E1: possible role in protection against oxidative DNA damage. *Carcinogenesis* 23: 67–72.

Giaccia, A.J. & Kastan, M.B. (1998) The complexity of p53 modulation: emerging patterns from divergent signals. *Genes* 12: 2973–2983.

Gluckman, E., Broxmeyer, H., Auerbach, A., Friedman, H., Douglas, G., Devergie, A., Esperou, H., Thierry, D., Socie, G., Lehn, P., Cooper, S., English, D., Kurtzberg, J., Bard, J. & Boyse, E. (1989) Hematopoietic reconstitution in a patient with Fanconi's anemia by means of umbilical-cord blood from an HLA identical sibling. *N Engl J* Med 321: 1174–1178.

Green, A.M. & Kupfer, G.M. (2009) Fanconi anemia. *Hematol Oncol Clin North Am.* 23:193-214.

Hadjur, S., Ung, K., Wadsworth, L., Dimmick, J., Rajcan-Separovic, E., Scott, R.W., Buchwald, M. & Jirik, F.R. (2001) Defective hematopoiesis and hepatic steatosis in mice with combined deficiencies of the genes encoding Fancc and Cu/Zn superoxide dismutase. *Blood* 98: 1003–1011.

Hakim, J. (1993) Reactive oxygen species and inflammation *C R Seances Soc Biol Fil.* 187(3):286-295.

Hammond, E. M., Dorie, M. J. & Giaccia, A. J. (2003) ATR/ATM targets are phosphorylated by ATR in response to hypoxia and ATM in response to reoxygenation. *J. Biol. Chem.* 278, 12207–12213.

Haneline, L.S., Broxmeyer, H.E., Cooper, S., Hangoc, G., Carreau, M., Buchwald, M. & Clapp, D.W. (1998) Multiple inhibitory cytokines induce deregulated progenitor growth and apoptosis in hematopoietic cells from FAC-/- mice. *Blood* 91: 4092–4098.

Haneline, L.S., Gobbett, T.A., Ramani, R., Carreau, M., Buchwald, M., Yoder, M.C. & Clapp, D.W. (1999) Loss of Fancc function results in decreased hematopoietic stem cell repopulating ability. *Blood* 94: 1–8.

Haneline, L.S., Li, X., Ciccone, S.L., Hong, P., Yang, Y., Broxmeyer, H.E., Lee, S.H., Orazi, A., Srour, E.F. & Clapp, D.W. (2003) Retroviralmediated expression of recombinant Fancc enhances the repopulating ability of Fancc-/- hematopoietic stem cells and decreases the risk of clonal evolution. *Blood* 101: 1299–1307.

Horejsi, Z., Collis, S.J., Boulton, S.J. (2009) FANCM-FAAP24 and HCLK2: roles in ATR signalling and the Fanconi anemia pathway. *Cell Cycle* 8:1133–1137.

Howlett, N.G., Taniguchi, T., Olson, S., Cox, B., Waisfisz, Q., De Die-Smulders, C., Persky, N., Grompe, M., Joenje, H., Pals, G., Ikeda, H., Fox, E.A. & D'Andrea, A.D. (2002) Biallelic inactivation of BRCA2 in Fanconi anemia. *Science* 297: 606–609.

Huang, H., Tindall, D.J. (2007) Dynamic FoxO transcription factors. *J Cell Sci.* 120:2479-2487.

Ibáñez, A., Río, P., Casado, J.A., Bueren, J.A., Fernández-Luna, J.L., Pipaón, C. (2009) Elevated levels of IL-1beta in Fanconi anaemia group A patients due to a constitutively active phosphoinositide 3-kinase-Akt pathway are capable of promoting tumour cell proliferation. *Biochem J.* 29; 422(1):161-170.

Ichijo, H., Nishida, E., Irie, K., ten Dijke, P., Saitoh, M., Moriguchi, T., Takagi, M., Matsumoto, K., Miyazono, K. & Gotoh, Y. (1997) Induction of apoptosis by ASK1, a mammalian MAPKKK that activates SAPK/JNK and p38 signaling pathways. *Science* 275: 90–94.

Joenje, H., Arwert, F., Eriksson, A.W., de Koning, H. & Oostra, A.B. (1987) Oxygen-dependence of chromosomal aberrations in Fanconi's anaemia. *Nature* 290: 142–143.

Joenje, H., Levitus, M., Waisfisz, Q., D' Andrea, A.D., Garcia-Higuera, I., Pearson, T., van Berkel, C.G., Rooimans, M.A., Morgan, N., Mathew, C.G. & Arwert, F. (2000) Complementation analysis in Fanconi anemia: Assignment of the reference. FA-H patient to group A. *Am J Hum Gene* 67: 759–762.

Jonkers, J., Meuwissen, R., van der Gulden, H., Peterse, H., van der Valk, M. & Bern, A. (2001) Synergistic tumor suppressor activity of BRCA2 and p53 in a conditional mouse model for breast cancer. *Nat Genet* 29: 418–425.

Kops, G.J., Dansen, T.B., Polderman, P.E., Saarloos, I., Wirtz, K.W., Coffer, P.J., Huang, T.T., Bos, J.L., Medema, R.H., Burgering, B.M. (2002) Forkhead transcription factor FOXO3a protects quiescent cells from oxidative stress. *Nature* 419(6904):316-321.

Jonsson, H., Allen, P., Peng, S.L. (2005) Inflammatory arthritis requires Foxo3a to prevent Fas ligand-induced neutrophil apoptosis. *Nat Med.* 11(6):666-671.

Kennedy, R.D. & D'Andrea, A.D. (2005) The Fanconi Anemia/BRCA pathway: new faces in the crowd. *Genes Dev* 19: 2925–2940.

Koh, P.S., Hughes, G.C., Faulkner, G.R., Keeble, W.W. & Bagby, G.C. (1999) The Fanconi anemia group C gene product modulates apoptotic responses to tumor necrosis factor- and Fas ligand but does not suppress expression of receptors of the tumor necrosis factor receptor superfamily. *Exp Hematol* 27: 1–8.

Konopleva, M. & Andreeff, M. (2007) Targeting the Leukemia Microenvironment. *Current Drug Targets,* 2007, *8,* 685-701.

Kruyt, F.A., Hoshino, T., Liu, J.M., Joseph, P., Jaiswal, A.K. & Youssoufian, H. (1998) Abnormal microsomal detoxification implicated in Fanconi anemia group C by interaction of the FAC protein with NADPH cytochrome P450 reductase. *Blood* 92: 3050–3056.

Kryston, T. B., Georgiev, A. & Georgakilas, A. G. (2011) *Mutat. Res.* 711, 193-201.

Kuper, H., Adami, H.O. & Trichopoulos, D. (2000) Infections as a major preventable cause of human cancer. *J Intern Med* 248:171–183.

Kutler, D.I., Wreesmann, V.B., Goberdhan, A., Ben-Prat, L., Satagopan, J., Ngai, I., Huvos, A.G., Giampietro, P., Levran, O., Pujara, K., Diotti, R., Carlson, D., Huryn, L.A., Auerbach, A.D. & Singh, B. (2003) Human papillomavirus DNA and p53 polymorphisms in squamous cell carcinomas from Fanconi anemia patients. *J Natl Cancer Inst* 95: 1718–1721.

Lensch, M.W., Rathbun, R.K., Olson, S.B., Jones, G.R. & Bagby, G.C. Jr. (1999) Selective pressure as an essential force in molecular evolution of myeloid leukemic clones: a view from the window of Fanconi anemia. *Leukemia* 13: 1784–1789.

Levitus, M., Rooimans, M.A., Steltenpool, J., Cool, N.F., Oostra, A.B., Mathew, C.G., Hoatlin, M.E., Waisfisz, Q., Arwert, F., De Winter, J.P. & Joenje, H. (2004) Heterogeneity in Fanconi anemia: evidence for two new genetic subtypes. *Blood* 103(7): 2498–2503.

Levran, O., Attwooll, C., Henry, R.T., Milton, K.L., Neveling, K., Rio, P., Batish, S.D., Kalb, R., Velleuer, E., Barral, S., Ott, J., Petrini, J., Schindler, D., Hanenberg, H. & Auerbach, A.D. (2005) The BRCA1-interacting helicase BRIP1 is deficient in Fanconi anemia. *Nat Genet* 37: 931–933.

Li, J., Sejas, D.P., Zhang, X., Qiu, Y., Nattamai, K.J., Rani, R., Rathbun, K.R., Geiger, H., Williams, D.A. & Bagby, G.C. & Pang, Q. (2007) TNF-α induces leukemic clonal evolution ex vivo in Fanconi anemia group C stem cells. *J Clin Invest* 117: 3283–3295.

Li, J., Du, W., Maynard, S., Andreassen, P.R. & Pang, Q. (2010) Oxidative stress-specific interaction between FANCD2 and FOXO3a. *Blood.* 115(8):1545-1548.

Li, X., Yang, Y., Yuan, J., Hong, P., Freie, B., Orazi, A., Haneline, L.S. & Clapp, D.W. (2004) Continuous in vivo infusion of interferon- gamma (IFN-gamma) preferentially reduces myeloid progenitor numbers and enhances engraftment of syngeneic wild-type cells in Fancc-/- mice. *Blood* 104: 1204– 1209.

Li, Y. & Youssoufian, H. (1997) MxA overexpression reveals a common genetic link in four Fanconi anemia complementation groups. *J Clin Invest* 100: 2873–2880.

Liu, J. (2000) Fanconi's anemia. In: Young NS, ed. *Bone Marrow Failure Syndromes*. 47–68.

Liu, T.X., Howlett, N.G., Deng, M., Langenau, D.M., Hsu, K., Rhodes, J., Kanki, J.P., D'Andrea, A.D. & Look, A.T. (2003) Knockdown of zebrafish Fancd2 causes developmental abnormalities via p53-dependent apoptosis. *Dev Cell* 5: 903–914.

Lohrum, M.A. & Vousden, K.H. (1999) Regulation and activation of p53 and its family members. *Cell Death Differ* 6: 1162– 1168.

Lo Ten Foe, J.R., Rooimans, M.A., Bosnoyan–Collins, L., Alon, N., Wijker, M., Parker, L., Lightfoot, J., Carreau, M., Callen, D.F., Savoia, A., Cheng, N.C., van Berkel, C.G., Strunk, M.H., Gille, J.J., Pals, G., Kruyt, F.A., Pronk, J.C., Arwert, F., Buchwald, M. & Joenje, H. (1996) Expression cloning of a cDNA for the major Fanconi anaemia gene, FAA. *Nature Gene* 14: 320–323.

Luna–Fineman, S., Shannon, K.M. & Lange, B.J. (1995) Childhood monosomy 7: epidemiology, biology, and mechanistic implications. *Blood* 85: 1985–1989.

Luke-Glaser, S., Luke, B., Grossi, S. & Constantinou, A. (2010) FANCM regulates DNA chain elongation, is stabilized by S-phase checkpoint signalling. *EMBO J.* 29: 795–805.

Ma, D.J., Li, S.J., Wang, L.S., Dai, J., Zhao, S.L & Zeng, R. (2009) Temporal and spatial profiling of nuclei-associated proteins upon TNF-alpha/NF-kappaB signaling. *Cell Res.* 19(5):651-664.

Macciò, A., Lai, P., Santona, M.C., Pagliara, L., Melis, G.B. & Mantovani, G. (1998) High serum levels of soluble IL-2 receptor, cytokines, and C-reactive protein correlate with impairment of T cell response in patients with advanced epithelial ovarian cancer. *Gynecol Oncol* 69: 248–252.

Macdougall, I.C. & Cooper, A.C. (2002) Erythropoitin resistence: the role of inflammation and pro-inflammatory cytokines. *Nephrol Dial Transplant* 17: 39–43.

Maciejewski, J.P., Selleri, C., Sato, T., Anderson, S. & Young, N.S. (1995) Increased expression of Fas antigen on bone marrow CD34_ cells of patients with aplastic anaemia. *Br J Haematol* 91: 245–252.

Mackay, I.R. & Rose, N.R. (2001) Autoimmunity and lymphoma: tribulations of B cells. *Nat Immunol* 2: 793–795.

Mantovani, G., Macciò, A., Pisano, M., Versace, R., Lai, P., Esu, S., Massa, E., Ghiani, M., Dessi, D., Melis, G.B. & Del Giacco, D.S. (1997) Tumor-associated lympho-monocytes from neoplastic effusions are immunologically defective in comparison with patient autologous PBMCs but are capable of releasing high amounts of various cytokines. *Int J Cancer* 71: 724–731.

Mantovani, G., Macciò, A., Madeddu, C., Mura, L., Gramigano, G., Lusso, M.R., Mulas, C., Mudu, M.C., Murgia, V., Camboni, P., Massa, E., Ferreli, L., Contu, P., Rinaldi, A., Sanjust, E., Atzei, D. & Elsener, B. (2002) Quantitative evaluation of oxidative stress, chronic inflammatory indices and leptin in cancer patients: correlation with stage and performance status. *Int J Cancer* 98: 84–91.

Marx, J. (2004) Cancer research. Inflammation and cancer: the link grows stronger. *Science* 306: 966–968.

Martin, O. A., Redon, C., Nakamura, A. J., Dickey, J. S., Georgakilas, A. G. & Bonner, W. M. (2011) *Cancer Res.* 71: 1-5.

Meetei, A.R., de Winter, J.P., Medhurst, A.L., Wallisch, M., Waisfisz, Q., van de Vrugt, H.J., Oostra, A.B., Yan, Z., Ling, C., Bishop, C.E., Hoatlin, M.E., Joenje, H. & Wang, W. (2003) A novel ubiquitin ligase is deficient in Fanconi anemia. *Nat Genet* 35: 165–170.

Meetei, A.R., Levitus, M., Xue, Y., Medhurst, A.L., Zwaan, M., Ling, C., Rooimans, M.A., Bier, P., Hoatlin, M., Pals, G., de Winter, J.P., Wang, W. & Joenje, H. (2004) X-linked inheritance of Fanconi anemia complementation group B. *Nat Gene* 36: 1219–1224.

Meetei, A.R., Medhurst, A.L., Ling, C., Xue, Y., Singh, T.R., Bier, P., Steltenpool, J., Stone, S., Dokal, I., Mathew, C.G,, Hoatlin, M., Joenje ,H., de Winter, J.P, & Wang, W. (2005) A human ortholog of archael DNA repair protein HEF is defective in Fanconi anemia complementation group M *Nat Genet* 37: 958–963.

Meindl, A., Hellebrand, H., Wiek, C., Erven, V., Wappenschmidt, B., Niederacher, D., Freund, M., Lichtner, P., Hartmann, L., Schaal, H., Ramser, J., Honisch, E., Kubisch, C., Wichmann, H.E., Kast, K., Deissler, H., Engel, C., Müller-Myhsok, B., Neveling, K., Kiechle, M., Mathew, C.G., Schindler, D., Schmutzler, R.K., Hanenberg, H. (2010) Germline mutations in breast and ovarian cancer pedigrees establish RAD51C as a human cancer susceptibility gene. *Nat Genet.* 42 (5): 410-414.

Miyamoto, K., Araki, K.Y., Naka, K., Arai, F., Takubo, K., Yamazaki, S., Matsuoka, S., Miyamoto, T., Ito, K., Ohmura, M., Chen, C., Hosokawa, K., Nakauchi, H., Nakayama, K., Nakayama, K.I., Harada, M., Motoyama, N., Suda, T. & Hirao, A. (2007) Foxo3a is essential for maintenance of the hematopoietic stem cell pool. *Cell Stem Cell.* 1(1):101-112.

Mukhopadhyay, S.S., Leung, K.S., Hicks, M.J., Hastings, P.J., Youssoufian, H. & Plon, S.E. (2006) Defective mitochondrial peroxiredoxin-3 results in sensitivity to oxidative stress in Fanconi anemia *J Cell Biol* 175: 225–235.

Nakamura, H., Nakamura, K. & Yodoi, J. (1997) Redox regulation of cellular activation. *Annu Rev Immunol* 15: 351–369.

Nakata, S., Matsumura, I., Tanaka, H., Ezoe, S., Satoh, Y., Ishikawa, J., Era, T. & Kanakura, Y. (2004) NF-kappa B family proteins proteins participate in multiple steps of hematopoiesis through elimination of reactive oxygen species. *J Biol Chem* 279: 55578–55586.

Nijnik, A., Woodbine, L., Marchetti, C., Dawson, S., Lambe, T., Liu, C., Rodrigues, N.P., Crockford, T.L., Cabuy, E., Vindigni, A., Enver, T., Bell, J.I., Slijepcevic, P., Goodnow, C.C., Jeggo, P.A. & Cornall, R.J. (2007) DNA repair is limiting for haematopoietic stem cells during ageing. *Nature.* 447(7145):686-690.

Otsuki, T., Nagakura, S., Wang, J., Bloom, M., Grompe, M. & Liu, J.M. (1999) Tumor necrosis factor- and CD95 ligation suppress erythropoiesis in Fanconi anemia C gene knockout mice. *J Cell Physiol* 179: 79–86.

Pagano, G., Degan, P., d'Ischia, M., Kelly, F. J., Nobili, B., Pallardó, F.V., Youssoufian, H. & Zatterale, A. (2005) Oxidative stress as a multiple effector in Fanconi anaemia clinical phenotype. *Eur J Haematol* 75: 93–100.

Pang, Q. Fagerlie, S., Christianson, T.A., Keeble, W., Faulkner, G., Diaz, J., Rathbun, R.K. & Bagby, G.C. (2000) The Fanconi anemia protein FANCC binds to and facilitates the activation of STAT1 by gamma interferon and hematopoietic growth factors. *Mol. Cell. Biol.* 20, 4724–4735.

Pang, Q., Keeble, W., Christianson, T.A., Faulkner, G.R. & Bagby, G.C. (2001) FANCC interacts with Hsp70 to protect hematopoietic cells from IFN-γ/TNF-α-mediated cytotoxicity. *EMBO J* 20: 4478–4489.

Pang, Q., Keeble, W., Diaz, J., Christianson, T.A., Fagerlie, S., Rathbun, K., Faulkner, G.R., O'Dwyer, M. & Bagby, G.C. Jr. (2001) Role of double-stranded RNA-dependent protein kinase in mediating hypersensitivity of Fanconi anemia complementation group C cells to interferon gamma, tumor necrosis factor-alpha, and double-stranded RNA. *Blood.* 2001 97(6):1644-1652.

Pang, Q., Christianson, T.A., Keeble, W., Koretsky, T. & Bagby, G,C. (2002) The anti-apoptotic function of Hsp70 in the interferon-inducible double-stranded RNA-dependent protein kinase-mediated death signaling pathway requires the Fanconi anemia protein, FANCC. *J Biol Chem.* 277(51):49638-49643.

Park, S.J., Ciccone, S.L., Beck, B.D., Hwang, B., Freie, B., Clapp, D.W. & Lee, S.H. (2004) Oxidative stress/damage induces multimerization and interaction of Fanconi anemia proteins. *J Biol Chem 279*: 30053–30059.

Potente, M., Urbich, C., Sasaki, K., Hofmann, W.K., Heeschen, C., Aicher, A., Kollipara, R., DePinho, R.A., Zeiher, A.M., Dimmeler, S. (2005) Involvement of Foxo transcription factors in angiogenesis and postnatal neovascularization *J Clin Invest.* 115(9):2382-2392.

Rathbun, R.K., Faulkner, G.R., Ostroski, M.H., Christianson, T.A., Hughes, G., Jones, G., Cahn, R., Maziarz, R., Royle, G., Keeble, W., Heinrich, M.C/, Grompe, M., Tower, P.A. & Bagby, G.C. (1997) Inactivation of the Fanconi anemia group C gene augments interferon-gamma-induced apoptotic responses in hematopoietic cells. *Blood* 90: 974–985.

Rathbun, R.K., Christianson, T.A., Faulkner, G.R., Jone, G., Keeble, W., O'Dwyer, M. & Bagby, G.C. (2000) Interferon—induced apoptotic responses of Fanconi anemia group C hematopoietic progenitor cells involve caspase 8-dependent activation of caspase 3 family members. *Blood* 96: 4204–4211.

Reid, S., Schindler, D., Hanenberg, H., Barker, K., Hanks, S., Kalb, R., Neveling, K., Kelly, P., Seal, S., Freund, M., Wurm, M., Batish, S.D., Lach, F.P., Yetgin, S., Neitzel, H.,

Ariffin, H., Tischkowitz, M., Mathew, C.G., Auerbach, A.D. & Rahman, N. (2006) Biallelic mutations in PALB2 cause Fanconi anemia subtype FA-N and predispose to childhood cancer. *Nat Genet* 39: 162–164.

Rossi, D.J., Bryder, D., Seita, J., Nussenzweig, A., Hoeijmakers, J., Weissman, I.L.(2007) Deficiencies in DNA damage repair limit the function of haematopoietic stem cells with age. *Nature.* 447(7145):725-729.

Rosselli, F., Sanceau, J., Wietzerbin, J. & Moustacchi, E. (1992) Abnormal lymphokine production: a novel feature of the genetic disease Fanconi anemia. I. Involvement of interleukin- 6. *Hum Genet* 89: 42–48.

Rosselli, F., Sanceau, J., Gluckman, E., Wietzerbin, J. & Moustacchi, E. (1994) Abnormal lymphokine production: a novel feature of the genetic disease Fanconi anemia. II. In vitro and in vivo spontaneous overproduction of tumor necrosis factor alpha. *Blood* 83: 1216–1225.

Rubin, C.M,, Arthur, D.C., Woods, W.G., Lange, B.J., Nowell, P.C., Rowley, J.D., Nachman, J., Bostrom, B., Baum, E.S., Suarez, C.R., Shah, N.R., Morgan, E., Mauer, H.S., McKenzie, S.E., Larson, R.A. & Le Beau, M.M. (1991) Therapy-related myelodysplastic syndrome and acute myeloid leukemia in children: correlation between chromosomal abnormalities and prior therapy. *Blood* 78: 2982–2988.

Saadatzadeh, M.R., Bijangi–Vishehsaraei, K., Hong, P., Bergmann, H. & Haneline, L.S. (2004) Oxidant hypersensitivity of Fanconi anemia type C-deficient cells is dependent on a redox- regulated apoptotic pathway. *J Biol Chem* 279: 16805–16812.

Scheller, J., Chalaris, A., Schmidt-Arras, D. & Rose-John, S. (2011) The pro- and anti-inflammatory properties of the cytokine interleukin-6. *Biochim Biophys Acta.* 1813(5):878-888.

Schindler, D. & Hoehn, H. (1988) Fanconi anemia mutation causes cellular susceptibility to ambient oxygen. *Am J Hum Genet* 43(4): 429–435.

Schultz, J.C. & Shahidi, N.T. (1993) Tumor necrosis factor-alpha overproduction in Fanconi's anemia. *Am J Hematol* 42:196–201.

Schwab, R.A., Blackford, A.N. & Niedzwiedz, W. (2010) ATR activation, replication fork restart are defective in FANCM-deficient cells. *EMBO J.* 29: 806–818.

Sedelnikova, O. A., Redon, C. E., Dickey, J. S., Nakamura, A. J., Georgakilas, A. G. & Bonner, W. M.(2010) *Mutat. Res.* 704, 152-159.

Sejas, D.P., Rani, R., Qiu, Y., Zhang, X., Fagerlie, S.R., Nakano, H., Williams, D.A. & Pang, Q. (2007) Inflammatory reactive oxygen species-mediated hematopoietic suppression in Fancc-deficient mice. *J Immunol* 178: 5277–5287.

Si, Y., Ciccone, S., Yang, F.C., Yuan, J., Zeng, D., Chen, S., van de Vrugt, H., Critser, J., Arwert, F., Haneline, L.S. & Clapp, D.W. (2006) Continuous in vivo infusion of interferon-gamma (IFNgamma) enhances engraftment of syngeneic wild-type cells in Fanca-/- and Fancg-/- mice. *Blood* 108: 4283–4287.

Singh, T.R., Saro, D., Ali, A.M., Zheng, X.F., Du, C.H., Killen, M.W., Sachpatzidis, A., Wahengbam, K., Pierce, A.J., Xiong, Y., Sung, P. & Meetei. A.R. (2010) MHF1-MHF2, a histone-fold-containing protein complex, participates in the Fanconi anemia pathway via FANCM. *Mol Cell.* 37:879–886.

Smogorzewska, A., Matsuoka, S., Vinciguerra, P., McDonald, E.R. 3rd, Hurov, K.E., Luo, J., Ballif, B.A., Gygi, S.P., Hofmann, K., D'Andrea, A.D. & Elledge, S.J. (2007)

Identification of the FANCI Protein, a Monoubiquitinated FANCD2 Paralog Required for DNA Repair. *Cell* 129: 1–13.

Somyajit, K., Subramanya, S., Nagaraju, G. (2010) RAD51C: a novel cancer susceptibility gene is linked to Fanconi anemia and breast cancer. *Carcinogenesis.* 31(12):2031-2038.

Stark, R., Andre, C., Thierry, D., Cherel, M., Galibert, F. & Gluckman, E. (1993) The expression of cytokine and cytokine receptor genes in long-term bone marrow culture in congenital and acquired bone marrow hypoplasias. *Br J Haematol* 83: 560–566.

Stoepker, C., Hain, K., Schuster, B., Hilhorst-Hofstee, Y., Rooimans, M.A., Steltenpool, J., Oostra, A.B., Eirich, K., Korthof, E.T., Nieuwint, A.W., Jaspers, N.G., Bettecken, T., Joenje ,H., Schindler, D., Rouse, J. & de Winter, J.P. (2011) SLX4, a coordinator of structure-specific endonucleases, is mutated in a new Fanconi anemia subtype. *Proc Natl Acad Sci U S A.* 108(16):6492-6496.

Strathdee, C.A., Gavish, H., Shannon, W.R. & Buchwald, M. (1992) Cloning of cDNAs for Fanconi's anaemia by functional complementation. *Nature* 356: 763–767.

Suematsu, N., Tsutsui, H., Wen, J., Kang, D., Ikeuchi, M., Ide, T., Hayashidani, S., Shiomi, T., Kubota, T., Hamasaki, N. & Takeshita, A. (2003) Oxidative stress mediates tumor necrosis factor-alpha-induced mitochondrial DNA damage and dysfunction in cardiac myocytes. *Circulation* 107:1418–1423.

Timmers, C., Taniguchi, T., Hejna, J., Reifsteck, C., Locas, L., Bruun, D., Thayer, M., Cox, B., Olson, S., D'Andrea, A.D., Moses, R. & Grompe, M. (2001) Positional cloning of a novel Fanconi anemia gene, FANCD2. *Mol Cell* 7: 241–248.

Tischkowitz, M.D. & Hodgson, S.V. (2003) Fanconi anaemia. *J Med Genet* 40: 1–10.

Tischkowitz, M. & Dokal, I. (2004) Fanconi anaemia and leukaemia—clinical and molecular aspects. *Br J Haematol* 126(2): 176–191.

Tothova, Z. & Gilliland, D.G. (2002) FoxO Transcription Factors and Stem Cell Homeostasis: Insights from the Hematopoietic System *Stem Cells.* 20(5):438-447.

Tothova, Z., Kollipara, R., Huntly, B.J., Lee, B.H., Castrillon, D.H., Cullen, D.E., McDowell, E.P., Lazo-Kallanian, S., Williams. I.R., Sears, C., Armstrong, S.A., Passegué, E., DePinho, R.A. & Gilliland, D.G. (2002) FoxOs are critical mediators of hematopoietic stem cell resistance to physiologic oxidative stress. *Cell.* 128(2):325-339.

Tsai, W.B., Chung, Y.M., Takahashi, Y., Xu, Z. & Hu, M.C. (2008) Functional interaction between FOXO3a and ATM regulates DNA damage response. *Nat Cell Biol.* 10(4):460-467

Turrel-Davin, F., Tournadre, A., Pachot, A., Arnaud, B., Cazalis, M.A,, Mougin, B. & Miossec, P. (2010) FoxO3a involved in neutrophil and T cell survival is overexpressed in rheumatoid blood and synovial tissue. *Ann Rheum Dis* 69:755-760.

Umeda, T. & Hino, O. (2002) Molecular aspects of human hepatocarcinogenesis mediated by inflammation: from hypercarcinogenic state to normo- or hypocarcinogenic state. *Oncology* 62: 38–42.

Ventura, J.J., Cogswell, P., Flavell, R.A., Baldwin, A.S. Jr & Davis, R.J. (2004) JNK potentiates TNF-stimulated necrosis by increasing the production of cytotoxic reactive oxygen species. *Genes Dev* 18: 2905–2915.

Wajant, H., Pfizenmaier, K. & Scheurich, P. (2003) Tumor necrosis factor signaling. *Cell Death Differ* 10: 45–65.

Walsh, C.E., Nienhuis, A.W., Samulski, R.J., Brown, M.G., Miller, J.L., Young, N.S. & Liu, J.M. (1994) Phenotypic correction of Fanconi anemia in human hematopoietic cells with a recombinant adeno-associated virus vector. *J Clin Invest* 94: 1440–1448.

Wang, J., Otsuki, T., Youssoufian, H., Foe, J.L., Kim, S., Devetten, M., Yu, J., Li, Y., Dunn, D. & Liu, J.M. (1998) Overexpression of the Fanconi anemia group C gene (FAC) protects hematopoietic progenitors from death induced by Fas-mediated apoptosis. *Cancer Res* 58: 3538–3541.

West, R.R., Stafford, D.A., White, A.D., Bowen, D.T. & Padua, R.A. (2000) Cytogenetic abnormalities in the myelodysplastic syndromes and occupational or environmental exposure. *Blood* 95: 2093–2097.

Whitney, M.A., Royle, G., Low, M.J., Kelly, M.A., Axthelm, M.K., Reifsteck, C., Olsen, S., Braun, R.E., Heinrich, M.C., Rathbun, R.K., Bagby, G.C. & Grompe, M. (1996) Germ cell defects and hematopoietic hypersensitivity to -interferon in mice with a targeted disruption of the Fanconi anemia C gene. *Blood* 88: 49–58.

Wilson, A., Laurenti, E., Oser, G., van der Wath, R.C., Blanco-Bose, W., Jaworski, M., Offner, S., Dunant, C.F., Eshkind, L., Bockamp, E., Lió, P., Macdonald, H.R. & Trumpp, A. (2008) Hematopoietic stem cells reversibly switch from dormancy to self-renewal during homeostasis and repair. *Cell.* 135(6):1118-1129.

Wong, J.C. & Buchwald, M. (2002) Disease model: Fanconi anemia. *Trends Mol Med.* 8(3):139-142.

Xia, B., Dorsman, J.C., Ameziane, N., de Vries, Y., Rooimans, M.A., Sheng, Q., Pals, G., Errami, A., Gluckman, E., Llera, J., Wang, W., Livingston, D.M., Joenje, H. & de Winter, J.P. (2006) Fanconi anemia is associated with a defect in the BRCA2 partner PALB2. *Nat Genet* 39: 159–161.

Yamamoto, K.N., Kobayashi, S., Tsuda, M., Kurumizaka, H., Takata, M., Kono, K., Jiricny, J., Takeda, S. & Hirota, K. (2011) Involvement of SLX4 in interstrand cross-link repair is regulated by the Fanconi anemia pathway. *Proc Natl Acad Sci U S A.* 108(16):6492-6496.

Yang, Y., Kuang, Y., Montes De Oca, R., Hays, T., Moreau, L., Lu, N., Seed, B. & D'Andrea, A.D. (2001) Targeted disruption of the murine Fanconi anemia gene, Fancg/Xrcc9. *Blood* 98, 3435–3440

Young, N.S. & Maciejewski, J. (1997) The pathophysiology of acquired aplastic anemia. *N. Engl. J. Med.* 336: 1365–1372.

Zhang, X., Li, J., Sejas, D.P., Rathbun, K.R., Bagby, G.C. & Pang, Q. (2004) The Fanconi anemia proteins functionally interact with the protein kinase regulated by RNA (PKR). *J Biol Chem.* 279(42):43910-43919.

Zhang, X., Li, J., Sejas, D.P. & Pang, Q. (2005) Hypoxia-reoxygenationinduces premature senescence in FA bone marrow hematopoietic cells. *Blood* 106: 75–85.

Zhang, X., Li, J., Sejas, D.P. & Pang, Q. (2005) The ATM/p53/p21 pathway influences cell fate decision between apoptosis and senescence in reoxygenated hematopoietic progenitor cells. *J Biol Chem 280*: 19635–19640.

Zhang, X., Sejas, D.P., Qiu, Y., Williams, D.A. & Pang, Q. (2007) Inflammatory ROS promote and cooperate with Fanconi anemia mutation for hematopoietic senescence. *J Cell Science* 120: 1572–1583.

Ziech, D., Franco, R., Georgakilas, A. G., Georgakila, S., Malamou-Mitsi, V., Schoneveld, O., Pappa, A. & Panayiotidis, M. I. (2010) Chem. *Biol. Interact.* 188: 334-339.

3

Staying a Step Ahead of Cancer

Somaira Nowsheen, Alexandros G. Georgakilas and Eddy S. Yang
University of Alabama at Birmingham
USA

1. Introduction

Despite decades of research, cancer continues to affect millions of people each year. However, the more we discover about cancer, the more we realize that no single therapeutic strategy can effectively treat it. As we learn about the aberrant signals and pathways which lead to cancer, prevention may be a more feasible strategy. Vaccines, chemo preventive compounds, and healthier lifestyle choices are our arms in the battle against this deadly disease. In this chapter we discuss the importance of cancer prevention, how chemoprevention can be our first line of defense, and consider the role of small molecules and vaccines in cancer prevention and therapy. Deciphering the role of early disease detection and understanding how biomarkers and epigenetics can be a tool against cancer is vital. Finally, tackling the causes of cancer is critical for eradicating this malignancy.

The process of carcinogenesis is extremely slow, offering ample opportunity for intervention and prevention. A mutation in the genome may lead to transformation to a precancerous lesion and eventually to cancer with unchecked cell growth. An untold number of genetic changes can trigger cells to become cancerous. Predicting the changes and the susceptible population is even more daunting.

Mutations, whether acquired or inherited and caused by endogenous and exogenous agents, result in oncogenic transformation. In the human genome, there are many different types of genes that control cell growth in a very systematic, precise way. Error in these genes leads to further alterations or mutations. An accumulation of many mutations in different genes occurring in a specific group of cells over time is required to cause malignancy. In general, mutations in two classes of genes, proto-oncogenes and tumor suppressor genes, lead to cancer.

1.1 Proto-oncogenes

Proto-oncogenes are typically responsible for promoting cell growth but alterations lead to transformation into oncogenes and promotion of tumor growth. Mutations in these genes are typically dominant in nature. Often, proto-oncogenes encode proteins that function to stimulate cell division, inhibit cell differentiation, and halt cell death. Oncogenes, however, typically exhibit increased production of these proteins, thus leading to increased cell division, decreased cell differentiation, and inhibition of cell death. These phenotypes typify cancer cells. Underlying genetic mechanisms associated with oncogene activation include point mutations, deletions, or insertions that lead to a hyperactive gene product. Other examples include alterations in the promoter region of a proto-oncogene that lead to increased transcription. Gene amplification events leading to extra chromosomal copies of a proto-oncogene may also lead to oncogenesis. Chromosomal translocation events that relocate a proto-oncogene to a new chromosomal site that leads to higher expression or lead to a fusion between a proto-oncogene and a second gene, which produces a fusion protein with oncogenic activity may lead to cancer as well.

1.2 Tumor suppressors

Tumor suppressor genes are also present in our cells to control cell growth and apoptosis. Exquisite control over these processes suppresses tumor development. Mutations in tumor suppressors, as mentioned above, can lead to carcinogenesis. Tumor suppressors are in place to oppose threats to the genome. p53, the guardian of the genome, is one of the most commonly mutated tumor suppressor genes in human cancer. p53, a transcription factor, plays a critical role in numerous signaling pathways, from development to maintaining genomic stability and cell death (Brosh and Rotter 2009). Mutant p53 has been shown to exhibit gain–of–function properties that drive tumor progression and metastasis (Brosh and Rotter 2009). p53 is a stress response protein that functions primarily as a tetrameric transcription factor which regulates a large number of genes in response to a variety of cellular insults, including oncogene activation and DNA damage. These signals activate p53 primarily through post-translational modifications that result in augmented p53 protein level and transactivation activity. Activated p53 suppresses cellular transformation mainly by inducing growth arrest, apoptosis, DNA repair and differentiation in damaged cells (Oren 2003). Not surprisingly, p53 function is almost always compromised in tumor cells. Mutations in p53, usually due to somatic mutations, are observed in approximately half of all human cancers and constitute a cornerstone in tumorigenesis (Hollstein et al. 1991, Vogelstein, Lane and Levine 2000).

1.3 Models of carcinogenesis

There are several models of carcinogenesis. One of the models proposed by Dr. Bert Vogelstein proposes the loss of function of tumor suppressors such as p53 which paves the way for genomic instability, changes in metabolism, insensitivity to apoptotic signals, invasiveness and motility. However, the nature of the causal link between early tumorigenic events and the induction of the p53-mediated checkpoints that constitute a barrier to tumor progression remains uncertain. Loss of p53 function occurs during the development of most, if not all, tumor types. The cascade of events starts with a mutation that inactivates tumor suppressor gene leading to hyper-proliferation of epithelial cells. The mutation may also inactivate DNA repair genes while mutation of proto-oncogene creates an oncogene. The same mutation may lead to a cascade of inactivation of several more tumor suppressor genes before resulting in cancer. For example in colon carcinogenesis, loss or mutation of APC gene leads to overexpression on cyclooxygenase (COX) genes, transforming the normal tissue to hyperproliferative epithelium, and resulting in early adenoma. Subsequent DNA hypomethylation leads to mutations such as in k-ras gene, and results in intermediate adenoma. Another mutation following this, such as loss or mutation of DCC or SMAD 4, results in late adenoma. Subsequent mutation in p53 leads to carcinogenesis. Further mutations result in metastasis and greater genomic instability. It is thus quite apparent that the perturbations necessary to form cancer are numerous and complex. **Figure 1** gives an overview of this model of carcinogenesis.

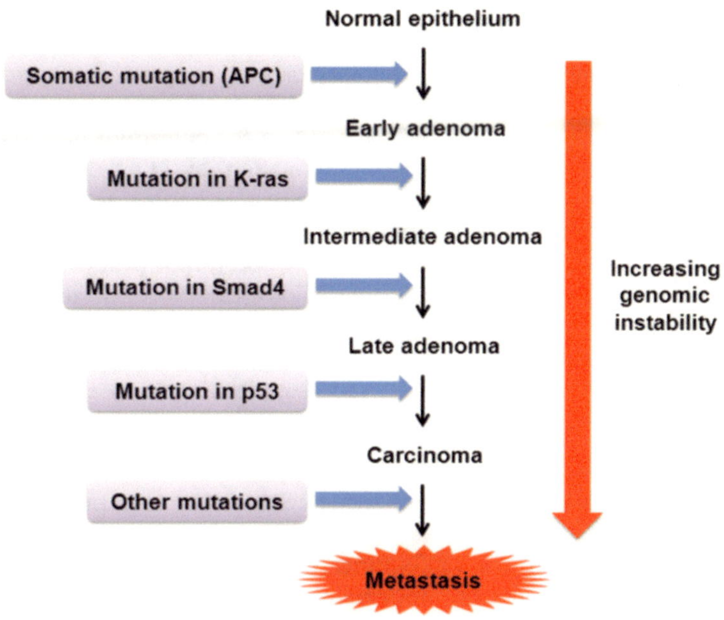

Fig. 1. The cascade of events that leads to colon carcinogenesis.

An alternate theory is Dr. Alfred Knudson's two-hit theory of cancer causation. This model accounts for both hereditary and non-hereditary cancer. Normal cells have two undamaged chromosomes, one from each parent, containing thousands of genes. People with a hereditary susceptibility to cancer inherit a damaged gene on one of the chromosomes. Thus, their first hit or mutation occurs at conception. Others receive the first hit in their lifetime. A subsequent damage to the same gene on the second chromosome may lead to cancer. Therefore, people with a hereditary susceptibility to cancer just need one hit during their lifetime to produce cancer. An overview of this model is given in **Figure 2**. This model is applicable for cancer such as retinoblastoma where inheritance of the first hit leads to a far greater chance of developing a second cancer causing mutation.

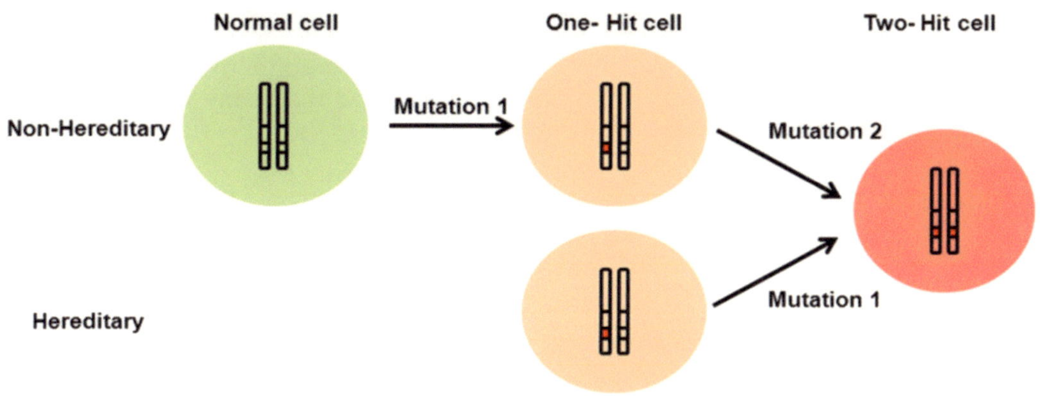

Fig. 2. The two-hit model of carcinogenesis.

2. Genomic instability and cancer

It should be noted that a state of genomic instability prevails in cancer. In certain cases, such as overexpression of licensing factors (hCdt1 and hCdc6), prolonged overexpression of these factors lead to a more aggressive phenotype, bypassing the antitumor barriers of accelerated senescence and apoptosis. The link between activation of DNA-damage response and tumorigenesis implies that continuous DNA damage checkpoint activation could lead to selective suppression of the DNA-damage response-induced antitumor barriers by inactivating mutations resulting in genomic instability and tumor progression (Bartkova et al. 2005, Bartkova et al. 2006, Gorgoulis et al. 2005, Di Micco et al. 2006, Halazonetis, Gorgoulis and Bartek 2008). Cells possessing re-replicated DNA above a critical threshold are typically neutralized by either senescence or apoptosis. However, cells with re-replicated elements below a critical threshold are prone to recombination processes leading to genomic instability. These events favor the selection of resilient cells and lead to therapeutic resistance (Liontos et al. 2007).

Proteins involved in DNA repair pathways have garnered attention because mutations causing dysfunction can lead to increased genetic instability and ultimately to increased cancer risk. Indeed, several studies have demonstrated alterations of these genes are associated with susceptibility to cancer (Berwick and Vineis 2000). Identification of factors associated with prognosis is an ever important process for both an escalation and de-escalation of therapies for appropriately selected patients. Additionally if alterations of these genes impact development of cancer, they are possible targets for therapy.

2.1 DNA damage and repair

The human body is under continuous attack from both external and internal insults which ultimately generates thousands of DNA lesions per day. But it has evolved its own defense mechanism to combat these lesions. The cellular response to DNA damage is critical for maintaining genomic integrity and for preventing carcinogenesis. Since DNA lesions can block genomic replication and transcription and lead to mutations it is imperative that DNA is repaired without any errors. Failure to repair any damage to the nucleic acid results in cell death in the form of apoptosis or necrosis. To combat threats posed by DNA damage, cells have evolved mechanisms, collectively termed the DNA-damage response, to detect DNA lesions, signal their presence, and promote DNA repair. Cells defective in these mechanisms generally display heightened sensitivity towards DNA-damaging agents. While this may be exploited for cancer therapy [e.g. poly ADP-ribose polymerase (PARP) inhibitors in breast cancer susceptibility protein (BRCA) deficient ovarian and breast tumors] it should also be noted that many such defects can lead to human disease, such as cancer.

2.2 DNA repair pathways

In an effort to repair the damaged DNA and avoid passing the damaged DNA onto the progeny cells, the cell has evolved several repair pathways. These repair pathways include base excision repair (BER), nucleotide excision repair (NER), double strand break (DSB) repair via homologous recombination (HR) or non-homologous end joining (NHEJ), and mismatch repair (MMR) (Polo and Jackson 2011, Stratton 2011, Stricker, Catenacci and Seiwert 2011). Though it is not clear what determines the choice of repair pathway, it is an area of active research.

Whereas some lesions are subject to direct protein-mediated reversal, most are repaired by a cascade of catalytic events mediated by multiple proteins. In MMR-mediated repair, detection of mismatches and insertion/deletion loops triggers a single-strand incision that is then worked upon by nuclease, polymerase and ligase enzymes. In BER-mediated repair, a damaged base is often recognized by a DNA glycosylase enzyme that mediates base removal before nuclease, polymerase and ligase proteins complete the repair in processes overlapping with those used in single strand break repair. In contrast, NER-mediated repair recognizes helix-distorting base lesions. It includes two sub-pathways that differ in the mechanism of lesion recognition: transcription-coupled NER, which specifically targets lesions that block transcription, and global-genome NER. A key aspect of NER is that the damage is excised as a 22–30-base oligonucleotide, producing single-stranded DNA that is acted upon by DNA polymerases and associated factors before ligation proceeds.

In NHEJ, DSBs are recognized by the Ku protein that then binds and activates the protein kinase DNA-PKcs, leading to recruitment and activation of end-processing enzymes, polymerases and DNA ligase IV. NHEJ repair, predominantly utilized in the repair of radiation induced DNA damage, is a highly efficient but error-prone process that often results in mutations in the repaired DNA. The NHEJ repair process is dependent on the DNA-dependent protein kinase (DNA-PK) catalytic subunit (DNA-PKcs), the Ku70/Ku80 heterodimer, and the XRCC4–ligase IV complex and ultimately rejoins the ends of DSBs with little or no homology. In response to radiation, DNA-PKcs is autophosphorylated at threonine 2609. This is required for the functional activation of the NHEJ repair pathway. Consistent with the role of NHEJ repair in the repair of radiation-induced DSBs, cells deficient in any NHEJ repair protein have been shown to be hypersensitive to radiation-mediated cytotoxicity (Iliakis et al. 2004, Yang et al. 2009, van Gent, Hoeijmakers and Kanaar 2001). A less-well-characterized Ku-independent NHEJ pathway, called micro-homology-mediated end-joining (MMEJ) or alternative end-joining, results in sequence deletions. Although both NHEJ and MMEJ are error-prone, they can operate in any phase of the cell cycle.

In contrast, HR is generally restricted to S and G2 because it uses sister-chromatid sequences as the template to mediate faithful repair. Although there are several HR sub-pathways, HR is always initiated by single strand DNA generation, which is promoted by various proteins including the MRE11–RAD50–NBS1 (MRN) complex. In events catalyzed by RAD51 and the breast-cancer susceptibility proteins BRCA1 and BRCA2, the single strand DNA then invades the undamaged template and, following the actions of polymerases, nucleases, helicases and other components, DNA ligation and substrate resolution occur. HR is also used to restart stalled replication forks and to repair inter-strand DNA crosslinks, the repair of which also involves the Fanconi anaemia protein complex. This high-fidelity, error-free process is also critical in the repair of lesions resulting from replicative stress (Yang et al. 2009, Jiang et al. 2011, Wang et al. 2010).

2.2.1 Cell cycle checkpoints

Checkpoints are also put in place throughout the cell cycle that halt further progression of DNA replication and cell division upon detection of damaged DNA. This can arrest the cell either transiently or permanently (senescence), as well as activate specific DNA repair pathways in response to certain types of DNA damage. Some of the proteins in these pathways are mutated or non-functional in human tumors causing cancer cells to be more reliant on an intact DNA repair pathway for survival. Key DNA damage signaling components in mammalian cells are the protein kinases ATM and ATR. ATM is recruited to and activated by DSBs. In contrast, ATR is recruited to and activated by replication protein A-coated double stranded DNA. Two of the best studied ATM/ATR targets are the protein kinases CHK1 and CHK2. Together with ATM and ATR, these proteins reduce cyclin-dependent kinase (CDK) activity by various mechanisms, often mediated by p53. Inhibition of CDKs slows down or arrests cell-cycle progression at the G1–S, intra-S and G2–M cell-cycle checkpoints. This allows more time for DNA repair before replication or mitosis. In parallel, ATM/ATR signaling enhances repair by a variety of methods: inducing DNA-repair proteins transcriptionally or post-transcriptionally, by recruiting repair factors to the damage-site, and by activating DNA-repair proteins by modulating their phosphorylation, acetylation, ubiquitylation or SUMOylation. The aforementioned proteins can be exploited for cancer therapy as well.

2.3 Epigenetic modifications in cancer

Both genotoxic and non-genotoxic mechanisms have been implicated in malignant transformation. Genotoxic mechanisms involve changes in genomic DNA sequences leading to mutations. On the other hand, non-genotoxic mechanisms modulate gene expression directly (Franco et al. 2008). Epigenetic pathway which involves changes in DNA methylation patterns and histone modifications is considered to be a non-genotoxic mechanism capable of modulating gene expression and thus promoting malignant transformation. Thus, it is vital to determine such epigenetic modifications in a way that we can expand on cancer biological marker development with clinical relevance (Franco et al. 2008). Epigenetic molecular marker development has been a hot topic in cancer research because of the ability to contribute to cancer diagnosis and/or prognosis due to their high sensitivity and specificity. A number of epigenetic modifications have been detected in critical genes involved in various cancers that can potentially serve as specific clinical biomarkers.

2.4 DNA hypomethylation and cancer

Promoter DNA hypomethylation modification has been observed for a number of genes including H-ras in prostate and thyroid cancers and cancer-testis antigen gene (CAGE) in prostate, breast, lung and laryngeal cancers. The X-inactive specific transcript (XIST) modification is observed in prostate cancer while erythropoietin (EPO) is found in prostate and breast cancers. Maspin changes are detected in ovarian, pancreatic and lung cancers. Changes in γ-Synuclein are prevalent in ovarian and breast cancers while c-myc modifications are found in breast and lung cancers. Urokinase-type plasminogen activator modification is observed in breast cancer, S100P in pancreatic cancer and Melanoma-associated antigen A (MAGE-A) in lung cancer (Ziech et al. 2010).

2.4.1 DNA hypermethylation and cancer

Promoter DNA hypermethylation modification has been associated with altered expression of critical genes associated with various cancers including BRCA1/BRCA2 in prostate, breast, pancreatic and ovarian cancers, Von Hippel–Lindau tumor suppressor (VHL) and p53 in breast cancer. A number of changes are observed in lung cancer including P16INK4a, H-cadherin, Death-associated protein kinase 1 (DAPK1), MDM2, and p53. Modification in p14ARF is observed in lung, esophageal and colorectal cancers while changes in hHML1 are seen in colorectal cancer. RASSF1A modification are present in lung and nasopharyngeal cancers (Ziech et al. 2010).

2.4.2 Modifications in chromatin structure in cancer

Besides changes in DNA methylation patterns, the chromatin has also been shown to regulate transcriptional activity. To this end, any modifications in core histone proteins (e.g. H2A, H2B, H3 and H4) can have an impact in the activation and/or repression of transcription. Such modifications can include, among others, methylation, acetylation, deacetylation, phosphorylation, and ubiquitination. Histone acetylation and/or deacetylation are observed in breast, prostate, colon, testicular, renal and pancreatic cancers. Histone demethylation is observed in breast, prostate, colon, testicular and esophageal cancers while histone H3 lysine 27 tri-methylation is observed in breast, ovarian, colon and pancreatic cancers. Histone H3 lysine 9 and/or Histone H4 lysine 20 tri-methylations are present in breast, lung and hepatocellular cancers. Histone H3 lysine 4 methylation is often observed in breast, ovarian, colorectal and hepatocellular cancers (Ziech et al. 2010).

2.5 BRCA1 and cancer

Perhaps, the most noted molecular marker for cancer is mutations in the BRCA family of genes. The BRCA family of proteins is essential for HR-mediated repair of DNA double strand breaks (Jackson and Bartek 2009, Bartek, Lukas and Lukas 2004, Wang et al. 2010, Jiang et al. 2011). As little as one unrepaired DNA double strand break is fatal to the cell (Yang et al. 2009, Aziz, Nowsheen and Georgakilas 2010). Thus, it is not surprising that certain mutations in the BRCA gene lead to an increased risk for breast cancer as part of a hereditary breast-ovarian cancer syndrome. Women with mutated BRCA1 or BRCA2 gene have up to a 60% risk of developing breast cancer (King et al. 2003, Graeser et al. 2009). Similarly, 55% increased risk of developing ovarian cancer is observed with BRCA1 mutations and about 25% for women with BRCA2 mutations (King et al. 2003). Research suggests hypermethylation of the BRCA1 promoter may be an inactivating mechanism for BRCA1 expression not only in breast and ovarian cancer but also lung and oral cancer (Esteller et al. 2000, Marsit et al. 2003). Due to the lack of reliable biomarkers, many women with breast cancer end up being over-treated or under-treated for the disease. Epigenetic modifications have been detected in critical genes involved in breast cancer that could potentially serve as specific clinical molecular markers. These include promoter DNA hypomethylation in c-myc, CAGE, Urokinase-type plasminogen activator, EPO and γ-Synuclein genes and promoter DNA hypermethylation in BRCA1, BRCA2, Von Hippel-Lindau tumor suppressor (VHL) and p53 genes (Ziech et al. 2010).

In addition to breast cancer, mutations in the BRCA1 gene also increase the risk of developing ovarian, fallopian tube, and prostate cancers (Brose et al. 2002, Thompson, Easton and the Breast Cancer Linkage 2002). Mutations in BRCA also increase the risk for a subset of leukemia and lymphoma (Friedenson 2007). Women having inherited a defective BRCA1 or BRCA2 gene have risks for breast and ovarian cancer that are so high and seem so selective that many mutation carriers choose to have prophylactic surgery. Promoter DNA hypomethylation in Maspin and γ-Synuclein genes and promoter DNA hypermethylation in BRCA1 and BRCA2 genes have been reported in ovarian cancer (Ziech et al. 2010). A number of epigenetic modifications have been detected in critical genes involved in pancreatic cancer that could potentially serve as specific clinical biomarkers including promoter DNA hypermethylation in BRCA1 and BRCA2 genes (Ziech et al. 2010). Thus, the tumor suppressor genes BRCA1 and BRCA2 are critical for the maintenance of our genome.

2.6 Mutations in DNA repair genes and cancer

Patients with underlying cellular defects in the response to DNA DSBs often exhibit genomic instability, increased cancer predisposition and radiation sensitivity. There are a number of other genetic disorders that predisposes an individual to cancer via defects in DNA repair pathways. For example, mutations in Ataxia telangiectasia mutated (ATM), a critical DNA repair protein, leads to Ataxia Telangiectasia (AT). ATM is a serine/threonine protein kinase that is recruited and activated by DNA DSB. It phosphorylates several key proteins that initiate activation of the DNA damage checkpoint, leading to cell cycle arrest, DNA repair or apoptosis. Several of these targets, including p53, CHK2 and H2AX are tumor suppressors (Shiloh 2003). Thus AT sufferers are predisposed to lymphoma, breast, brain, stomach, bladder, pancreas, lung, ovaries, T cell prolymphocytic leukemia, B cell chronic lymphocytic leukemia and sporadic colon cancers (Aziz et al. 2010). They are also extremely sensitive to radiation, a source of DNA damage (Alderton 2007).

Nijmegen breakage syndrome (NBS) is a rare autosomal recessive congenital disorder causing chromosomal instability and DNA repair deficiency. NBS1 codes for a protein that stops cell cycle progression following DNA damage and interacts with FANCD2 that can activate the BRCA1/BRCA2 pathway of DNA repair (Stavridi and Halazonetis 2005). Thus, mutations in the NBS1 gene lead to higher levels of cancer, primarily lymphoma (Aziz et al. 2010). Similarly, Lynch syndrome is marked by defects in MMR genes such as MSH1, MSH2, MSH6, and PMS2 (Vasen and de Vos tot Nederveen Cappel 2011). This leads to increased incidence of colorectal cancer, cancers of the stomach, small intestine, liver, gallbladder ducts, upper urinary tract, brain, skin, prostate, endometrium and ovary (Aziz et al. 2010). Li-Fraumeni patients demonstrate mutations in Chk2 and p53 and defects in MMR. They have a higher incidence of osteosarcoma (Aziz et al. 2010). Werner syndrome, on the other hand, is marked by mutations in WRN and Rad51 genes leading to deficiency in HR- and NHEJ mediated DSB repair. This syndrome leads to a number of cancers including osteosarcoma, colon, rectal, lung, stomach, prostate, breast, thyroid and soft tissue sarcomas (Aziz et al. 2010). Xeroderma Pigmentosum is marked by mutations in XPD gene, defects in NER-mediated repair and higher incidence of skin cancer (Aziz et al. 2010). Bloom is caused by mutations in Blm gene and leads to leukemia, lymphoma, melanoma, and bladder cancer due to defects in HR-mediated repair (Aziz et al. 2010). Mutations in RECQL4, a key BER and HR-repair protein, leads to Rothmund Thompson, Baller Gerold and Rapadilino syndromes which are marked by predisposition to osteosarcoma (Aziz et al.

2010). Mutations in the FANC gene, a marker of Fanconi anemia, leads to deficient DNA crosslink repair and subsequent increased risk of acute myeloid leukemia, head and neck cancer, gynecological malignancies, and gastrointestinal squamous cell carcinoma (Aziz et al. 2010). DNA Lig4 deficiency, a mutation in a key NHEJ repair protein, leads to pancreatic and lung cancers (Aziz et al. 2010). Other defects in NHEJ mediated repair pathways, e.g. Rag1 and Rag2 or Artemis, lead to an increased incidence of lymphoma. XCIND and RS-SCID syndromes are characterized by the aforementioned defects (Aziz et al. 2010). Mutations in XLF, a marker of Cernunnos deficiency and a key NHEJ-mediated repair protein, lead lymphoma while defects in ATR, a key DSB repair protein, lead to ATR-Seckel syndrome which predisposes the individual to leukemia (Aziz et al. 2010).

Another protein, OGG1, an enzyme involved in DNA repair, has been shown to have predictive value for lung cancer (Hatt et al. 2008). OGG1 levels can be easily assayed in blood samples and low levels correlate with higher chance of developing lung cancer. In a recent study, 40% of people with lung cancer had low levels of the enzyme compared to 4% of healthy individuals (Paz-Elizur et al. 2003).

2.7 Other modifications in cancer

Progression of any cancer is accompanied by genetic alteration(s) which leads to altered protein structure and function. In the last several years, the association between human papilloma virus (HPV) and head and neck cancer has been solidified (Wansom et al. 2010, Albers et al. 2005, Sirianni et al. 2004, Sirianni, Wang and Ferris 2005, Kumar et al. 2007, Kumar et al. 2008, Sisk et al. 2002). Interestingly, HPV associated head and neck cancers exhibit better prognosis and appear to respond better to chemo-radiation. Saliva or serum of head and neck cancer patients can be analyzed for p53, EGFR, and HPV status and microsatellite alterations. In addition, a number of epigenetic modifications have been detected in critical genes involved in this particular cancer type that could potentially serve as specific clinical biological markers. These include promoter DNA hypomethylation in H-ras and CAGE genes in thyroid and laryngeal cancers respectively and promoter DNA hypermethylation in p14ARF and RASSF1A genes in esophageal and nasopharyngeal cancers respectively (Ziech et al. 2010).

3. The role of lifestyle choices in cancer

Billions of dollars are spent each year to research new therapeutic strategies against cancer. Still, millions of people die from the disease each year. Thus, successful prevention appears to be the better option and requires attacking the root causes of the disease. The best way to control cancer is to prevent it from happening in the first place. Geographic and economic differences in cancer incidence and mortality are striking. The types of cancer vary greatly between the developed and developing countries. Lung, prostate, breast and colorectal cancer are common in the developed countries like the US while ovarian, cervical, hepatocellular, and head and neck cancer are wide-spread in the poorer nations (Ott et al. 2011). **Table 1** lists the common cancers and their associated risk factors which can be avoided to prevent these malignancies.

Risk factor	Cancer
Tobacco	• Bladder • Head and neck • Lung
Human papillomavirus	• Cervical • Head and neck
Hepatitis	• Hepatocellular
Weight/ Diet	• Breast • Cervix • Colon • Esophagus • Gall-bladder • Kidney • Liver • Ovary • Pancreas • Prostate • Stomach • Uterus
Alcohol	• Breast • Colorectal • Esophageal • Liver • Lung • Melanoma • Oral • Pharyngeal • Stomach

Table 1. Preventable cancers and their risk factors.

3.1 HPV

Of note, persistent HPV infections are now recognized as one of the causes of cancer. HPV is the cause of essentially all cervical cancers, as well as most cases of anal cancer. Genital HPV infection also causes some cancers of the vulva, vagina, and penis. In addition, oral HPV infection causes some cancers of the oropharynx and head and neck (Lowy and Munger 2010). HPV-induced cancers often have viral sequences integrated into the cellular DNA. Some of the HPV genes, such as E6 and E7, act as oncogenes that promote tumor growth and malignant transformation. E6/E7 proteins inactivate two tumor suppressor proteins, p53 (inactivated by E6) and retinoblastoma (RB) (inactivated by E7) (Dyson et al. 1989, Sherr and McCormick 2002, Storey et al. 1998, Werness, Levine and Howley 1990). As mentioned before, p53 is a tumor suppressor gene that arrests the cell cycle, prevents cell growth and stimulates apoptosis in the presence of DNA damage (Vogelstein et al. 2000). p53 also upregulates p21 which blocks the formation of the Cyclin D/Cdk4 complex, thereby preventing the phosphorylation of RB and, in turn, halting cell cycle progression by preventing the activation of E2F (Sherr and McCormick 2002). E6 has a close relationship with E6-associated protein (E6-AP) which is involved in the ubiquitin ligase pathway. E6-AP binds ubiquitin to p53, thereby flagging it for proteosomal degradation (Werness et al. 1990). In contrast, E7 competes for RB binding, freeing the transcription factor E2F to transactivate its targets, thus pushing the cell cycle forward (Dyson et al. 1989). Most HPV infections are cleared rapidly by the immune system and do not progress to cancer. Since the process of transforming normal cells into cancerous ones is slow, cancer occurs in people with persistent HPV infection.

3.2 Alcohol

Alcohol, a carcinogen, also causes a plethora of cancers (Wang et al. 2011, Chang, Straif and Guha 2011, Land et al. 2011, Pelucchi et al. 2008, Thomas 1995). Increased alcohol consumption has been linked to breast, liver, stomach, colorectal, melanoma, lung, and other cancers. Alcohol is thought to stimulate tumor growth by fuelling the production of growth factors that stimulate angiogenesis (Pelucchi et al. 2011). In addition, alcohol suppresses immune activity. Thus, alcohol should only be consumed in moderation.

3.3 Smoking

Cigarette smoking leads to lung cancer since smoking exposes the individual to multiple DNA-damaging carcinogens and mutagens that result in mutations in critical genes that control cellular growth (Gonzalez et al. 2011, Hymowitz 2011, Lam and Minna 2011, Pesch et al. 2011, Proctor et al. 2011, Shields 2011). Moreover, smokers are exposed to multiple tumor promoting substances and inflammatory agents that exacerbate the process. Effective tobacco control led by clean air legislation, taxation, and anti-tobacco advertising is gradually contributing to decreased lung cancer incidence ((CDC) 2011, Bajoga et al. 2011, Ballbe et al. 2011, Kasza et al. 2011, King et al. 2011a, King et al. 2011b, Mage et al. 2011, Walsh et al. 2011). Thorough understanding of the biochemical, genetic and behavioral mechanisms of smoking can help us identify people who have a particularly high susceptibility to tobacco promoted cancers. These individuals can then be targeted for novel prevention measures, such as a nicotine vaccination and chemoprevention. Other simple individual steps that can help against developing cancer include vaccination (discussed in detail in a subsequent section) and screening for cervical cancer and hepatitis B, avoidance of excessive sun exposure for skin cancer, and limiting alcohol consumption for head and neck cancer and liver cancer (Pelucchi et al. 2008, Thomas 1995, Herrero et al. 2011, Chang et al. 2011, Pelucchi et al. 2011, No et al. 2011). Education and public outreach are immensely critical in this field. To this end, as research resources are allocated on cancer prevention, simultaneously there is a need to support scientific research to better understand the specific causes and mechanisms of cancers. Effort to identify susceptible individuals and target them for preventive interventions is necessary.

3.4 Diet

A number of studies have examined the impact of diet on cancer risk. Both the quantity and quality of food plays a role in cancer, with the former thought to be more critical. Some foods do contain anticancer compounds. Phytonutrients, often found in pungent and bitter vegetables, include resveratrol in grapes and curcumin in turmeric (Azari et al. 2009, Feeney 2004, Greenlee, Hershman and Jacobson 2009, Holst and Williamson 2008, Kale, Gawande and

Kotwal 2008, Kaur, Agarwal and Agarwal 2009, Lanzotti 2006, Mates et al. 2011, Mattoo et al. 2010, McGrath and Spigelman 2008, Neto 2007, Surh 2008, Wahlqvist and Lee 2007, Wenefrida et al. 2009). Other molecules, including sulforaphane and genistein, an isoflavone found in soybeans, are currently being tested as pharmaceutical agents in cancer prevention (Ali et al. 2005, Caetano et al. 2006, Takahashi et al. 2006, Shenouda et al. 2004). A healthy balanced diet with these nutrients can help prevent cancer. The barriers to the effectiveness of these phytonutrients lie in the genome and microbiomes. For instance, consumption of a known amount of the phytonutrient sulforaphane does not guarantee absorption of a predicted amount of anti-cancer molecule since differences in the glutathione S transferase M1 gene influences the metabolic rate of sulforaphane, a phytonutrient present in broccoli. The faster it is metabolized, the faster it is expelled from the body (Chung et al. 2000, Gasper et al. 2005, Gross-Steinmeyer et al. 2010, Joseph et al. 2004, Lampe 2007, Lampe 2009, McWalter et al. 2004, Riedl, Saxon and Diaz-Sanchez 2009, Ritz, Wan and Diaz-Sanchez 2007, Traka et al. 2008, Wan and Diaz-Sanchez 2007). Similarly, a number of the nutrients, e.g. isoflavones from soy, cannot be absorbed without the aid of microbes in the intestine (Di Cagno et al. 2010, Ding and Shah 2010, Rekha and Vijayalakshmi 2010, Szliszka et al. 2011, Szliszka and Krol 2011). Nonetheless, a healthy diet can reduce the chances of developing cancer.

Diet plays a vital role in the promotion of prostate cancer (Nelson, De Marzo and Isaacs 2003). Increased total fat intake, animal fat intake, and consumption of red meat have been associated with an increased risk of developing prostate cancer. In addition, the level of consumption of red meat correlates with the risk of prostate cancer (Giovannucci et al. 1993). Cooking meat at high temperatures or broiling on charcoal grills causes heterocyclic aromatic amine and polycyclic aromatic hydrocarbon carcinogens to form (Gross et al. 1993). Substantiating the claim, one such heterocyclic amine carcinogen, 2-amino-1-methyl-6-phenylimidazo[4,5-b]pyridine, causes prostate cancer when fed to rats (Shirai et al. 1997). On the other hand, antioxidant carotenoid lycopene found in tomatoes, isothiocyanate sulforaphane found in cruciferous vegetables, as well as other micronutrients may protect against prostate cancer by reducing oxidative genomic damage (Chan and Giovannucci 2001, Cohen, Kristal and Stanford 2000). Other antioxidants, such as vitamin E, isothiocyanate sulforaphane and selenium, may also reduce the risk of prostate cancer (Nelson et al. 2003, Hoque et al. 2001, Cohen et al. 2000, Heinonen et al. 1998). Factors involved in inflammation and angiogenesis, such as NFκB and vascular endothelial growth factor (VEGF) pathways, have been reported to be critical regulators in prostate carcinogenesis (Heymach et al. 2011).

The association between diet and breast cancer risk has been investigated extensively and has led to some recommendations for cancer prevention. Maintaining a healthy weight reduces the risk for breast cancer. Excess weight and weight gain in adult life are related to higher risk of postmenopausal breast cancer, and weight loss after menopause is associated with substantially reduced risk. Moderate levels of alcohol consumption increase the risk for breast cancer. Interestingly, this effect can be mitigated by adequate folate intake (Kim et al. 2011, Linos, Holmes and Willett 2007, Linos and Willett 2009, Linos and Willett 2007). Emerging research suggests that dietary intake of fiber and nuts during adolescence influences subsequent risk of breast disease and may suggest a viable means for breast cancer prevention (Linos et al. 2010, Su et al. 2010, Holmes et al. 2009). Since breast cancer is a heterogeneous disease and dietary factors may differentially affect certain breast cancer subtypes future studies should therefore attempt to characterize associations according to tumor characteristics.

A significant association between body mass index and higher cancer-induced mortality has been reported (**Table 1**) (Lampe 2007, Teucher, Rohrmann and Kaaks 2009, Boniol and Autier 2010, Gotay 2010, Khan, Afaq and Mukhtar 2010, Land et al. 2011, Lanzotti 2006, Li et al. 2011a). Specifically, a correlation between being overweight (excess body fat) and cancers of the esophagus, colon, liver, gall-bladder, pancreas, kidney, breast, uterus, cervix, ovary, prostate and stomach has been observed. But researchers have yet to fully decipher the link between being overweight and cancer. The mechanism likely depends on the type of malignancy. For instance, abdominal fat pressing on the stomach causes acid to splash up into the esophagus leading to tissue damage, which can ultimately result in esophageal cancer (Etemadi et al. 2011, Hall and Crowe 2011, Kong et al. 2011, Lagergren 2011, Li et al. 2011b, Olsen et al. 2011, Rutegard et al. 2011, Ryan et al. 2011). Estrogen, produced by fat cells, appears to play a role in endometrial cancer and breast cancer in postmenopausal women since it fuels cellular growth of estrogen receptor positive cancers (Bradlow et al. 2011, Colonna, Douglas Case and Lawrence 2011, Creighton et al. 2011, Perks and Holly 2011, Rondini et al. 2011, Sikalidis and Varamini 2011, Subbaramaiah et al. 2011, Willyard 2011, Yang et al. 2010). Androgen promotes some forms of prostate cancer as well (Aggarwal, Ryan and Chan 2011, Capitanio et al. 2011, Hoda et al. 2010, Ribeiro et al. 2010). Similarly, obesity promotes production of excess insulin which can promote growth of cancer. Interestingly, blockade of these receptors using antibodies and small molecular inhibitors have been shown to stop cancer cell proliferation. For example, Tamoxifen, an antagonist of the estrogen receptor, is currently used for the treatment of both early and advanced estrogen receptor positive breast cancer (University 2011, Amir et al. 2011, Braems et al. 2011, Cuzick et al. 2011, Doughty 2011, Fleeman et al. 2011, Gandhi and Verma 2011, Garrido et al. 2011, Goetz et al. 2011, Kilic et al. 2011, Kiyotani et al. 2011, Lin, Zhang and Manson 2011, Obiorah and Jordan 2011, Teunissen et al. 2011). Furthermore, it has also been approved by the FDA as a chemo preventative agent in women adjudged to be at high-risk of developing breast cancer (University 2011, Amir et al. 2011, Cuzick et al. 2011, Goetz et al. 2011). Similarly, people on metformin treatment to control their insulin level appear to have a lower risk of developing breast and pancreatic cancer (Papanas, Maltezos and Mikhailidis 2010, Rozengurt, Sinnett-Smith and Kisfalvi 2010, Suh and Kim 2011, Vigneri et al. 2009).

Regular physical activity cuts down on the risk of cancer as well. One proposed theory is that active people tend to digest their food faster, decreasing the chance of absorption of any carcinogenic products that happen to be going through the colon to be in contact with the mucosal lining (Azcárate-Peril, Sikes and Bruno-Bárcena 2011). In the same way, improved lung function limits exposure to airborne carcinogens, decreasing the risk of cancer. Interestingly, physically active individuals had lower estrogen levels compared to sedentary women, reducing their chance of developing the disease (Eliassen et al. 2010, Kossman et al. 2011, Lynch, Neilson and Friedenreich 2010, Phipps et al. 2011, Suzuki et al. 2011, Winzer et al. 2011). Thus, it is clear that simple healthy lifestyle choices can help reduce the chances of developing cancer.

3.5 Prophylactic surgery

A more drastic measure to prevent cancer is prophylactic surgery. It involves removal of as much of the at-risk tissue as possible in order to reduce the chance of developing cancer.

Bilateral prophylactic mastectomy (removal of healthy breasts) and prophylactic salpingo-oophorectomy (removal of healthy fallopian tubes and ovaries) do not, however, offer a guarantee against developing cancer. Because not all at-risk tissue can be removed by these procedures, some women have developed breast cancer, ovarian cancer, or primary peritoneal carcinomatosis even after prophylactic surgery.

Additionally, there are instances where despite strict lifestyles, cancer unfortunately will still develop. In these situations where prevention has failed, the next effective strategy is early detection of disease, which can improve the chance of beating cancer. Regular screening for cancer increases the chance of catching the disease early, while it is still treatable. Screening does not, however, change the risk of developing cancer. For example, breast cancer can be screened by mammography and clinical breast exams. Studies are currently under way to test the effectiveness of other breast cancer screening methods, such as magnetic resonance imaging (MRI), in women with BRCA1 or BRCA2 mutations. For ovarian cancer, surveillance methods include transvaginal ultrasound, blood tests for CA-125 antigen, and clinical exams. Similarly, prostate cancer screening includes assaying prostate specific antigen (PSA) levels and digital rectal exam for lumps in the prostate. High PSA levels and lumps may be indicative of cancer but infection and inflammation may falsely elevate PSA levels as well. Routine colonoscopy to look for early signs of cancer is recommended at age 50 or earlier if there is a family history of colorectal cancer, a personal history of inflammatory bowel disease, or other risk factors. These strategies help in diagnosing cancer at its early stages.

The most effective steps to curb cancer are low-cost and low-tech. For example, giving up smoking and losing weight can drastically reduce the chances of developing cancer. Smoking has long been known to be a risk factor while obesity has more recently been recognized as one. Together they account for roughly half of all cancer cases (Ott et al. 2011, Brand et al. 2011, Land et al. 2011, Li et al. 2011a, Boniol and Autier 2010, Giovannucci et al. 2010, Gotay 2010, Khan et al. 2010, Teucher et al. 2009). Since these habits are easier said than done, policies that make unhealthy lifestyle choices difficult and expensive while making healthier ones easier and cheaper will be a step in the right direction. In addition, a number of clinical compounds have also been proposed to reduce the risk of carcinogenesis. These are discussed in detail below.

4. Chemo preventative strategies against cancer

A number of chemo preventative compounds have been proposed to reduce the risk of tumorigenesis (**Table 2**). A chemoprevention agent that blocks the very first step of tumorigenesis would be best. The next sections will discuss various pathways which can be targeted to potentially prevent cancer.

4.1 Inflammation

Dysregulation of cell proliferation and apoptosis evasion are major determinants of the evolution of neoplasia and tumor growth, the hallmarks of cancer (Hanahan and Weinberg 2000). As tumors move to a progressed state and possibly metastasis, it is generally accepted that there is further induction of genetic and genomic alterations which has been synonymous with an increase in DNA mutations and further loss of homeostasis primarily

Cancer	Drug	Notes	Reference
Breast	Tamoxifen	• Selective estrogen receptor modulator	(Vogel et al. 2006)
	Raloxifene	• Selective estrogen receptor modulator	(Vogel et al. 2006)
Cervical/vulvar/anal	HPV vaccine	• Promotes immune response to prevent HPV infection	(Einstein et al. 2009, Heard 2011, Saslow et al. 2007, Wheeler et al. 2011)
Esophageal	Porfimer sodium and photodynamic therapy with omeprazole	• Lodges in precancerous cells and upon exposure to light produces reactive species of oxygen • Kills surrounding cancer cells	(Overholt, Panjehpour and Haydek 1999, Overholt et al. 2007, Panjehpour and Overholt 2006)
Skin	Fluorouracil	• Interferes with DNA synthesis • Results in cell death	(Madan, Lear and Szeimies 2010)
	5-aminolevulinic acid in combination with Porfimer sodium and photodynamic therapy	• Lodges in precancerous cells and upon exposure to light produces reactive species of oxygen • Kills surrounding cancer cells	(Madan et al. 2010)
	Imiquimod	• Enhances immune response • Promotes apoptosis	(Madan et al. 2010)
Prostate	Finasteride	• An inhibitor of 5α-reductase • Inhibits the conversion of testosterone to dihydrotestosterone • Prevents or delays the appearance of prostate cancer • Possible benefit and a reduced risk of urinary problems must be weighed against sexual side effects and the increased risk of high-grade prostate cancer.	(Thompson et al. 2003)

Table 2. Chemo preventative drugs currently approved by the FDA.

via inflammation-based pathways (Colotta et al. 2009, Solinas et al. 2010, Klein and Glazer 2010). Inflammatory chemokines and cytokines such as *CCL2, CCL18,* and others have been implicated in such processes (Chen et al. 2011, Bonecchi, Locati and Mantovani 2011, Redon et al. 2010). It has been suggested that the tumor surrounding may contribute to tumor proliferation. Tumors have the ability to alter their stroma and support the development of both tumor cells and non-malignant cells (Polyak, Haviv and Campbell 2009). The tumor eventually escapes from the host immune system via activation of one or several molecular mechanisms that lead to inhibition of immune cell functions or to apoptosis of anti-tumor effector cells (Schreiber, Old and Smyth 2011). The ability to block tumor escape hinges on a better understanding of cellular and molecular pathways operating in the tumor microenvironment. Monitoring the change(s) in the tumor stroma such as those occurring in the mesenchymal stem cells within tumor stroma via molecular and cellular profiles as the tumor progresses allows for identification of cell or protein targets for cancer prevention and therapy (Karnoub et al. 2007). Increasingly, cancer treatments are being modified to include tumor surrounding as a therapeutic target, since the non-malignant cells are more genetically stable and less likely to evolve into drug resistant phenotypes. For example, aspirin inhibits COX-1, while Celebrex inhibits COX-2 (Chan, Ogino and Fuchs 2007, Harris et al. 2005, Cooper et al. 2010, Ghosh et al. 2010, Harris 2007, Koehne and Dubois 2004, Reddy 2007, Reddy and Rao 2005, Smith et al. 1998). COX-1 is produced in tissues throughout the body, and is known to mediate the production of prostaglandins, chemical messengers that control a number of physiological functions, such as lowering blood pressure, regulating body temperature and controlling inflammation (Kundu and Fulton 2002, Smith et al. 1998, Pereira, Medeiros and Dinis-Ribeiro 2009). COX-2, on the other hand, is strictly regulated and tends to spike during inflammation and other stress (Cesario, Rocca and Rutella 2011). Abundance of COX-2 has been linked to the growth and proliferation of cancerous and pre-cancerous cells (Cesario et al. 2011, Khan et al. 2011). Inhibiting the COX pathways can alter cancerous and precancerous cells by decreasing angiogenesis and cell growth (Banu et al. 2007, Half, Sun and Sinicrope 2007, Ishizaki et al. 2006, Sheng et al. 1997, Suh et al. 2009, Tuynman et al. 2008, Zhang et al. 2009). In addition, COX inhibition enhances apoptosis and enables the immune system to recognize and target the cells for destruction (Hida et al. 2000, Ding, Tong and Adrian 2000, Hsu et al. 2000, Souza et al. 2000). While COX-2 inhibitors are still a promising drug for chemoprevention, they have not been approved as a standard chemo preventative agent yet. This is, in part, due to increased risk of stroke, gastrointestinal bleeding, and heart attack following administration of these agents (Marnett 2009, Menter, Schilsky and DuBois 2010, Psaty and Furberg 2005). Nevertheless, a number of clinical trials evaluating the clinical efficacy of aspirin in decreasing the risk of colon, lung, prostate and brain cancer are currently in progress (Rothwell et al. 2011). Five year follow up data suggests that aspirin dramatically reduces the risk of death from solid tumors and gastrointestinal cancers. The latent period before an effect on deaths was about 5 years for esophageal, pancreatic, brain, and lung cancer, but was more delayed for stomach, colorectal, and prostate cancer. For lung and esophageal cancer, benefit was confined to adenocarcinomas. Benefit was unrelated to aspirin dose as long as the administered dose was 75 mg or upwards. Benefit was unrelated to sex or smoking, but increased with age (Rothwell et al. 2011).

Emerging research suggests that other systemic anti-inflammatory drugs may have anti-tumorigenic potential as well. For example, statins, which were initially developed for cholesterol management, has been shown to disrupt the growth and proliferation of cancer cells such as prostate cancer (Kochuparambil et al. 2011). This has been verified in clinical trials as well where the use of statin drugs was linked with a reduced risk of advanced, especially metastatic or fatal, prostate cancer (Platz et al. 2006).

4.2 Estrogen signaling

Other small molecules, such as metformin and tamoxifen, demonstrate anti-tumor activity against breast cancer (Goodwin, Ligibel and Stambolic 2009, Jiralerspong et al. 2009, Osborne 1998). Raloxifene and tamoxifen have been shown to cut down the risk of estrogen-receptor positive breast cancers by as much as 50% (Vogel et al. 2006). Tamoxifen, a selective estrogen receptor modulator, has demonstrated benefit when used alone as well as in combination with chemotherapy to treat advanced breast cancer. It reduces circulating insulin-like growth factor-1, inhibits angiogenesis, and induces apoptosis (Li et al. 2009). It is also efficacious in reducing tumor recurrence and prolonging survival when administered as postoperative adjuvant therapy in stages I and II disease. In a randomized breast cancer prevention clinical trial to evaluate the worth of taking tamoxifen for the prevention of breast cancer in women considered to be at increased risk for the disease, tamoxifen prevented the appearance of a substantial number of breast cancers (Fisher et al. 1998). Tamoxifen administered daily for at least 5 years prevented invasive breast cancer in women at increased risk (Fisher et al. 1998). Women who took tamoxifen also had fewer diagnoses of noninvasive breast tumors, such as lobular carcinoma in situ. The study found that though tamoxifen reduced the occurrence of estrogen receptor-positive tumors, it had no effect on the occurrence of estrogen receptor-negative tumors (Fisher et al. 2005). Tamoxifen is available in the United States for the reduction of breast cancer incidence in high-risk premenopausal and postmenopausal women.

Raloxifene, another selective estrogen receptor modulator, has successfully been tested for the treatment and prevention of osteoporosis. Raloxifene hydrochloride is a selective estrogen receptor modulator that binds to estrogen receptors to competitively block estrogen-induced DNA transcription (Grese et al. 1997, Brzozowski et al. 1997). An evaluation of breast cancer incidence in women treated with raloxifene for the prevention of osteoporosis showed a 75% decrease in invasive breast cancer, and, as with tamoxifen, only the estrogen receptor positive disease is reduced (Martino et al. 2004, Cummings et al. 1999). These data emphasize the fact that these drugs target the estrogen receptor-mediated growth mechanism. These data validate the original hypothesis that a non-steroidal anti-estrogen in the same class as tamoxifen could be used not only to prevent osteoporosis but also to prevent breast cancer as a beneficial side effect.

4.3 Androgen signaling

Similar to other cancers, prostate cancer chemoprevention involves the use of natural and synthetic agents that inhibit or reverse the development of precancerous lesions or delay progression of these lesions to invasive disease. Since androgens are involved in the development of prostate cancer, they are an obvious chemotherapeutic target. Finasteride, an inhibitor of 5α-reductase, inhibits the conversion of testosterone to dihydrotestosterone, the primary androgen in the prostate (Thompson et al. 2003). A phase III trial for prostate cancer prevention, the Prostate Cancer Prevention Trial using the drug finasteride, suggested that this chemopreventive agent can reduce the risk of developing prostate cancer (Thompson et al. 2003). In this clinical trial, 18,882 men 55 years of age or older with a normal digital rectal examination and a prostate-specific antigen level of 3.0 ng per milliliter or lower were randomly assigned to treatment with Finasteride (5 mg per day) or placebo for seven years. The primary end point was the prevalence of prostate cancer during the seven years of the study and a 24% reduction in incidence of prostate cancer was observed in the treatment arm. However, the incidence of high-grade tumors was higher in men receiving finasteride compared to those on placebo (Thompson et al. 2003).

4.4 Vitamin D

Another molecule that has shown great chemopreventive potential is vitamin D. Vitamin D promotes the differentiation and apoptosis of cancer cells, slowing down their proliferation. It has been previously reported that Vitamin D has anti-proliferative effects in prostate cancer and mechanism of action involves nuclear exclusion of cyclin dependent kinase 2 (CDK2) and increase in p27 levels, an inhibitor of CDK2. This results in G1 cell cycle arrest of tumor cells (Yang and Burnstein 2003, Yang et al. 2002). Supplemental vitamin D intake or synthesis of vitamin D has the potential to reduce the incidence and death rates of colon, breast, prostate, and ovarian cancers (Manson, Mayne and Clinton 2011). A number of studies have established the association between vitamin D and its metabolites and cancer. It has long been observed that cancer rates were lower among people living in southern latitudes compared to similar groups in northern latitudes. Long-term studies have confirmed the efficacy of moderate intake of vitamin D in reducing cancer risk and, when administered with calcium, in reducing the incidence of fractures. Calcitriol, the hormonally active form of vitamin D, is being actively evaluated in clinical trials as an anti-cancer agent (Crescioli et al. 2004, Scher et al. 2011). Besides anti-proliferative, pro-apoptotic, and pro-differentiating actions on various malignant cells and decreasing tumor growth in vivo, calcitriol also exhibits several anti-inflammatory effects including suppression of prostaglandin action, inhibition of p38 stress kinase signaling, and the subsequent production of pro-inflammatory cytokines and inhibition of NF-κB signaling (Krishnan et al. 2011). Calcitriol also decreases the expression of aromatase, the enzyme that catalyzes estrogen synthesis in breast cancer, both by a direct transcriptional repression and indirectly by reducing prostaglandins, which are major stimulators of aromatase transcription (Diaz et al. 2009, Swami et al. 2011, Zanatta et al. 2011, Krishnan et al. 2009). Other important effects include the suppression of tumor angiogenesis, invasion, and metastasis (Krishnan and Feldman 2010, Krishnan and Feldman 2009, So et al. 2010, Krishnan et al. 2010, Chung et al. 2009, Ma, Trump and Johnson 2010). These calcitriol actions provide a basis for its potential use in cancer therapy and chemoprevention.

As mentioned above, calcium supplementation has great anti-tumorigenic potential as well (Lappe et al. 2007). Multiple theories exist on the mechanism of anti-tumor activity of calcium. Calcium binds to bile acids and fatty acids in the gastrointestinal tract to form insoluble complexes known as calcium soaps. This reduces the ability of the acids to damage cells in the lining of the colon and stimulate cell proliferation to repair the damage (Newmark, Wargovich and Bruce 1984, Pence 1993, Suzuki and Mitsuoka 1992, Wargovich, Lynch and Levin 1991). Calcium may also act directly to reduce cell proliferation in the lining of the colon or cause proliferating colon cells to undergo differentiation, which, in turn, leads to a reduction in cell proliferation (Boyce and Ham 1983, Hennings et al. 1980).

Finally, calcium may also improve signaling within cells and cause tumor cells to differentiate and undergo cell death (Varani 2011, Roberts-Thomson, Curry and Monteith 2011, Fedirko et al. 2009, Peterlik, Grant and Cross 2009).

4.5 Retinoids

Retinoids such as all-trans retinoic acid and 9-cis retinoic acid are derivatives of vitamin A that play a pivotal role in a diverse group of biologic processes including cellular proliferation, differentiation, apoptosis, and development (Sporn and Roberts 1983). Retinoic acids have been studied intensively for their anticancer effects, which are exerted through a wide range of mechanisms. All-trans-retinoic acid-based differentiation therapy which slows proliferation and induces differentiation is utilized in acute promyelocytic leukemia (Reichman et al. 1997). Relapse of this subtype of leukemia is often associated with acquired resistance to retinoid maturation induction. In addition to leukemia, retinoids have been shown to be efficacious in the prevention of breast, cervical, neural, and hematological cancers (Casillas et al. 2003, Choi et al. 2000, Ding et al. 2002, Sanborn et al. 2000).

hTERT up-regulation has long been known as a key element in tumorigenesis, vital to the immortality of cancer cells. Treatment with the retinoid 9cUAB30, a synthetic analog of 9-cis-retinoic acid, leads to downregulation of hTERT expression, decrease in telomerase activity, and induction of apoptosis of leukemic cells (Love et al. 2008). The compound has also demonstrated beneficial effects against breast cancer (Hansen et al. 2007). These findings strongly support the use of 9cUAB30 as a chemo preventative agent. A first in human pharmacokinetic study with this compound was recently completed and further research is currently underway.

4.6 Potential chemo preventative agents

A number of other compounds have shown promise based on anti-cancer effects and low toxicity. With most solid-tumor cancers, the biggest threat is not the tumor itself but its ability to metastasize. Genistein, a soy isoflavone has been promising in preventing metastasis of prostate cancer by preventing the activation of the focal adhesion kinase and decreasing the levels of matrix metalloproteinase-2 (MMP-2) (Li et al. 2006, Huang et al. 2005, Kumi-Diaka et al. 2010, El Touny and Banerjee 2009, Xu et al. 2009).

Curcumin, a molecule derived from turmeric, has potential anti-cancer activity as well (Wilken et al. 2011). Curcumin inhibits proliferation and induces apoptosis in cancer cells via suppression of the AKT pathway (Wong et al. 2011, Sun et al. 2010, Duarte et al. 2010, Saini et al. 2011, Prakobwong et al. 2011, Zanotto-Filho et al. 2011, Sreekanth et al. 2011). Moreover, it decreases cell growth via inactivation of NF-κB, preventing DNA binding, nuclear translocation, and p65 phosphorylation. Curcumin also suppresses activation of STAT-3 as indicated by decreased phosphorylation and inhibition of JAK1 phosphorylation (Rajasingh et al. 2006, Zhang et al. 2010, Saydmohammed, Joseph and Syed 2010, Bill et al. 2010). Moreover, curcumin induces expression of peroxisome proliferator activated receptor gamma and upregulates death receptors, DR4 and DR5. Curcumin also inhibits expression of cell survival proteins such as Bcl-2, Bcl-xl, XIAP, cFLIP, cIAP-1, cIAP-2, and survivin, and proteins linked to cell proliferation, such as cyclin D1 and c-Myc (Bava et al. 2010, Glienke et al. 2010, Prakobwong et al. 2011, Watson et al. 2009, Fossey et al. 2011). The growth inhibitory effects of curcumin are enhanced in the IKK deficient cells, the enzyme required for NF-κB activation (Prakobwong et al. 2011). Thus, curcumin mediates its anti-proliferative and apoptotic effects through activation of multiple cell signaling pathways, and thus its anti-tumor activity is under active research. Curcumin blocks a number of targets involved in tumor initiation, promotion, and progression, and is considered a promising chemopreventive agent. Thus, among others, a phase II trial of curcuminoids' effect on cellular proliferation, apoptosis and COX-2 expression in the colorectal mucosa of subjects with recently resected sporadic adenomatous polyps is currently ongoing. Further research is warranted to evaluate the efficacy of cucumin in other cancers.

5. Vaccines for cancer prevention

Cancer vaccines have been developed to boost the immune system to fend off cancer. These vaccines or biological response modifiers work by stimulating or restoring the immune system's ability to fight infections and disease. There are two broad types of cancer vaccines: preventive (or prophylactic) vaccines, which are intended to prevent cancer from developing in healthy people; and treatment (or therapeutic) vaccines, which are intended to treat an existing cancer by strengthening the body's natural defenses against the cancer. The FDA has approved two types of vaccines to prevent cancer: vaccines against the hepatitis B virus, which can cause liver cancer, and vaccines against human papillomavirus types 16 and 18, which are responsible for more than 50% of cervical cancer cases (Lehtinen et al. 2011, Wheeler et al. 2011, El-Serag 2011). Furthermore, researchers are developing treatment vaccines against many types of cancer and testing them in clinical trials.

Table 3 lists the current anti-cancer vaccines either in clinical trial or approved for clinical use. HPV types 16 and/or 18 also cause some vaginal, vulvar, anal, penile, and oropharyngeal cancers (D'Souza et al. 2007, Heard 2011, Wattleworth 2011). The FDA approved vaccines Gardasil and Cervarix protect against HPV 16 and 18 infections which cause cervical cancer (Roden and Wu 2006, Einstein et al. 2009, Saslow et al. 2007). Gardasil is approved for use in females to prevent cervical cancer and some vulvar and vaginal cancers caused by HPV types 16 and 18. It is also approved for use in males and females to prevent anal cancer and precancerous anal lesions caused by these HPV types. Cervarix is approved for use in females ages 10 to 25 to prevent cervical cancer caused by HPV types 16 and 18. All prophylactic vaccines work through the induction of virus-neutralizing antibodies and reduction of the number of cells that are infected after viral infection. This prevents the clinical disease associated with infection. Successful vaccines immunologically mimic the infections they prevent. This primes the adaptive immune system to recall specific effector functions on interaction with the infectious agent in the future. This restimulation process boosts immunity and induces protection against future viral infection. These vaccines are considered to be molecularly targeted because they generate immune responses against specific proteins; that is, the L1 HPV viral capsid protein (for Cervarix and Gardasil) and the hepatitis B surface antigen (for hepatitis B vaccine) (Frederick and Huh 2008, Herzog et al. 2008, Huh, Kendrick and Alvarez 2007, Huh and Roden 2008, Kendrick, Huh and Alvarez 2006, Kirby, Huh and Alvarez 2002, Myers et al. 2008). The HPV vaccines are manufactured from purified L1 structural proteins by recombinant technology. L1 viral capsid proteins are the same protein against which antibodies are made in the natural immune response to HPV. These proteins self-assemble spontaneously to form

Type	Cancer	Vaccine
Therapeutic	Kidney	• Oncophage
	Prostate	• Provenge • DC-Vax Prostate • Onyvax-P
	Melanoma	• Oncophage • M-vax • Uvidem • M3TK • CYT004-MelQbG10 • MAGE-A3 antigen-specific cancer immunotherapeutic
	Leukemia	• GRNVAC1 • GVAX leukemia
	Bladder	• Bexidem
	Colorectal	• Collidem • IMA901IMA910
	Breast	• INGN 225 • NeuVax • Ii-Key/HER2/neu cancer vaccine
	Lung	• INGN 225 • Lucanix • IDM-2101 • Stimuvax • GV1001
	Brain	• Oncophage • DC-Vax Brain • HSPPC-96 Oncophage • CDX-110
	Ovarian	• CVac
	Pancreatic	• GVAX pancreatic • GV1001
	Lymphoma	• Biovax ID
	Renal	• IMA901IMA910
	Liver	• GV1001
Preventive	Cervical	• HPV vaccine (Gardasil and Cervarix)
	Vaginal	• HPV vaccine (Gardasil and Cervarix)
	Vulvar	• HPV vaccine (Gardasil and Cervarix)
	Anal	• HPV vaccine (Gardasil and Cervarix)
	Penile	• HPV vaccine (Gardasil and Cervarix)
	Oropharyngeal	• HPV vaccine (Gardasil and Cervarix)
	Liver	• Hepatitis B
	Colorectal	• MUC1 - poly-ICLC

Table 3. Preventive and therapeutic cancer vaccines either in clinical trial or approved for clinical use.

noninfectious virus-like particles that induce a protective host immune response. Because the virus-like particles contain the same epitopes as naturally occurring HPV, the immune system mounts a primary immune response to the vaccine, enabling a stronger and faster secondary immune response if naturally exposed to the same HPV types (Huh et al. 2007). The difference in the immune response generated by vaccination and natural infection is attributable to high immunogenicity of virus like particles inducing much higher concentrations of neutralizing antibodies to L1. In addition, higher antigen dose in the virus like particles and direct exposure of capsids to systemic immune responses are also observed. One of the challenges in vaccine formulation is balancing immunogenicity and toxicity. Addition of aluminum adjuvants to these vaccines helped to stimulate an immune response by acting as vehicles or immunomodulators. These vehicles transport antigen to lymphoid tissues or cause formation of an antigen depot at the site of injection. Immunomodulators help activate innate and adaptive immunity and increased immunogenicity of the vaccine (Huh et al. 2007, Huh and Roden 2008). The mechanisms by which these vaccines induce protection have not been fully defined but involve cellular immunity and neutralizing immunoglobulin G antibodies. HPV vaccines are designed for prophylactic use only; they do not clear existing HPV infection or treat HPV-related disease. Data from clinical trials utilizing these vaccines suggest that molecular targeting through immunization against infectious agents related to neoplasia is a successful way to prevent or treat early steps of host cell damage that can otherwise lead to cancer.

The FDA has also approved a cancer preventive vaccine that protects against HBV infection. Chronic HBV infection can lead to liver cancer. The original HBV vaccine was approved in 1981, making it the first cancer preventive vaccine to be successfully developed and marketed (Poland and Jacobson 2004). Today, most children in the United States are vaccinated against HBV shortly after birth.

6. Conclusion

With more and more people being diagnosed with cancer every day, undoubtedly, more effort needs to be vested in cancer prevention and therapy. Research organizations are starting to infuse a prevention ethos into their medical approach. Prevention messages are being added to the patient consultation process. A crosstalk between multiple disciplines such as psychology, molecular genetics, epidemiology, and medicine is needed for progressing cancer prevention and therapy.

7. References

(CDC), C. f. D. C. a. P. (2011) State smoke-free laws for worksites, restaurants, and bars--United States, 2000-2010. *MMWR Morb Mortal Wkly Rep*, 60, 472-5.

Aggarwal, R. R., C. J. Ryan & J. M. Chan (2011) Insulin-like growth factor pathway: A link between androgen deprivation therapy (ADT), insulin resistance, and disease progression in patients with prostate cancer? *Urol Oncol*.

Albers, A., K. Abe, J. Hunt, J. Wang, A. Lopez-Albaitero, C. Schaefer, W. Gooding, T. L. Whiteside, S. Ferrone, A. DeLeo & R. L. Ferris (2005) Antitumor activity of human papillomavirus type 16 E7-specific T cells against virally infected squamous cell carcinoma of the head and neck. *Cancer Res*, 65, 11146-55.

Alderton, G. (2007) Radiation sensitivity: Tolerance is not a virtue. *Nat Rev Cancer,* 7, 230-231.

Ali, A. A., M. T. Velasquez, C. T. Hansen, A. I. Mohamed & S. J. Bhathena (2005) Modulation of carbohydrate metabolism and peptide hormones by soybean isoflavones and probiotics in obesity and diabetes. *J Nutr Biochem,* 16, 693-9.

Amir, E., B. Seruga, S. Niraula, L. Carlsson & A. Ocana (2011) Toxicity of adjuvant endocrine therapy in postmenopausal breast cancer patients: a systematic review and meta-analysis. *J Natl Cancer Inst,* 103, 1299-309.

Azari, R., Y. Tadmor, A. Meir, M. Reuveni, D. Evenor, S. Nahon, H. Shlomo, L. Chen & I. Levin (2009) Light signaling genes and their manipulation towards modulation of phytonutrient content in tomato fruits. *Biotechnol Adv,* 28, 108-18.

Azcárate-Peril, M. A., M. Sikes & J. M. Bruno-Bárcena (2011) The intestinal microbiota, gastrointestinal environment and colorectal cancer: a putative role for probiotics in prevention of colorectal cancer? *American Journal of Physiology - Gastrointestinal and Liver Physiology,* 301, G401-G424.

Aziz, K., S. Nowsheen & A. G. Georgakilas (2010) Nanotechnology in cancer therapy: targeting the inhibition of key DNA repair pathways. *Curr Mol Med,* 10, 626-39.

Bajoga, U., S. Lewis, A. McNeill & L. Szatkowski (2011) Does the introduction of comprehensive smoke-free legislation lead to a decrease in population smoking prevalence? *Addiction,* 106, 1346-54.

Ballbe, M., G. Nieva, S. Mondon, C. Pinet, E. Bruguera, E. Salto, E. Fernandez & A. Gual (2011) Smoke-free policies in psychiatric services: identification of unmet needs. *Tob Control.*

Banu, N., A. Buda, S. Chell, D. Elder, M. Moorghen, C. Paraskeva, D. Qualtrough & M. Pignatelli (2007) Inhibition of COX-2 with NS-398 decreases colon cancer cell motility through blocking epidermal growth factor receptor transactivation: possibilities for combination therapy. *Cell Prolif,* 40, 768-79.

Bartek, J., C. Lukas & J. Lukas (2004) Checking on DNA damage in S phase. *Nat Rev Mol Cell Biol,* 5, 792-804.

Bartkova, J., Z. Horejsi, K. Koed, A. Kramer, F. Tort, K. Zieger, P. Guldberg, M. Sehested, J. M. Nesland, C. Lukas, T. Orntoft, J. Lukas & J. Bartek (2005) DNA damage response as a candidate anti-cancer barrier in early human tumorigenesis. *Nature,* 434, 864-70.

Bartkova, J., N. Rezaei, M. Liontos, P. Karakaidos, D. Kletsas, N. Issaeva, L. V. Vassiliou, E. Kolettas, K. Niforou, V. C. Zoumpourlis, M. Takaoka, H. Nakagawa, F. Tort, K. Fugger, F. Johansson, M. Sehested, C. L. Andersen, L. Dyrskjot, T. Orntoft, J. Lukas, C. Kittas, T. Helleday, T. D. Halazonetis, J. Bartek & V. G. Gorgoulis (2006) Oncogene-induced senescence is part of the tumorigenesis barrier imposed by DNA damage checkpoints. *Nature,* 444, 633-7.

Bava, S. V., C. N. Sreekanth, A. K. Thulasidasan, N. P. Anto, V. T. Cheriyan, V. T. Puliyappadamba, S. G. Menon, S. D. Ravichandran & R. J. Anto (2010) Akt is upstream and MAPKs are downstream of NF-kappaB in paclitaxel-induced survival signaling events, which are down-regulated by curcumin contributing to their synergism. *Int J Biochem Cell Biol,* 43, 331-41.

Berwick, M. & P. Vineis (2000) Markers of DNA repair and susceptibility to cancer in humans: an epidemiologic review. *J Natl Cancer Inst,* 92, 874-97.

Bill, M. A., J. R. Fuchs, C. Li, J. Yui, C. Bakan, D. M. Benson, Jr., E. B. Schwartz, D. Abdelhamid, J. Lin, D. G. Hoyt, S. L. Fossey, G. S. Young, W. E. Carson, 3rd, P. K. Li & G. B. Lesinski (2010) The small molecule curcumin analog FLLL32 induces apoptosis in melanoma cells via STAT3 inhibition and retains the cellular response to cytokines with anti-tumor activity. *Mol Cancer,* 9, 165.

Bonecchi, R., M. Locati & A. Mantovani (2011) Chemokines and cancer: A fatal attraction. *Cancer cell,* 19, 434-435.

Boniol, M. & P. Autier (2010) Prevalence of main cancer lifestyle risk factors in Europe in 2000. *Eur J Cancer,* 46, 2534-44.

Boyce, S. T. & R. G. Ham (1983) Calcium-Regulated Differentiation of Normal Human Epidermal Keratinocytes in Chemically Defined Clonal Culture and Serum-Free Serial Culture. *J Investig Dermatol,* 81, 33s-40s.

Bradlow, H. L., D. W. Sepkovic, N. Telang & R. Tiwari (2011) Adipocyte-derived factor as a modulator of oxidative estrogen metabolism: implications for obesity and estrogen-dependent breast cancer. *In Vivo,* 25, 585-8.

Braems, G., H. Denys, O. De Wever, V. Cocquyt & R. Van den Broecke (2011) Use of Tamoxifen Before and During Pregnancy. *Oncologist.*

Brand, J. S., M. F. Chan, M. Dowsett, E. Folkerd, N. J. Wareham, R. N. Luben, Y. T. van der Schouw & K. T. Khaw (2011) Cigarette smoking and endogenous sex hormones in postmenopausal women. *J Clin Endocrinol Metab,* 96, 3184-92.

Brose, M. S., T. R. Rebbeck, K. A. Calzone, J. E. Stopfer, K. L. Nathanson & B. L. Weber (2002) Cancer Risk Estimates for BRCA1 Mutation Carriers Identified in a Risk Evaluation Program. *Journal of the National Cancer Institute,* 94, 1365-1372.

Brosh, R. & V. Rotter (2009) When mutants gain new powers: news from the mutant p53 field. *Nat Rev Cancer,* 9, 701-713.

Brzozowski, A. M., A. C. W. Pike, Z. Dauter, R. E. Hubbard, T. Bonn, O. Engstrom, L. Ohman, G. L. Greene, J.-A. Gustafsson & M. Carlquist (1997) Molecular basis of agonism and antagonism in the oestrogen receptor. *Nature,* 389, 753-758.

Caetano, B., L. Le Corre, N. Chalabi, L. Delort, Y. J. Bignon & D. J. Bernard-Gallon (2006) Soya phytonutrients act on a panel of genes implicated with BRCA1 and BRCA2 oncosuppressors in human breast cell lines. *Br J Nutr,* 95, 406-13.

Capitanio, U., N. Suardi, A. Briganti, A. Gallina, F. Abdollah, G. Lughezzani, A. Salonia, M. Freschi & F. Montorsi (2011) Influence of obesity on tumour volume in patients with prostate cancer. *BJU Int.*

Casillas, M. A., S. L. Brotherton, L. G. Andrews, J. M. Ruppert & T. O. Tollefsbol (2003) Induction of endogenous telomerase (hTERT) by c-Myc in WI-38 fibroblasts transformed with specific genetic elements. *Gene,* 316, 57-65.

Cesario, A., B. Rocca & S. Rutella (2011) The interplay between indoleamine 2,3-dioxygenase 1 (IDO1) and cyclooxygenase (COX)-2 in chronic inflammation and cancer. *Curr Med Chem,* 18, 2263-71.

Chan, A. T., S. Ogino & C. S. Fuchs (2007) Aspirin and the Risk of Colorectal Cancer in Relation to the Expression of COX-2. *New England Journal of Medicine,* 356, 2131-2142.

Chan, J. M. & E. L. Giovannucci (2001) Vegetables, fruits, associated micronutrients, and risk of prostate cancer. *Epidemiologic Reviews,* 23, 82-86.

Chang, J. S., K. Straif & N. Guha (2011) The role of alcohol dehydrogenase genes in head and neck cancers: a systematic review and meta-analysis of ADH1B and ADH1C. *Mutagenesis*.

Chen, J., Y. Yao, C. Gong, F. Yu, S. Su, J. Chen, B. Liu, H. Deng, F. Wang, L. Lin, H. Yao, F. Su, Karen S. Anderson, Q. Liu, Mark E. Ewen, X. Yao & E. Song (2011) CCL18 from tumor-associated macrophages promotes breast cancer metastasis via PITPNM3. *Cancer Cell,* 19, 541-555.

Choi, S. H., H. K. Kang, E. O. Im, Y. J. Kim, Y. T. Bae, Y. H. Choi, K. H. Lee, H. Y. Chung, H. K. Chang & N. D. Kim (2000) Inhibition of cell growth and telomerase activity of breast cancer cells in vitro by retinoic acids. *Int J Oncol,* 17, 971-6.

Choy, A., L. C. Barr, J. W. Serpell & M. Baum (1993) Radiation-induced sarcoma of the retained breast after conservative surgery and radiotherapy for early breast cancer. *Eur J Surg Oncol,* 19, 376-7.

Chung, F. L., C. C. Conaway, C. V. Rao & B. S. Reddy (2000) Chemoprevention of colonic aberrant crypt foci in Fischer rats by sulforaphane and phenethyl isothiocyanate. *Carcinogenesis,* 21, 2287-91.

Chung, I., G. Han, M. Seshadri, B. M. Gillard, W. D. Yu, B. A. Foster, D. L. Trump & C. S. Johnson (2009) Role of vitamin D receptor in the antiproliferative effects of calcitriol in tumor-derived endothelial cells and tumor angiogenesis in vivo. *Cancer Res,* 69, 967-75.

Cohen, J. H., A. R. Kristal & J. L. Stanford (2000) Fruit and Vegetable Intakes and Prostate Cancer Risk. *Journal of the National Cancer Institute,* 92, 61-68.

Colonna, S. V., L. Douglas Case & J. A. Lawrence (2011) A retrospective review of the metabolic syndrome in women diagnosed with breast cancer and correlation with estrogen receptor. *Breast Cancer Res Treat.*

Colotta, F., P. Allavena, A. Sica, C. Garlanda & A. Mantovani (2009) Cancer-related inflammation, the seventh hallmark of cancer: links to genetic instability. *Carcinogenesis,* 30, 1073-1081.

Cooper, K., H. Squires, C. Carroll, D. Papaioannou, A. Booth, R. F. Logan, C. Maguire, D. Hind & P. Tappenden (2010) Chemoprevention of colorectal cancer: systematic review and economic evaluation. *Health Technol Assess,* 14, 1-206.

Creighton, C. J., Y. H. Sada, Y. Zhang, A. Tsimelzon, H. Wong, B. Dave, M. D. Landis, H. D. Bear, A. Rodriguez & J. C. Chang (2011) A gene transcription signature of obesity in breast cancer. *Breast Cancer Res Treat.*

Crescioli, C., P. Ferruzzi, A. Caporali, M. Scaltriti, S. Bettuzzi, R. Mancina, S. Gelmini, M. Serio, D. Villari, G. B. Vannelli, E. Colli, L. Adorini & M. Maggi (2004) Inhibition of prostate cell growth by BXL-628, a calcitriol analogue selected for a phase II clinical trial in patients with benign prostate hyperplasia. *European Journal of Endocrinology,* 150, 591-603.

Cummings, S. R., S. Eckert, K. A. Krueger, D. Grady, T. J. Powles, J. A. Cauley, L. Norton, T. Nickelsen, N. H. Bjarnason, M. Morrow, M. E. Lippman, D. Black, J. E. Glusman, A. Costa & V. C. Jordan (1999) The Effect of Raloxifene on Risk of Breast Cancer in Postmenopausal Women. *JAMA: The Journal of the American Medical Association,* 281, 2189-2197.

Cuzick, J., A. DeCensi, B. Arun, P. H. Brown, M. Castiglione, B. Dunn, J. F. Forbes, A. Glaus, A. Howell, G. von Minckwitz, V. Vogel & H. Zwierzina (2011) Preventive therapy for breast cancer: a consensus statement. *Lancet Oncol,* 12, 496-503.

D'Souza, G., A. R. Kreimer, R. Viscidi, M. Pawlita, C. Fakhry, W. M. Koch, W. H. Westra & M. L. Gillison (2007) Case Control Study of Human Papillomavirus and Oropharyngeal Cancer. *New England Journal of Medicine,* 356, 1944-1956.

Di Cagno, R., F. Mazzacane, C. G. Rizzello, O. Vincentini, M. Silano, G. Giuliani, M. De Angelis & M. Gobbetti (2010) Synthesis of isoflavone aglycones and equol in soy milks fermented by food-related lactic acid bacteria and their effect on human intestinal Caco-2 cells. *J Agric Food Chem,* 58, 10338-46.

Di Micco, R., M. Fumagalli, A. Cicalese, S. Piccinin, P. Gasparini, C. Luise, C. Schurra, M. Garre, P. G. Nuciforo, A. Bensimon, R. Maestro, P. G. Pelicci & F. d'Adda di Fagagna (2006) Oncogene-induced senescence is a DNA damage response triggered by DNA hyper-replication. *Nature,* 444, 638-42.

Diaz, L., N. Noyola-Martinez, D. Barrera, G. Hernandez, E. Avila, A. Halhali & F. Larrea (2009) Calcitriol inhibits TNF-alpha-induced inflammatory cytokines in human trophoblasts. *J Reprod Immunol,* 81, 17-24.

Ding, W. K. & N. P. Shah (2010) Enhancing the biotransformation of isoflavones in soymilk supplemented with lactose using probiotic bacteria during extended fermentation. *J Food Sci,* 75, M140-9.

Ding, X. Z., W. G. Tong & T. E. Adrian (2000) Blockade of cyclooxygenase-2 inhibits proliferation and induces apoptosis in human pancreatic cancer cells. *Anticancer research,* 20, 2625-31.

Ding, Z., A. G. Green, X. Yang, G. Chernenko, S. C. Tang & A. Pater (2002) Retinoic acid inhibits telomerase activity and downregulates expression but does not affect splicing of hTERT: correlation with cell growth rate inhibition in an in vitro cervical carcinogenesis/multidrug-resistance model. *Exp Cell Res,* 272, 185-91.

Doughty, J. C. (2011) When to start an aromatase inhibitor: now or later? *J Surg Oncol,* 103, 730-8.

Duarte, V. M., E. Han, M. S. Veena, A. Salvado, J. D. Suh, L. J. Liang, K. F. Faull, E. S. Srivatsan & M. B. Wang (2010) Curcumin enhances the effect of cisplatin in suppression of head and neck squamous cell carcinoma via inhibition of IKKbeta protein of the NFkappaB pathway. *Mol Cancer Ther,* 9, 2665-75.

Dyson, N., P. M. Howley, K. Munger & E. Harlow (1989) The human papilloma virus-16 E7 oncoprotein is able to bind to the retinoblastoma gene product. *Science,* 243, 934-937.

Einstein, M. H., M. Baron, M. J. Levin, A. Chatterjee, R. P. Edwards, F. Zepp, I. Carletti, F. J. Dessy, A. F. Trofa, A. Schuind, G. Dubin & H. P. V. S. Group (2009) Comparison of the immunogenicity and safety of Cervarix and Gardasil human papillomavirus (HPV) cervical cancer vaccines in healthy women aged 18-45 years. *Human vaccines,* 5, 705-19.

El-Serag, H. B. (2011) Hepatocellular Carcinoma. *New England Journal of Medicine,* 365, 1118-1127.

El Touny, L. H. & P. P. Banerjee (2009) Identification of a biphasic role for genistein in the regulation of prostate cancer growth and metastasis. *Cancer Res,* 69, 3695-703.

Eliassen, A. H., S. E. Hankinson, B. Rosner, M. D. Holmes & W. C. Willett (2010) Physical activity and risk of breast cancer among postmenopausal women. *Arch Intern Med,* 170, 1758-64.

Esteller, M., J. M. Silva, G. Dominguez, F. Bonilla, X. Matias-Guiu, E. Lerma, E. Bussaglia, J. Prat, I. C. Harkes, E. A. Repasky, E. Gabrielson, M. Schutte, S. B. Baylin & J. G. Herman (2000) Promoter Hypermethylation and BRCA1 Inactivation in Sporadic Breast and Ovarian Tumors. *Journal of the National Cancer Institute,* 92, 564-569.

Etemadi, A., A. Golozar, F. Kamangar, N. D. Freedman, R. Shakeri, C. Matthews, F. Islami, P. Boffetta, P. Brennan, C. C. Abnet, R. Malekzadeh & S. M. Dawsey (2011) Large body size and sedentary lifestyle during childhood and early adulthood and esophageal squamous cell carcinoma in a high-risk population. *Ann Oncol.*

Fedirko, V., R. M. Bostick, W. D. Flanders, Q. Long, E. Sidelnikov, A. Shaukat, C. R. Daniel, R. E. Rutherford & J. J. Woodard (2009) Effects of vitamin d and calcium on proliferation and differentiation in normal colon mucosa: a randomized clinical trial. *Cancer Epidemiol Biomarkers Prev,* 18, 2933-41.

Feeney, M. J. (2004) Fruits and the prevention of lifestyle-related diseases. *Clin Exp Pharmacol Physiol,* 31 Suppl 2, S11-3.

Fisher, B., J. P. Costantino, D. L. Wickerham, R. S. Cecchini, W. M. Cronin, A. Robidoux, T. B. Bevers, M. T. Kavanah, J. N. Atkins, R. G. Margolese, C. D. Runowicz, J. M. James, L. G. Ford & N. Wolmark (2005) Tamoxifen for the Prevention of Breast Cancer: Current Status of the National Surgical Adjuvant Breast and Bowel Project P-1 Study. *Journal of the National Cancer Institute,* 97, 1652-1662.

Fisher, B., J. P. Costantino, D. L. Wickerham, C. K. Redmond, M. Kavanah, W. M. Cronin, V. Vogel, A. Robidoux, N. Dimitrov, J. Atkins, M. Daly, S. Wieand, E. Tan-Chiu, L. Ford, N. Wolmark, B. other National Surgical Adjuvant & I. Bowel Project (1998) Tamoxifen for Prevention of Breast Cancer: Report of the National Surgical Adjuvant Breast and Bowel Project P-1 Study. *Journal of the National Cancer Institute,* 90, 1371-1388.

Fleeman, N., C. Martin Saborido, K. Payne, A. Boland, R. Dickson, Y. Dundar, A. Fernandez Santander, S. Howell, W. Newman, J. Oyee & T. Walley (2011) The clinical effectiveness and cost-effectiveness of genotyping for CYP2D6 for the management of women with breast cancer treated with tamoxifen: a systematic review. *Health Technol Assess,* 15, 1-102.

Fossey, S. L., M. D. Bear, J. Lin, C. Li, E. B. Schwartz, P. K. Li, J. R. Fuchs, J. Fenger, W. C. Kisseberth & C. A. London (2011) The novel curcumin analog FLLL32 decreases STAT3 DNA binding activity and expression, and induces apoptosis in osteosarcoma cell lines. *BMC Cancer,* 11, 112.

Franco, R., O. Schoneveld, A. G. Georgakilas & M. I. Panayiotidis (2008) Oxidative stress, DNA methylation and carcinogenesis. *Cancer Lett.,* 266, 6-12

Frederick, P. J. & W. K. Huh (2008) Evaluation of the interim analysis from the PATRICIA study group: efficacy of a vaccine against HPV 16 and 18. *Expert Rev Anticancer Ther,* 8, 701-5.

Friedenson, B. (2007) The BRCA1/2 pathway prevents hematologic cancers in addition to breast and ovarian cancers. *BMC Cancer,* 7, 152.

Gandhi, S. & S. Verma (2011) Early breast cancer in the older woman. *Oncologist,* 16, 479-85.

Garrido, J. M., E. Manuela, P. J. Garrido, A. M. Oliveira-Brett & F. Borges (2011) An electrochemical outlook on tamoxifen biotransformation: current and future prospects. *Curr Drug Metab,* 12, 372-82.

Gasper, A. V., A. Al-Janobi, J. A. Smith, J. R. Bacon, P. Fortun, C. Atherton, M. A. Taylor, C. J. Hawkey, D. A. Barrett & R. F. Mithen (2005) Glutathione S-transferase M1 polymorphism and metabolism of sulforaphane from standard and high-glucosinolate broccoli. *Am J Clin Nutr,* 82, 1283-91.

Ghosh, N., R. Chaki, V. Mandal & S. C. Mandal (2010) COX-2 as a target for cancer chemotherapy. *Pharmacol Rep,* 62, 233-44.

Giovannucci, E., D. M. Harlan, M. C. Archer, R. M. Bergenstal, S. M. Gapstur, L. A. Habel, M. Pollak, J. G. Regensteiner & D. Yee (2010) Diabetes and cancer: a consensus report. *CA Cancer J Clin,* 60, 207-21.

Giovannucci, E., E. B. Rimm, G. A. Colditz, M. J. Stampfer, A. Ascherio, C. C. Chute & W. C. Willett (1993) A Prospective Study of Dietary Fat and Risk of Prostate Cancer. *Journal of the National Cancer Institute,* 85, 1571-1579.

Glienke, W., L. Maute, J. Wicht & L. Bergmann (2010) Curcumin inhibits constitutive STAT3 phosphorylation in human pancreatic cancer cell lines and downregulation of survivin/BIRC5 gene expression. *Cancer Invest,* 28, 166-71.

Goetz, M. P., D. J. Schaid, D. L. Wickerham, S. Safgren, T. Mushiroda, M. Kubo, A. Batzler, J. P. Costantino, V. G. Vogel, S. Paik, E. E. Carlson, D. A. Flockhart, N. Wolmark, Y. Nakamura, R. M. Weinshilboum, J. N. Ingle & M. M. Ames (2011) Evaluation of CYP2D6 and Efficacy of Tamoxifen and Raloxifene in Women Treated for Breast Cancer Chemoprevention: Results from the NSABP P1 and P2 Clinical Trials. *Clin Cancer Res,* 17, 6944-6951.

Gonzalez, M., J. M. Vignaud, C. Clement-Duchene, A. Luc, P. Wild, O. Bertrand, L. Thiberville, Y. Martinet, J. Benichou & C. Paris (2011) Smoking, Occupational Risk Factors, and Bronchial Tumor Location: A Possible Impact for Lung Cancer Computed Tomography Scan Screening. *J Thorac Oncol.*

Goodwin, P. J., J. A. Ligibel & V. Stambolic (2009) Metformin in Breast Cancer: Time for Action. *Journal of Clinical Oncology,* 27, 3271-3273.

Gorgoulis, V. G., L. V. Vassiliou, P. Karakaidos, P. Zacharatos, A. Kotsinas, T. Liloglou, M. Venere, R. A. Ditullio, Jr., N. G. Kastrinakis, B. Levy, D. Kletsas, A. Yoneta, M. Herlyn, C. Kittas & T. D. Halazonetis (2005) Activation of the DNA damage checkpoint and genomic instability in human precancerous lesions. *Nature,* 434, 907-13.

Gotay, C. C. (2010) Cancer prevention: major initiatives and looking into the future. *Expert Rev Pharmacoecon Outcomes Res,* 10, 143-54.

Graeser, M. K., C. Engel, K. Rhiem, D. Gadzicki, U. Bick, K. Kast, U. G. Froster, B. Schlehe, A. Bechtold, N. Arnold, S. Preisler-Adams, C. Nestle-Kraemling, M. Zaino, M. Loeffler, M. Kiechle, A. Meindl, D. Varga & R. K. Schmutzler (2009) Contralateral Breast Cancer Risk in BRCA1 and BRCA2 Mutation Carriers. *Journal of Clinical Oncology,* 27, 5887-5892.

Greenlee, H., D. L. Hershman & J. S. Jacobson (2009) Use of antioxidant supplements during breast cancer treatment: a comprehensive review. *Breast Cancer Res Treat,* 115, 437-52.

Grese, T. A., J. P. Sluka, H. U. Bryant, G. J. Cullinan, A. L. Glasebrook, C. D. Jones, K. Matsumoto, A. D. Palkowitz, M. Sato, J. D. Termine, M. A. Winter, N. N. Yang & J. A. Dodge (1997) Molecular determinants of tissue selectivity in estrogen receptor modulators. *Proceedings of the National Academy of Sciences,* 94, 14105-14110.

Gross-Steinmeyer, K., P. L. Stapleton, J. H. Tracy, T. K. Bammler, S. C. Strom & D. L. Eaton (2010) Sulforaphane- and phenethyl isothiocyanate-induced inhibition of aflatoxin B1-mediated genotoxicity in human hepatocytes: role of GSTM1 genotype and CYP3A4 gene expression. *Toxicol Sci,* 116, 422-32.

Gross, G. A., R. J. Turesky, L. B. Fay, W. G. Stillwell, P. L. Skipper & S. R. Tannenbaum (1993) Heterocyclic aromatic amine formation in grilled bacon, beef and fish and in grill scrapings. *Carcinogenesis,* 14, 2313-2318.

Halazonetis, T. D., V. G. Gorgoulis & J. Bartek (2008) An oncogene-induced DNA damage model for cancer development. *Science,* 319, 1352-5.

Half, E., Y. Sun & F. A. Sinicrope (2007) Anti-EGFR and ErbB-2 antibodies attenuate cyclooxygenase-2 expression and cooperatively inhibit survival of human colon cancer cells. *Cancer Lett,* 251, 237-46.

Hall, E. H. & S. E. Crowe (2011) Environmental and lifestyle influences on disorders of the large and small intestine: implications for treatment. *Dig Dis,* 29, 249-54.

Hanahan, D. & R. A. Weinberg (2000) The hallmarks of cancer. *Cell,* 100, 57-70.

Hansen, N. J., R. C. Wylie, S. M. Phipps, W. K. Love, L. G. Andrews & T. O. Tollefsbol (2007) The low-toxicity 9-cis UAB30 novel retinoid down-regulates the DNA methyltransferases and has anti-telomerase activity in human breast cancer cells. *Int J Oncol,* 30, 641-50.

Harris, R. E. (2007) Cyclooxygenase-2 (cox-2) and the inflammogenesis of cancer. *Subcell Biochem,* 42, 93-126.

Harris, R. E., J. Beebe-Donk, H. Doss & D. Burr Doss (2005) Aspirin, ibuprofen, and other non-steroidal anti-inflammatory drugs in cancer prevention: a critical review of non-selective COX-2 blockade (review). *Oncol Rep,* 13, 559-83.

Hatt, L., S. Loft, L. Risom, P. MÃ¸ller, M. SÃ¸rensen, O. Raaschou-Nielsen, K. Overvad, A. TjÃ¸nneland & U. Vogel (2008) OGG1 expression and OGG1 Ser326Cys polymorphism and risk of lung cancer in a prospective study. *Mutation Research/Fundamental and Molecular Mechanisms of Mutagenesis,* 639, 45-54.

Heard, I. (2011) Human papillomavirus, cancer and vaccination. *Curr Opin HIV AIDS,* 6, 297-302.

Heinonen, O. P., L. Koss, D. Albanes, P. R. Taylor, A. M. Hartman, B. K. Edwards, J. Virtamo, J. K. Huttunen, J. Haapakoski, N. Malila, M. Rautalahti, S. Ripatti, H. MÃ¤enpÃ¤Ã¤, L. Teerenhovi & M. Virolainen (1998) Prostate Cancer and Supplementation With Î±-Tocopherol and Î²-Carotene: Incidence and Mortality in a Controlled Trial. *Journal of the National Cancer Institute,* 90, 440-446.

Hennings, H., D. Michael, C. Cheng, P. Steinert, K. Holbrook & S. H. Yuspa (1980) Calcium regulation of growth and differentiation of mouse epidermal cells in culture. *Cell,* 19, 245-254.

Herrero, J. I., F. Pardo, D. D'Avola, F. Alegre, F. Rotellar, M. Iñarrairaegui, P. Martí, B. Sangro & J. Quiroga (2011) Risk factors of lung, head and neck, esophageal, and kidney and urinary tract carcinomas after liver transplantation: The effect of smoking withdrawal. *Liver Transplantation,* 17, 402-408.

Herzog, T. J., W. K. Huh, L. S. Downs, J. S. Smith & B. J. Monk (2008) Initial lessons learned in HPV vaccination. *Gynecol Oncol,* 109, S4-11.

Heymach, J. V., T. J. Shackleford, H. T. Tran, S.-Y. Yoo, K.-A. Do, M. Wergin, P. Saintigny, R. T. Vollmer, T. J. Polascik, D. C. Snyder, M. T. Ruffin, S. Yan, M. Dewhirst, A. B. Kunnumakkara, B. B. Aggarwal & W. Demark-Wahnefried (2011) Effect of Low-Fat Diets on Plasma Levels of NF-kB Regulated Inflammatory Cytokines and Angiogenic Factors in Men with Prostate Cancer. *Cancer Prevention Research,* 4, 1590-1598.

Hida, T., K.-i. Kozaki, H. Muramatsu, A. Masuda, S. Shimizu, T. Mitsudomi, T. Sugiura, M. Ogawa & T. Takahashi (2000) Cyclooxygenase-2 Inhibitor Induces Apoptosis and Enhances Cytotoxicity of Various Anticancer Agents in Non-Small Cell Lung Cancer Cell Lines. *Clinical Cancer Research,* 6, 2006-2011.

Hoda, M. R., A. Hamza, K. Fischer, S. Wagner, J. Schneider, H. Heynemann & P. Fornara (2010) Obesity as a risk factor for prostate cancer: role for adipocytokines and involvement of tyrosine kinase pathway. *Aktuelle Urol,* 41, 178-83.

Hollstein, M., D. Sidransky, B. Vogelstein & C. C. Harris (1991) P53 MUTATIONS IN HUMAN CANCERS. *Science,* 253, 49-53.

Holmes, M. D., W. Y. Chen, S. E. Hankinson & W. C. Willett (2009) Physical activity's impact on the association of fat and fiber intake with survival after breast cancer. *Am J Epidemiol,* 170, 1250-6.

Holst, B. & G. Williamson (2008) Nutrients and phytochemicals: from bioavailability to bioefficacy beyond antioxidants. *Curr Opin Biotechnol,* 19, 73-82.

Hoque, A., D. Albanes, S. Lippman, M. Spitz, P. Taylor, E. Klein, I. Thompson, P. Goodman, J. Stanford, J. Crowley, C. Coltman & R. Santella (2001) Molecular epidemiologic studies within the Selenium and Vitamin E Cancer Prevention Trial (SELECT). *Cancer Causes and Control,* 12, 627-633.

Hsu, A.-L., T.-T. Ching, D.-S. Wang, X. Song, V. M. Rangnekar & C.-S. Chen (2000) The Cyclooxygenase-2 Inhibitor Celecoxib Induces Apoptosis by Blocking Akt Activation in Human Prostate Cancer Cells Independently of Bcl-2. *Journal of Biological Chemistry,* 275, 11397-11403.

Huang, X., S. Chen, L. Xu, Y. Liu, D. K. Deb, L. C. Platanias & R. C. Bergan (2005) Genistein inhibits p38 map kinase activation, matrix metalloproteinase type 2, and cell invasion in human prostate epithelial cells. *Cancer Res,* 65, 3470-8.

Huh, W. K., J. E. Kendrick & R. D. Alvarez (2007) New advances in vaccine technology and improved cervical cancer prevention. *Obstet Gynecol,* 109, 1187-92.

Huh, W. K. & R. B. Roden (2008) The future of vaccines for cervical cancer. *Gynecol Oncol,* 109, S48-56.

Hymowitz, N. (2011) Smoking and cancer: a review of public health and clinical implications. *J Natl Med Assoc,* 103, 695-700.

Iliakis, G., H. Wang, A. R. Perrault, W. Boecker, B. Rosidi, F. Windhofer, W. Wu, J. Guan, G. Terzoudi & G. Pantelias (2004) Mechanisms of DNA double strand break repair and chromosome aberration formation. *Cytogenetic and Genome Research,* 104, 14-20.

Ishizaki, T., K. Katsumata, A. Tsuchida, T. Wada, Y. Mori, M. Hisada, H. Kawakita & T. Aoki (2006) Etodolac, a selective cyclooxygenase-2 inhibitor, inhibits liver metastasis of colorectal cancer cells via the suppression of MMP-9 activity. *Int J Mol Med,* 17, 357-62.

Jackson, S. P. & J. Bartek (2009) The DNA-damage response in human biology and disease. *Nature,* 461, 1071-1078.

Jiang, J., E. S. Yang, G. Jiang, S. Nowsheen, H. Wang, T. Wang, Y. Wang, D. Billheimer, A. B. Chakravarthy, M. Brown, B. Haffty & F. Xia (2011) p53-dependent BRCA1 nuclear export controls cellular susceptibility to DNA damage. *Cancer Res,* 71, 5546-57.

Jiralerspong, S., S. L. Palla, S. H. Giordano, F. Meric-Bernstam, C. Liedtke, C. M. Barnett, L. Hsu, M.-C. Hung, G. N. Hortobagyi & A. M. Gonzalez-Angulo (2009) Metformin and Pathologic Complete Responses to Neoadjuvant Chemotherapy in Diabetic Patients With Breast Cancer. *Journal of Clinical Oncology,* 27, 3297-3302.

Joseph, M. A., K. B. Moysich, J. L. Freudenheim, P. G. Shields, E. D. Bowman, Y. Zhang, J. R. Marshall & C. B. Ambrosone (2004) Cruciferous vegetables, genetic polymorphisms in glutathione S-transferases M1 and T1, and prostate cancer risk. *Nutr Cancer,* 50, 206-13.

Kale, A., S. Gawande & S. Kotwal (2008) Cancer phytotherapeutics: role for flavonoids at the cellular level. *Phytother Res,* 22, 567-77.

Karnoub, A. E., A. B. Dash, A. P. Vo, A. Sullivan, M. W. Brooks, G. W. Bell, A. L. Richardson, K. Polyak, R. Tubo & R. A. Weinberg (2007) Mesenchymal stem cells within tumour stroma promote breast cancer metastasis. *Nature,* 449, 557-563.

Kasza, K. A., A. J. Hyland, A. Brown, M. Siahpush, H. H. Yong, A. D. McNeill, L. Li & K. M. Cummings (2011) The effectiveness of tobacco marketing regulations on reducing smokers' exposure to advertising and promotion: findings from the International Tobacco Control (ITC) Four Country Survey. *Int J Environ Res Public Health,* 8, 321-40.

Kaur, M., C. Agarwal & R. Agarwal (2009) Anticancer and cancer chemopreventive potential of grape seed extract and other grape-based products. *J Nutr,* 139, 1806S-12S.

Kendal, W. S. & G. Nicholas (2007) A Population-Based Analysis of Second Primary Cancers After Irradiation for Rectal Cancer. *American Journal of Clinical Oncology,* 30, 333-339 10.1097/01.coc.0000258084.55036.9e.

Kendrick, J. E., W. K. Huh & R. D. Alvarez (2006) Novel methods to treat and prevent human papillomavirus infection. *Expert Rev Anti Infect Ther,* 4, 593-600.

Khan, N., F. Afaq & H. Mukhtar (2010) Lifestyle as risk factor for cancer: Evidence from human studies. *Cancer Lett,* 293, 133-43.

Khan, Z., N. Khan, R. P. Tiwari, N. K. Sah, G. B. Prasad & P. S. Bisen (2011) Biology of Cox-2: an application in cancer therapeutics. *Curr Drug Targets,* 12, 1082-93.

Kilic, N., M. E. Myrick, S. M. Schmid & U. Gueth (2011) Eligibility, Compliance and Persistence of Sequential Therapy with Aromatase Inhibitors following 2-3 Years of Tamoxifen in Endocrine Adjuvant Breast Cancer Therapy. *Oncology,* 81, 151-157.

Kim, E. H., W. C. Willett, T. Fung, B. Rosner & M. D. Holmes (2011) Diet quality indices and postmenopausal breast cancer survival. *Nutr Cancer,* 63, 381-8.

King, B. A., A. J. Hyland, R. Borland, A. McNeill & K. M. Cummings (2011a) Socioeconomic variation in the prevalence, introduction, retention, and removal of smoke-free policies among smokers: findings from the International Tobacco Control (ITC) Four Country Survey. *Int J Environ Res Public Health,* 8, 411-34.

King, B. A., M. C. Mahoney, K. M. Cummings & A. J. Hyland (2011b) Intervention to promote smoke-free policies among multiunit housing operators. *J Public Health Manag Pract,* 17, E1-8.

King, M.-C., J. H. Marks, J. B. Mandell & G. The New York Breast Cancer Study (2003) Breast and Ovarian Cancer Risks Due to Inherited Mutations in BRCA1 and BRCA2. *Science,* 302, 643-646.

Kirby, T. O., W. Huh & R. Alvarez (2002) Immunotherapy of ovarian cancer. *Expert Opin Biol Ther,* 2, 409-17.

Kiyotani, K., T. Mushiroda, Y. Nakamura & H. Zembutsu (2011) Pharmacogenomics of tamoxifen: roles of drug metabolizing enzymes and transporters. *Drug Metab Pharmacokinet.*

Klein, T. J. & P. M. Glazer (2010) The Tumor Microenvironment and DNA Repair. *Semin. Radiat. Oncol.* , 20, 282-287.

Kleinerman, R. A., J. D. Boice, Jr., H. H. Storm, P. Sparen, A. Andersen, E. Pukkala, C. F. Lynch, B. F. Hankey & J. T. Flannery (1995) Second primary cancer after treatment for cervical cancer. An international cancer registries study. *Cancer,* 76, 442-52.

Kochuparambil, S. T., B. Al-Husein, A. Goc, S. Soliman & P. R. Somanath (2011) Anticancer Efficacy of Simvastatin on Prostate Cancer Cells and Tumor Xenografts Is Associated with Inhibition of Akt and Reduced Prostate-Specific Antigen Expression. *Journal of Pharmacology and Experimental Therapeutics,* 336, 496-505.

Koehne, C. H. & R. N. Dubois (2004) COX-2 inhibition and colorectal cancer. *Semin Oncol,* 31, 12-21.

Kong, C. Y., K. J. Nattinger, T. J. Hayeck, Z. B. Omer, Y. C. Wang, S. J. Spechler, P. M. McMahon, G. S. Gazelle & C. Hur (2011) The Impact of Obesity on the Rise in Esophageal Adenocarcinoma Incidence: Estimates from a Disease Simulation Model. *Cancer Epidemiol Biomarkers Prev.*

Kossman, D. A., N. I. Williams, S. M. Domchek, M. S. Kurzer, J. E. Stopfer & K. H. Schmitz (2011) Exercise Lowers Estrogen and Progesterone Levels in Premenopausal Women at High Risk of Breast Cancer. *J Appl Physiol.*

Krishnan, A. V. & D. Feldman (2009) Molecular pathways mediating the anti-inflammatory effects of calcitriol: implications for prostate cancer chemoprevention and treatment. *Endocr Relat Cancer,* 17, R19-38.

--- (2010) Mechanisms of the anti-cancer and anti-inflammatory actions of vitamin D. *Annu Rev Pharmacol Toxicol,* 51, 311-36.

Krishnan, A. V., D. Feldman, D. L. Trump & C. S. Johnson. 2011. Anti-inflammatory Activity of Calcitriol in Cancer

Vitamin D and Cancer. 53-71. Springer New York.

Krishnan, A. V., S. Swami, L. Peng, J. Wang, J. Moreno & D. Feldman (2009) Tissue-selective regulation of aromatase expression by calcitriol: implications for breast cancer therapy. *Endocrinology,* 151, 32-42.

Krishnan, A. V., D. L. Trump, C. S. Johnson & D. Feldman (2010) The role of vitamin D in cancer prevention and treatment. *Endocrinol Metab Clin North Am,* 39, 401-18, table of contents.

Kumar, B., K. G. Cordell, J. S. Lee, M. E. Prince, H. H. Tran, G. T. Wolf, S. G. Urba, F. P. Worden, D. B. Chepeha, T. N. Teknos, A. Eisbruch, C. I. Tsien, J. M. Taylor, N. J. D'Silva, K. Yang, D. M. Kurnit, C. R. Bradford & T. E. Carey (2007) Response to therapy and outcomes in oropharyngeal cancer are associated with biomarkers including human papillomavirus, epidermal growth factor receptor, gender, and smoking. *Int J Radiat Oncol Biol Phys,* 69, S109-11.

Kumar, B., K. G. Cordell, J. S. Lee, F. P. Worden, M. E. Prince, H. H. Tran, G. T. Wolf, S. G. Urba, D. B. Chepeha, T. N. Teknos, A. Eisbruch, C. I. Tsien, J. M. Taylor, N. J. D'Silva, K. Yang, D. M. Kurnit, J. A. Bauer, C. R. Bradford & T. E. Carey (2008) EGFR, p16, HPV Titer, Bcl-xL and p53, sex, and smoking as indicators of response to therapy and survival in oropharyngeal cancer. *J Clin Oncol,* 26, 3128-37.

Kumi-Diaka, J., K. Merchant, A. Haces, V. Hormann & M. Johnson (2010) Genistein-selenium combination induces growth arrest in prostate cancer cells. *J Med Food,* 13, 842-50.

Kundu, N. & A. M. Fulton (2002) Selective Cyclooxygenase (COX)-1 or COX-2 Inhibitors Control Metastatic Disease in a Murine Model of Breast Cancer. *Cancer Research,* 62, 2343-2346.

Lagergren, J. (2011) Influence of obesity on the risk of esophageal disorders. *Nat Rev Gastroenterol Hepatol,* 8, 340-7.

Lam, D. C. & J. D. Minna (2011) How do we safely get people to stop smoking? *Cancer Prev Res (Phila),* 4, 1724-7.

Lampe, J. W. (2007) Diet, genetic polymorphisms, detoxification, and health risks. *Altern Ther Health Med,* 13, S108-11.

--- (2009) Interindividual differences in response to plant-based diets: implications for cancer risk. *Am J Clin Nutr,* 89, 1553S-1557S.

Land, S. R., W. M. Cronin, D. L. Wickerham, J. P. Costantino, N. J. Christian, W. M. Klein & P. A. Ganz (2011) Cigarette smoking, obesity, physical activity, and alcohol use as predictors of chemoprevention adherence in the national surgical adjuvant breast and bowel project p-1 breast cancer prevention trial. *Cancer Prev Res (Phila),* 4, 1393-400.

Lanzotti, V. (2006) The analysis of onion and garlic. *J Chromatogr A,* 1112, 3-22.

Lappe, J. M., D. Travers-Gustafson, K. M. Davies, R. R. Recker & R. P. Heaney (2007) Vitamin D and calcium supplementation reduces cancer risk: results of a randomized trial. *The American Journal of Clinical Nutrition,* 85, 1586-1591.

Lehtinen, M., J. Paavonen, C. M. Wheeler, U. Jaisamrarn, S. M. Garland, X. Castellsague, S. R. Skinner, D. Apter, P. Naud, J. Salmeron, S. N. Chow, H. Kitchener, J. C. Teixeira, J. Hedrick, G. Limson, A. Szarewski, B. Romanowski, F. Y. Aoki, T. F. Schwarz, W. A. Poppe, N. S. De Carvalho, M. J. Germar, K. Peters, A. Mindel, P. De Sutter, F. X. Bosch, M. P. David, D. Descamps, F. Struyf & G. Dubin (2011) Overall efficacy of HPV-16/18 AS04-adjuvanted vaccine against grade 3 or greater cervical intraepithelial neoplasia: 4-year end-of-study analysis of the randomised, double-blind PATRICIA trial. *Lancet Oncol.*

Li, C., L. S. Balluz, C. A. Okoro, T. W. Strine, J. M. Lin, M. Town, W. Garvin, W. Murphy, W. Bartoli & B. Valluru (2011a) Surveillance of certain health behaviors and conditions among states and selected local areas --- Behavioral Risk Factor Surveillance System, United States, 2009. *MMWR Surveill Summ,* 60, 1-250.

Li, Y., O. Kucuk, M. Hussain, J. Abrams, M. L. Cher & F. H. Sarkar (2006) Antitumor and antimetastatic activities of docetaxel are enhanced by genistein through regulation of osteoprotegerin/receptor activator of nuclear factor-kappaB (RANK)/RANK ligand/MMP-9 signaling in prostate cancer. *Cancer Res,* 66, 4816-25.

Li, Z., L. Carrier, A. Belame, A. Thiyagarajah, V. Salvo, M. Burow & B. Rowan (2009) Combination of methylselenocysteine with tamoxifen inhibits MCF-7 breast cancer xenografts in nude mice through elevated apoptosis and reduced angiogenesis. *Breast Cancer Research and Treatment,* 118, 33-43.

Li, Z., W. Li, L. Song & W. Zhu (2011b) Cilia, adenomatous polyposis coli and associated diseases. *Oncogene.*

Lin, J. H., S. M. Zhang & J. E. Manson (2011) Predicting adherence to tamoxifen for breast cancer adjuvant therapy and prevention. *Cancer Prev Res (Phila),* 4, 1360-5.

Linos, E., M. D. Holmes & W. C. Willett (2007) Diet and breast cancer. *Curr Oncol Rep,* 9, 31-41.

Linos, E. & W. Willett (2009) Meat, dairy, and breast cancer: do we have an answer? *Am J Clin Nutr,* 90, 455-6.

Linos, E. & W. C. Willett (2007) Diet and breast cancer risk reduction. *J Natl Compr Canc Netw,* 5, 711-718.

Linos, E., W. C. Willett, E. Cho & L. Frazier (2010) Adolescent diet in relation to breast cancer risk among premenopausal women. *Cancer Epidemiol Biomarkers Prev,* 19, 689-96.

Liontos, M., M. Koutsami, M. Sideridou, K. Evangelou, D. Kletsas, B. Levy, A. Kotsinas, O. Nahum, V. Zoumpourlis, M. Kouloukoussa, Z. Lygerou, S. Taraviras, C. Kittas, J. Bartkova, A. G. Papavassiliou, J. Bartek, T. D. Halazonetis & V. G. Gorgoulis (2007) Deregulated Overexpression of hCdt1 and hCdc6 Promotes Malignant Behavior. *Cancer Research,* 67, 10899-10909.

Love, W. K., J. T. Deangelis, J. B. Berletch, S. M. Phipps, L. G. Andrews, W. J. Brouillette, D. D. Muccio & T. O. Tollefsbol (2008) The Novel Retinoid, 9cUAB30, Inhibits Telomerase and Induces Apoptosis in HL60 Cells. *Transl Oncol,* 1, 148-52.

Lowy, D. R. & K. Munger (2010) Prognostic Implications of HPV in Oropharyngeal Cancer. *New England Journal of Medicine,* 363, 82-84.

Lynch, B. M., H. K. Neilson & C. M. Friedenreich (2010) Physical activity and breast cancer prevention. *Recent Results Cancer Res,* 186, 13-42.

Ma, Y., D. L. Trump & C. S. Johnson (2010) Vitamin D in combination cancer treatment. *J Cancer,* 1, 101-7.

Madan, V., J. T. Lear & R.-M. Szeimies (2010) Non-melanoma skin cancer. *The Lancet,* 375, 673-685.

Mage, C., A. O. Goldstein, S. Colgan, B. Skinner, K. D. Kramer, J. Steiner & A. H. Staples (2011) Secondhand smoke policies at state and county fairs. *N C Med J,* 71, 409-12.

Manson, J. E., S. T. Mayne & S. K. Clinton (2011) Vitamin D and Prevention of Cancer - Ready for Prime Time? *New England Journal of Medicine,* 364, 1385-1387.

Marnett, L. J. (2009) Mechanisms of Cyclooxygenase-2 Inhibition and Cardiovascular Side Effectsâ€"The Plot Thickens. *Cancer Prevention Research,* 2, 288-290.

Marsit, C. J., M. Liu, H. H. Nelson, M. Posner, M. Suzuki & K. T. Kelsey (2003) Inactivation of the Fanconi anemia//BRCA pathway in lung and oral cancers: implications for treatment and survival. *Oncogene,* 23, 1000-1004.

Martino, S., J. A. Cauley, E. Barrett-Connor, T. J. Powles, J. Mershon, D. Disch, R. J. Secrest, S. R. Cummings & C. I. For the (2004) Continuing Outcomes Relevant to Evista: Breast Cancer Incidence in Postmenopausal Osteoporotic Women in a Randomized Trial of Raloxifene. *Journal of the National Cancer Institute,* 96, 1751-1761.

Mates, J. M., J. A. Segura, F. J. Alonso & J. Marquez (2011) Anticancer antioxidant regulatory functions of phytochemicals. *Curr Med Chem,* 18, 2315-38.

Mattoo, A. K., V. Shukla, T. Fatima, A. K. Handa & S. K. Yachha (2010) Genetic engineering to enhance crop-based phytonutrients (nutraceuticals) to alleviate diet-related diseases. *Adv Exp Med Biol,* 698, 122-43.

McGrath, D. R. & A. D. Spigelman (2008) Putative mechanisms of action for indole-3-carbinol in the prevention of colorectal cancer. *Expert Opin Ther Targets,* 12, 729-38.

McWalter, G. K., L. G. Higgins, L. I. McLellan, C. J. Henderson, L. Song, P. J. Thornalley, K. Itoh, M. Yamamoto & J. D. Hayes (2004) Transcription factor Nrf2 is essential for induction of NAD(P)H:quinone oxidoreductase 1, glutathione S-transferases, and glutamate cysteine ligase by broccoli seeds and isothiocyanates. *J Nutr,* 134, 3499S-3506S.

Menter, D. G., R. L. Schilsky & R. N. DuBois (2010) Cyclooxygenase-2 and Cancer Treatment: Understanding the Risk Should Be Worth the Reward. *Clinical Cancer Research,* 16, 1384-1390.

Mills, T. D., S. J. Vinnicombe, C. A. Wells & R. Carpenter (2002) Angiosarcoma of the Breast After Wide Local Excision and Radiotherapy for Breast Carcinoma. *Clinical Radiology,* 57, 63-66.

Myers, E., W. K. Huh, J. D. Wright & J. S. Smith (2008) The current and future role of screening in the era of HPV vaccination. *Gynecol Oncol,* 109, S31-9.

Nelson, W. G., A. M. De Marzo & W. B. Isaacs (2003) Prostate Cancer. *New England Journal of Medicine,* 349, 366-381.

Neto, C. C. (2007) Cranberry and blueberry: evidence for protective effects against cancer and vascular diseases. *Mol Nutr Food Res,* 51, 652-64.

Newmark, H. L., M. J. Wargovich & W. R. Bruce (1984) Colon cancer and dietary fat, phosphate, and calcium: a hypothesis. *J Natl Cancer Inst,* 72, 1323-5.

No, J. H., M.-K. Kim, Y.-T. Jeon, Y.-B. Kim & Y.-S. Song (2011) Human papillomavirus vaccine: Widening the scope for cancer prevention. *Molecular Carcinogenesis,* 50, 244-253.

Obiorah, I. & V. C. Jordan (2011) Progress in endocrine approaches to the treatment and prevention of breast cancer. *Maturitas.*

Olsen, C. M., N. Pandeya, A. C. Green, P. M. Webb & D. C. Whiteman (2011) Population attributable fractions of adenocarcinoma of the esophagus and gastroesophageal junction. *Am J Epidemiol,* 174, 582-90.

Oren, M. (2003) Decision making by p53: life, death and cancer. *Cell Death and Differentiation,* 10, 431-442.

Osborne, C. K. (1998) Tamoxifen in the Treatment of Breast Cancer. *New England Journal of Medicine,* 339, 1609-1618.

Ott, J. J., A. Ullrich, M. Mascarenhas & G. A. Stevens (2011) Global cancer incidence and mortality caused by behavior and infection. *Journal of Public Health,* 33, 223-233.

Overholt, B. F., M. Panjehpour & J. M. Haydek (1999) Photodynamic therapy for Barrett's esophagus: follow-up in 100 patients. *Gastrointest Endosc,* 49, 1-7.

Overholt, B. F., K. K. Wang, J. S. Burdick, C. J. Lightdale, M. Kimmey, H. R. Nava, M. V. Sivak, Jr., N. Nishioka, H. Barr, N. Marcon, M. Pedrosa, M. P. Bronner, M. Grace & M. Depot (2007) Five-year efficacy and safety of photodynamic therapy with Photofrin in Barrett's high-grade dysplasia. *Gastrointest Endosc,* 66, 460-8.

Panjehpour, M. & B. F. Overholt (2006) Porfimer sodium photodynamic therapy for management of Barrett's esophagus with high-grade dysplasia. *Lasers Surg Med,* 38, 390-5.

Papanas, N., E. Maltezos & D. P. Mikhailidis (2010) Metformin and cancer: licence to heal? *Expert Opin Investig Drugs,* 19, 913-7.

Paz-Elizur, T., M. Krupsky, S. Blumenstein, D. Elinger, E. Schechtman & Z. Livneh (2003) DNA Repair Activity for Oxidative Damage and Risk of Lung Cancer. *Journal of the National Cancer Institute,* 95, 1312-1319.

Pelucchi, C., S. Gallus, W. Garavello, C. Bosetti & C. La Vecchia (2008) Alcohol and tobacco use, and cancer risk for upper aerodigestive tract and liver. *Eur J Cancer Prev,* 17, 340-4.

Pelucchi, C., I. Tramacere, P. Boffetta, E. Negri & C. L. Vecchia (2011) Alcohol Consumption and Cancer Risk. *Nutrition and Cancer,* 63, 983-990.

Pence, B. C. (1993) Role of calcium in colon cancer prevention: experimental and clinical studies. *Mutat Res,* 290, 87-95.

Pereira, C., R. M. Medeiros & M. J. Dinis-Ribeiro (2009) Cyclooxygenase polymorphisms in gastric and colorectal carcinogenesis: are conclusive results available? *Eur J Gastroenterol Hepatol,* 21, 76-91.

Perks, C. M. & J. M. Holly (2011) Hormonal mechanisms underlying the relationship between obesity and breast cancer. *Endocrinol Metab Clin North Am,* 40, 485-507, vii.

Pesch, B., B. Kendzia, P. Gustavsson, K. H. Jockel, G. Johnen, H. Pohlabeln, A. Olsson, W. Ahrens, I. M. Gross, I. Broske, H. E. Wichmann, F. Merletti, L. Richiardi, L. Simonato, C. Fortes, J. Siemiatycki, M. E. Parent, D. Consonni, M. T. Landi, N. Caporaso, D. Zaridze, A. Cassidy, N. Szeszenia-Dabrowska, P. Rudnai, J. Lissowska, I. Stucker, E. Fabianova, R. S. Dumitru, V. Bencko, L. Foretova, V. Janout, C. M. Rudin, P. Brennan, P. Boffetta, K. Straif & T. Bruning (2011) Cigarette smoking and lung cancer - relative risk estimates for the major histological types from a pooled analysis of case-control studies. *Int J Cancer.*

Peterlik, M., W. B. Grant & H. S. Cross (2009) Calcium, vitamin D and cancer. *Anticancer Res,* 29, 3687-98.

Phipps, A. I., R. T. Chlebowski, R. Prentice, A. McTiernan, M. L. Stefanick, J. Wactawski-Wende, L. H. Kuller, L. L. Adams-Campbell, D. Lane, M. Vitolins, G. C. Kabat, T. E. Rohan & C. I. Li (2011) Body size, physical activity, and risk of triple-negative and estrogen receptor-positive breast cancer. *Cancer Epidemiol Biomarkers Prev,* 20, 454-63.

Platz, E. A., M. F. Leitzmann, K. Visvanathan, E. B. Rimm, M. J. Stampfer, W. C. Willett & E. Giovannucci (2006) Statin Drugs and Risk of Advanced Prostate Cancer. *Journal of the National Cancer Institute,* 98, 1819-1825.

Poland, G. A. & R. M. Jacobson (2004) Prevention of Hepatitis B with the Hepatitis B Vaccine. *New England Journal of Medicine,* 351, 2832-2838.

Polo, S. E. & S. P. Jackson (2011) Dynamics of DNA damage response proteins at DNA breaks: a focus on protein modifications. *Genes Dev,* 25, 409-33.

Polyak, K., I. Haviv & I. G. Campbell (2009) Co-evolution of tumor cells and their microenvironment. *Trends Genet.* , 25, 30-38.

Prakobwong, S., S. C. Gupta, J. H. Kim, B. Sung, P. Pinlaor, Y. Hiraku, S. Wongkham, B. Sripa, S. Pinlaor & B. B. Aggarwal (2011) Curcumin suppresses proliferation and

induces apoptosis in human biliary cancer cells through modulation of multiple cell signaling pathways. *Carcinogenesis,* 32, 1372-80.
Proctor, I., V. Sharma, M. Khoshzaban & A. Winstanley (2011) Does smoking kill? A study of death certification and smoking. *J Clin Pathol.*
Psaty, B. M. & C. D. Furberg (2005) COX-2 Inhibitors - Lessons in Drug Safety. *New England Journal of Medicine,* 352, 1133-1135.
Quilty, P. M. & G. R. Kerr (1987) Bladder cancer following low or high dose pelvic irradiation. *Clinical Radiology,* 38, 583-585.
Rajasingh, J., H. P. Raikwar, G. Muthian, C. Johnson & J. J. Bright (2006) Curcumin induces growth-arrest and apoptosis in association with the inhibition of constitutively active JAK-STAT pathway in T cell leukemia. *Biochem Biophys Res Commun,* 340, 359-68.
Reddy, B. S. (2007) Strategies for colon cancer prevention: combination of chemopreventive agents. *Subcell Biochem,* 42, 213-25.
Reddy, B. S. & C. V. Rao (2005) Chemoprophylaxis of colon cancer. *Curr Gastroenterol Rep,* 7, 389-95.
Redon, C., J. S. Dickey, A. Nakamura, I. Kareva, D. Naf, S. Nowsheen, T. B. Kryston, W. M. Bonner, A. G. Georgakilas & O. A. Sedelnikova (2010) Tumors induce complex DNA damage in distant proliferative tissues *in vivo. Proc. Natl. Acad. Sci. USA,* 107, 17992-17997.
Reichman, T. W., J. Albanell, X. Wang, M. A. S. Moore & G. P. Studzinski (1997) Downregulation of telomerase activity in HL60 cells by differentiating agents is accompanied by increased expression of telomerase-associated protein. *Journal of Cellular Biochemistry,* 67, 13-23.
Rekha, C. R. & G. Vijayalakshmi (2010) Isoflavone phytoestrogens in soymilk fermented with beta-glucosidase producing probiotic lactic acid bacteria. *Int J Food Sci Nutr,* 62, 111-20.
Ribeiro, A. M., S. Andrade, F. Pinho, J. D. Monteiro, M. Costa, C. Lopes, A. P. Aguas & M. P. Monteiro (2010) Prostate cancer cell proliferation and angiogenesis in different obese mice models. *Int J Exp Pathol,* 91, 374-86.
Riedl, M. A., A. Saxon & D. Diaz-Sanchez (2009) Oral sulforaphane increases Phase II antioxidant enzymes in the human upper airway. *Clin Immunol,* 130, 244-51.
Ritz, S. A., J. Wan & D. Diaz-Sanchez (2007) Sulforaphane-stimulated phase II enzyme induction inhibits cytokine production by airway epithelial cells stimulated with diesel extract. *Am J Physiol Lung Cell Mol Physiol,* 292, L33-9.
Roberts-Thomson, S. J., M. C. Curry & G. R. Monteith (2011) Plasma membrane calcium pumps and their emerging roles in cancer. *World J Biol Chem,* 1, 248-53.
Roden, R. & T. C. Wu (2006) How will HPV vaccines affect cervical cancer? *Nat Rev Cancer,* 6, 753-763.
Romanenko, A., K. Morimura, H. Wanibuchi, M. Wei, W. Zaparin, W. Vinnichenko, A. Kinoshita, A. Vozianov & S. Fukushima (2003) Urinary bladder lesions induced by persistent chronic low-dose ionizing radiation. *Cancer Science,* 94, 328-333.
Rondini, E. A., A. E. Harvey, J. P. Steibel, S. D. Hursting & J. I. Fenton (2011) Energy balance modulates colon tumor growth: Interactive roles of insulin and estrogen. *Mol Carcinog,* 50, 370-82.

Rothwell, P. M., F. G. R. Fowkes, J. F. F. Belch, H. Ogawa, C. P. Warlow & T. W. Meade (2011) Effect of daily aspirin on long-term risk of death due to cancer: analysis of individual patient data from randomised trials. *The Lancet,* 377, 31-41.

Rozengurt, E., J. Sinnett-Smith & K. Kisfalvi (2010) Crosstalk between insulin/insulin-like growth factor-1 receptors and G protein-coupled receptor signaling systems: a novel target for the antidiabetic drug metformin in pancreatic cancer. *Clin Cancer Res,* 16, 2505-11.

Rutegard, M., P. Lagergren, H. Nordenstedt & J. Lagergren (2011) Oesophageal adenocarcinoma: the new epidemic in men? *Maturitas,* 69, 244-8.

Ryan, A. M., M. Duong, L. Healy, S. A. Ryan, N. Parekh, J. V. Reynolds & D. G. Power (2011) Obesity, metabolic syndrome and esophageal adenocarcinoma: epidemiology, etiology and new targets. *Cancer Epidemiol,* 35, 309-19.

Saini, S., S. Arora, S. Majid, V. Shahryari, Y. Chen, G. Deng, S. Yamamura, K. Ueno & R. Dahiya (2011) Curcumin modulates microRNA-203-mediated regulation of the Src-Akt axis in bladder cancer. *Cancer Prev Res (Phila),* 4, 1698-709.

Sanborn, C. K., A. O'Connor, R. S. Sawin, K. Moore, M. J. Dehart & K. S. Azarow (2000) Comparison of telomerase levels before and after differentiation of two cell lines of human neuroblastoma. *J Surg Res,* 93, 206-10.

Saslow, D., P. E. Castle, J. T. Cox, D. D. Davey, M. H. Einstein, D. G. Ferris, S. J. Goldie, D. M. Harper, W. Kinney, A.-B. Moscicki, K. L. Noller, C. M. Wheeler, T. Ades, K. S. Andrews, M. K. Doroshenk, K. G. Kahn, C. Schmidt, O. Shafey, R. A. Smith, E. E. Partridge & F. Garcia (2007) American Cancer Society Guideline for Human Papillomavirus (HPV) Vaccine Use to Prevent Cervical Cancer and Its Precursors. *CA: A Cancer Journal for Clinicians,* 57, 7-28.

Saydmohammed, M., D. Joseph & V. Syed (2010) Curcumin suppresses constitutive activation of STAT-3 by up-regulating protein inhibitor of activated STAT-3 (PIAS-3) in ovarian and endometrial cancer cells. *J Cell Biochem,* 110, 447-56.

Scher, H. I., X. Jia, K. Chi, R. de Wit, W. R. Berry, P. Albers, B. Henick, D. Waterhouse, D. J. Ruether, P. J. Rosen, A. A. Meluch, L. T. Nordquist, P. M. Venner, A. Heidenreich, L. Chu & G. Heller (2011) Randomized, Open-Label Phase III Trial of Docetaxel Plus High-Dose Calcitriol Versus Docetaxel Plus Prednisone for Patients With Castration-Resistant Prostate Cancer. *Journal of Clinical Oncology,* 29, 2191-2198.

Schreiber, R. D., L. J. Old & M. J. Smyth (2011) Cancer immunoediting: integrating immunity's roles in cancer suppression and promotion. *Science,* 331, 1565-1570.

Senkus, E., T. Konefka, M. Nowaczyk & J. Jassem (2000) Second lower genital tract squamous cell carcinoma following cervical cancer. *Acta Obstetricia et Gynecologica Scandinavica,* 79, 765-770.

Sheng, H., J. Shao, S. C. Kirkland, P. Isakson, R. J. Coffey, J. Morrow, R. D. Beauchamp & R. N. DuBois (1997) Inhibition of human colon cancer cell growth by selective inhibition of cyclooxygenase-2. *J Clin Invest,* 99, 2254-9.

Shenouda, N. S., C. Zhou, J. D. Browning, P. J. Ansell, M. S. Sakla, D. B. Lubahn & R. S. MacDonald (2004) Phytoestrogens in Common Herbs Regulate Prostate Cancer Cell Growth in Vitro. *Nutrition and Cancer,* 49, 200-208.

Sherr, C. J. & F. McCormick (2002) The RB and p53 pathways in cancer. *Cancer Cell,* 2, 103-112.

Shields, P. G. (2011) Long-term Nicotine Replacement Therapy: Cancer Risk in Context. *Cancer Prev Res (Phila),* 4, 1719-23.

Shiloh, Y. (2003) ATM and related protein kinases: safeguarding genome integrity. *Nat Rev Cancer,* 3, 155-168.

Shirai, T., M. Sano, S. Tamano, S. Takahashi, M. Hirose, M. Futakuchi, R. Hasegawa, K. Imaida, K. Matsumoto, K. Wakabayashi, T. Sugimura & N. Ito (1997) The prostate: A target for carcinogenicity of 2-amino-1-methyl-6-phenylimidazo[4,5-b]pyridine (PhIP) derived from cooked foods. *Cancer Research,* 57, 195-198.

Sikalidis, A. K. & B. Varamini (2011) Roles of Hormones and Signaling Molecules in Describing the Relationship Between Obesity and Colon cancer. *Pathol Oncol Res,* 17, 785-90.

Sirianni, N., P. K. Ha, M. Oelke, J. Califano, W. Gooding, W. Westra, T. L. Whiteside, W. M. Koch, J. P. Schneck, A. DeLeo & R. L. Ferris (2004) Effect of human papillomavirus-16 infection on CD8+ T-cell recognition of a wild-type sequence p53264-272 peptide in patients with squamous cell carcinoma of the head and neck. *Clin Cancer Res,* 10, 6929-37.

Sirianni, N., J. Wang & R. L. Ferris (2005) Antiviral activity of Cidofovir on a naturally human papillomavirus-16 infected squamous cell carcinoma of the head and neck (SCCHN) cell line improves radiation sensitivity. *Oral Oncol,* 41, 423-8.

Sisk, E. A., S. G. Soltys, S. Zhu, S. G. Fisher, T. E. Carey & C. R. Bradford (2002) Human papillomavirus and p53 mutational status as prognostic factors in head and neck carcinoma. *Head Neck,* 24, 841-9.

Smith, C. J., Y. Zhang, C. M. Koboldt, J. Muhammad, B. S. Zweifel, A. Shaffer, J. J. Talley, J. L. Masferrer, K. Seibert & P. C. Isakson (1998) Pharmacological analysis of cyclooxygenase-1 in inflammation. *Proceedings of the National Academy of Sciences,* 95, 13313-13318.

So, J. Y., H. J. Lee, A. K. Smolarek, S. Paul, C. X. Wang, H. Maehr, M. Uskokovic, X. Zheng, A. H. Conney, L. Cai, F. Liu & N. Suh (2010) A novel Gemini vitamin D analog represses the expression of a stem cell marker CD44 in breast cancer. *Mol Pharmacol,* 79, 360-7.

Solinas, G., F. Marchesi, C. Garlanda, A. Mantovani & P. Allavena (2010) Inflammation-mediated promotion of invasion and metastasis. *Cancer Metastasis Rev.,* 29, 243-8.

Sountoulides, P., N. Koletsas, D. Kikidakis, K. Paschalidis & N. Sofikitis (2011) Secondary malignancies following radiotherapy for prostate cancer. *Ther Adv Urol,* 2, 119-25.

Souza, R. F., K. Shewmake, D. G. Beer, B. Cryer & S. J. Spechler (2000) Selective Inhibition of Cyclooxygenase-2 Suppresses Growth and Induces Apoptosis in Human Esophageal Adenocarcinoma Cells. *Cancer Research,* 60, 5767-5772.

Sporn, M. B. & A. B. Roberts (1983) Role of retinoids in differentiation and carcinogenesis. *Cancer Res,* 43, 3034-40.

Sreekanth, C. N., S. V. Bava, E. Sreekumar & R. J. Anto (2011) Molecular evidences for the chemosensitizing efficacy of liposomal curcumin in paclitaxel chemotherapy in mouse models of cervical cancer. *Oncogene,* 30, 3139-52.

Stavridi, E. S. & T. D. Halazonetis (2005) Nbs1 moving up in the world. *Nat Cell Biol,* 7, 648-650.

Storey, A., M. Thomas, A. Kalita, C. Harwood, D. Gardiol, F. Mantovani, J. Breuer, I. M. Leigh, G. Matlashewski & L. Banks (1998) Role of a p53 polymorphism in the development of human papilloma-virus-associated cancer. *Nature,* 393, 229-234.

Stratton, M. R. (2011) Exploring the genomes of cancer cells: progress and promise. *Science,* 331, 1553-8.

Stricker, T., D. V. Catenacci & T. Y. Seiwert (2011) Molecular profiling of cancer--the future of personalized cancer medicine: a primer on cancer biology and the tools necessary to bring molecular testing to the clinic. *Semin Oncol,* 38, 173-85.

Su, X., R. M. Tamimi, L. C. Collins, H. J. Baer, E. Cho, L. Sampson, W. C. Willett, S. J. Schnitt, J. L. Connolly, B. A. Rosner & G. A. Colditz (2010) Intake of fiber and nuts during adolescence and incidence of proliferative benign breast disease. *Cancer Causes Control,* 21, 1033-46.

Subbaramaiah, K., L. R. Howe, P. Bhardwaj, B. Du, C. Gravaghi, R. K. Yantiss, X. K. Zhou, V. A. Blaho, T. Hla, P. Yang, L. Kopelovich, C. A. Hudis & A. J. Dannenberg (2011) Obesity is associated with inflammation and elevated aromatase expression in the mouse mammary gland. *Cancer Prev Res (Phila),* 4, 329-46.

Suh, S. & K. W. Kim (2011) Diabetes and cancer: is diabetes causally related to cancer? *Diabetes Metab J,* 35, 193-8.

Suh, Y., F. Afaq, J. J. Johnson & H. Mukhtar (2009) A plant flavonoid fisetin induces apoptosis in colon cancer cells by inhibition of COX2 and Wnt/EGFR/NF-kappaB-signaling pathways. *Carcinogenesis,* 30, 300-7.

Suit, H., S. Goldberg, A. Niemierko, M. Ancukiewicz, E. Hall, M. Goitein, W. Wong & H. Paganetti (2007) Secondary Carcinogenesis in Patients Treated with Radiation: A Review of Data on Radiation-Induced Cancers in Human, Non-human Primate, Canine and Rodent Subjects. *Radiation Research,* 167, 12-42.

Sun, Z. J., G. Chen, W. Zhang, X. Hu, Y. Liu, Q. Zhou, L. X. Zhu & Y. F. Zhao (2010) Curcumin dually inhibits both mammalian target of rapamycin and nuclear factor-kappaB pathways through a crossed phosphatidylinositol 3-kinase/Akt/IkappaB kinase complex signaling axis in adenoid cystic carcinoma. *Mol Pharmacol,* 79, 106-18.

Surh, Y. J. (2008) NF-kappa B and Nrf2 as potential chemopreventive targets of some anti-inflammatory and antioxidative phytonutrients with anti-inflammatory and antioxidative activities. *Asia Pac J Clin Nutr,* 17 Suppl 1, 269-72.

Suzuki, K. & T. Mitsuoka (1992) Effect of low-fat, high-fat, and fiber-supplemented high-fat diets on colon cancer risk factors in feces of healthy subjects. *Nutr Cancer,* 18, 63-71.

Suzuki, R., M. Iwasaki, S. Yamamoto, M. Inoue, S. Sasazuki, N. Sawada, T. Yamaji, T. Shimazu & S. Tsugane (2011) Leisure-time physical activity and breast cancer risk defined by estrogen and progesterone receptor status--the Japan Public Health Center-based Prospective Study. *Prev Med,* 52, 227-33.

Swami, S., A. V. Krishnan, J. Y. Wang, K. Jensen, L. Peng, M. A. Albertelli & D. Feldman (2011) Inhibitory effects of calcitriol on the growth of MCF-7 breast cancer xenografts in nude mice: selective modulation of aromatase expression in vivo. *Horm Cancer,* 2, 190-202.

Szliszka, E., Z. P. Czuba, A. Mertas, A. Paradysz & W. Krol (2011) The dietary isoflavone biochanin-A sensitizes prostate cancer cells to TRAIL-induced apoptosis. *Urol Oncol.*

Szliszka, E. & W. Krol (2011) Soy isoflavones augment the effect of TRAIL-mediated apoptotic death in prostate cancer cells. *Oncol Rep,* 26, 533-41.

Takahashi, Y., J. A. Lavigne, S. D. Hursting, G. V. Chandramouli, S. N. Perkins, Y. S. Kim & T. T. Wang (2006) Molecular signatures of soy-derived phytochemicals in androgen-responsive prostate cancer cells: a comparison study using DNA microarray. *Mol Carcinog,* 45, 943-56.

Teucher, B., S. Rohrmann & R. Kaaks (2009) Obesity: focus on all-cause mortality and cancer. *Maturitas,* 65, 112-6.

Teunissen, S. F., H. Rosing, M. D. Seoane, L. Brunsveld, J. H. Schellens, A. H. Schinkel & J. H. Beijnen (2011) Investigational study of tamoxifen phase I metabolites using chromatographic and spectroscopic analytical techniques. *J Pharm Biomed Anal,* 55, 518-26.

Thomas, D. B. (1995) Alcohol as a cause of cancer. *Environ Health Perspect,* 103 Suppl 8, 153-60.

Thompson, D., D. F. Easton & C. the Breast Cancer Linkage (2002) Cancer Incidence in BRCA1 Mutation Carriers. *Journal of the National Cancer Institute,* 94, 1358-1365.

Thompson, I. M., P. J. Goodman, C. M. Tangen, M. S. Lucia, G. J. Miller, L. G. Ford, M. M. Lieber, R. D. Cespedes, J. N. Atkins, S. M. Lippman, S. M. Carlin, A. Ryan, C. M. Szczepanek, J. J. Crowley & C. A. Coltman (2003) The Influence of Finasteride on the Development of Prostate Cancer. *New England Journal of Medicine,* 349, 215-224.

Traka, M., A. V. Gasper, A. Melchini, J. R. Bacon, P. W. Needs, V. Frost, A. Chantry, A. M. Jones, C. A. Ortori, D. A. Barrett, R. Y. Ball, R. D. Mills & R. F. Mithen (2008) Broccoli consumption interacts with GSTM1 to perturb oncogenic signalling pathways in the prostate. *PLoS One,* 3, e2568.

Tuynman, J. B., L. Vermeulen, E. M. Boon, K. Kemper, A. H. Zwinderman, M. P. Peppelenbosch & D. J. Richel (2008) Cyclooxygenase-2 inhibition inhibits c-Met kinase activity and Wnt activity in colon cancer. *Cancer Res,* 68, 1213-20.

University, E. C. a. O. H. S. (2011) Medications To Reduce the Risk of Primary Breast Cancer in Women.

van Gent, D. C., J. H. J. Hoeijmakers & R. Kanaar (2001) Chromosomal stability and the DNA double-stranded break connection. *Nat Rev Genet,* 2, 196-206.

Varani, J. (2011) Calcium, calcium-sensing receptor and growth control in the colonic mucosa. *Histol Histopathol,* 26, 769-79.

Vasen, H. F. A. & W. H. de Vos tot Nederveen Cappel (2011) Cancer: Lynch syndrome-how should colorectal cancer be managed? *Nat Rev Gastroenterol Hepatol,* 8, 184-186.

Vigneri, P., F. Frasca, L. Sciacca, G. Pandini & R. Vigneri (2009) Diabetes and cancer. *Endocr Relat Cancer,* 16, 1103-23.

Vogel, V. G., J. P. Costantino, D. L. Wickerham, W. M. Cronin, R. S. Cecchini, J. N. Atkins, T. B. Bevers, L. Fehrenbacher, E. R. Pajon, J. L. Wade, A. Robidoux, R. G. Margolese, J. James, S. M. Lippman, C. D. Runowicz, P. A. Ganz, S. E. Reis, W. McCaskill-Stevens, L. G. Ford, V. C. Jordan, N. Wolmark, B. for the National Surgical Adjuvant & P. Bowel (2006) Effects of Tamoxifen vs Raloxifene on the Risk of Developing Invasive Breast Cancer and Other Disease Outcomes. *JAMA: The Journal of the American Medical Association,* 295, 2727-2741.

Vogelstein, B., D. Lane & A. J. Levine (2000) Surfing the p53 network. *Nature,* 408, 307-310.

Wahlqvist, M. L. & M. S. Lee (2007) Regional food culture and development. *Asia Pac J Clin Nutr,* 16 Suppl 1, 2-7.

Walsh, R. A., C. L. Paul, L. Paras, F. Stacey & F. Tzelepis (2011) Workplace-related smoking in New South Wales: extent of bans, public attitudes and relationships with relapse. *Health Promot J Austr,* 22, 85-90.

Wan, J. & D. Diaz-Sanchez (2007) Antioxidant enzyme induction: a new protective approach against the adverse effects of diesel exhaust particles. *Inhal Toxicol,* 19 Suppl 1, 177-82.

Wang, H., E. S. Yang, J. Jiang, S. Nowsheen & F. Xia (2010) DNA damage-induced cytotoxicity is dissociated from BRCA1's DNA repair function but is dependent on its cytosolic accumulation. *Cancer Res,* 70, 6258-67.

Wang, S., M. Xu, F. Li, X. Wang, K. Bower, J. Frank, Y. Lu, G. Chen, Z. Zhang, Z. Ke, X. Shi & J. Luo (2011) Ethanol promotes mammary tumor growth and angiogenesis: the involvement of chemoattractant factor MCP-1. *Breast Cancer Research and Treatment,* 1-12.

Wansom, D., E. Light, F. Worden, M. Prince, S. Urba, D. B. Chepeha, K. Cordell, A. Eisbruch, J. Taylor, N. D'Silva, J. Moyer, C. R. Bradford, D. Kurnit, B. Kumar, T. E. Carey & G. T. Wolf (2010) Correlation of cellular immunity with human papillomavirus 16 status and outcome in patients with advanced oropharyngeal cancer. *Arch. Otolaryngol. Head Neck Surg.,* 136, 1267-73.

Wargovich, M. J., P. M. Lynch & B. Levin (1991) Modulating effects of calcium in animal models of colon carcinogenesis and short-term studies in subjects at increased risk for colon cancer. *Am J Clin Nutr,* 54, 202S-205S.

Watson, J. L., A. Greenshields, R. Hill, A. Hilchie, P. W. Lee, C. A. Giacomantonio & D. W. Hoskin (2009) Curcumin-induced apoptosis in ovarian carcinoma cells is p53-independent and involves p38 mitogen-activated protein kinase activation and downregulation of Bcl-2 and survivin expression and Akt signaling. *Mol Carcinog,* 49, 13-24.

Wattleworth, R. (2011) Human papillomavirus infection and the links to penile and cervical cancer. *J Am Osteopath Assoc,* 111, S3-10.

Wenefrida, I., H. S. Utomo, S. B. Blanche & S. D. Linscombe (2009) Enhancing essential amino acids and health benefit components in grain crops for improved nutritional values. *Recent Pat DNA Gene Seq,* 3, 219-25.

Werness, B. A., A. J. Levine & P. M. Howley (1990) Association of human papillomavirus types 16 and 18 E6 proteins with p53. *Science,* 248, 76-79.

Wheeler, C. M., X. Castellsague, S. M. Garland, A. Szarewski, J. Paavonen, P. Naud, J. Salmeron, S. N. Chow, D. Apter, H. Kitchener, J. C. Teixeira, S. R. Skinner, U. Jaisamrarn, G. Limson, B. Romanowski, F. Y. Aoki, T. F. Schwarz, W. A. Poppe, F. X. Bosch, D. M. Harper, W. Huh, K. Hardt, T. Zahaf, D. Descamps, F. Struyf, G. Dubin & M. Lehtinen (2011) Cross-protective efficacy of HPV-16/18 AS04-adjuvanted vaccine against cervical infection and precancer caused by non-vaccine oncogenic HPV types: 4-year end-of-study analysis of the randomised, double-blind PATRICIA trial. *Lancet Oncol.*

Wijnmaalen, A., B. van Ooijen, B. N. van Geel, S. C. Henzen-Logmans & A. D. Treurniet-Donker (1993) Angiosarcoma of the breast following lumpectomy, axillary lymph node dissection, and radiotherapy for primary breast cancer: three case reports and a review of the literature. *Int J Radiat Oncol Biol Phys,* 26, 135-9.

Wilken, R., M. Veena, M. Wang & E. Srivatsan (2011) Curcumin: A review of anti-cancer properties and therapeutic activity in head and neck squamous cell carcinoma. *Molecular Cancer,* 10, 12.

Willyard, C. (2011) Lifestyle: Breaking the cancer habit. *Nature,* 471, S16-7.

Winzer, B. M., D. C. Whiteman, M. M. Reeves & J. D. Paratz (2011) Physical activity and cancer prevention: a systematic review of clinical trials. *Cancer Causes Control,* 22, 811-26.

Wong, T. F., T. Takeda, B. Li, K. Tsuiji, M. Kitamura, A. Kondo & N. Yaegashi (2011) Curcumin disrupts uterine leiomyosarcoma cells through AKT-mTOR pathway inhibition. *Gynecol Oncol,* 122, 141-8.

Xu, L., Y. Ding, W. J. Catalona, X. J. Yang, W. F. Anderson, B. Jovanovic, K. Wellman, J. Killmer, X. Huang, K. A. Scheidt, R. B. Montgomery & R. C. Bergan (2009) MEK4 function, genistein treatment, and invasion of human prostate cancer cells. *J Natl Cancer Inst,* 101, 1141-55.

Yang, E. S. & K. L. Burnstein (2003) Vitamin D Inhibits G1 to S Progression in LNCaP Prostate Cancer Cells through p27Kip1 Stabilization and Cdk2 Mislocalization to the Cytoplasm. *Journal of Biological Chemistry,* 278, 46862-46868.

Yang, E. S., C. A. Maiorino, B. A. Roos, S. R. Knight & K. L. Burnstein (2002) Vitamin D-mediated growth inhibition of an androgen-ablated LNCaP cell line model of human prostate cancer. *Molecular and Cellular Endocrinology,* 186, 69-79.

Yang, E. S., H. Wang, G. Jiang, S. Nowsheen, A. Fu, D. E. Hallahan & F. Xia (2009) Lithium-mediated protection of hippocampal cells involves enhancement of DNA-PKâ€"dependent repair in mice. *The Journal of Clinical Investigation,* 119, 1124-1135.

Yang, X. R., J. Chang-Claude, E. L. Goode, F. J. Couch, H. Nevanlinna, R. L. Milne, M. Gaudet, M. K. Schmidt, A. Broeks, A. Cox, P. A. Fasching, R. Hein, A. B. Spurdle, F. Blows, K. Driver, D. Flesch-Janys, J. Heinz, P. Sinn, A. Vrieling, T. Heikkinen, K. Aittomaki, P. Heikkila, C. Blomqvist, J. Lissowska, B. Peplonska, S. Chanock, J. Figueroa, L. Brinton, P. Hall, K. Czene, K. Humphreys, H. Darabi, J. Liu, L. J. Van 't Veer, F. E. van Leeuwen, I. L. Andrulis, G. Glendon, J. A. Knight, A. M. Mulligan, F. P. O'Malley, N. Weerasooriya, E. M. John, M. W. Beckmann, A. Hartmann, S. B. Weihbrecht, D. L. Wachter, S. M. Jud, C. R. Loehberg, L. Baglietto, D. R. English, G. G. Giles, C. A. McLean, G. Severi, D. Lambrechts, T. Vandorpe, C. Weltens, R. Paridaens, A. Smeets, P. Neven, H. Wildiers, X. Wang, J. E. Olson, V. Cafourek, Z. Fredericksen, M. Kosel, C. Vachon, H. E. Cramp, D. Connley, S. S. Cross, S. P. Balasubramanian, M. W. Reed, T. Dork, M. Bremer, A. Meyer, J. H. Karstens, A. Ay, T. W. Park-Simon, P. Hillemanns, J. I. Arias Perez, P. Menendez Rodriguez, P. Zamora, J. Benitez, Y. D. Ko, H. P. Fischer, U. Hamann, B. Pesch, T. Bruning, C. Justenhoven, H. Brauch, D. M. Eccles, W. J. Tapper, S. M. Gerty, E. J. Sawyer, I. P. Tomlinson, A. Jones, M. Kerin, N. Miller, N. McInerney, H. Anton-Culver, A. Ziogas, et al. (2010) Associations of breast cancer risk factors with tumor subtypes: a pooled analysis from the Breast Cancer Association Consortium studies. *J Natl Cancer Inst,* 103, 250-63.

Zanatta, L., H. Bouraima-Lelong, C. Delalande, F. R. Silva & S. Carreau (2011) Regulation of aromatase expression by 1alpha,25(OH)2 vitamin D3 in rat testicular cells. *Reprod Fertil Dev,* 23, 725-35.

Zanotto-Filho, A., E. Braganhol, M. I. Edelweiss, G. A. Behr, R. Zanin, R. Schroder, A. Simoes-Pires, A. M. Battastini & J. C. Moreira (2011) The curry spice curcumin selectively inhibits cancer cells growth in vitro and in preclinical model of glioblastoma. *J Nutr Biochem*.

Zhang, C., B. Li, X. Zhang, P. Hazarika, B. B. Aggarwal & M. Duvic (2010) Curcumin selectively induces apoptosis in cutaneous T-cell lymphoma cell lines and patients' PBMCs: potential role for STAT-3 and NF-kappaB signaling. *J Invest Dermatol,* 130, 2110-9.

Zhang, M. Z., J. Xu, B. Yao, H. Yin, Q. Cai, M. J. Shrubsole, X. Chen, V. Kon, W. Zheng, A. Pozzi & R. C. Harris (2009) Inhibition of 11beta-hydroxysteroid dehydrogenase type II selectively blocks the tumor COX-2 pathway and suppresses colon carcinogenesis in mice and humans. *J Clin Invest,* 119, 876-85.

Ziech, D., R. Franco, A. Pappa, V. Malamou-Mitsi, S. Georgakila, A. G. Georgakilas & M. I. Panayiotidis (2010) The role of epigenetics in environmental and occupational carcinogenesis. *Chem. Biol. Interact.,* 188, 334-339.

4

Kaiso and Prognosis of Cancer in the Current Epigenetic Paradigm

Jaime Cofre
Federal University of Santa Catarina (UFSC), Molecular Embryology and Cancer Laboratory, Florianopolis, SC, Brazil

1. Introduction

The term cancer is used generically to represent a set of more than 100 diseases, including malignant tumors from different locations. The understanding, diagnosis and management of malignancies require scientific knowledge and experiences ranging from the knowledge of the complex epigenetic mechanisms (intracellular regulation) to the individual lifestyle choice in different societies. Therefore, cancer prevention, prognosis and control are issues of profound importance to global public health.

Cancer appears as a major public health problem both in developed and developing countries. According to the latest report from the International Agency for Research on Cancer (IARC) / WHO (Boyle & Levin, 2008), the overall impact of cancer more than doubled in 30 years. About 12 million cancer cases and 7 million cancer deaths are estimated to have occurred in 2008. Of these, lung cancer had the greatest incidence rate (1.52 million new cases), followed by breast cancer (1.29 million cases) and colorectal cancer (1.15 million cases). Due to poor prognosis, lung cancer was the leading cause of death (1.31 million), followed by stomach cancer (780,000 deaths) and liver cancer (699,000 deaths About one million new cancer cases and 589,000 cancer deaths are estimated to have occurred in South America, Central America and in the Caribbean. Prostate cancer was the most common cancer in men, followed by lung, stomach and colon and rectum. Breast cancer was the most common cancer in women, followed by cancers of the cervix, colon and rectum, stomach and lung (Boyle & Levin, 2008).

The continued population growth and ageing significantly affect the impact of cancer in the world, which is greater in developing and under-developed countries. Half of the world's new cancer cases and about two thirds of cancer deaths are estimated to have occurred in 2008 in these countries (Farmer et al., 2010). Therefore, it is essential that resources and efforts are directed towards guiding strategies for cancer prevention, diagnosis and treatment.

In this particular chapter the strategies for prevention, diagnosis and treatment in the current epigenetic scenario of the new molecular mechanisms proposed for the development of cancer will be discussed.

2. Epigenetics

Epigenetics is the study of heritable changes in phenotype or gene expression caused by mechanisms other than changes in DNA sequence. The molecular mechanisms of epigenetic inheritance and its relationship with the expression of chromatin include three interrelated processes, namely DNA methylation, genomic imprinting and histone modifications (Kouzarides, 2007). Through small chemical molecules called methyl groups, which bind covalently with DNA or histones, the epigenetic processes improve the ability of genome to store and transmit biological information beyond the known structure and sequence of genetic material.

In recent years we have faced a new paradigm, a view more focused on the cell and on the search for information layers outside of the cell nucleus and even of the DNA as the center for information of the cell. These layers of epigenetic information transcend embryogenesis and cancer development processes, as follows.

3. The embryogenesis as an epigenetic process

The importance of epigenetics in experimental biology is decisively felt in the process of cell differentiation. The information and epigenetic marks are essential to determine which cell is phenotypically different from any other cell as a result of embryogenesis. This allows us to reprogram a somatic cell and transform it based on epigenetic principles, in a cell with characteristics of pluripotent stem cells. These cells are called ips cells (induced pluripotent stem cells)(Takahashi et al., 2007). In the Ips cells the DNA has not been changed or modified and the pluripotent state can be inherited during each cell division. This indicates that the changes in the machinery of epigenetic information, rather than genetic material, play a decisive role in controlling differentiation.

4. The cancer as an epigenetic process

The process of cancer development involves genomic changes identified as genetic and also changes in the epigenetic information (Jones & Baylin, 2002; Hake et al., 2004; McGarvey et al., 2008). Altered DNA methylation patterns have been described and histone modifications in cancer cells may occur at different stages of tumor development and contribute to the development and progression of cancer (Galm et al., 2006; McGarvey et al., 2008).

Historically, the first evidence has emerged that the contribution of epigenetics to cancer development comes from nuclear transfer experiments. Nuclear transfer provides a tool for selective reprogramming of the epigenetic state of a cell genome, without changing their genetic constitution, with the purpose of assessing the role of epigenetics in tumorigenesis.

Experiments with frogs have shown that renal carcinoma nuclei can be reprogrammed to support embryonic development at the tadpole stage (McKinnell et al. 1969). Similar results were also obtained with nuclei from medulloblastoma in mice (Li et al. 2003). Therefore, the nuclei of cancer cells can be reprogrammed through a process of nuclear transfer.

Another experimental approach was also based on nuclear transfer with blastocyst formation. However, it included the creation of explants from the inner cell mass in "in vitro" culture to develop embryonic stem cell lines (Hochedlinger et al., 2004). These embryonic stem cells were used to confirm the origin of the tumor clone and test the initial conservation of the tumorigenic capacity of these cells originated by tumor cores. In these experiments it has been unequivocally demonstrated that the clones derived from cancer cells and that the nuclei of cancer cells (leukemia, lymphoma and breast cancer) were able to sustain the embryonic development until the preimplantation blastocyst stage. It has also been demonstrated that the oocyte cytoplasm is able to reprogram the epigenetic state of some nuclei of tumor cells, transforming these cells into pluripotent and also enabling them to sustain the differentiation of multiple somatic cell types such as melanocytes, lymphocytes and fibloblasts. Therefore, the cancer state is an epigenetic cell state susceptible of change regardless of the DNA alterations (Feinberg, 2008).

The role of epigenetics was also confirmed by studying cohorts of twins and analyzing the concordance in cancer between monozygotic and dizygotic twins, and, thus, providing information about whether family patterns are influenced by environmental or genetic patterns. If the concordance in cancer is greater between monozygotic twins (who share 100% of the genes) than between dizygotic twins (who share in average 50% of the segregated genes) the genetic effects are probably more important. On the other hand, if the concordance rate is similar in both types of twins, then the environmental effects are probably more important. Thus, the use of statistics to analyze large populations of twins allows us to estimate the magnitude of environmental and genetic effects on susceptibility to sporadic cancer.

This retrospective study has shown that hereditary factors make a minor contribution to susceptibility to most types of neoplasms, indicating that the environment plays a major role in sporadic cancer in populations living in the study areas (Lichtenstein et al., 2000). The study, on the other hand, stresses that some types of cancer, such as prostate and colorectal cancers are more influenced by genetic factors than previously thought.

Thus, even more important aspects related to diseases are being reworked, and cancer may no longer be categorized as a disease based on genetics alone, and all the data indicate that most commonly diagnosed cancers in the world have primarily environmental or epigenetic origin. Except for some types of cancer considered hereditary, familial adenomatous polyposis, colorectal cancer and prostate cancer, the contribution of hereditary factors to the development of cancer is thought to be relatively small.

5. How the epigenetics affects genetics

The DNA methylation takes place only at cytosine bases that are located 5′ to a guanosine in a CpG dinucleotide. This dinucleotide is actually underrepresented in the genome, but short regions, known as CpG islands, are rich in CpG content. Most CpG islands are found in the proximal promoter regions of almost half of the genes in the mammalian genome and are, generally, unmethylated in normal cells. In cancer, however, the hypermethylation of these promoter regions is now the most well categorized epigenetic change to occur in tumours, it is found in virtually every type of human neoplasm and is associated with the inappropriate transcriptional silencing of genes, involving tumour-suppressor genes.

These tumour suppressor genes are predicted to be important for tumorigenesis, but seem not to be frequently mutated and *de novo* hypermethylation of CpG islands in the promoters of *MLH1* (mutL homologue 1, colon cancer, non-polyposis type 2) (Herman et al., 1998) and

Author	Organ/tissue	Genes studied	Altered genes-aberrant methylation-aberrant Distribution (p)
Herman et al., 1995	Many Cancers	p16	p16 - Hypermethylation (the first evidence)
Herman et al., 1998	Colorectal	hMLH1	hMLH1-Hypermethylation ($p < .001$)
Esteller et al., 2000	Breast, Ovary	BRCA1	BRCA1- Hypermethylation ($p < .0002$)
Esteller et al., 2000	Colorectal	hMGMT	MGMT (k-RAS)-Hypermethylation ($p= .002$)
Cho et al., 2003	Stomach	CAGE	CAGE- Hypomethylation
Russo et al., 2005	Lung/Blood	p16/DAPK	p16/DAPK - Hypermethylation ($p = .001$)
Sinha et al., 2009	Tongue	p16	p16- Hypermethylation ($p =.0361$)
Tanemura et al., 2009	Skin	RASSF1A	RASSF1A- Hypermethylation ($p < .005$)
Daí et al., 2009	Lung	Kaiso	kaiso- Cyoplasmic distribution ($p = .005$)
Kim et al., 2010	Intestine	p16/MINT31	Hypermethylation- p16 ($p < .0001$) MINT31 ($p < .004$)
Muggerud t al., 2010	Breast	RASSF1A	RASSF1A- Hypermethylation ($p < .001$)
Taghavi et al., 2010	Esophagus	p16	p16 - Hypermethylation ($p <.001$)

Table 1. Summary of epigenetic modifications associated with human cancers (prospective and retrospective studies).

MGMT (O^6-methylguanine-DNA methyltransferase) (Esteller et al., 2000b), seems to be that leads to their inactivation. Hypermethylation of the promoter of *MLH1* can lead to microsatellite instability, and hypermethylation of the promoter of *MGMT* leads to increased G →A transitions. Additionally, there is a growing list, of other tumour suppressor genes in which promoter hypermethylation is the only mechanism for the loss of function of these genes in tumorigenesis: breast cancer 1, early onset (BRCA1) (Esteller et al., 2000a), von Hippel–Lindau syndrome (VHL)(Herman et al., 1994), p16 (Herman et al., 1995; Russo et al., 2005; Sinha et al., 2009; Kim et al., 2010; Taghavi et al., 2010), death associate protein (DAP) kinase 1 (DAPK1) (Russo et al., 2005), and *RASSF1A* (Tanemura et al., 2009; Muggerud et al., 2010), which encodes a protein of unknown function that can bind to the *RAS* oncogene (Table 1).

The epigenetic modifications can also be induced by environmental and occupational exposures thus contributing to carcinogenesis. A good example is the methylation changing the absorption wavelength of cytosine, into the range of incident sunlight, resulting in CC →TT mutations, which commonly occur in skin cancers (Pfeifer et al., 2000). So, tobacco smoke has been estimated to account for 30% of all cancer deaths and 85% of lung cancer deaths due to the presence of thousands of mutagenic compounds, including polycyclic aromatic hydrocarbons and nitrosamines. In this case, methylated CpGs are also preferred binding sites for benzo(a)pyrene diol epoxide and other carcinogens that are found in tobacco smoke (Yoon et al., 2001). These cause DNA adducts and G →T transversion mutations, which are often found in the aerodigestive tumours of smokers (Ziech et al., 2010). On the other hand, one of the most well established occupational carcinogenic agents is asbestos along with a growing list of tumorigenic agents that include: wood-dust particulates, solvents, paints, dye products, gasoline, petroleum-based mixtures, benzenes, mineral oils, phthalates and metal ions (Ziech et al., 2010). For these agents, the free radical-induced damage is suggested to be involved in aberrant epigenetic changes observed during the carcinogenic process. The understanding of epigenetic alterations has become clearer the mechanism by which lifestyle choice like smoking and drinking, diet, environment and infections affecting the DNA tissue-specific cells and altering the behavior of cells in this tissue.

Finally, besides DNA hypermethylation, cancer cells have also been shown to undergo dramatic global hypomethylation (Ehrlich, 2002; Cho et al., 2003) and changes in the organization of the histone protein complex that would serve as epigenetic biomarkers indicative of the carcinogenic process (He and Lehming, 2003). Many references in the literature published in the last years reviewed the importance of alterations in DNA methylation and histone modifications for better cancer diagnostics and therapeutic strategies (Jones and Baylin, 2002; Ziech et al., 2010; table 1). Further review of this subject is not within the scope of this chapter, which is aimed to show the role of proteins, like Kaiso, which interact with methylated DNA and participate in the establishment of cancer, as we shall see later in this chapter.

6. The epigenetics and proteomics walking together toward the diagnosis and prognosis of cancer, in the current epigenetic context

A major challenge faced by cancer therapy is to be able to predict the early stage of the disease in order to provide an appropriate treatment for the patient (Ludwig and Weinstein, 2005). In this regard, the molecular biomarkers have been useful for distinguishing different subtypes of patients with different clinical profiles and at all stages of disease, expanding our prognostic ability (Seligson et al., 2005).

Over the past decades high-throughput technologies including genomics, epigenome, transcriptome and proteomics have been applied to improve our understanding of cancer pathogenesis in order to develop strategies aimed to improve cancer treatment (Seligson, 2005; Ocak et al., 2009). The ultimate goal of these technologies is to help develop noninvasive methods for specific and sensitive diagnosis and facilitate prediction of the response of a patient to a given therapy, as well as help identify potential therapeutic targets (Ueda et al., 2011).

The most important technologies used in the study of cancer are proteomics and epigenomics that help understand that cancer cell phenotype is primarily determined by proteins, and, thus, a genomic or transcriptome approach of the disease are extremely limited. This can be said because it is known that i. levels and protein expression have a low correlation with mRNA levels, ii. proteins undergo post-translational modifications that may alter its function, iii. in the same cell can express different proteins using a mechanism of differential splicing from the same mRNA and very important as we shall see iv. the same protein may have a different function depending on the cellular compartment where it is located. Therefore, the protein detection techniques, including immunohistochemistry (IMH), in this new context, are of vital importance for understanding cellular processes and disease emergence.

In order to better understand the cancer cell and the development of cancer, proteomic information projects have been created based on epigenetics in which proteins and their interactions with the epigenome inside the cell become the key aspect in the understanding of how cancer cells work (Stefanska et al., 2011; Jerónimo et al., 2011). Therefore, knowledge of machinery and all the protein interactions established by them may be important for the prognosis of the tumor and the development of a proper drug to fight cancer and to determine the mechanisms of the disease.

A good example is the study of the proteins of the methyl-CpG-binding domain (MBD) that "read" and interpret the signals in DNA methylation and are critical mediators of various epigenetic processes. We currently know that the family of MBD proteins is formed by five MBD1 and MeCP2 -4 members. There is also a member of non-classical MBD protein called Kaiso that uses a "zinc finger" domain to bind to methylated DNA and mediate transcriptional repression. The factor Kaiso and its partner p120ctn are considered similar to the β-catenin-TCF/LEF (T-cell factor / Lymphoid Enhancing factor) pair that regulate genes of canonical Wnt pathways, with the peculiarity that Kaiso (the difference in TCF/LEF) can interact with the epigenome in cancer development. As usually, hypermethylation is a recognized gene silencing mechanism in processes of tumorigenesis and drug resistance. Obviously, the MBD protein and Kaiso could be important modulators of tumorigenesis and excellent therapeutic targets for developing anti-cancer therapies (Sansom et el., 2007). Therefore, the role of protein detection methods in the diagnosis, prognosis and even in the development of therapies against cancer is unquestionable in the current epigenetic scenery of disease etiology (Yoshimura et al., 2011).

7. The multifunctional protein and its relation to cellular compartments

A single protein can have different functions in a cell and these functions concern the compartment where they are located. One of the best documented examples is that transglutaminase 2 (TG2) may act as a transglutaminase, G-protein kinase, protein disulfide isomerase or as an adapter protein. These multiple biochemical activities are involved in a wide variety of cellular processes such as differentiation, cell death, inflammation, cell migration and others. The specific microhabitats and subcellular compartments of location of the plasma membrane, cytoplasm, nucleus, mitochondria, or extracellular space are important in the development of different biochemical activities by the same protein structure (Park et al., 2010).

Thus, in our search for a drug target, e.g., cancer, we must always know the location of a given protein in the cell and be aware of how this cell places these proteins in different micro environments, and that more often than not these different functions may occur simultaneously. So part of the strategy to find the correct pharmacological targets is the previous understanding of the structure and the establishment of subcellular microenvironments inside the cells and the better knowledge of the complex and dynamic subcellular compartmentalization that will be further explained.

Therefore, immunohistochemistry provides information that cannot be obtained in any other way, which is the relationship between the pathological state and the dimension of the altered compartment (Oliver and Jamur, 2009; Dabbs, 2010), of great relevance to the establishment of the cancer diagnosis, as we shall see soon.

8. The multifunctional proteins, compartments and cancer

Surprisingly, over the past few decades multifunctional proteins provided the basis of the study of some diseases, including cancer. Alterations and aberrations of the multifunctional proteins regarding their distribution and subcellular localization have been used to diagnose the pathological state. I will consider briefly connexins, β-catenin and kaiso as examples of these proteins and their role in cancer development.

9. Connexins

Connexins can be channels of intercellular communication or proteins that trigger processes of proliferation or apoptosis, depending on the cellular context (Goodenough & Paul, 2003).

Traditionally, it was believed that the role of connexins in cancer development was related to its role in intercellular communication channel or gap junctional intercellular communication activity (GJIC). In fact, cancer was the first disease to be associated with connexin disorders (Loewenstein, 1979). The evidence was mainly related to the use of tumor-promoting agents (non-mutagenic carcinogens) and mitogens that decreased the activity of connexin-mediated intercellular communication (Budunova & Williams, 1994) and, on the other hand, antineoplastic agents or chemicals promoting cell coupling through these proteins (King & Bertram, 2005). It was also shown that tumor-derived cells were deficient in expression of connexins (Lee et al., 1992; Laird et al., 1999) and that studies of overexpression of these proteins showed decrease in cellular proliferation (Yamasaki & Naus, 1996). This created a favorable scenario that could lead one to believe that the decrease in expression of connexins and, thus, intercellular communication, was related to cell proliferation and tumor progression.

The most important work on the change in concepts regarding these channels of communication was the transfection of connexin43 that makes it possible reversing the neoplastic phenotype of a strain of human glioblastoma cells and that showed that phenotypic reversion was associated with a cytoplasmic localization of connexins without increasing the ability to establish intercellular communication between cells (Huang et al, 1998). Therefore, a new concept has arisen, according to which connexins could have two different functions not necessarily connected: (i) intercellular communication in the plasma membrane and (ii) direct modulation of cell growth control in cell cytoplasm.

Concerning the connexin role in regulating cell proliferation, two hypotheses have been developed: 1) a downregulation of connexins from the plasma membrane is an indirect result of the activation of MAPK (mitogen-activated protein kinase) and Akt (phosphoinositide-activated kinase) and 2) they act as negative regulators of intercellular junctions (Kojima et al., 2004). However, other lines of evidence indicated that the connexins were directly involved in the regulation of cell growth and that its downregulation would contribute to (and not be a consequence of) the loss of cell cycle control (Vinken et al., 2006).

A detailed study supporting this latter idea used transfection of connexin 43 in human osteosarcoma cells, which inhibited cell proliferation without restoring intercellular communication (Zhang et al., 2001). In this model direct connexin 43 changes the expression of p27/Kip1 (the cyclin-dependent kinase inhibitor). Importantly, Cx43, or at least the carboxy terminal tail of this protein has been localized within the nucleus with the use of immunohistochemistry, confirming an intracellular regulatory role (Dang et al., 2003; Cofre & Abdelhay, 2007).

In primary breast tumors, immunohistochemistry can clearly detect the cytoplasmic expression of connexins 43 and 26, being a commonly used diagnostic test for this stage of the disease (Kanczuga-koda et al., 2006). However, immunohistochemistry shows that in the same metastatic tumor cells taken from the lymph node, the expression of connexin43 and 26 changes and has now expanded, though in the plasma membrane. This increased expression in the cell membrane is considered the earliest event in the process of metastasis

(Kanczuga-koda et al., 2006). The important diagnostic value of IMH is evident in the resolution stage of the disease.

Although the role of connexins in the process of metastasis is controversial because some studies indicate that connexin expression is inversely proportional to metastatic capacity of a primary tumor (Nicolson et al., 1988), other studies reveal that connexins might be involved in metastasis (Carystinos et al., 2001).

At least it is clear that, unlike previously thought, connexins have a tumor suppressor function, but not from a classical point of view, since there are no mutations of this protein associated with carcinogenesis. So, they seem to have different effects on different stages of carcinogenesis, (depending on the connexin isoform or cell type in which it is expressed). Connexins seem to favor cell proliferation when they are downregulated (cytoplasmic localization) and increase the potential for invasion and metastasis when they are overexpressed (initially in the plasma membrane) (for a review of this literature sees Crespin et al., 2008). As we shall see at the end of this chapter, this issue needs to be clarified for a better understanding of subcellular compartmentalization and mechanisms of regulation of intracellular signaling.

10. β-catenin

The decisive factor in paradigm change regarding proteins with various compartments inside the cell and its relationship with the processes of disease establishment was β-catenin. The protein β-catenin is a transcriptional factor with nuclear function and also a structural component of tight junctions (adherens junctions) in the plasma membranes of the cell. The role of cell adhesion was the first to be characterized and such role is possible because β-catenin interacts with cadherins and with the actin cytoskeleton via an adapter protein α-catenin (Kemler, 1993)(Figure 1a). The transcriptional function developed as part of the intracellular pathways of the canonical Wnt. In the nucleus β-catenin acts as a cofactor along with TCF/LEF in the upregulation of a variety of oncogenes including cyclin D1 and c-myc (Figure 1d). The canonical Wnt/Wingless signaling pathway plays an important role in embryonic development and tumorigenesis (Morin, 1999; Polakis, 2000; Bienz, 2005).

The transcriptional role of β-catenin is very interesting because it involves translocation from the cytoplasm to the nucleus and initiates the expression of its target genes within it (Nusse, 1997; Akiyama, 2000). In the absence of Wnt binding a macromolecular complex formed by the cytoplasmic protein APC (adenomatous polyposis coli), Axin and disheveled (DSH) stimulate the phosphorylation of β-catenin. Directly responsible for this phosphorylation is the protein casein kinase 1 (CK1) and glycogen synthase kinase 3 (GSK3). Β-catenin phosphorylated is destined to a ubiquitin-mediated degradation of β-catenin (Figure 1 b). So, in the absence of Wnt signaling levels of β-catenin are kept low by the action of Gsk3 and CK1 (Clevers, 2006; McDonald et al., 2009).

Translocation of β-catenin only happens when the receptors of the canonical Wnt pathways are activated and the macromolecular complex is recruited to the plasma membrane proteins with CK1 and GSK3 and thus could not phosphorylate β-catenin (Figure 1 c). The key point in this model is that the activation of canonical pathway leads to stabilization of β catenin. Therefore, Wnt signaling would finally prevent β-catenin degradation, which could then translocate to the nucleus and perform its transcriptional activity (Clevers, 2006). As we shall see later, this classical interpretation may change when additional information on subcellular compartmentalization is gained.

In clinical practice aberrant changes in the expression of β-catenin in the nucleus have made it possible to suggest the use of this molecule as a complement to the differential diagnosis of various cancers, including cancers of the gastrointestinal tract, lung and tumors of gynecological origin (Montgomery & Folpe, 2005). Also, the absence or loss of nuclear expression of β-catenin expression associated with strong cytoplasmic P-cadherin was associated with melanoma aggressiveness and poor patient survival, establishing an important prognostic value in these types of cancer for β-catenin (Bachmann et al., 2005).

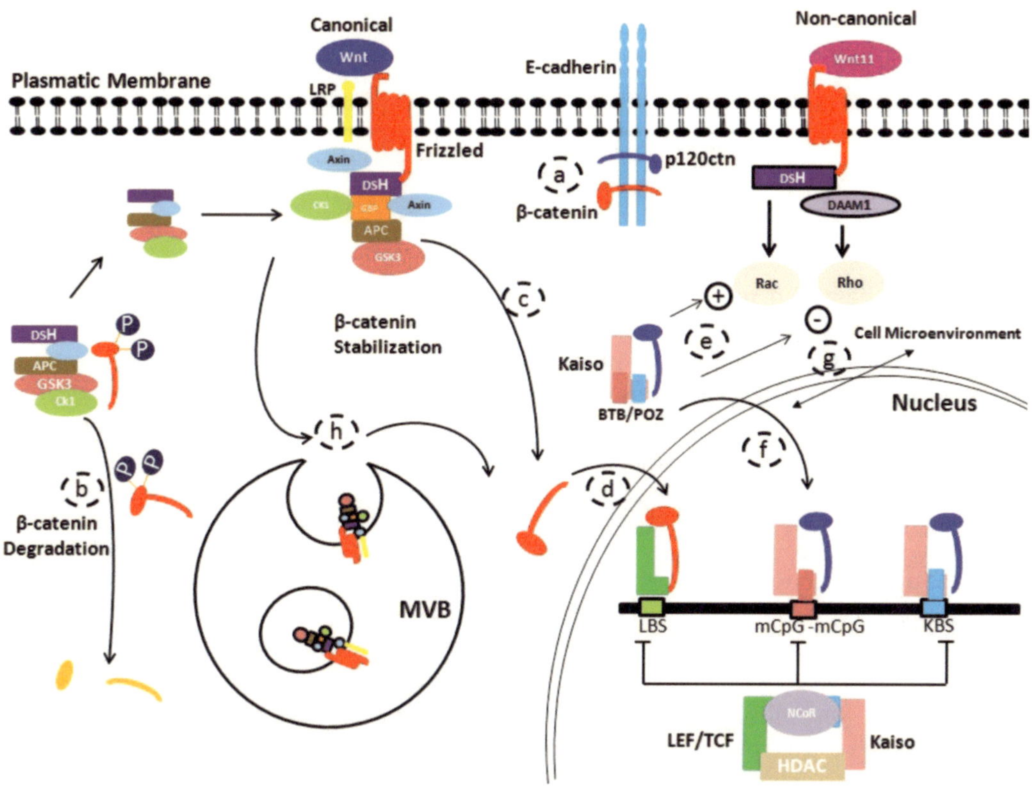

Fig. 1. Canonical and non-canonical Wnt signaling pathway. Crosstalk between Kaiso, Kaiso–p120ctn, β-catenin and Endossomal compartments. a. In the absence of Wnt ligands or in the case of high E-cadherin concentrations, β-catenin and p120ctn associate with E-cadherin, promoting intercellular adhesion. b. In the absence of Wnt binding, a macromolecular complex formed by the cytoplasmic protein APC (adenomatous polyposis coli), Axin and disheveled (DSH) stimulate the phosphorylation of β-catenin. Directly responsible for this phosphorylation is the protein casein kinase 1 (CK1) and glycogen synthase kinase 3 (GSK3). B-catenin phosphorylated is destined to a ubiquitin-mediated degradation of β-catenin. c. The activation of canonical pathway leads to stabilization of β catenin. Therefore, Wnt signaling would finally prevent β-catenin degradation, which could then (d.) translocate to the nucleus, and perform its transcriptional activity, associate with lymphoid enhancer-binding protein (LEF)/T-cell factor (TCF). e. If E-cadherin is mutated or

downregulated, p120ctn become at least partly cytoplasmic. Cytoplasmic p120ctn is stable and modulates small GTPases by stimulating RAC and inhibiting RHO. Both small GTPases are stimulated by non-canonical Wnt signalling. f. Kaiso translocate into the nucleus and within the nucleus kaiso associates with co-repressors (N-CoR) and histone deacetylases (HDAC) and represses genes harbouring KBS (Kaiso-binding sites) or methylated CpG (mCpG) islands in their regulatory domain. Likewise, a NCoR complex with lymphoid enhancer-binding protein (LEF)/T-cell factor (TCF) represses genes with a LEF binding sequence (LBS). g. Translocation of Kaiso in the nucleus and vice versa is mainly under the influence of microenvironmental factors. h. The protein complexes involving the Wnt receptor, Gsk3 and CK1 (among others), are then taken inside the lumen of the multivesicular bodies (MVBs), separating Gsk3 from their cytoplasmic substrates and it also produces the stabilization of β-catenin. APC, adenometous polyposis coli protein; BTB/POZ, broad-complex, tramtrak and bric-a-brac/poxvirus and zinc finger domain; DAAM1, Dishevelled-associated activator of morphogenesis 1; GBP, GSK3-binding protein; LRP, LDL-receptor-related protein (Wnt co-receptor). Wnt signalling pathway modified from Van Roy & McCrea, 2005.

11. Kaiso

This protein has been recently considered revolutionary due to its multifunctional role, modulating cytoplasmic processes and fulfilling transcriptional functions. It has the specific ability to interact with methylated DNA configuring an interesting pharmacological target for molecules that participate in the interphase of the epigenome. It is also known to be decisive in the process of tumorigenesis, and cytoplasmic accumulation of this protein, such as detection by IMH, plays an important role in the prognosis of some cancers. Because of these important reasons, the impact produced by this protein in a new scenario in epigenetic cancer shall deserve greater consideration.

Kaiso protein (encoded by the zinc finger and broad-complex, tramtrack and bric-a-brac (BTB)-domain-containing 33 gene ZBTB33) is a transcriptional factor that has a BTB/POX domain for the protein-protein interaction in the amino-terminal portion and a "Zinc Finger" domain for interaction with DNA in the carboxyl-terminal portion (Collins et al., 2001; Daniel & Reynolds, 1999). Due to the aforementioned characteristics Kaiso is member of a subfamily of "zinc finger" proteins known as POZ-ZF (Daniel & Reynolds, 1999). Most members of this subfamily (POZ-ZF) transcriptional factors including, Kaiso, BCL-6, PLZF, HIC-1, FAZF, APM1, MIZ-1, ZBTB7 and champignon are involved in the process of cancer development (Bardwell & Treisman, 1994; Albagli et al., 1995; Wales et al., 1995; Schneider et al., 1997; Reuter et al., 1998; Hoatlin et al., 1999; Maeda et al., 2005a).

Kaiso protein interacts specifically with p120 catenin (p120ctn), a member of the armadillo family that owns β-catenin (Daniel & Reynolds, 1999). β-catenin and p120ctn are very similar molecules possessing the two i. domains of interaction with the cytosolic portion of cadherins and ii. the ability to translocate from the cytoplasm to the nucleus (Reynolds & Roczniak-Ferguson, 2004). A p120ctn is a regulator of the kaiso function and it is known that in the nucleus of the cell they directly modulate the action of canonical Wnt pathways and target genes of β-catenin, which is another indication of the importance of Kaiso in the development of cancer (Daniel, 2007).

The genes transcriptionally regulated by Kaiso are matrilysin (Spring et al., 2005), c-myc and cyclin D1 (Van Roy & McCrea, 2005), all of them widely known for their involvement in cell proliferation and metastasis and all also regulated by the domain "Zinc finger" of Kaiso (Daniel, 2007). Gene Wnt11 is another important and well- known regulatory target, which belongs to the non-canonical Wnt pathways (Kim et al., 2004).

The non-canonical Wnt pathways are involved in cell polarity and cell movements of epithelial-mesenchymal transition observed during gastrulation, and also during the process of metastasis (Wallingford et al., 2002; Veeman et al., 2003). The cytoplasmic molecules involved in the transduction of non-canonical Wnt pathway are DSH (Dishevelled) and DAAM1 (Dishevelled-associated activator of morphogenesis 1) (Habas et al., 2001) that through two independent and parallel pathways lead to activation of GTPases, Rho (Marlow et al., 2002; Habas et al., 2001) and Rac (Habas et al., 2003)(Figure 1 e). Ultimately, the activation of a kinase assorted to the Rho called ROCK would be responsible for the reorganization of the cytoskeleton (Veeman et al., 2003). p120ctn regulates the cell cytoplasm proteins Rho and Rac (Van Roy & McCrea, 2005) and Kaiso would be indirectly related to processes that involve reorganization of the cytoskeleton during metastasis.

The Kaiso protein, unlike other members of the subfamily, appears to be the only factor with bimodal features in their interaction with DNA, being able to interact specifically with methylated CpG island sites and with consensus DNA sequences CTGCNA (Prokhortchouk et al., 2001; Daniel et al., 2002) (Figure 1 f). These interactions are important for the epigenetic silencing of tumor suppressor genes, which is an essential role of Kaiso in colon cancer development processes (Lopes et al., 2008).

Regarding epigenetic silencing, the Kaiso protein also acts as a histone-deacetylase-dependent transcriptional repressor (Daniel, 2007). The HDAC (histone deacetylase) catalyzes the deacetylation of histones and these changes facilitate more closed chromatin conformation and restrict gene transcription. The HDAC acts as a protein complex with corepressors recruited. Some of them are directly recruited by Kaiso as NCOR1 (nuclear receptor co-repressor 1) (Yoon et al., 2003) and SIN3A (Van Roy & McCrea, 2005) (Figure 1f).

The information on repression of target genes of the canonical and non-canonical Wnt pathways, associated with cancer (including matrilysin and Wnt11) can lead us to think that the role of Kaiso in the healthy cell is that of a tumor suppressor gene.

12. Kaiso and tumorigenesis

Almost all the members of the POZ-ZF family were found to be involved in cancer development. BCL-6 and PLZF are oncoproteins linked to non-Hodgkin's lymphoma and acute promyelocytic leukemia, respectively (Chen et al., 1994; Onizuka et al., 1995). FAZF and ZBTB7 are related to Fanconi's anemia and several other human cancers (Hoatlin et al., 1999; Maeda et al., 2005b; Dai et al., 2002; Pessler et al., 1997). On the other hand, ICH-6 and APM1 are candidate tumor suppressors in various human cancers (Schneider et al., 1997; Albagli, 2003).

Like other members of the subfamily POZ-ZF, the Kaiso protein has been implicated in cancer and the first indirect evidence emerged because the target genes of the Kaiso protein

(MTA2, MMP2, and siamois CiclinD1) are linked to cell proliferation or metastasis tumor, providing a good indication of the importance, though indirect, of Kaiso in tumorigenesis processes.

More consistent and direct data about the participation of Kaiso in the cancer development process have been recently obtained, when it has been found that Kaiso inhibits activation mediated by β-catenin of the Mmp7 gene (also known as matrilysin), which is well known for metastatic spread (Spring et al., 2005). Recently another study suggests that Kaiso can regulate TCF/LEF1-activity, via modulating HDAC1 and beta-catenin-complex formation (Iioka et al., 2009) (Figure 1f). This shows that Kaiso can directly regulate the signaling pathway of canonical Wnt / β-catenin widely known for its involvement in human tumors. Other evidence also showed that Kaiso rescues the dorsalization of the mesoderm produced by β-catenin and siamois in Xenopus laevis (Park et al., 2005). Siamois is a high mobility group (HMG)-box transcription factor that promotes the dorsalization of the mesoderm of amphibians and is a well-known target of the canonical Wnt pathway involving TCF/LEF. The Kaiso overexpression decreases the ability of TCF/LEF to interact with β-catenin, which implies that Kaiso and TCF/LEF are associated in the nucleus (Van Roy & McCrea, 2005). Other target genes of canonical Wnt pathway, such as Fos, Myc and CCND1 also appear to be directly regulated by Kaiso. On the other hand, the non-canonical Wnt pathways would also be modulated by Kaiso, at least in Xenopus, where it has been demonstrated that Kaiso depletion directly directly activates the Wnt11 promoter (Kim et al, 2004).

However, there is still controversy regarding the Kaiso's oncogenic or tumor suppressor role. As aforementioned, it is known that matrilysin and Wnt11 are repressed by Kaiso, and, thus, it is believed that it might act as a tumor suppressor (Dai et al., 2009). Nevertheless, Kaiso could also act as a methylation-dependent oncogene, repressing the tumor suppressor gene CDKN2A and providing increased survival of colon cancer cells (Lopes et al., 2008). The epigenetic silencing role of kaiso was approached to produce a depletion of Kaiso (by RNA interference) and an increased expression of the tumor suppressor gene CDKN2 was found, which did not affect the DNA methylation levels. As a result, the colon cancer cells were more susceptible to cell death mediated by chemotherapy (Lopes et al., 2008). It is then possible to assess the importance of kaiso as a possible therapeutical target to improve the efficiency of the current cancer treatments.

13. Subcellular localization of Kaiso and prognosis of cancer

As expected for a transcriptional factor, the Kaiso protein is often found in the nucleus of several tumor or non-tumor derived mammalian cell lines (Daniel, 2007). Recent studies using immunohistochemistry analysis of normal and tumor tissue revealed that Kaiso protein is predominantly localized in the cytoplasm of the cell or is totally absent, though (Soubry et al., 2005).

This seems to be unusual because Kaiso has a signal "NLS" highly conserved and required for any protein with nuclear localization. Moreover, Kaiso uses classical nuclear transport mechanisms through interaction with Importin α/β nuclear (Kelly et al., 2004). One possible explanation is that Kaiso, like other proteins or factors that normally reside in the cytoplasm, require a post-translational modification, to be targeted and translocated to the cell nucleus.

However, 2009 data has shown for the first time that the subcellular localization of Kaiso in the cytoplasm of a cell is directly associated with the poor prognosis of patients with lung cancer (non-small cell), and around 85 to 95% of lung cancers are non-small cell (Dai et al., 2009). Such data shows a direct relationship between the clinical profile of patients with pathological expression of Kaiso. Therefore, evidence of changes in subcellular localization seems to be relevant to the diagnosis and prognosis of various types of human tumors.

14. Analysis of the subcellular location of Kaiso in Mielode Chronic Leukemia (CML)

Data obtained by our group in collaboration with the laboratory of stem cells of the Brazilian National Cancer Institute (INCA of Rio de Janeiro), headed by Dr. Eliana Abdelhay, shows the subcellular distribution of Kaiso by immunofluorescence on cell lines K562, used as a model of CML in the blastic phase. As it can be seen in Figure 2a, the expression of Kaiso is clearly cytoplasmic (Cofre, J., personal communications). As expected, cytoplasmic expression is significantly reduced when using the duplex for inhibition of Kaiso (Rnai) 48 hours after transfection (Figure 2b). As a control, we used the β-tubulin marker and demonstrated that the duplex Kaiso does not modify the expression of this marker after transfection for 48 hours (Figure 2 c and d) .

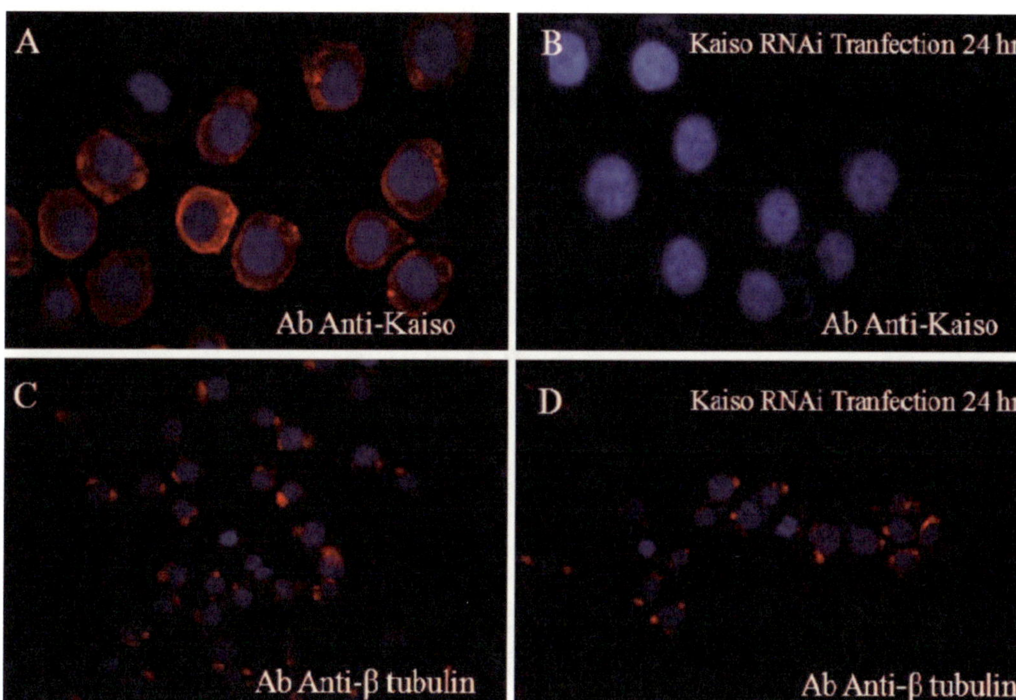

Fig. 2. Immunofluorescence analysis of kaiso expression. A.Kaiso was expressed in the cytoplasm of K562 cells (a human erythroleukemic line). B. siRNA-Kaiso efficiently down-regulates cytoplasm expression after 48 hours transfection. As a control, we used the marker beta-tubulin and showed that siRNA-Kaiso does not modify the expression of this marker after 48 hours transfection.

These results are promising, first because they make it possible to relate the LMC disease to the presence of cytoplasmic Kaiso, and second, because the molecule may have a diagnostic value of clinical interest, not only in LMC, but also in other types of leukemia.

15. The new view of cellular compartments

Another noteworthy aspect is that the cellular compartments are currently the object of many discussions in experimental biology, and we are witnessing a reconceptualization of these compartments, which involves the way they are structured and work, as well as their possible relationships with disease development at the cellular level.

It is logical to think that since a cell is in a process of constant division, for any given cell division, the elements in the nucleus and the cytoplasm are mixed, and at this important moment for cellular functioning, the cytoplasmic and nuclear components share the same general compartment that is the cytoplasm of the cell under division. According to this view, there is a very tenuous separation between the cytoplasm and the nucleus of a cell, and the sub compartments generated inside the cytoplasm are what really matters in a cell. Although many scenarios of the separation of specific functions have been detected inside the nucleus (Zhao et al., 2009; Spector & Lamond, 2011), none of these microenvironments would be maintained in cells in the process of cell division.

These new sub compartments that are important for the understanding of the mechanisms of diseases such as cancer are the networks of endocytic membrane represented by a system of interconnected membranous organelles and endosomes that are responsible for the selection of destination and transport of various types of macromolecules from the extracellular milieu into the cell and within the cell. A recent discovery reveals that the process of endocytosis and endosomes would be crucial for the maintenance of cellular homeostasis, ensuring the compartmentalization of transduction processes of intracellular signals (Scita & Di Fiore, 2010). It is now widely accepted that systems of endocytic membrane trafficking and intracellular signaling are closely interconnected and endosomes could act as signaling platforms (Hupalowska & Miaczynska, 2011).

The main endosomal compartment that regulates intracellular signaling processes would be the so-called multivesicular bodies (MVB). It would have a specific role in the sequestration of receptors activated in the membrane that by means of an intracellular mechanism of endocytosis would be placed inside the lumen of the MVB, unable to access the components of intracellular signaling, which would reduce and negatively regulate the signaling pathway of these receptors (Katzmann et al., 2002; Raiborg & Stenmark, 2009).

Surprisingly, this compartment can also play a role in positive regulation of certain signaling pathways through sequestration of inhibitors (Taelman et al., 2010). Because of its important role in cancer, it is worth mentioning that the Gsk3 and CK1 promoted by the Wnt signaling pathways would be hidden in internal vesicles inside the MVB. The protein complexes involving the Wnt receptor, Gsk3 and CK1 (among others), are then taken inside the lumen of the MVB, separating Gsk3 from their cytoplasmic substrates (Figure 1h). Consequently, in the absence of Gsk3, which is now inside the MVB, β-catenin would be stabilized in the cytoplasm, translocate into the nucleus and activate transcription.

The endosomal compartments are, thus, a trapping mechanism of enzyme and receptors, and it is believed that it produces the stabilization of many cellular proteins. Coincidentally, as discussed in the chapter, proteins as connexin and Kaiso, which are essential for the diagnosis and prognosis of cancer, are always accumulated in the cytoplasm in cancer cells.

This knowledge of endosomal compartments can be of paramount importance for the understanding of the molecular mechanisms by which diseases such as cancer initiate. For example, in the case of specific connexins, the tumor suppressor role could be related to the sequestration of these proteins in MVB during the onset of this tumor. Other related studies have proposed connexins as platforms for sequestering signaling proteins, suggesting that connexins might directly sequester MAPK (Mitogen-Activated Protein Kinase), CDK (Cyclin-dependent kinase), and Src (Proto-oncogene tyrosine-protein kinase) by SH2 and SH3 domains of the carboxyl terminal tail of Cx43 and, thus, act as a tumor suppressor (Cofre & Bermudez, 2011).

No studies have shown the association of connexins and endosomal compartments, and yet such studies could help understand the controversy of the expression of connexins in the plasma membrane during early metastasis, which can be related to deregulation mechanisms of cellular physiology of the endocytic compartment.

16. Future directions

Therefore, a view focused on subcellular compartments and proteins modulating the epigenome can provide a greater understanding of the biology of malignant cells, as well as improve our approach to cancer treatment. It is known that cancer treatment is dictated by the stage of the disease, and that cancer treatment is more effective during the chronic phase of the disease. Unfortunately, clinical and molecular tests cannot predict disease progression, which can create an obstacle to diagnosis: the inability to identify subtypes of patients most likely to benefit from specific treatment options for specific stages of the disease, which would make it possible to offer a therapy targeted to a given cancer patient.

Finally, the understanding of this new biology of disease progression can provide markers for clinical diagnosis and different approximations for better therapeutic strategies. Also, there is always hope that we'll be able to identify proteins and signaling pathways that may be useful as reliable prognostic markers of the disease and therapeutic targets in the near future.

17. Acknowledgment

The author thanks Dr. João Menezes for his contribution in the immunofluorescence of Kaiso, Dra. Eliana Abdelhay and Luciana Pizzatti for critical discussion of the results of cytoplasmic expression of Kaiso. The study was supported by Brazilian National Cancer Institute (INCA of Rio de Janeiro).

18. References

Akiyama, T. (2000). Wnt/beta-catenin signaling. *Cytokine Growth Factor Rev.*, Vol.11, No.4, (December 2000), pp.273-282, ISSN 1359-6101.

Albagli, O.; Dhordain, P.; Deweindt, C.; Lecocq, G. & Leprince, D. (1995). The BTB/ POZ domain: a new protein-protein interaction motif common to DNA and actin-binding proteins. *Cell Growth Differ.*, Vol. 6, No.9, (September 1995), pp.1193–1198, ISSN 1044-9523.

Bachmann, I.M.; Straume, O.; Puntervoll, H. E.; Kalvenes, M.B. & Akslen, L. A. (2005). Importance of P-cadherin, beta-catenin, and Wnt5a/frizzled for progression of melanocytic tumors and prognosis in cutaneous melanoma. *Clin Cancer Res*, vol. 11, No. 24 part 1, (December 2005), pp. 8606-8614, ISSN 1078-0432.

Bardwell, V. J. & Treisman, R. (1994). The POZ domain: a conserved protein-protein interaction motif. *Genes Dev.*, Vol. 8, No.14, (July 1994), pp.1664–1677, ISSN 0890-9369.

Bienz, M. (2005).beta-Catenin: a pivot between cell adhesion and Wnt signalling. *Curr Biol.*, vol.15, No.2, (January 2005). pp.R64-R67, ISSN 0960-9822.

Boyle, P. & Levin, B (2008). *World Cancer Report 2008*, International Agency for Research on Cancer, ISBN 978-928-3204-23-7, Lyon, France.

Budunova, I. V. & Williams, G. M. (1994). Cell culture assays for chemicals with tumor-promoting or tumor-inhibiting activity based on the modulation of intercellular communication. *Cell Biol Toxicol*, Vol. 10, No. 2, (april 1994), pp. 71–116, ISSN 0742-2091.

Carystinos, G.D.; Bier, A. & Batist, G. (2001). The role of connexin-mediated cell-cell communication in breast cancer metastasis. *J Mammary Gland Biol Neoplasia*, Vol.6, No.4, (October 2001), pp. 431–440, ISSN 1083-3021.

Chen, Z.; Guidez, F.; Rousselot, P.; Agadir, A.; Chen, S.J.; Wang, Z.Y.; Degos, L.; Zelent, A.; Waxman, S. & Chomienne, C. (1994). PLZF-RAR alpha fusion proteins generated from the variant t(11;17)(q23;q21) translocation in acute promyelocytic leukemia inhibit ligand-dependent transactivation of wildtype retinoic acid receptors. *Proc. Natl. Acad. Sci. U. S. A.*, Vol.91, No.3, (February 1994), pp.1178–1182, ISSN 0027-8424.

Cho, B.; Lee, H.; Jeong, S.; Bang, Y. J.; Lee, H. J.; Hwang, K. S.; Kim, H. Y.; Lee, Y.S.; Kang, G. H. & Jeoung, D. I. (2003). Promoter hypomethylation of a novel cancer/testis antigen gene CAGE is correlated with its aberrant expression and is seen in premalignant stage of gastric carcinoma. *Biochem Biophys Res Commun.*, Vol. 307, No. 1, (July 2003), pp. 52-63, ISSN 0006-291X.

Clevers, H. (2006). Wnt/beta-catenin signaling in development and disease. *Cell*, Vol. 127, No.3, (November 2006), pp. 469–480, ISSN 0092-8674.

Cofre, J. & Abdelhay, E. (2007). Connexins in the early development of the African clawed frog Xenopus laevis (Amphibia): The role of the connexin43 carboxyl terminal tail in the establishment of the dorso-ventral axis, *Genet. Mol. Biol.*, Vol. 30, No.2, pp. 483-493, ISSN 1415-4757.

Cofre, J. & Bermudez R. (2011). Conexinas: Canais de Comunicação ou Supressores de Tumores?, In: *Discussão de novos paradigmas, Vida Embriologia e Evolução*, J. Cofre & K. Saalfeld (Eds), pp. 175-189, Editoraufsc, ISBN 978-853-2804-93-8, Florianópolis, Brazil.

Collins, T.; Stone, J. R. & Williams, A. J. (2001). All in the family: the BTB/POZ, KRAB, and SCAN domains. *Molecular and cellular biology*, vol. 21, No.11, (June 2001), pp.3609-3615, ISSN 0270-7306.

Crespin, S.; Defamie, N.; Cronier, L. & Mesnil, M. (2008). Connexins and Carcinogenesis, In: *Connexins: A Guide*, A. Harris & D. Locke, (eds.), pp. 529-542, Springer-Verlag, ISBN 978-193-4115-46-6, New York, USA.

Dabbs, D. J. (2010). Diagnostic Immunohistochemistry: Theranostic and Genomic Applications, Saunders, ISBN 978-141-6057-66-6, Philadelphia, USA.

Dai, M.S.; Chevallier, N.; Stone, S.; Heinrich, M.C.; McConnell, M.; Reuter, T.; Broxmeyer, H.E.; Licht, J.D.; Lu, L. & Hoatlin, M.E. (2002). The effects of the Fanconi anemia zinc finger (FAZF) on cell cycle, apoptosis, and proliferation are differentiation stage-specific. *J. Biol. Chem.*, Vol.277, No.29, (May 2002), pp. 26327–26334, ISSN 0021-9258.

Dai, S.D.; Wang, Y.; Miao, Y.; Zhao, Y.; Zhang, Y.; Jiang, G.Y.; Zhang, P.X.; Yang, Z.Q. & Wang, E.H. (2009). Cytoplasmic Kaiso is associated with poor prognosis in non-small cell lung cancer. *BMC Cancer*, Vol.9, pp. 178-189, ISSN 1471-2407.

Daniel, J.M. & Reynolds, A. B. (1999). The catenin p120(ctn) interacts with Kaiso, a novel BTB/POZ domain zinc finger transcription factor. *Mol Cell Biol*, vol.19, No.5, (May 1999), pp.3614-3623, ISSN 0270-7306.

Daniel, J.M.; Spring, C.M.; Crawford, H.C.; Reynolds, A.B. & Baig, A. (2002). The p120(ctn)-binding partner Kaiso is a bi-modal DNA-binding protein that recognizes both a sequence-specific consensus and methylated CpG dinucleotides. *Nucleic Acids Res.*, Vol. 30, No.13, (July 2002), pp. 2911–2919, ISSN 1362-4962.

Daniel, J. M. (2007). Dancing in and out of the nucleus p120^{ctn} and the transcription factor kaiso. *Biochimica Biophysica Ac*ta, Vol.1773, No.1, (January 2007), pp.59-68, ISSN 0006-3002.

Dang, X.; Doble, B. W. & Kardami, E. (2003).The carboxy-tail of connexin-43 localizes to the nucleus and inhibits cell growth. *Mol Cell Biochem.*, Vol.242, No.1-2, (January 2003), pp.35–38, ISSN 0300-8177.

Ehrlich, M. (2002). DNA methylation in cancer: too much, but also too little. *Oncogene*, vol. 21, No. 35, (August 2002), pp. 5400-5413, ISSN 0950-9232.

Esteller, M.; Silva, J. M.; Dominguez, G.; Bonilla, F.; Matias-Guiu, X.; Lerma, E.; Bussaglia, E.; Prat, J.; Harkes, I. C.; Repasky, E. A.; Gabrielson, E.; Schutte, M.; Baylin, S. B. & Herman, J. G. (2000a). Promoter hypermethylation and BRCA1 inactivation in sporadic breast and ovarian tumors. *J Natl Cancer Inst.*, Vol.92,No.7, (April 2000), pp.564-569, ISSN 0027-8874.

Esteller, M.; Toyota, M.; Sanchez-Cespedes, M.; Capella, G.; Peinado, M. A.; Watkins, D. N.; Issa, J. P.; Sidransky, D.; Baylin, S. B. & Herman, J. G. (2000b). Inactivation of the DNA repair gene O6-methylguanine-DNA methyltransferase by promoter hypermethylation is associated with G to A mutations in K-ras in colorectal tumorigenesis. *Cancer Res.*, Vol. 60, No.9, (May 2000), pp. 2368-2371, ISSN 0008-5472.

Farmer, P.; Frenk, J.; Knaul, F. M.; Shulman, L. N.; Alleyne, G.; Armstrong, L.; Atun, R.; Blayney, D.; Chen, L.; Feachem, R.; Gospodarowicz, M.; Gralow, J.; Gupta, S.; Langer, A.; Lob-Levyt, J.; Neal, C.; Mbewu, A.; Mired, D.; Piot, P.; Reddy, K. S.; Sachs, J. D.; Sarhan, M. & Seffrin, J. R. (2010). Expansion of cancer care and control in countries of low and middle income: a call to action. *Lancet*, vol.376, No. 9747, (August 2010), pp. 1186-1193, ISSN 1474-547X.

Feinberg, A. P. (2008). Epigenetics at the Epicenter of Modern Medicine. *JAMA.*, Vol. 299, No. 11, PP. 1345-1350, ISSN 1538-3598.Galm, O.; Herman, J. G. & Baylin, S. B. (2006).The fundamental role of epigenetics in hematopoietic malignancies. *Blood Rev.*, vol. 20, No.1, (February 2005), pp. 1-13, ISSN 0268-960X.

Goodenough, D. A. & Paul, D. L. (2003). Beyond the gap: functions of unpaired connexon channels.*Nat Rev Mol Cell Biol.*, vol. 4, No.4, (April 2003), pp.285-294, ISSN 1471-0072

Habas, R.; Kato, Y. & He, X. (2001). Wnt/Frizzled activation of Rho regulates vertebrate gastrulation and requires a novel Formin homology protein Daam1. *Cell*, Vol. 107, No.7, (December 2001), pp.843-854, ISSN 0092-8674.

Habas, R.; Dawid, .IB. & He, X. (2003). Coactivation of Rac and Rho by Wnt/Frizzled signaling is required for vertebrate gastrulation. *Genes Dev.*, Vol. 17, No.2, (January 2003), pp. 295-309, ISSN 0890-9369.

Hake, S.B.; Xiao, A. & Allis, C. D. (2004. Linking the epigenetic 'language' of covalent histone modifications to cancer. *Br J Cancer*, vol. 90, No. 4, (February 2004), pp. 761-769, ISSN 0007-0920.

He, H. & Lehming, N. (2003). Global effects of histone modifications. *Brief Funct Genomic Proteomic.*, Vol. 2, No. 3, (October 2003), pp. 234-243, ISSN 1473-9550.

Herman, J. G.; Latif, F.; Weng, Y.; Lerman, M. I.; Zbar, B.; Liu, S.; Samid, D.; Duan, D. S.; Gnarra, J. R.; Linehan, W. M. & Baylin, S. B. (1994). Silencing of the VHL tumor-suppressor gene by DNA methylation in renal carcinoma. *Proc Natl Acad Sci U S A.*, Vol. 91, No. 21, (October 1994), pp. 9700-9704, ISSN 0027-8424.

Herman, J.G.; Merlo, A.; Mao, L.; Lapidus, R.G.; Issa, J.P.; Davidson, N.E.; Sidransky, D. & Baylin, S. B. (1995). Inactivation of the CDKN2/p16/MTS1 gene is frequently associated with aberrant DNA methylation in all common human cancers. *Cancer Res.*, Vol. 55, No. 20, (October 1995), pp. 4525-4530, ISSN 0008-5472.

Herman, J. G.; Umar, A.; Polyak, K.; Graff, J. R.; Ahuja, N.; Issa, J. P.; Markowitz, S.; Willson, J. K.; Hamilton, S. R.; Kinzler, K. W.; Kane, M. F.; Kolodner, R. D.; Vogelstein, B.; Kunkel, T. A. & Baylin, S. B. Incidence and functional consequences of hMLH1 promoter hypermethylation in colorectal carcinoma. *Proc Natl Acad Sci U S A.*, vol. 95, No. 12, (June 1998), pp. 6870-6875, ISSN 0027-8424.

Hoatlin, M. E.; Zhi, Y.; Ball, H.; Silvey, K.; Melnick, A.; Stone, S.; Arai, S.; Hawe, N.; Owen, G.; Zelent, A. & Licht. J. D. (1999). A novel BTB/POZ transcriptional repressor protein interacts with the Fanconi Anemia Group C protein and PLZF. *Blood*,Vol. 94, No.11, (December 1999), pp. 3737–3747, ISSN 0006-4971.

Hochedlinger, K.; Blelloch, R.; Brennan, C.;Yamada, Y.; Kim, M.; Chin, L. & Jaenisch, R. (2004). Reprogramming of a melanoma genome by nuclear transplantation. *Genes Dev.*, Vol. 18, pp. 1875–1885, ISSN 0890-9369.

Huang, R. P.; Fan, Y.; Hossain, M. Z.; Peng, A.; Zeng, Z. L. & Boynton, A. L. (1998). Reversion of the neoplastic phenotype of human glioblastoma cells by connexin 43 (Cx43). *Cancer Res.*, vol.58, No.22, (November 1998), pp.5089–5096, ISSN 0008-5472.

Hupalowska, A. & Miaczynska, M. (2011).The New Faces of Endocytosis in Signaling, In: *Traffic*, 1.08.2011.,Availablefrom:http://onlinelibrary.wiley.com/doi/10.1111/j.16000854.2011.01249.x/pdf.

Iioka, H.; Doerner, S.K. & Tamai, K. (2009). Kaiso is a bimodal modulator for Wnt/beta-catenin signaling. *FEBS Lett.*, Vol. 583, No. 4, (January 2009), pp. 627-632, ISSN 1873-3468.

Jerónimo, C.; Bastian, P. J.; Bjartell, A.; Carbone, G. M.; Catto, J.W.; Clark, S. J.; Henrique, R.; Nelson, W. G. & Shariat, S.F. (2011). Epigenetics in prostate cancer: biologic and clinical relevance. Eur Urol., vol. 60, No. 4, (June 2011), pp. 753-766, ISSN 1873-7560.

Jones, P. A. & Baylin, S. B. (2002).The fundamental role of epigenetic events in cancer. Nat Rev Genet., vol. 3, No 6, (June 2002), pp. 415-428, ISSN 1471-0056

Kanczuga-Koda, L.; Sulkowski, S.; Lenczewski, A.; Koda, M.; Wincewicz, A.; Baltaziak, M. & Sulkowska, M.(2006).Increased expression of connexins 26 and 43 in lymph node metastases of breast cancer. *J Clin Pathol*, vol. 59, No.4, (April 2006), pp.429–433, ISSN 0021-9746.

Katzmann, D.J.; Odorizzi, G. & Emr, S.D. (2002). Receptor downregulation and multivesicular-body sorting. *Nat Rev Mol Cell Biol*, Vol. 3, No.12, (December 2002), pp. 893–905, ISSN 1471-0072.

Kelly, K. F.; Otchere, A. A.; Graham, M. & Daniel, J. M. (2004). Nuclear import of the BTB/POZ transcriptional regulator Kaiso. *J Cell Science*, Vol. 117, No.(Pt 25), (December 2004), pp. 6143-6152, ISSN 0021-9533.

Kemler, R. (1993). From cadherins to catenins: cytoplasmic protein interactions and regulation of cell adhesion, *Trends Genet*, vol. 9, No.9, (September 1993), pp.317–321, ISSN 0168-9525.

Kim, S.W.; Park, J.I., Spring, C.M.; Sater, A.K.; Ji, H.; Otchere, A.A.; Daniel, J.M. & McCrea, P.D. (2004). Non-canonical Wnt signals are modulated by the Kaiso transcriptional repressor and p120-catenin. *Nature cell biology*, Vol. 6, No.12, (November 2004), pp. 1212-1220, ISSN 1465-7392.

Kim, J.C.; Choi, J.S.; Roh, S.A.; Cho, D.H.; Kim, T.W. & Kim, Y.S. (2010). Promoter methylation of specific genes is associated with the phenotype and progression of colorectal adenocarcinomas. *Ann Surg Oncol.*, Vol. 17, No. 7, (January 2010), pp. 1767-1776, ISSN 1534-4681.

King, T. J & Bertram, J. S. (2005). Connexins as targets for cancer chemoprevention and chemotherapy. *Biophys Biochim Acta*, vol. 1719, No. 1-2, (October 2005), pp.146–160, ISSN 0006-3002.

Kojima, T.; Yamamoto, T.; Lan, M.; Murata, M.; Takano, K.; Go, M.; Ichimiya, S.; Chiba, H. & Sawada, N. (2004). Inhibition of MAP kinase activity moderates changes in expression and function of Cx32 but not claudin-1 during DNA synthesis in primary cultures of rat hepatocytes. *Med Electron Microsc.*, vol. 37, No.2, (June 2004),pp.101–113, ISSN 0918-4287.

Kouzarides, T. (2007). Chromatin modifications and their function. *Cell*, Vol. 128, No. 4, (february 2007), pp. 693-705, ISSN 0092-8674.

Laird, D. W.; Fistouris, P.; Batist, G.; Alpert, L.; Huynh, H. T.; Carystinos, G. D. & Alaoui-Jamali, M. A. (1999). Deficiency of connexin 43 gap junctions is an independent marker for breast tumors. *Cancer Res*, vol. 59, No.16, (August 1999), pp. 4104-4110, ISSN 0008-5472.

Lee, S.W.; Tomasetto, C.; Paul, D.; Keyomarsi. K. & Sager, R. (1992). Transcriptional down-regulation of gap-junction proteins blocks junctional communication in human mammary tumor cell lines. *J Cell Biol*, vol.118, No.5, (September 1992), pp. 1213–1221, ISSN 0021-9525

Li, L.; Connelly, M.C.; Wetmore, C.; Curran, T. & Morgan, J. I. (2003). Mouse embryos cloned from brain tumors. *Cancer Res.*, Vol. 63, pp. 2733–2736, ISSN 0008-5472.

Lichtenstein, P.; Holm, N. V.; Verkasalo, P. K.; Iliadou, A.; Kaprio, J.; Koskenvuo, M.; Pukkala, E.; Skytthe, A. & Hemminki, K. (2000). Environmental and heritable factors in the causation of cancer-analyses of cohorts of twins from Sweden, Denmark, and Finland. *N Engl J Med.*, vol. 343, No. 2, (July 2000), pp. 78-85, ISSN 0028-4793.

Loewenstein, W. R. (1979). Junctional intercellular communication and the control of growth. *Biophys Biochim Acta*, vol. 560, No. 1, (February 1979), pp.1–65, ISSN 0006-3002.

Lopes, E.C.; Valls, E.; Figueroa, M.E.; Mazur, A.; Meng, F.G.; Chiosis, G.; Laird, P.W.; Schreiber-Agus, N.; Greally, J.M.; Prokhortchouk, E. & Melnick, A. (2008). Kaiso contributes to DNA methylation-dependent silencing of tumor suppressor genes in colon cancer cell lines. *Cancer research*, Vol.68, No.18, (September 2008), pp. 7258-7263, ISSN 1538-7445.

Ludwig JA, Weinstein JN. Biomarkers in cancer staging, prognosis and treatment selection. Nat Rev Cancer, Vol. 5, No. 11, (November 2005), pp. 845-856, ISSN 1474-175X.

MacDonald, B.T.; Tamai, K. & He, X. (2009). Wnt/beta-catenin signaling: components, mechanisms, and diseases. *Dev Cell*, Vol.17, No.1, (July 2009), pp.9–26, ISSN 1878-1551.

Maeda, T.; Hobbs, R. M.; Merghoub, T.; Guernah, I.; Zelent, A.; Cordon-Cardo, C.; Teruya-Feldstein, J. & Pandolfi, P. P. (2005a). Role of the proto-oncogene Pokemon in cellular transformation and ARF repression. *Nature*, Vol. 433, No 7023, (January 2005), pp.278–285, ISSN 1476-4687.

Maeda, T.; Hobbs, R.M. & Pandolfi, P.P. (2005b). The transcription factor Pokemon: a new key player in cancer pathogenesis. *Cancer Res.*, Vol.65, No.19, (October 2005), pp. 8575–8578, ISSN 0008-5472.

Marlow, F.; Topczewski, J.; Sepich, D. & Solnica-Krezel, L. (2002). Zebrafish Rho kinase 2 acts downstream of Wnt11 to mediate cell polarity and effective convergence and extension movements. *Curr Biol.*, Vol.12, No.11, (June 2002), pp. 876-884, ISSN 0960-9822.

McGarvey KM, Van Neste L, Cope L, Ohm JE, Herman JG, Van Criekinge W, Schuebel KE, Baylin SB. (2008). Defining a chromatin pattern that characterizes DNA-hypermethylated genes in colon cancer cells. Cancer Res., vol. 68, No. 14, (July 2008), pp. 5753-5759, ISSN 1538-7445.

McKinnell, R.G.; Deggins, B. A. & Labat, D.D. (1969). Transplantation of pluripotential nuclei from triploid frog tumors. *Science* 165: 394–396, ISSN 0036-8075.

Montgomery, E. & Folpe, A. L. (2005). The diagnostic value of beta-catenin immunohistochemistry, Adv Anat Pathol, vol. 12, No. 6, (November 2005), pp. 350-366, ISSN 1072-4109.

Morin, P. J. (1999). beta-Catenin signaling and cancer. *BioEssays*, vol. 21, No.12, (December 1999), pp.1021-1030, ISSN 0265-9247.

Muggerud, A.A.; Rønneberg, J. A.; Wärnberg, F.; Botling, J.; Busato, F.; Jovanovic, J.; Solvang, H.; Bukholm, I.; Børresen-Dale, A. L.; Kristensen, V. N.; Sørlie, T. & Tost, J. (2010). Frequent aberrant DNA methylation of ABCB1, FOXC1, PPP2R2B and PTEN in ductal carcinoma in situ and early invasive breast cancer. Breast Cancer Res., Vol. 12, No. 1, (January 2010), pp. R13, ISSN 1465-542X.

Nicolson, G. L.; Dulski, K. M. & Trosko, J. E. (1988). Loss of intercellular junctional communication correlates with metastatic potential in mammary adenocarcinoma cells. *Proc Natl Acad Sci USA*, vol.85, No.2, (January 1988), pp.473–476, ISSN 0027-8424.

Nusse, R. (1997). A versatile transcriptional effector of Wingless signaling. *Cell*, vol.89, No. 3, (may 1997), pp. 321–323, ISSN 0092-8674.

Ocak, S.; Sos, M. L.; Thomas, R. K. & Massion, P. P. (2009).High-throughput molecular analysis in lung cancer: insights into biology and potential clinical applications. *Eur Respir J.*, Vol. 34,No. 2,(August 2009), pp. 489-506, ISSN 1399-3003.

Oliver, C. & Jamur, M. C. (2009). Immunocytochemical Methods and Protocols, Humana Press, ISBN 978-158-8294-63-0, New York, USA

Onizuka, T.; Moriyama, M.; Yamochi, T.; Kuroda, T.; Kazama, A.; Kanazawa, N.; Sato, K.; Kato, T.; Ota, H. & Mori, S. (1995). BCL-6 gene product, a 92- to 98-kD nuclear phosphoprotein, is highly expressed in germinal center B cells and their neoplastic counterparts. *Blood*, Vol. 86, No.1, (July 1995), pp. 28–37, ISSN 0006-4971.

Park, J. I.; Kim, S.W.; Lyons, J.P.; Ji, H.; Nguyen. T.T.; Cho, K.; Barton, M.C.; Deroo, T.; Vleminckx, K.; Moon, R.T. & McCrea, P.D. (2005). Kaiso/p120-catenin and TCF/beta-catenin complexes coordinately regulate canonical Wnt gene targets. *Dev Cell*, Vol. 8, No.6, (June 2005), pp. 843-854, ISSN 1534-5807.

Park, D.; Choi, S. S. & Ha, K-S. (2010). Transglutaminase 2: a multi-functional protein in multiple subcellular compartments. *Amino Acids*, vol.39, No. 3, (february 2010), pp. 619–631, ISNN 1438-2199.

Pessler, F.; Pendergrast, P.S. & Hernandez, N. (1997). Purification and characterization of FBI-1, a cellular factor that binds to the human immunodeficiency virus type 1 inducer of short transcripts. Mol. Cell. Biol., Vol. 17, No.7, (July 1997), pp. 3786–3798, ISSN 0270-7306.

Pfeifer, G. P.; Tang, M. & Denissenko, M. F. (2000). Mutation hotspots and DNA methylation. *Curr Top Microbiol Immunol.*, Vol. 249, pp. 1-19, ISSN 0070-217X.

Polakis, P. (2000). Wnt signaling and cancer, *Genes Dev.*, vol.14, No.15, (August 2000), pp. 1837–1851, ISSN 0890-9369.

Prokhortchouk, A.; Hendrich, B.; Jorgensen, H.; Ruzov, A.; Wilm, M.; Georgiev, G.; Bird, A. & Prokhortchouk, E. (2001). The p120 catenin partner Kaiso is a DNA methylation-dependent transcriptional repressor. *Genes Dev.*, Vol.15, No.13, (July 2001), pp.1613–1618, ISSN 0890-9369.

Raiborg, C. & Stenmark, H. (2009). The ESCRT machinery in endosomal sorting of ubiquitylated membrane proteins. *Nature*, Vol.458, No7237, (March 2009), pp.445–452, ISSN 1476-4687.

Reuter, S.; Bartelmann, M.; Vogt, M.; Geisen, C.; Napierski, I.; Kahn, T.; Delius, H.; Lichter, P.; Weitz, S.; Korn, B. & Schwarz, E. (1998). APM-1, a novel human gene, identified by aberrant co-transcription with papillomavirus oncogênese in a cervical carcinoma cell line, encodes a BTB/POZ-zinc finger protein with growth inhibitory activity. *EMBO J.*, Vol. 17, No.1, (January 1998), pp. 215–222, ISSN 0261-4189.

Reynolds, A. B. & Roczniak-Ferguson, A. (2004). Emerging roles for p120-catenin in cell adhesion and cancer. *Oncogene*, Vol.23, No.48, (October 2004), pp.7947–7956, ISSN 0950-9232.

Russo, A. L.; Thiagalingam, A.; Pan, H.; Califano, J.; Cheng, K. H.; Ponte, J. F.; Chinnappan, D.; Nemani, P.; Sidransky, D. & Thiagalingam, S. (2005). Differential DNA hypermethylation of critical genes mediates the stage-specific tobacco smoke-induced neoplastic progression of lung cancer. Clin Cancer Res., Vol. 11, No. 7, (April 2005), pp. 2466-2470, ISSN 1078-0432.

Sansom, O. J.; Maddison, K. & Clarke, A. R. (2007). Mechanisms of disease: methyl-binding domain proteins as potential therapeutic targets in cancer. *Nat Clin Pract Oncol.*, vol. 4, No. 5, (May 2007), pp. 305-135, ISNN 1743-4262.

Schneider, A.; Peukert, K.; Eilers, M. & Hanel, F. (1997). Association of Myc with the zinc-finger protein Miz-1 defines a novel pathway for gene regulation by myc. *Curr. Top. Microbiol. Immunol.*, Vol.224, pp.137–146, ISSN 0070-217X.

Scita, G. & Di Fiore, P.P. (2010). The endocytic matrix. *Nature*, Vol.463, No.7280, (January 2010), pp.464–473, ISSN 1476-4687.

Seligson, D.B.; Horvath, S.; Shi, T.; Yu, H.; Tze, S.; Grunstein, M. & Kurdistani, S. K. (2005). Global histone modification patterns predict risk of prostate cancer recurrence. *Nature*, vol. 435, No 7046, (June 2005), pp. 1262-1266, ISSN 1476-4687.

Seligson, D. B. (2005). The tissue micro-array as a translational research tool for biomarker profiling and validation. *Biomarkers*, vol. 10, suppl 1, (November 2005), pp. S77-S82, ISSN 1354-750X.

Sinha, P.; Bahadur, S.; Thakar, A.; Matta, A.; Macha, M.; Ralhan, R. & Gupta, S. D. (2009). Significance of promoter hypermethylation of p16 gene for margin assessment in carcinoma tongue. *Head Neck.*, Vol. 31, No. 11, (November 2009), pp. 1423-1430, ISSN 1097-0347.

Soubry, A.; van Hengel, J.; Parthoens, E.; Colpaert, C.; Van Marck, E.; Waltregny, D.; Reynolds, A.B. & van Roy, F. (2005). Expression and nuclear location of the transcriptional repressor Kaiso is regulated by the tumor microenvironment. Cancer Res., Vol.65, No.6, (March 2005), pp. 2224 -2233, ISSN 0008-5472.

Spector, D.L. & Lamond, A.I. (2011). Nuclear speckles. *Cold Spring Harb Perspect Biol.*, Vol. 3, No. 2, (February 2011), pp. a000646, ISSN 1943-0264.

Spring , C. M.; Kelly, K. F.; O'Kelly, I.; Graham, M.; Crawford, H.C. & Daniel, J. M. (2005).The catenin p120ctn inhibits Kaiso-mediated transcriptional repression of the beta-catenin/TCF target gene matrilysin. *Experimental cell research*, Vol.305, No.2, (May 2005), pp.253-265, ISSN 0014-4827.

Stefanska, B.; Huang, J.; Bhattacharyya, B.; Suderman, M.; Hallett, M.; Han, Z. G. & Szyf, M.(2011). Definition of the landscape of promoter DNA hypomethylation in liver cancer. *Cancer Res.*, vol. 71, No. 17, (July 2011),pp. 5891-5903, ISSN 1538-7445.

Taelman, V.F.; Dobrowolski, R.; Plouhinec, J.L.; Fuentealba, L.C.; Vorwald, P.P.; Gumper, I.; Sabatini, D.D. & De Robertis, E.M. (2010). Wnt signaling requires sequestration of glycogen synthase kinase 3 inside multivesicular endosomes. *Cell*, Vol.143, No.7,(December 2010), pp.1136–1148, ISSN 1097-4172.

Taghavi, N.; Biramijamal, F.; Sotoudeh, M.; Khademi, H.; Malekzadeh, R.; Moaven, O.; Memar, B.; A'rabi, A. & Abbaszadegan, M.R. (2010). p16INK4a hypermethylation and p53, p16 and MDM2 protein expression in esophageal squamous cell carcinoma. *BMC Cancer.*, Vol. 10, (April 2010), pp. 138, ISSN 1471-2407.

Takahashi, K.; Tanabe, K.; Ohnuki, M.; Narita, M.; Ichisaka, T.; Tomoda, K. & Yamanaka, S. (2007). Induction of pluripotent stem cells from adult human fibroblasts by defined factors. *Cell*, Vol. 131, No 5, (November2007), pp. 861-872, ISSN 0092-8674

Tanemura, A.; Terando, A.M.; Sim, M.S.; van Hoesel, A. Q.; de Maat, M. F.; Morton, D.L. & Hoon, D.S. (2009). CpG island methylator phenotype predicts progression of malignant melanoma. *Clin Cancer Res.*, Vol. 15, No. 5, (February 2009), pp. 1801-1807, ISSN 1078-0432.

Ueda, K.; Saichi, N.; Takami, S.; Kang, D.; Toyama, A.; Daigo, Y.; Ishikawa, N.; Kohno, N.; Tamura, K.; Shuin, T.; Nakayama, M.; Sato, T. A.; Nakamura,. Y. & Nakagawa, H. (2011). A comprehensive peptidome profiling technology for the identification of early detection biomarkers for lung adenocarcinoma. *PLoS One*, Vol. 6, No. 4, (april 2011), pp. e18567, ISSN 1932-6203.

Van Roy, F.M. & McCrea, P.D. (2005). A role for Kaiso-p120ctn complexes in cancer? *Nat Rev Cancer*, Vol. 5, No.12, (December 2005), pp. 956-964, ISSN 1474-175X

Veeman, M.T.; Axelrod, J.D. & Moon, R.T. (2003). A second canon. Functions and mechanisms of β-catenin-independent Wnt signaling. *Dev Cell*, Vol. 5, No.3, (Setember 2003), pp. 367-377, ISSN 1534-5807.

Vinken, M.; Vanhaecke, T.; Papeleu, P.; Snykers, S.; Henkens, T. & Rogiers, V. (2006). Connexins and their channels in cell growth and cell death. *Cell Signal*, vol. 18, No.5, (September 2005), pp.592–600, ISSN 0898-6568.

Wales, M. M.; Biel, M. A.; Deiry, W. E.; Nelkin, B. D.; Issa, J.-P.; Cavenee, W. K.; Kuerbitz, S. J. & Baylin, S. B. (1995). p53 activates expression of HIC-1, a new candidate tumor suppressor gene on 17p13.3. *Nat. Med.*, Vol.1, No.6, (June 1995), pp. 570–576, ISSN 1078-8956.

Wallingford, J.B.; Fraser, S.E. & Harland, R.M. (2002). Convergent extension: the molecular control of polarized cell movement during embryonic development. *Dev Cell*, Vol.2, No.6, (June 2002), pp.695-706, ISSN 1534-5807.

Yamasaki, H. & Naus, C. C. (1996). Role of connexin genes in growth control. Carcinogenesis, Vol.17, No.6, (June 1996),pp.1199–1213, ISSN 0143-3334.

Yoon, J.H.; Smith, L.E.; Feng, Z.; Tang, M.; Lee, C.S. & Pfeifer, G.P. (2001). Methylated CpG dinucleotides are the preferential targets for G-to-T transversion mutations induced by benzo[a]pyrene diol epoxide in mammalian cells: similarities with the p53 mutation spectrum in smoking-associated lung cancers. *Cancer Res.*, Vol. 61, No. 19, (October 2001), pp. 7110-7117, ISSN 0008-5472.

Yoon, H. G.; Chan, D. W.; Reynolds, A. B.; Qin, J. & Wong, J. M. (2003). N-CoR mediates DNA methylation-dependent repression through a methyl CpG binding protein Kaiso. *Mol. Cell*, Vol.12, No.3, (September 2003), pp. 723–734, ISSN 1097-2765.

Yoshimura, T.; Nagahara, M.; Kuo, C.; Turner, R. R.; Soon-Shiong, P. & Hoon, D. S. (2011). Lymphovascular invasion of colorectal cancer is correlated to SPARC expression in the tumor stromal microenvironment. Epigenetics, Vol. 6 No. 8, (august 2011), pp.1001-1011, ISSN 1559-2308.

Zhao, R.; Bodnar, M.S. & Spector, D.L. (2009). Nuclear neighborhoods and gene expression. *Curr Opin Genet Dev.*, Vol. 19, No.2, (March 2009), pp.172-179, ISSN 1879-0380.

Zhang, Y. W.; Morita, I.; Ikeda, M.; Ma, K. W. & Murota, S. (2001). Connexin43 suppresses proliferation of osteosarcoma U2OS cells through post-transcriptional regulation of p27. *Oncogene*, vol.20, No.31, (July 2001), pp. 4138–4149, ISSN 0950-9232.

Ziech, D.; Franco, R.; Pappa, A.; Malamou-Mitsi, V.; Georgakila, S.; Georgakilas, A. G. & Panayiotidis, M.I. (2010). The role of epigenetics in environmental and occupational carcinogenesis. *Chem Biol Interact.*, Vol. 188, No. 2, (July 2010), pp. 340-349, ISSN 1872-7786.

5

Targeting Molecular Pathways for Prevention of High Risk Breast Cancer: A Model for Cancer Prevention

Shayna Showalter and Brian J. Czerniecki
Department of Surgery and the Rena Rowan Breast Center, Abramson Cancer Center, Perelman School of Medicine, University of Pennsylvania, Philadelphia, PA, USA

1. Introduction

1.1 Role of vaccines in disease prevention and cancer prevention

Vaccine therapy is traditionally designed to be given prophylactically in order to prevent infectious diseases. Vaccines formulated against pathogens known to cause disease have been successfully created and implementation policies have been effective in the prevention and eradication of many life-threatening diseases. A well-know example of the success that is possible with a well constructed vaccine and an efficient vaccination strategy is the poliomyelitis vaccine. Poliomyelitis was first documented in the late 19th century and it quickly reached the level of causing annual global endemics. The vaccine was introduced in the United States in 1955 and was associated with an immediate reduction in the disease and eventual the elimination of wild-type polioviruses in the United States by 1972. Subsequent global expansion of polio vaccination has resulted in a drastic reduction of documented cases of the disease as well as eradication of wild type 2 poliovirus [1].

A natural next step after the development of prophylactic vaccines to prevent infectious disease was the emergence of vaccines used against specific infectious agents that are known to cause cancer. An estimated 12% of human cancers are attributable to viral infections [2]. Viral infections that are known to cause cancer include human papillomavirus (HPV), hepatitis B virus (HBV), hepatitis C virus (HCV), Epstein-Barr virus (EBV), and Kaposi's sarcoma-associated herpes virus (KSHV). Safe and effective vaccines have been developed against two oncovirus, HPV to prevent HPV-associated cervical carcinoma and HBV to prevent HBV-associated hepatocellular carcinoma.

1.2 Primary versus secondary prevention

A small number of cancers are directly associated with exposure to an oncovirus. Vaccinating against these viruses and preventing infection and subsequent cancer formation is referred to as 'primary cancer prevention'. This term also encompasses the theoretic potential of vaccinating against non-infectious cancers prior to tumorigenesis. Most cancers do not have a direct link to one specific pathogen. Therefore, experimental cancer vaccines are designed to stimulate an immune response against pathogens from established tumors. The creation of a vaccine against an established tumor, either invasive or pre-invasive, is referred to as 'secondary cancer prevention'. The goal of secondary cancer prevention is to use active specific immunotherapy to eradicate cancer cells without causing harm to healthy tissues. Successful secondary cancer prevention can have of a number of goals including inhibiting the evolution of pre-invasive to invasive disease, impeding the progression of disease and the formation of metastases, and increasing patient survival.

1.3 Breast cancer background and potential for vaccine therapy

Breast cancer remains the most common non-skin cancer diagnosis and the second leading cause of cancer related death in women [3]. Major improvements in the surgical and adjuvant treatment of breast cancer during recent decades have resulted in improved disease-free and overall survival for breast cancer patients. Morbidity from surgery, chemotherapy and radiation is substantial and even with optimal current treatments approximately 40,000 women a year succumb to breast cancer [3].

A general challenge to constructing an effective cancer vaccine is that all tumor cells contain self-antigens that vary from normal tissue by mutation or expression level and therefore cancer cells are able to evade immune surveillance. It is essential to find tissue and tumor specific molecules that are capable of stimulating an immune response. Vaccination efforts are often focused on high risk cancers where the clinical impact can be the greatest. Immunotherapy, which involves actively manipulating the immune system to target tumors, promises the potential for a safe and effective adjuvant treatment for patients with high risk breast cancer.

1.4 Molecular phenotypes of breast cancer

Elucidation of the molecular basis of carcinogenesis has identified that breast cancer and probably all solid tumors exist as discrete molecular subtypes rather than a single disease. Breast cancer is a heterogeneous disease and several microarray profiling studies have identified distinct subtypes of breast tumors that are associated with different clinical outcomes [4-7]. The implications of classifying tumors based on gene profiling are both therapeutic and predictive. Gene expression profiling facilitates both the prediction of patient outcome and the selection of patients that will benefit from specific adjuvant therapies.

Breast tumors are typically classified into five distinct genetic subtypes based on immunphenotype and the expression of the following receptors; estrogen (ER), progesterone (PR), human epidermal growth factor receptor-2/neu (HER-2), cytokeratin 5/6 (CK5/6) and epidermal growth factor (EGFR). *Luminal A* cancers are ER positive and/or PR positive, HER-2 negative and Grades 1 or 2. *Luminal B* cancers are (a) ER positive and/or PR positive and HER-2 positive or (b) ER positive and/or PR positive and HER-2 negative and high grade. *HER-2 type* cancers stain negative for ER and PR and positive for HER-2. *Basal-like* tumors have no staining for ER, PR and HER-2, but do stain positive for CK 5/6 and/or EGFR. Tumors that have no staining for all 5 markers are referred to as *Unclassified* [4, 8, 9]. These molecular phenotypes of breast carcinoma can be delineated with routine immunohistochemical markers. Substantial differences in the survival of patients with different subtypes have been reported. Luminal A tumors have a significantly better 5- and

10- year survival compared to Luminal B, HER-2, Basal-like and unclassified tumors [4]. In addition, certain ductal carcinoma in situ (DCIS) lesions over express HER-2, which results in a more rapid progression to invasive disease [11] and higher risk of recurrence [10, 13].

Anti-estrogen therapy is used for primary and secondary prevention of luminal tumors, but there are currently no similar options for prevention of the high risk tumors (Luminal B, Basal, HER-2). Trastuzumab is a human epidermal HER-2-targeted monoclonal antibody that has been shown to decrease recurrence and improve survival when used in the adjuvant setting combined with chemotherapy to treat patients with invasive disease that over-express the HER-2 protein [14]. The effect of trastuzumab has been postulated to be mediated by antibody-dependent cytotoxicity (ADCC) [15]. Unfortunately, this regimen is often not curative [14, 16] and patients can become resistant to therapy and ultimately fail [17] . A protein in the HER family would be an ideal target for a breast cancer vaccine. The HER family of tyrosine receptor kinases of which HER-1, HER-2, HER-3 and HER-4 are members make intriguing targets as these molecules are implicated in HER-2 and Basal-type breast cancers and also play a significant role in the development of some of the Luminal-type breast cancers.

2. Cancer and the immune response

The immune system is a complex and overlapping cellular network that protects against foreign pathogens and closely regulates self-tolerance. The innate system represents the first line of defense to tissue injury and foreign pathogens. It is comprised of natural barriers, cytokines, neutrophils, macrophages, dendritic cells (DCs), and natural killer (NK) cells [18, 19]. The innate response also includes the activation of the complement pathway. The early, antigen-nonspecific response of the innate immune system is necessary for the activation of the adaptive immune system which is comprised of B- and T- lymphocytes that express antigen-specific receptors and are ultimately responsible for producing and maintaining immunologic memory [20].

2.1 Cancer response to the immune system: exploitation and evasion and editing

In order for cancer cells to survive they must be able to either evade the immune system or to exploit it in a way that causes immune cells to actually enhance tumor growth. The immune response to neoplastic development is often described as paralleling the body's response to inflammation. It can be simplistically divided into an 'acute' and 'chronic' reaction. Epithelial cancer progression and eradication, similar to an inflammatory reaction, are regulated by both the innate and adaptive immune systems [21]. The specific immune cells involved paradoxically enhance and eliminate carcinogenesis. Accumulated data from animal and human studies has shown that the acute immune response to tumor growth is an anti-neoplastic process, comprised of CD8+ T cells, T_H1 cells and NK cells [22].

Continued epithelial cancer development leads to dysregulation between the two subsets of the immune system and excessive activation results in an immune response that is similar to the body's response to chronic inflammation. Chronic activation of innate immune cells is associated with an ongoing infiltration cells that facilitate the survival of neoplastic cell survival by stimulating angiogenesis, inflammation and proliferation [19-23]. The chronic activation of the innate immune system also directly contributes to cancer development by suppressing the anti-tumor adaptive immune response (CD8+ T cells, T_H1 cells, NK cells) and allowing tumor cells to escape from surveillance. One type of innate immune cells, myeloid suppressor cells, are known to accumulate in the peripheral blood of patients with cancer [24, 25]. Myeloid suppressor cells directly inhibit T lymphocytes and therefore inhibit the anti-tumor environment produced by innate immune cells [25, 26]. These cells also promote tumor growth by assisting in angiogenesis [27].

In addition to suppressing the anti-tumor effects of the adaptive immune system, chronic activation of the cells of the innate immune (B cells, T_H2 cells) response actually promotes tumor development [21]. Multiple population based studies have definitively linked chronic inflammatory conditions with the development of certain cancers. For example *Helibacter pylori* infection and gastric cancer, inflammatory bowel disease and colon cancer, and hepatitis and hepatocellular carcinoma [28-30]. Subsequent studies that revealed an inverse relationship between long-term usage of anti-inflammatory medications and a decreased cancer risk support the support the direct association between chronic inflammation and cancer development [31]. Through a variety of cellular mediators, chemokines and cytokines, innate immune cells and T_H2 cells are able to create a pro-tumor microenvironment that favors cell proliferation, genomic instability and malignant conversion [32].

In addition to exploiting the immune system to stimulate tumor growth, cancer cells must also be able to evade the immune response. Prolonged activation of the innate immune cells results in subsequent suppression of the anti-tumor adaptive immune response, therefore allowing tumors cells to avoid specific immune surveillance. Neoplastic lesions attract regulatory T cells that suppress cytotoxic T cells [33]. Furthermore, cancer cells avoid immune surveillance by over expression or mutation of self-peptides. These non-foreign antigens are only weakly immunogenic and thus evade the host immune response or do not induce an immune specific response in the same way that a completely foreign antigen would.

Growing tumors are phenotypically sculpted by the immune system. One of the risks of cancer immunotherapy is that it can result in 'immunoediting', whereby the immune response sculpts cancer cells into a more aggressive phenotype [34, 35]. Surviving tumor cells acquire the ability to evade immune recognition through selective pressures that favor the survival and reproduction of cancer cells that lack the selected antigen. In considering an immunotherapy target it is important to select an antigen that is central to the survival of the tumor cell or that contributes to the aggressiveness of the disease. Therefore, when the cells adapt, only variants that do not express the antigen will survive. This creates a tumor that consists of cells that are unable to survive or that have a phenotype that is associated with a better clinical prognosis [36]. This process of immunoediting explains in part why targeting only single antigens has resulted in limited clinical success.

2.2 General potential for vaccine therapy

The intimate relationship between cancer and the immune system illustrates the potential for an effective immunotherapeutic agent, such as a cancer vaccine, to harness the immune system and then to manipulate the immune cells to create a strong anti-tumor environment. Traditional vaccines are designed to be prophylactic. The immunogens in the vaccines are administered prior to disease exposure and effective immunity is created before infection. In contrast, cancer vaccines are intended to stimulate active immunity only after tumors cells are already present and established. Oftentimes, vaccines are not given until the cancer has spread systemically. Also, unlike bacteria or other microbes for which vaccines are used, all tumor cells also express antigens that are very similar to established self-antigens. The ideal vaccine target would be an antigen that is present only on cancer cells and not on normal cells. Since this is uncommon, one of the largest challenges in vaccine development is breaking immune tolerance without inducing autoimmune reaction that would be harmful to healthy tissues. Several vaccine approaches have been established for a multitude of cancers in both early and late stages.

3. Immune response in relation to invasive and in situ breast cancer

Breast cancer, both the *in situ* and invasive forms, is an ideal target for vaccine therapy since this disease creates a significant public health burden. There is potential for vaccines to inhibit the progression of in situ disease into invasive cancer. The ultimate goal would be to prevent the formation of breast cancer altogether. Central to success of using immunotherapy to treat breast cancer is that breast tumors have already been established to be relatively immunogenic and the growing tumors are subject to immunosurveillance. Tumor antigens that are over-expressed or mutated in breast cancer cells initiate the development of a tumor-specific adaptive immune response [23, 37, 38]. T-cells that recognize these antigens have been isolated from breast cancer patients [39, 40]. As further evidence that the cell-mediated immune reaction has an important role in breast cancer development and clinical outcome, lymphocyte infiltration has been shown to be associated with improved survival in breast cancer patients [41]. Recent data by Mahmoud *et al* confirmed that the presence of an efficient T-cell-mediated immune response is associated with breast cancer outcomes [42]. This study, a retrospective review of immunohistochemical staining from nearly 2000 patients with invasive breast cancer who received standard surgical and adjuvant treatment revealed that a higher number of $CD8^+$ T lymphocytes infiltrating the tumor of adjacent stroma was independently associated with longer survival in patients with invasive breast cancers.

In addition to being immunogenic, other aspects of breast cancer make it a good model for the development of a high-impact cancer vaccine, especially for patients with early stage disease. First, solid tumor cancer vaccines have had limited success when used to treat advanced or metastatic disease [43]. Breast cancer is most frequently treated with surgery and radiation therapy, which greatly decreases the disease burden, even in advanced cases. This tumor debulking provides a greater potential for disease eradication by competent immune cells. Second, the typical slow growing nature of most breast cancers allows for the expansion of immune cells over time with repeated vaccine boosters. Therefore, effective levels of active and immune competent cells can be achieved before the disease becomes systemic.

Although most cancer vaccines have been developed to treat metastatic and systemic disease, there are a number of theoretical benefits to instead delivering vaccine therapy to patients with limited, microscopic cancer burden (as neoadjuvant therapy) in the absence of bulky disease. For instance, immune-competent patients would be able to produce a significant response comprised of antigen-competent T-cells that can rapidly expand when presented with low antigen levels of early disease or early recurrence [44]. In addition, patients with early stage breast cancer do not require aggressive adjuvant therapy. The immune response in vaccinated patients with early stage cancers will not be compromised by the limitations of these cytotoxic treatments, most importantly the long-term reductions in functioning B and T lymphocytes [45-47]. There has therefore been a shift in the field of immunotherapy towards the treatment of patients with minimal disease and the prevention breast cancer formation.

3.1 Immunotherapy and ductal carcinoma in situ

With the increasing use of screening mammography, DCIS, the pre-invasive form of breast cancer, has become the most frequently diagnosed breast malignancy. DCIS is a heterogeneous disease both in terms of nuclear grade and expression of cell-surface receptors. DCIS is the non-obligate precursor of invasive ductal carcinoma. Low-grade DCIS may develop into invasive cancer slowly or not all. In contrast, high-grade DCIS almost always develops into invasive disease and often requires more aggressive surgical and adjuvant therapy [48].

Currently, in most clinical practices, DCIS lesions are examined for the over-expression of ER and PR. Interest in the correlation between the molecular biology of DCIS and its clinical aggressiveness has led to staining for other markers. The additional information about potential antigen targets on DCIS is useful to guide development of novel adjuvant vaccines against DCIS. Specifically, for the past 6 years we have routinely stained all of the tumors from our DCIS patients for the over-expression of HER-2. Other biologic markers that are may have prognostic significance include HER 1-4, Ki67, p21, bcl-2, p16 and COX-2, c-myc and survivin [10, 13, 49].

Multiple recent studies have concentrated on determining molecular phenotypes for DCIS similar to those described for invasive breast cancer. In 2010 *Tamimi et al* published a large case series of DCIS and invasive breast tumors that were analyzed using tissue microarray and immunostaining for ER, PR, HER-2, CK 5/6 and EGFR. The authors concluded that the same 5 molecular phenotypes used to describe invasive cancer were all identified among the cases of DCIS. The prevalence of the lesions was not consistent between the DCIS and invasive tumors; the Luminal A phenotype was significantly more frequent among the invasive cancers and the Luminal B and HER-2 molecular phenotypes were more frequent in DCIS. The triple negative (Basal-like) phenotype is very uncommon in DCIS [50]. This is consistent with other studies that show a higher prevalence of HER-2 over expression in DCIS compared to invasive breast cancer [51-53]. Additional work has expanded the traditional molecular profiling to incorporate many more biomarkers that have been found to be biologically relevant to invasive breast cancer, including p53, bcl-2 and P-cadherin. Bcl-2 was found to be one of the most common genes to be up regulated in the well-differentiated sample of DCIS [53] and has also been reported to be a predictor of good prognosis in invasive breast cancers [54].

DCIS is a particularly attractive vaccine target because the elimination of this disease prevents the subsequent development of invasive breast cancer. In addition, a novel neoadjuvant vaccine would be ideal to reduce size of these lesions prior to surgery. This could theoretically decrease the amount of breast tissue required to obtain clear margins during surgical excision and could also prevent the risk of subsequent recurrence. In general, DCIS patients are often otherwise healthy and are therefore able to mount an immune response to vaccination. The long latency period between the diagnosis of *in situ* disease and the development of invasive breast cancer, as well as the minimal disease burden of DCIS, provides an ideal therapeutic window to administer preventative vaccines. This strategy of treating early disease is applicable to early invasive breast cancer as well as to other cancers with indolent courses or those that are diagnosed in early stages, such as prostate and colon cancers, chronic leukemia and lymphomas [48, 55].

4. Selection of a tumor antigen target

The selection of an appropriate target tumor antigen is paramount to the success of any cancer vaccine. The ideal vaccine would stimulate a significant immune response without causing autoimmunity and without a detrimental side effect profile. One strategy to avoid autoimmunity and to enhance the specificity of the vaccine is to target tumor antigens that are overexpressed in cancer cells but have minimal expression in normal cells. As mentioned in a previous section, one challenge to targeting oncogenic molecules is that these tumor associated antigens are usually only weakly immunogenic and are therefore capable of evading the immune response, or the immune system can immunoedit the tumors leaving behind antigen negative tumor cells. Many of the breast cancer tumor antigens are also overexpressed in other cancers of epithelial cell origin (colon cancer and ovarian cancer). Previously targeted peptides in the experimental production of vaccines against breast cancer include Mucin (MUC)-1, Her-2, carcinoembryonic antigen (CEA), and survivin [56-58].

4.1 The EGF receptor family

The epidermal growth factor receptor (EGFR) family is a group of four related transmembrane receptor tyrosine kinases that have been implicated in the development of a multiple solid malignancies and have subsequently been targeted in a variety of novel therapeutics [59]. The EGFR family consists of HER-1 (also known as ERBB1), HER-2 (ERBB2), HER-3 (ERBB3) and HER-4 (ERBB4). These receptors bind 13 different ligands and form a number of different dimers between the family members. Ligand binding and dimerazation initiates various intracellular signaling pathways that affect numerous cellular processes involved in cell survival and proliferation. The oncogenic effects of the EGFR proteins result from amplification, over expression or mutation [60]. Refer to Fig. 1.

4.2 HER-1, HER-3, HER-4

HER-1 is a non-tissue specific peptide that has been implicated in the oncogenesis of multiple malignancies including breast, colorectal, pancreatic adenocarcinoma, brain glioma multiforme and non-small cell lung cancer [60]. The Food and Drug Administration (FDA) recently approved the use of a novel HER-1 directed tyrosine kinase inhibitor, erlotinab, in conjunction with other established medications for the treatment of advanced pancreatic and non-small cell lung cancers [61]. In addition, cetuximab is an anti-HER-1 monoclonal antibody that has been approved to treat patients with advanced colorectal cancer [62]. Although no anti-tumor vaccines have been formulated that are directed against HER-1, it is a feasible possibility to target this protein in order to develop an anti-HER-1 T cell response.

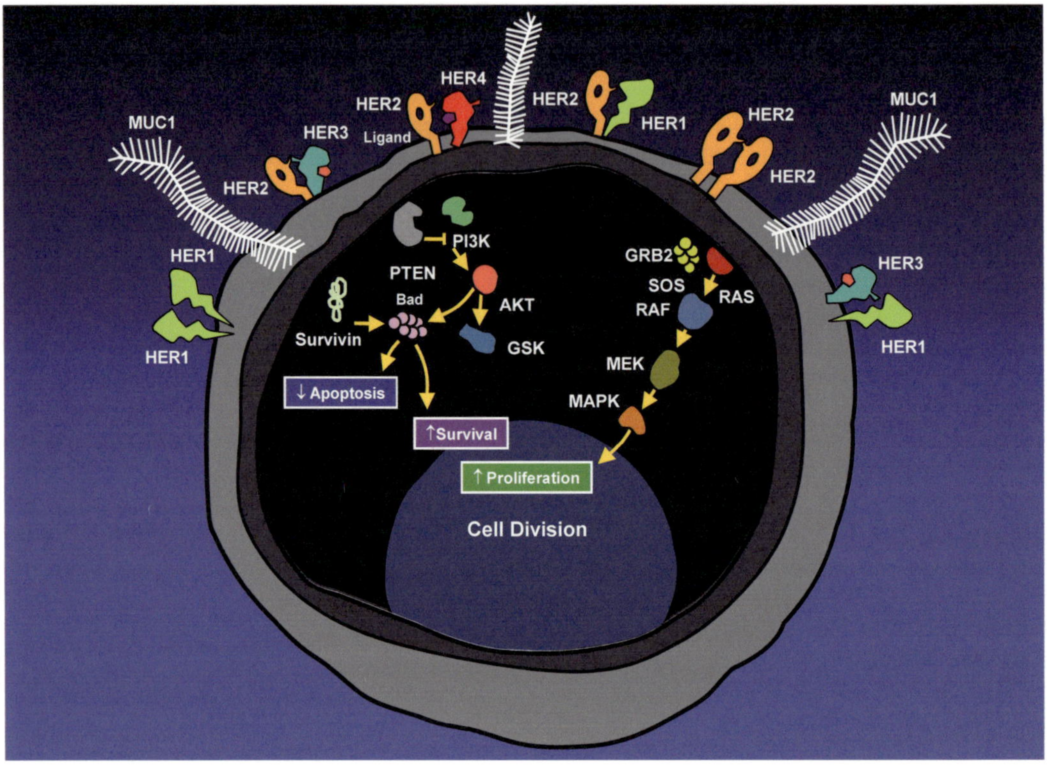

Fig. 1. The EGF receptor family.

HER-3 has a more ambiguous role in tumorigenesis compared to the other members of the EGFR family. It is frequently expressed in breast, ovarian and lung cancers [62-64]. The role of HER-4 in relationship to tumor development is also not clear. HER-4 mutations have recently been shown to augment proliferation and cell survival in melanomas. Agents that target HER-4 may be found to be effective against melanoma and other cancers [60].

4.3 HER-2

The HER-2 protein is a well established target of immunotherapy in breast cancer. The proto-oncogene HER-2 is found on chromosome 17q and encodes a transmembrane tyrosine kinase growth factor receptor. HER-2 over expression occurs in ovarian, pancreatic, gastric, lung and head/neck cancers [65-68]. Twenty to thirty percent of breast cancers have been found to amplify the HER-2 gene or overexpress the HER-2 protein, which portends a poorer prognosis and higher risk of recurrence in patients with both invasive and in situ disease [69].

HER-2 represents an ideal target for antigen-specific vaccines used to treat breast cancer. Over expression of this protein is immunogenic as it induces a T cell immune response causing HER-2 specific antibodies to be present in the serum of breast cancer patient [70].

The feasibility of HER-2 targeted vaccines has been demonstrated in animal models [71]. In addition, a number of phase I and II trials using HER-2 based vaccines of all types have been performed in patients with high risk breast cancer. The vaccines in all of these studies were well tolerated and caused minimal toxicity [18].

5. Development of dendritic cell vaccines for the treatment and prevention of cancer

The concept of producing a vaccine aimed at specific breast cancer antigens is theoretically straightforward although the details and execution are obviously complex to carry out. There are several different vaccine approaches under investigation for the treatment of early and late stage breast cancer (dendritic cells, whole tumor cells, peptide-based and viral-based) [72, 73]. Breast cancer vaccines utilizing all of these different strategies are in various stages of development [18, 38, 72-74]. A comprehensive review of the published data on all breast cancer vaccines is beyond the scope of this chapter.

The advent of dendritic cell (DC) vaccines, propelled by the ability to culture human DC cells, has provided promise for a novel vaccine strategies [75]. Despite preclinical evidence and high expectations for the potential effectiveness of DC-based cancer vaccines, initial results of clinical trials were somewhat disappointing with discordant tumor response rates [43, 76, 77]. However, continued interest in therapeutic possibilities of DC vaccines has led to recent successes and promising data in breast and other cancers. The efficacy of DC vaccines continues to improve as efforts have been made to optimize DC vaccines and circumvent tumor escape mechanisms.

5.1 Dendritic cells

DC vaccines represent one of a number of strategies for vaccinating patients against tumor-associated antigens. DCs are the most powerful of the APCs and are the primary means by which naïve T cells become immunized to specific antigens. DCs are unique in their ability to activate both the innate and adaptive immune systems. Immature DCs arise from progenitors in the bone marrow and then enter the blood stream and circulate throughout the peripheral tissues where they are exposed to foreign antigens. After capturing antigens, DCs undergo a maturation process that ultimately guides their travel to secondary lymphoid tissues. Once in the regional lymph nodes, the DCs process the captured antigen and then display the antigen as a peptide on their MHC molecules. DCs present the peptides to naïve T cells resulting in T lymphocyte expansion and differentiation.

In addition to T cell stimulation, contact with DCs causes activation of B lymphocytes which leads them to differentiate into plasma cells that subsequently release antibodies targeted against the initial pathogen. After antigen exposure, DCs also release cytokines which can activate the cells of the innate immune system, including eosinophils, macrophages, and NK cells. In this way, DCs are capable of activating both the innate and adaptive immunity and are central to the communication between the two immune systems [36, 78-80].

5.2 Production and adminstration of DC vaccines

No standard protocol exists for the production of DC vaccines, but there are some general components that are often involved. First, the DCs are collected from the patient via leukapheresis and then activated *ex vivo* with the specific tumor antigen and human granulocyte-macrophage colony-stimulating factor (GM-CSF). The activated DCs are then reintroduced to the patient in order to stimulate a T cell response. We have developed a DC vaccine targeting HER-2 and used to treat patients with DCIS. The production process will be briefly described.

First, peripheral blood monocytes are obtained by leukapheresis followed by elutriation under good clinical practice conditions. Monocytes are then cultured overnight in monocyte-macrophage serum-free medium GM-CSF and interleukin (IL)-4. Immature DCs are next pulsed with HER-2 MHC II binding peptides, extracellular and intracellular domain peptides for 12 hours. In order to potentiate the benefits of signaling infectious non-self at the time of vaccine administration, we then sequentially culture the cells with interferon-gamma (IFN-γ) and bacterial lipopolysaccharcharide (LPS), a TLR agonist, prior to pulsing with MHC class I peptides. As mentioned previously, TLR stimulation leads to cytokine release and DC maturation. This activation strategy assures that the DC are able to robustly secrete IL-12 which maximizes their ability to produce IFN-γ and a functional T cell response [55].

The major technical disadvantage to the use of DC vaccines relates to the *ex-vivo* nature of their generation. A number of obstacles must be dealt with in order to make the process successful and efficient [36, 81]. Most importantly, the production of DC must be made individually for each patient. The process is dependent on access to leukapheresis facilities at the treatment center. Leukapheresis is complex procedure that does not always generate consistent results. The procedure is associated with minimal patient morbidity including, brief electrolyte imbalances, minimal risk of infection and vascular injury. Another important consideration in the production of DC vaccines is the financial burden of manufacturing and administering such an individualized treatment. Sipuleucel-T, the only cancer vaccine that is currently approved by the FDA, is priced at $31,000 and is typically given three times, making a complete treatment cost $93,000. This is one of the most expensive cancer therapies ever approved [77, 82].

We advocate injecting the vaccines directly into distal lymph nodes. It has been shown that only a proportion of peripherally administered DCs migrate to regional lymph nodes [83]. Using ultrasound guidance to inject the cultured DCs directly into distal lymph nodes assures that a predetermined and defined quantity of antigen-loaded DC cells are delivered to the site of T-cell sensitization, thus allowing the vaccine to activate an adaptive immune response. This method also synchronizes peak IL-2 secretion to occur when the DCs are close to T cells. Vaccinating patients prior to surgical resection also allows us to have the opportunity to review the histopathological effects of vaccination on the tumor cells [36].

In April 2010, the FDA approved the first cancer vaccine. This individualized DC vaccine, Sipuleucel-T (Provenge; Dendreon Corp.), is approved for use in men with metastatic castration-resistant prostate cancer. Similar to other DC vaccines, the production of Sipuleucel-T begins with leukaphoresis and the isolation of peripheral blood mononuclear cells. The DCs are then activated by exposure to a recombinant fusion protein (prostatic acid phosphatase and GM-CSF). The treated cells are re-infused into the patient. This process is repeated every two weeks for a total of three treatments [84].

The results from initial trials reported a 41 % relative reduction in the risk of death and a trend toward increased survival in the men treated with Sipuleucel-T compared to the men in the placebo group [85, 86]. The IMPACT study, a double-blind, placebo-controlled, multicenter trial involving 512 men with metastatic castration-resistant prostate cancer, was designed with overall survival as the primary endpoint. Of note, these men were either asymptomatic or minimally symptomatic, representing a patient population that is at an earlier stage and therefore more likely to be amenable to immunotherapy. Compared with the placebo arm, patients in the Sipuleucel-T arm achieved a 22% relative reduction in the risk of death. This represented a 4.1 month increase in median overall survival between the placebo and Sipuleucel-T arms. There was no significant difference achieved in the prostate-specific antigen response or time to progression between the two arms. Sipuleucel-T was well tolerated [84].

6. DC vaccination in breast cancer

Successful reduction of HER-2 over expressing tumors requires activation of both the innate and adaptive immune responses [87]. As described, DCs are unique in their ability to elicit responses from tumor-specific effector and memory T cells. Numerous strategies exist that aim to introduce tumor antigens into DCs in order to generate vaccines (loading individual tumor peptides, transfer of tumor-specific DNA or RNA through lipofection or viral vectors, whole tumor cell fusion). An early DC vaccine strategy for breast cancer involved the production of DC/tumor cell fusion vaccines. Avigen *et al* conducted a trial in which 16 patients with metastatic breast cancer were injected with a fusion vaccine using tumor cells obtained from a biopsy and DCs acquired from leukapheresis [88]. Three patients had a significant clinical response. Unfortunately the efficacy of fusion cell generation is less than 45% and multiple patients were not able to receive the full course of vaccines due to limited yield.

In 2007, Park *et al* published data from a phase I study in which they treated 18 metastatic breast cancer patients with Lapuleucel-T (Dendreon Corp), a vaccine produced in a similar fashion as sipuleucel-T, although a HER-2 fusion protein is used [89]. The study was designed to evaluate the safety and immunologic activity of the novel agent. The therapy was well tolerated. Significant immune responses were stimulated (as measured by lymphocyte proliferation and IFN-γ enzyme-linked immunospot assays). The therapy was also associated with tumor response and extended disease stabilization. Further trials are warranted to determine the efficacy in patients with earlier stage disease and in combination with other anti-HER-2 therapies.

Another DC vaccine approach that is being explored is Adevexin (Introgen Therapuetics), made form leukapheresed APCs that are transfected with a replication-impaired adenoviral vector that brings the p53 gene under control of a cytomegalovirus promoter [90]. This vaccine is not specifically anti-HER-2, but instead works under the theory that p53 restoration can be used to treat cancer. This vaccine triggers p53-specific T-cell responses against cancer cells with mutant p53 and has proven to be safe and synergistically effective in a number of tumor types.

Currently other anti-HER-2 DC vaccines trials are recruiting patients and results of these trials are pending [74]. We are conducting a clinical trial with a novel DC vaccine designed to treat DCIS patients with lesions that overexpress HER-2. No other DC-based vaccines have been designed specifically to treat HER-2 expressing DCIS tumors. We anticipate a significant reduction in disease burden in our patients after a complete vaccine course. We hope that this vaccine will also be preventative in terms of both disease recurrence and rate of transformation into invasive breast cancer.

Our strategy of vaccine production utilizes both MHC I and II peptides as well as ex vivo activation with IFN-γ and LPS to yield polarized DC cells that induce a unique set of soluble factors including high levels of IL-12 and Th1 chemokines not elicited through traditional vaccines methods. This innovative DC vaccine strategy called Immune Conditioning by Activated Innate Transfer (ICAIT) uses monocyte-derived DCs that are activated with and a special clinical-grade TLR 4 ligand, LPS and IFN-γ (ICAIT-DC). This unique DC activation method gives the DCs qualities that are not found in the so-called "gold-standard" DCs used in prior vaccine trials. The "gold standard" DC vaccines, activated with TNF, IL-6, PGE2, IL-1β, have the potential to simulate aseptic inflammation [91]. In contrast, ICAIT-DCs produce high levels of factors that specifically enhance aspects of anti-tumor immunity such as NK cells which augment tumor rejection, and TNF and IL-12 which are anti-angiogenic [55, 92]. ICAIT-DCs also have the distinct ability to influence the quality of sensitized T cells and can condition T cells for recognition of HER-2 expressing tumors. Lastly, ICAIT-DCs posses a killer function that enables them to lyse breast cancer cells.

Our DC vaccine is unique in its design against DCIS rather than invasive breast cancer. Our first neoadjuvant trial involved treating patients with HER-2 expressing DCIS tumors. The patients were treated with a course of four weekly intranodal injections of ICAIT-DCs that had been pulsed with HER-2 derived proteins. This approach yielded promising results that have positive implications for the treatment and prevention of high risk breast cancers. Specifically, 85% of ICAIT-treated patients developed immune responses to at least one of the HER-2 peptides. Eleven of the 22 patients with residual DCIS treated with the vaccine in our initial studies showed loss of HER-2 expression and tumor regression. The immunized patients developed a specific immune response against the HER-derived peptides and presented high levels of CD4+ and CD8+ T lymphocytes. These results have potential positive implications not only for prognosis but also in terms of breast-conserving surgery [55]. Five of the 27 patients had no evidence of remaining disease. The vaccination was most effective in patients with hormone-independent DCIS as 40% of ER negative HER-2 positive patients had no residual disease whereas only 5% of ER positive HER-2 positive had no residual disease. The vaccine appeared to alter the phenotype of the remaining DCIS in the patients that were found to have residual disease. The rate of change to a different post-vaccination phenotype was significantly different between the ER positive and ER negative patients. 43.8% of the patients that were initially ER positive and HER-2 positive phenotype converted to ER positive and HER-2 negative phenotype. In comparison, 50% of the patients that initially had tumors that were ER negative and HER-2 positive changed to the ER negative and HER-2 negative phenotype. These results supported the safety and efficacy of the DC based HER-2 vaccine. The vaccine induced a decline or eradication of HER-2 expression (work not yet published).

7. Future direction and prevention

There are a number of molecules that have been discovered to be present in breast carcinomas that have not yet been exploited to their fullest potential. The future directions for the development of breast cancer vaccines should focus not only on targeting molecules that are specific tumor related antigens, but also to the downstream signaling pathways involved in tumorigenesis. For example, recent work has elucidated the role of survivin (Figure 1), a protein in the anti-apoptotic family. Blocking the expression of survivin, was found to have a direct role in the initiation of apoptosis of breast cancer cells [93]. Up-regulation of survivin is also directly linked to HER-2 over expression [94]. A novel anti-survivin based therapy in combination with an anti-HER-2 DC vaccine is an exciting possibility to treat and possibly prevent breast cancers.

Another promising possibility is to develop immune responses against other HER family members including HER-1 and HER-3. HER-3 has no ligand binding sites but intracellular signaling moieties and can partner with HER-2 and HER-1. HER-3 signaling may lead to HER-2 resistance thus developing vaccines against these targets may supplement HER-2 vaccines to make them better preventive agents eliminating vaccine escapes.

MUC-1(Figure 1), an epithelial glycoprotein that is over expressed in may breast cancers, is another molecule that has yet to be fully exploited as an anti-cancer drug target. This molecule has been implicated in tumor invasion and metastases [95]. MUC-1 pulsed DC based vaccine trials for patients with pancreatic and biliary carcinomas are currently underway and the clinical efficacy of these vaccines is not known at this time [96]. MUC-1 is another molecule that could potentially used to target breast cancers.

There is immeasurable potential for vaccine therapy to be used in immunocompetent patients with minimal disease to prevent disease progression and recurrence. Even more exciting is the potential to treat patients with no disease at all. Forty percent of the participants in our recent vaccine trial converted from ER positive HER-2 positive to ER positve HER-2 negative suggesting that HER-2 vaccines can direct or steer tumors to more favorable phenotypes. The ultimate goal is therefore to produce a vaccine that could prevent breast cancer formation altogether. The development of successful breast cancer prevention would be applicable to other solid tumor malignancies such as colorectal, head and neck cancer, lung cancer, gastric cancer and other GI malignancies.

8. References

[1] Nathanson, N. and O.M. Kew, *From emergence to eradication: the epidemiology of poliomyelitis deconstructed.* Am J Epidemiol. 172(11): p. 1213-29.
[2] Schiller, J.T. and D.R. Lowy, *Vaccines to prevent infections by oncoviruses.* Annu Rev Microbiol. 64: p. 23-41.
[3] Jemal, A., et al., *Global cancer statistics.* CA Cancer J Clin. 61(2): p. 69-90.
[4] Dawood, S., et al., *Defining breast cancer prognosis based on molecular phenotypes: results from a large cohort study.* Breast Cancer Res Treat. 126(1): p. 185-92.
[5] Sorlie, T., et al., *Gene expression patterns of breast carcinomas distinguish tumor subclasses with clinical implications.* Proc Natl Acad Sci U S A, 2001. 98(19): p. 10869-74.
[6] Sorlie, T., et al., *Repeated observation of breast tumor subtypes in independent gene expression data sets.* Proc Natl Acad Sci U S A, 2003. 100(14): p. 8418-23.
[7] van 't Veer, L.J., et al., *Gene expression profiling predicts clinical outcome of breast cancer.* Nature, 2002. 415(6871): p. 530-6.

[8] Perou, C.M., et al., *Molecular portraits of human breast tumours.* Nature, 2000. 406(6797): p. 747-52.

[9] Sotiriou, C. and L. Pusztai, *Gene-expression signatures in breast cancer.* N Engl J Med, 2009. 360(8): p. 790-800.

[10] Holmes, P., et al., *Prognostic markers and long-term outcomes in ductal carcinoma in situ of the breast treated with excision alone.* Cancer.

[11] Roses, R.E., et al., *HER-2/neu overexpression as a predictor for the transition from in situ to invasive breast cancer.* Cancer Epidemiol Biomarkers Prev, 2009. 18(5): p. 1386-9.

[12] Panet-Raymond, V., et al., *Clinicopathologic factors of the recurrent tumor predict outcome in patients with ipsilateral breast tumor recurrence.* Cancer. 117(10): p. 2035-43.

[13] Kerlikowske, K., et al., *Biomarker expression and risk of subsequent tumors after initial ductal carcinoma in situ diagnosis.* J Natl Cancer Inst. 102(9): p. 627-37.

[14] Carlson, R.W., et al., *Invasive breast cancer.* J Natl Compr Canc Netw. 9(2): p. 136-222.

[15] Lee, S.C., et al., *Natural killer (NK):dendritic cell (DC) cross talk induced by therapeutic monoclonal antibody triggers tumor antigen-specific T cell immunity.* Immunol Res. 50(2-3): p. 248-54.

[16] Madarnas, Y., et al., *Adjuvant/neoadjuvant trastuzumab therapy in women with HER-2/neu-overexpressing breast cancer: a systematic review.* Cancer Treat Rev, 2008. 34(6): p. 539-57.

[17] Haffty, B.G., et al., *Locoregional relapse and distant metastasis in conservatively managed triple negative early-stage breast cancer.* J Clin Oncol, 2006. 24(36): p. 5652-7.

[18] Anderson, K.S., *Tumor vaccines for breast cancer.* Cancer Invest, 2009. 27(4): p. 361-8.

[19] DeNardo, D.G. and L.M. Coussens, *Inflammation and breast cancer. Balancing immune response: crosstalk between adaptive and innate immune cells during breast cancer progression.* Breast Cancer Res, 2007. 9(4): p. 212.

[20] de Visser, K.E. and L.M. Coussens, *The interplay between innate and adaptive immunity regulates cancer development.* Cancer Immunol Immunother, 2005. 54(11): p. 1143-52.

[21] Coussens, L.M. and Z. Werb, *Inflammation and cancer.* Nature, 2002. 420(6917): p. 860-7.

[22] Johansson, M., et al., *Immune cells as anti-cancer therapeutic targets and tools.* J Cell Biochem, 2007. 101(4): p. 918-26.

[23] Disis, M.L. and K.H. Park, *Immunomodulation of breast cancer via tumor antigen specific Th1.* Cancer Res Treat, 2009. 41(3): p. 117-21.

[24] Almand, B., et al., *Increased production of immature myeloid cells in cancer patients: a mechanism of immunosuppression in cancer.* J Immunol, 2001. 166(1): p. 678-89.

[25] Serafini, P., et al., *Derangement of immune responses by myeloid suppressor cells.* Cancer Immunol Immunother, 2004. 53(2): p. 64-72.

[26] Gabrilovich, D.I., et al., *Mechanism of immune dysfunction in cancer mediated by immature Gr-1+ myeloid cells.* J Immunol, 2001. 166(9): p. 5398-406.

[27] Yang, L., et al., *Expansion of myeloid immune suppressor Gr+CD11b+ cells in tumor-bearing host directly promotes tumor angiogenesis.* Cancer Cell, 2004. 6(4): p. 409-21.

[28] Ernst, P.B. and B.D. Gold, *The disease spectrum of Helicobacter pylori: the immunopathogenesis of gastroduodenal ulcer and gastric cancer.* Annu Rev Microbiol, 2000. 54: p. 615-40.

[29] Kuper, H., H.O. Adami, and D. Trichopoulos, *Infections as a major preventable cause of human cancer.* J Intern Med, 2000. 248(3): p. 171-83.

[30] Shacter, E. and S.A. Weitzman, *Chronic inflammation and cancer.* Oncology (Williston Park), 2002. 16(2): p. 217-26, 229; discussion 230-2.
[31] Peek, R.M., Jr., S. Mohla, and R.N. DuBois, *Inflammation in the genesis and perpetuation of cancer: summary and recommendations from a national cancer institute-sponsored meeting.* Cancer Res, 2005. 65(19): p. 8583-6.
[32] Tlsty, T.D. and L.M. Coussens, *Tumor stroma and regulation of cancer development.* Annu Rev Pathol, 2006. 1: p. 119-50.
[33] Zou, W., *Immunosuppressive networks in the tumour environment and their therapeutic relevance.* Nat Rev Cancer, 2005. 5(4): p. 263-74.
[34] Dunn, G.P., L.J. Old, and R.D. Schreiber, *The three Es of cancer immunoediting.* Annu Rev Immunol, 2004. 22: p. 329-60.
[35] Dunn, G.P., et al., *Cancer immunoediting: from immunosurveillance to tumor escape.* Nat Immunol, 2002. 3(11): p. 991-8.
[36] Koski, G.K., et al., *Reengineering dendritic cell-based anti-cancer vaccines.* Immunol Rev, 2008. 222: p. 256-76.
[37] Boon, T., et al., *Tumor antigens recognized by T lymphocytes.* Annu Rev Immunol, 1994. 12: p. 337-65.
[38] Mittendorf, E.A., G.E. Peoples, and S.E. Singletary, *Breast cancer vaccines: promise for the future or pipe dream?* Cancer, 2007. 110(8): p. 1677-86.
[39] Disis, M.L., et al., *Existent T-cell and antibody immunity to HER-2/neu protein in patients with breast cancer.* Cancer Res, 1994. 54(1): p. 16-20.
[40] Jerome, K.R., N. Domenech, and O.J. Finn, *Tumor-specific cytotoxic T cell clones from patients with breast and pancreatic adenocarcinoma recognize EBV-immortalized B cells transfected with polymorphic epithelial mucin complementary DNA.* J Immunol, 1993. 151(3): p. 1654-62.
[41] Menard, S., et al., *Lymphoid infiltration as a prognostic variable for early-onset breast carcinomas.* Clin Cancer Res, 1997. 3(5): p. 817-9.
[42] Mahmoud, S.M., et al., *Tumor-Infiltrating CD8+ Lymphocytes Predict Clinical Outcome in Breast Cancer.* J Clin Oncol. 29(15): p. 1949-55.
[43] Draube, A., et al., *Dendritic cell based tumor vaccination in prostate and renal cell cancer: a systematic review and meta-analysis.* PLoS One. 6(4): p. e18801.
[44] Disis, M.L., et al., *Effect of dose on immune response in patients vaccinated with an her-2/neu intracellular domain protein--based vaccine.* J Clin Oncol, 2004. 22(10): p. 1916-25.
[45] Hakim, F.T., et al., *Constraints on CD4 recovery postchemotherapy in adults: thymic insufficiency and apoptotic decline of expanded peripheral CD4 cells.* Blood, 1997. 90(9): p. 3789-98.
[46] Mellios, T., H.L. Ko, and J. Beuth, *Impact of adjuvant chemo- and radiotherapy on the cellular immune system of breast cancer patients.* In Vivo. 24(2): p. 227-30.
[47] Rotstein, S., et al., *Long term effects on the immune system following local radiation therapy for breast cancer. I. Cellular composition of the peripheral blood lymphocyte population.* Int J Radiat Oncol Biol Phys, 1985. 11(5): p. 921-5.
[48] Czerniecki, B.J., R.E. Roses, and G.K. Koski, *Development of vaccines for high-risk ductal carcinoma in situ of the breast.* Cancer Res, 2007. 67(14): p. 6531-4.
[49] Altintas, S., et al., *Prognostic significance of oncogenic markers in ductal carcinoma in situ of the breast: a clinicopathologic study.* Breast J, 2009. 15(2): p. 120-32.

[50] Tamimi, R.M., et al., *Comparison of molecular phenotypes of ductal carcinoma in situ and invasive breast cancer.* Breast Cancer Res, 2008. 10(4): p. R67.

[51] Zafrani, B., et al., *Mammographically-detected ductal in situ carcinoma of the breast analyzed with a new classification. A study of 127 cases: correlation with estrogen and progesterone receptors, p53 and c-erbB-2 proteins, and proliferative activity.* Semin Diagn Pathol, 1994. 11(3): p. 208-14.

[52] Evans, A.J., et al., *Correlations between the mammographic features of ductal carcinoma in situ (DCIS) and C-erbB-2 oncogene expression. Nottingham Breast Team.* Clin Radiol, 1994. 49(8): p. 559-62.

[53] Clark, S.E., et al., *Molecular subtyping of DCIS: heterogeneity of breast cancer reflected in pre-invasive disease.* Br J Cancer. 104(1): p. 120-7.

[54] Dawson, S.J., et al., *BCL2 in breast cancer: a favourable prognostic marker across molecular subtypes and independent of adjuvant therapy received.* Br J Cancer. 103(5): p. 668-75.

[55] Czerniecki, B.J., et al., *Targeting HER-2/neu in early breast cancer development using dendritic cells with staged interleukin-12 burst secretion.* Cancer Res, 2007. 67(4): p. 1842-52.

[56] Otto, K., et al., *Lack of toxicity of therapy-induced T cell responses against the universal tumour antigen survivin.* Vaccine, 2005. 23(7): p. 884-9.

[57] Morse, M.A., et al., *Immunotherapy with autologous, human dendritic cells transfected with carcinoembryonic antigen mRNA.* Cancer Invest, 2003. 21(3): p. 341-9.

[58] Brossart, P., et al., *Induction of cytotoxic T-lymphocyte responses in vivo after vaccinations with peptide-pulsed dendritic cells.* Blood, 2000. 96(9): p. 3102-8.

[59] Hynes, N.E. and G. MacDonald, *ErbB receptors and signaling pathways in cancer.* Curr Opin Cell Biol, 2009. 21(2): p. 177-84.

[60] Lee, M.K.t., A. Sharma, and B.J. Czerniecki, *It's all in for the HER family in tumorigenesis.* Expert Rev Vaccines. 9(1): p. 29-34.

[61] Mendelsohn, J. and J. Baselga, *Epidermal growth factor receptor targeting in cancer.* Semin Oncol, 2006. 33(4): p. 369-85.

[62] Harding, J. and B. Burtness, *Cetuximab: an epidermal growth factor receptor chemeric human-murine monoclonal antibody.* Drugs Today (Barc), 2005. 41(2): p. 107-27.

[63] Tanner, B., et al., *ErbB-3 predicts survival in ovarian cancer.* J Clin Oncol, 2006. 24(26): p. 4317-23.

[64] Engelman, J.A., et al., *ErbB-3 mediates phosphoinositide 3-kinase activity in gefitinib-sensitive non-small cell lung cancer cell lines.* Proc Natl Acad Sci U S A, 2005. 102(10): p. 3788-93.

[65] Slamon, D.J., et al., *Studies of the HER-2/neu proto-oncogene in human breast and ovarian cancer.* Science, 1989. 244(4905): p. 707-12.

[66] Williams, T.M., et al., *Expression of c-erbB-2 in human pancreatic adenocarcinomas.* Pathobiology, 1991. 59(1): p. 46-52.

[67] Holbro, T., G. Civenni, and N.E. Hynes, *The ErbB receptors and their role in cancer progression.* Exp Cell Res, 2003. 284(1): p. 99-110.

[68] Ibrahim, S.O., et al., *Expression of c-erbB proto-oncogene family members in squamous cell carcinoma of the head and neck.* Anticancer Res, 1997. 17(6D): p. 4539-46.

[69] Ross, J.S. and J.A. Fletcher, *The HER-2/neu Oncogene in Breast Cancer: Prognostic Factor, Predictive Factor, and Target for Therapy.* Oncologist, 1998. 3(4): p. 237-252.

[70] Disis, M.L., et al., *High-titer HER-2/neu protein-specific antibody can be detected in patients with early-stage breast cancer.* J Clin Oncol, 1997. 15(11): p. 3363-7.
[71] Park, J.M., et al., *Early role of CD4+ Th1 cells and antibodies in HER-2 adenovirus vaccine protection against autochthonous mammary carcinomas.* J Immunol, 2005. 174(7): p. 4228-36.
[72] Shumway, N.M., et al., *Therapeutic breast cancer vaccines: a new strategy for early-stage disease.* BioDrugs, 2009. 23(5): p. 277-87.
[73] Soliman, H., *Developing an effective breast cancer vaccine.* Cancer Control. 17(3): p. 183-90.
[74] Ladjemi, M.Z., et al., *Anti-HER2 vaccines: new prospects for breast cancer therapy.* Cancer Immunol Immunother. 59(9): p. 1295-312.
[75] Romani, N., et al., *Proliferating dendritic cell progenitors in human blood.* J Exp Med, 1994. 180(1): p. 83-93.
[76] Palucka, K., H. Ueno, and J. Banchereau, *Recent developments in cancer vaccines.* J Immunol. 186(3): p. 1325-31.
[77] Gulley, J.L. and C.G. Drake, *Immunotherapy for prostate cancer: recent advances, lessons learned, and areas for further research.* Clin Cancer Res. 17(12): p. 3884-91.
[78] Dallal, R.M. and M.T. Lotze, *The dendritic cell and human cancer vaccines.* Curr Opin Immunol, 2000. 12(5): p. 583-8.
[79] Palucka, K. and J. Banchereau, *Dendritic cells: a link between innate and adaptive immunity.* J Clin Immunol, 1999. 19(1): p. 12-25.
[80] Palucka, K., et al., *Dendritic cells and immunity against cancer.* J Intern Med. 269(1): p. 64-73.
[81] Andrews, D.M., E. Maraskovsky, and M.J. Smyth, *Cancer vaccines for established cancer: how to make them better?* Immunol Rev, 2008. 222: p. 242-55.
[82] Chambers, J.D. and P.J. Neumann, *Listening to Provenge--what a costly cancer treatment says about future Medicare policy.* N Engl J Med. 364(18): p. 1687-9.
[83] De Vries, I.J., et al., *Effective migration of antigen-pulsed dendritic cells to lymph nodes in melanoma patients is determined by their maturation state.* Cancer Res, 2003. 63(1): p. 12-7.
[84] Kantoff, P.W., et al., *Sipuleucel-T immunotherapy for castration-resistant prostate cancer.* N Engl J Med. 363(5): p. 411-22.
[85] Higano, C.S., et al., *Integrated data from 2 randomized, double-blind, placebo-controlled, phase 3 trials of active cellular immunotherapy with sipuleucel-T in advanced prostate cancer.* Cancer, 2009. 115(16): p. 3670-9.
[86] Small, E.J., et al., *Placebo-controlled phase III trial of immunologic therapy with sipuleucel-T (APC8015) in patients with metastatic, asymptomatic hormone refractory prostate cancer.* J Clin Oncol, 2006. 24(19): p. 3089-94.
[87] Wiedermann, U., et al., *A virosomal formulated Her-2/neu multi-peptide vaccine induces Her-2/neu-specific immune responses in patients with metastatic breast cancer: a phase I study.* Breast Cancer Res Treat. 119(3): p. 673-83.
[88] Avigan, D., et al., *Fusion cell vaccination of patients with metastatic breast and renal cancer induces immunological and clinical responses.* Clin Cancer Res, 2004. 10(14): p. 4699-708.
[89] Park, J.W., et al., *Treatment with autologous antigen-presenting cells activated with the HER-2 based antigen Lapuleucel-T: results of a phase I study in immunologic and clinical activity in HER-2 overexpressing breast cancer.* J Clin Oncol, 2007. 25(24): p. 3680-7.

[90] Senzer, N. and J. Nemunaitis, *A review of contusugene ladenovec (Advexin) p53 therapy.* Curr Opin Mol Ther, 2009. 11(1): p. 54-61.
[91] Lombardi, V., et al., *Human dendritic cells stimulated via TLR7 and/or TLR8 induce the sequential production of Il-10, IFN-gamma, and IL-17A by naive CD4+ T cells.* J Immunol, 2009. 182(6): p. 3372-9.
[92] Albini, A., et al., *Angiostatin anti-angiogenesis requires IL-12: the innate immune system as a key target.* J Transl Med, 2009. 7: p. 5.
[93] Gritsko, T., et al., *Persistent activation of stat3 signaling induces survivin gene expression and confers resistance to apoptosis in human breast cancer cells.* Clin Cancer Res, 2006. 12(1): p. 11-9.
[94] Siddiqa, A., et al., *Expression of HER-2 in MCF-7 breast cancer cells modulates anti-apoptotic proteins Survivin and Bcl-2 via the extracellular signal-related kinase (ERK) and phosphoinositide-3 kinase (PI3K) signalling pathways.* BMC Cancer, 2008. 8: p. 129.
[95] Wierecky, J., M. Mueller, and P. Brossart, *Dendritic cell-based cancer immunotherapy targeting MUC-1.* Cancer Immunol Immunother, 2006. 55(1): p. 63-7.
[96] Lepisto, A.J., et al., *A phase I/II study of a MUC1 peptide pulsed autologous dendritic cell vaccine as adjuvant therapy in patients with resected pancreatic and biliary tumors.* Cancer Ther, 2008. 6(B): p. 955-964.

Section 2

Dietary and Lifestyle Patterns in Cancer Prevention

6

Lifestyle Changes May Prevent Cancer

Budimka Novaković, Jelena Jovičić and Maja Grujičić
University of Novi Sad, Faculty of Medicine
Serbia

1. Introduction

Cancer development is a result of interactions among environmental and hereditary factors (Kim, 2006). The majority of genetic abnormalities, which increase the risk of cancer are not hereditary, but a result of DNA damage occurring during lifetime. The causes of DNA damage include internal (nutrient metabolism, cell hormones) and/or external factors (diet, insufficient physical activity, tobacco use, exposure to chemical agents and radiation) (International Life Sciences Institute [ILSI], 2005; World Cancer Research Fund [WCRF], 2007; Kryston et al., 2011). Epidemiological studies have shown that diet and lifestyle are the most important external factors implicated in the development of malignant diseases (ILSI, 2005; WCRF & AICR, 2007; Go et al., 2003).

Why the same environmental factors cause different changes in human genome among individuals is a question for scientists searching unique combinations of factors leading to cancer (Brower, 2011). There is a growing body of evidence that many cancers are not caused by mutations in genes, but by chemical modifications that alter the way genes function. Chemical modifications of genes are called epigenetic changes. Epidemiological studies have shown that diet and lifestyle may cause such changes (Brower, 2011).

According to World Cancer Report (Boyle & Levin, 2008) 12.4 million new cases of cancer were reported in 2008. Malignant diseases accounted for 7.6% of all deaths during the same year and estimations are that in 2030, cancers will be responsible for 17.0% of deaths worldwide. The number of new cases is expected to rise, especially in developing countries (Boyle & Levin, 2008).

In total, malignancies account for 83 million disability-adjusted life years (DALYs). The estimated global economic loss from cancer is US$ 895.2 billion, measured by the economic value of DALYs (American Cancer Society & Livestrong, 2010).

The aforementioned data, coupled with rising health care expenditures for cancer patients, led to cancer being seen not only as a health problem, but also as a political issue (WHO, 2011a, 2011b). Identification of cancers as the leading non-communicable diseases [NCDs], together with cardiovascular diseases, type 2 diabetes and chronic obstructive pulmonary diseases, was followed by an initiative to include NCDs among the global development goals that will succeed the Millennium Development Goals in 2015 (The NCD Alliance, 2011).

Scientists around the world declared war on cancer (Waldorp, 2011). Preventive medicine has been recognized as the most promising field in reducing the risk of malignant diseases development. As diet and lifestyle are believed to be the most important external factors implicated in cancer development, nutrition care process [NCP] (American Dietetic Association [ADA], 2006a, 2008) and medical nutrition prevention [MNP] are considered the most important tools in cancer risk management (Key et al., 2004; Béliveau & Gingras, 2007).

NCP and MNP can be used to reduce the potential of nutrition misinformation to increase the cancer risks in populations and individuals who are inadequately educated about healthy food and lifestyle choices (ADA, 2006b).

Registered dietitians are well aware of dietary reference values and safe upper limits for nutrients intake in different population groups, but these recommendations neglect genetic differences in population subgroups. Therefore, special scientific disciplines - nutrigenetics and nutrigenomics - study the effects of different foods and food constituents on gene expression (Fenech et al., 2011). There is a distinct difference between nutrigenetics and nutrigenomics. Nutrigenetics studies effects of genetic variations on body response to diet and nutrition, while nutrigenomics studies health effects of gene alterations influenced by food constituents (Milner, 2006a). Both disciplines aim to determine the optimal nutrient intake and nutrient combinations (called nutriom) in order to sustain the genome and support the physiological processes of gene expression, metabolism and cell functioning. These findings are expected to be used in cancer risk reduction in dietetic practice (Milner, 2006a).

2. Risk factors related to lifestyle and the possibility of cancer prevention

Many lifestyle factors are related to cancer risks, but at the same time they are highly preventable or modifiable.

2.1 Body composition

Nutrition transitions, taking place in developing countries since the 20th century, toward more energy-dense foods, associated with insufficient physical activity, resulted in pandemic prevalence of overweight and obesity (Popkin, 1995). Overweight and obesity are metabolic disorders and the leading causes of NCDs. Worldwide, 4.8% of all deaths and 2.3% of DALYs are attributable to overweight and obesity (WHO, 2009a).

Overweight and obesity are associated with increased risk of some cancer localizations (Calle et al., 2003; Lagergren, 2011; Fontham & Su, 2008; Stoll, 2002; Ma et al., 2008). Visceral adiposity and central obesity are risk factors for some cancers (AICR & WCRF, 2009). Fat mapping (adipotopography) is an emerging biomedical field dealing with localization and amount of intra-abdominal adipose tissue [IAAT] in the human body. Subjects with higher amount of intra-abdominal adipose tissue are at greater risk for insulin resistance, diabetes and cancer (Thomas et al., 2011). The recommended body-mass index [BMI] for cancer risk reduction is 21.5 kg/m^2 on a population scale, and between 18.5 kg/m^2 and 25.0 kg/m^2 on individual level (AICR & WCRF, 2009; Food and Agriculture Organization of the United Nations [FAO], 2004). Individuals with BMI within the physiological range, but with high-risk waist circumference [WC], are classified as thin-on-the-outside, fat-on-the-inside [TOFI] phenotype (Thomas et al., 2011) and they are at greater risk of certain cancer localizations. TOFI is a pathological phenomenon, synonymous with "metabolically obese", whereas thin-on-the-outside, thin-on-the-inside [TOTI] is an acronym for healthy adipose tissue distribution (Thomas et al., 2011).

TOFI phenotype may be used to explain the rising incidence of cancers in developing countries. Rapid economic growth and social transitions happening in these countries affect dietary and other lifestyle choices. Energy-dense foods become easily accessible to consumers, while the level of physical activity decreases, promoting overweight and obesity (Popkin, 2001).

Higher amount of IAAT or visceral adiposity is usually related to increased serum levels of insulin-like growth factor [IGF-1], insulin, leptin, sex hormones and adipocytokines (tumor necrosis factor-alpha [TNF-α], interleukin-6 [IL-6], C-reactive protein [CRP], adiponectin, resistin, visfatin, apelin), all known as cancer and type 2 diabetes risk factors (Donohoe et al., 2011; Bon, 2008; Redinger, 2008). Epidemiological studies show that type 2 diabetes patients are at higher risk for developing many types of cancer. There is an ongoing effort in research of shared risk factors for cancer and type 2 diabetes supported by the American Diabetes Association and the American Cancer Society. This research strives to find a biological link between cancer and type 2 diabetes, as well as to explain whether diabetes mellitus therapy affects the risk for cancer development (Giovannucci et al., 2010).

Taller individuals are more likely to get cancer, due to cells being stimulated by IGF-1 and growth hormone continuously, increasing the possibility of DNA replication error, some of which may lead to malignant alterations (Hernandez et al., 2009).

Overweight and obesity are usually the result of external factors, and are therefore, preventable and treatable (WHO, 2005, 2008a) risk factors for some cancers (Table 1).

Cancer site	USA [%]	UK [%]	Brazil [%]	China [%]
Endometrium	70	56	52	34
Esophagus	69	75	60	44
Mouth, pharynx & larynx	63	67	63	44
Stomach	47	45	41	33
Colon	45	43	37	17
Pancreas	39	41	34	14
Breast	38	42	28	20
Lung	36	33	36	38
Kidney	24	19	13	8
Gallbladder	21	16	10	6
Liver	15	17	6	6
Prostate	11	20	n/a	n/a
Total for these cancers combined	34	39	30	27
Total for all cancers	24	26	19	20

Table 1. Estimated percentage of cancers that could be prevented by healthy diet, regular physical activity and healthy weight in selected countries based on the conclusions of the 2007 WCRF/AICR Diet and Cancer Report (n/a – exposure data not available). Adapted from AICR & WCRF, 2009.

According to Fair & Montgomery, "nutritional energy intake is a modifiable factor in the energy balance-cancer linkage". Animal studies showed that reduction of energy intake by 10.0 to 40.0% decreases cell proliferation, by increasing apoptosis due to insufficient angiogenesis (Fair & Montgomery, 2009). Although known to have anticarcinogenic potential, decreased energy intake alone cannot reduce the risk of cancer, since energy expenditure depends highly on the physical activity level. Regular physical activity helps weight loss, reduction of IAAT, serum insulin, IGF-1 and adipocytokines levels, hence reducing the risk of cancer (WHO, 2008a).

Body mass reduction and maintenance of healthy body mass calls for accurate determination of daily energy requirements (Table 2), depending on age, gender and physical activity levels (U.S. Department of Agriculture [USDA] & U.S. Department of Health and Human Services, 2011).

		Physical Activity Level		
Gender	**Age [years]**	**Sedentary [kcal/day]**	**Moderately active [kcal/day]**	**Active [kcal/day]**
Child (female and male)	2-3	1000-1200[a]	1000-1400[a]	1000-1400[a]
Female[b]	4-8	1200-1400	1400-1600	1400-1600
	9-13	1400-1600	1600-2000	1800-2400
	14-18	1800	2000	2400
	19-30	1800-2000	2000-2200	2400
	31-50	1800	2000	2200
	51+	1600	1800	2000-2200
Male	4-8	1200-1400	1400-1600	1600-2000
	9-13	1600-1800	1800-2200	2000-2600
	14-18	2000-2400	2400-2800	2800-3200
	19-30	2400-2600	2600-2800	3000
	31-50	2200-2400	2400-2600	2800-3000
	51+	2000-2200	2200-2400	2400-2800

Table 2. Estimated calorie needs per day by age, gender and physical activity level (a. The calorie ranges accommodate needs of different ages within the group. Children and adolescents need more calories at older ages, and adults need less calories at older ages.; b. Not including pregnant and breastfeeding females.) Adapted from: U.S. Department of Agriculture [USDA] & U.S. Department of Health and Human Services, 2011.

High waist circumference (WC) values increase the cancer risks, and they are undoubtedly related to all-cause mortality in middle aged men and women (Bigaard et al., 2005). Health risks of high waist circumference values in adolescence and young adulthood are similar to those of middle aged individuals. Efforts are being made to standardize WC reference data in accordance with age, gender, body height and ethnicity. Standardization of WC by BMI, site of waist measurement, meal timing and phase of respiration are suggested (Wang, 2006). According to Wang the "unit for WC standardization that investigators will accept logically and mathematically and that would increase the use of WC measurement in the clinical field" should be similar to the percentile system used in children's growth rate nomograms, or T-score used in bone density evaluation (Wang, 2006). Cut-off values of WC by gender and ethnicity are shown in table 3.

Country/Ethnic group	Gender	Waist circumference
Europids[a] In the USA, the ATP III values (102 cm male, 88 cm female are likely to continue to be used for clinical purposes)	Male	> 94 cm
	Female	> 80 cm
South Asians Based on Chinese, Malay and Asian-Indian population	Male	> 90 cm
	Female	> 80 cm
Japanese	Use South Asian recommendations until more specific data are available	
Ethnic South and Central Americans	Use South Asian recommendations until more specific data are available	
Sub-Saharan Africans	Use European recommendations until more specific data are available	
Eastern Mediterranean and Middle East (Arab) populations	Use European recommendations until more specific data are available	

Table 3. Cut-off values of waist circumference by gender and ethnicity excluding children younger than 6 years (a. In future epidemiological studies of populations of Europid origin, prevalence should be given using both European and North American cut-points to allow better comparisons). Table adapted from IDF, 2006.

Key recommendations for long term maintenance of healthy body mass are as follows (Grace, 2011):

1. Being physically active (at least 60 minutes of moderate physical activity daily),
2. Choosing low energy and low fat foods,
3. Eating breakfast regularly,
4. Monitoring body mass,
5. Catching body mass gain before it turns into overweight or obesity,
6. Establishing a consistent healthy diet and proper lifestyle choices.

2.2 Cancer protective diet versus diet-related cancer risk

Nutrition is the source of life. Healthy diet with optimal nutrients intake prevents nutrient deficiency and helps to maintain or improve health. Types of nutrients and their amounts sufficient for sustaining life and maintaining good health are well known and recommendations for nutrients intake are given according to age, gender, pregnancy or lactation (Smolin & Grosvenor, 2010). A number of factors (e.g. genetic background, physical activity level) affect individual's optimal nutrients intake, so it is still not possible for dietitians to practice personalized nutrition.

The inter-individual variability of responses to different food constituents is being scrutinized (Simopoulos & Milner, 2010). The scientific position that genetic predisposition to complex diseases is a result of small variations of a large number of genes and their ability to interact with specific ecological factors is strongly supported in available literature. Therefore, results of nutrigenomic and nutrigenetic research could, through practical and clinical use of new knowledge, reduce the risk for malignant alterations and help control the burden of cancer as the second most common cause of death in the world (Kinsella & He, 2009; WHO, 2011c). It is expected that nutrigenetics and nutrigenomics will shed some light on the complex relations between nutritional molecules, genetic variations and the biological system, thus facilitating the concept of personalized nutrition. Development of nutrition guides intended for individual use depends on agricultural production and food availability (Simopoulos & Milner, 2010).

At this moment, only population-based nutrition guides exist. They first appeared in early 20th century (USDA, 2002). The first significant guide was the Exchange List for Meal Planning (American Diabetic Association & ADA, 2003) and it was followed by globally accepted MyPyramid (USDA, 2011a). In June 2011, USDA published the enhanced version of nutrition guide called ChooseMyPlate (USDA, 2011b), based on Dietary Guidelines for Americans, published earlier in 2011 (USDA & U.S. Department of Health and Human Services, 2011). The use of nutritional guides is still encouraged in dietetics practice, because they can help manage cancer risks by changing diet and lifestyle.

No specific food can be labelled as anticarcinogenic, but certain food constituents have the potential to reduce cancer risks (WCRF & AICR, 2007; WHO, 2003). Diet rich in fresh vegetables, fruits and low in red and processed meat has been referred to as chemoprotective, while foods with high glycemic indices and sweetened beverages have been linked to hyperinsulinemia, overweight, obesity and increased cancer risks (WCRF & AICR, 2007; Kushi et al., 2006).

2.2.1 Grains and grain products

The amount of nutrients in cereals and cereal products depends on the degree of refinement and processing. Dietary fibers, antioxidants, phenols, lignans and phytoestrogens, present in whole grain products may reduce the risk for some types of cancer (Schatzkin et al., 2007). Dietary fibers are defined as partially or completely indigestible carbohydrates consisting of 3 or more monosaccharide units (Gray, 2006). "Isolated indigestible carbohydrates shown to have beneficial physiological effects in humans" are called functional fibers (Institute of Medicine, 2005). The fiber content of carbohydrates, determines the food's glycemic index [GI] (Smolin & Grosvenor, 2010; Gray, 2006; Barclay, 2008). Foods labelled with "low GI" on nutrition claims (good sources of dietary fibers) are recommended for risk reduction of certain cancers (Barclay, 2008; Buttriss & Stokes, 2008). Nutrition (and health) claims have enormous potential for chronic diseases risk reduction and health promotion and improvement, but better education of consumers on this issue is necessary (Buttriss & Stokes, 2008; Jovičić et al., 2010; Bonsmann et al., 2010). Key recommendation concerning grains and grain products category is to pay attention to the GI and dietary fiber content per 100 g or per serving of foods.

2.2.2 Fruits and vegetables

During the last decade of the 20th century, scientists started emphasizing that high intake of fruits and vegetables may reduce cancer risks. That is why the "5-A-Day" program was developed by the American National Cancer Institute (Havas et al., 1994), but later studies failed to back up the optimistic findings from the 90s (Boffeta et al., 2010; Willet, 2010; Cancer Council Australia, 2007). There is an ongoing effort to find specific fruits and vegetables and their constituents (or their interactions) that are responsible for cancer risk reduction (Table 4).

Organisation Review	**Highest Evidence Convincing**	**Moderate Evidence Probable**	**Lower Evidence Possible / Limited**
WCRF/ AICR (2007)		Mouth (f&v) Pharynx (f&v) Larynx (f&v) Oesophagus (f&v) Stomach (f&v) Lung (f)	Nasopharynx (f&v) Colon & rectum (f&v) Pancreas (f) Liver (f) Lung (v) Ovary (v) Endometrium (v)
IARC (2003)		Oesophagus (f&v) Stomach (f) Colon & rectum (v)	Mouth (f&v) Pharynx (f&v) Larynx (f&v) Kidney (f&v) Colon & rectum (f) Bladder (f) Stomach (v) Lung (v) Ovary (v)
WHO/ FAO (2003)		Oral Cavity (f&v) Oesophagus (f&v) Stomach (f&v) Colon & rectum (f&v)	
COMA (1998)	Oesophagus (f&v)	Stomach (f&v) Colon & rectum (v)	Breast (f&v)
WCRF/ AICR (1997)	Mouth (f&v) Pharynx (f&v) Oesophagus (f&v) Stomach (f&v) Colon & rectum (v) Lung (f&v)	Larynx (f&v) Pancreas (f&v) Breast (f&v) Bladder (f&v)	Ovaries (f&v) Cervix (f&v) Endometrium (f&v) Thyroid (f&v) Liver (v) Prostate (v) Kidney (v)

Table 4. Conclusions from the major cancer prevention reports regarding the cancer protective effect of fruit (f) and vegetables (v). Used with permission of Cancer Council Australia (www.cancer.org.au) (Cancer Council Australia, 2007).

Fruits and vegetables contain dietary fibers, vitamins, minerals and other bioactive molecules, as well as a large percentage of water which makes them low-energy foods. Replacing high-energy dense foods with fruits and vegetables may lead to body mass reduction and, consequently, to cancer risk reduction (Willet, 2010; Cancer Council Australia, 2007; Slimani & Margetts, 2009; Novaković et al., 2010).

Nutritional and health benefits of indigestible oligosaccharides contained in fruits and vegetables are being pointed out in scientific journals. Oligosaccharides are dietary fibers which are generally highly fermentable. Some oligosaccharides, namely fructooligosaccharides, inulin and lactulose are valued for their prebiotic properties (Gray, 2006; Roberfroid et al., 2010; Mujal et al., 2009). High-energy dense nutrition is low in indigestible oligosaccharides and other dietary fibers. Chronic high fat intake and low dietary fiber intake may lead to gut microflora changes, specifically to Bifidobacterium spp. number decrease (Cani & Delzenne, 2009). Altered microflora may play an important role in obesity initiation and homeostasis perturbation (Cani et al., 2007a; Cani et al., 2009;

Heilbronn & Campbell, 2008). Lipopolysaccharides [LPS] from Gram negative bacteria (in altered gut microflora) promote secretion of inflammatory cytokines. LPS pass through intestinal wall, travel by chylomicrons to target organs where they promote inflammation-induced metabolic disorders (obesity, insulin resistance, macrophage infiltration into adipose tissue, liver steatosis). Bifidobacterium spp. as an important actor in healthy gut microflora, decreases the levels of intestinal endotoxins and enhances mucosal barrier function (Tuohy et al., 2005). Increasing the intake of prebiotics may be a beneficial strategy in keeping the number of Bifidobacterium spp. optimal and gut microflora healthy and functional, reducing low-grade inflammation (Tohuy et al., 2005; Cani et al., 2007b). According to Goodlad et al. "prebiotic dietary fibers may also modulate other targets prone to influence metabolic disorders associated with obesity, such as gut peptides" (Goodlad et al., 1987). Decreasing low-grade inflammation and beneficially influencing the body mass, prebiotics (together with probiotics) may be a factor in cancer risk reduction (Grey, 2006; Tuohy et al., 2005; Cani et al., 2007a; Goodlad et al., 1987; World Gastroenterology Organisation, 2008; Donaldson, 2004; Yan & Polk, 2010). Jain et al. indicated that certain synbiotics (combinations of prebiotics and probiotics) are more efficient in vivo than in either treatment alone, but that more research is needed to identify the most potent synbiotics (Jain et al., 2010).

2.2.3 Milk and dairy products

Milk and dairy products are sources of many essential nutrients, e.g. amino acids, fatty acids, lactose, vitamin D, vitamin A, vitamin B_{12}, calcium, potassium and they are prerequisites for growth and development, as well as for optimal bone health (USDA & U.S. Department of Health and Human Services, 2011; Smolin & Grosvenor, 2010). The strength of evidence suggesting that intake of milk and dairy products is associated with reduced cardiovascular and type 2 diabetes risks and blood pressure lowering is moderate (Smolin & Grosvenor, 2010; Huth & al., 2006). A large number of epidemiological studies were conducted in order to explore the relations between milk and dairy products consumption and cancer risks, but the results were largely equivocal (Huth & al., 2006; Quigley, 2011; Järvinen, 2011; Van der Pols et al., 2007). Chronic excessive intake of dairy fat can promote development of malignancies, but certain fatty acids from milk, like conjugated linoleic acid [CLA] can inhibit cancer growth. Vitamin D_3 may reduce the risk of prostate cancer. Calcium from milk and dairy products may have protective properties against colon cancer, while bovine lactoferrin from whey may inhibit colon carcinogenesis (Tsuda et al., 2000; Aune et al., 2011).

The aforementioned contradictory results do not undermine the importance of milk and dairy products in daily diet. Dietary Guidelines for Americans, 2010 recommendations for dairy intake are in accordance with cancer risk reduction (USDA & U.S. Department of Health and Human Services, 2011; Smolin & Grosvenor, 2010).

2.2.4 Protein foods

ChooseMyPlate nutrition guide classifies meat, fish, eggs and their products, legumes, nuts and seeds as protein foods (USDA, 2011b). Proteins have not been linked with increase in obesity, diabetes or cancer risks (WHO, 2007a; Joslin Diabetes Center & Joslin Clinic, 2007), but foods from this group are rich sources of fats, oils and other substances that might affect cancer risks (Smolin & Grosvenor, 2010; USDA, 2011b).

The majority of case-control studies suggested a positive link between meat consumption and colorectal cancer risk (WCRF & AICR, 2007; Gonzalez, 2006; Chan et al., 2011).

Globally, meat and meat products account for 8.0% of the daily energy intake (FAO, 2011). On account of essential amino acids, fatty acids, vitamin B_{12}, folates, iron, copper and zinc content, meat should be consumed on a daily basis. The amount and the percentage of fat in consumed meat, as well as the type of processing correlate with the incidence of colorectal malignancies (Gonzalez, 2006; Chan et al., 2011; Cross & Sinha, 2004). Risk factors associated with consumption of meat and meat products include nitrates, nitrites, N-nitroso compounds, heterocyclic amines and polycyclic aromatic carbohydrates. Iron is also considered to be a risk factor, because of its prooxidative properties (WCRF & AICR, 2007; Cross & Sinha, 2004; Eichholzer & Gutzwiller, 1998; Lanou & Svenson, 2010; Butler et al., 2003; Zheng et al., 2009). The overall evidence supports limiting red and processed meat intake in order to reduce the risk of colorectal cancer (WCRF & AICR, 2007; Key et al., 2004; Béliveau & Gingras, 2007; Kushi, 2006).

Dietary fatty acid composition plays a role in the process of carcinogenesis and tumor proliferation (WCRF & AICR, 2007; Fenech et al., 2011; WHO, 2008a; FAO, 2004; USDA & U.S. Department of Health and Human Services, 2011; Chan & Giovannucci, 2010; Hu et al., 2011a). The single most prominent issue responsible for global increase of total dietary fat and saturated fatty acids intake is the process of hydrogenation of oils (USDA & U.S. Department of Health and Human Services, 2011; Van Stuyvenberg, 1969). Total hydrogenation transforms unsaturated fatty acids from fish oil and plant oils to saturated fatty acids, while partial hydrogenation produces unsaturated trans-fatty acids. When consumed, trans-fatty acids act as saturated (USDA & U.S. Department of Health and Human Services, 2011; Van Stuyvenberg, 1969). WCRF (WCRF & AICR, 2007) and North Carolina Colon Cancer Study (Vinikoor et al., 2009) claim that specific effects of trans-fatty acids on cancer risk is not known, since positive correlation linking trans-fatty acids intake and overall cancer prevalence was detected using mailed food questionnaires (Hu et al., 2011b).

Data on health effects of fatty fish intake, the correlation between fatty fish intake and gastric cancer (Wu et al., 2011), breast cancer (Terry et al., 2003; Murff et al., 2011), prostate cancer (Terry et al., 2003; Allen et al., 2004) and colorectal cancer (Aune et al., 2009a; Vinikoor et al., 2009; Daniel et al., 2009) are inconsistent (Daniel et al., 2009). Long-chain polyunsaturated fatty acids from fish are seen as promising nutrients in cancer prevention, but currently there is not enough supportive scientific evidence. On the other hand, intake of α-linolenic acid might be a risk factor for cancer (Daniel et al., 2009; Colquhoun et al., 2009). New studies, both experimental and epidemiological, are necessary to shed more light on these findings.

The link between eggs consumption and cancer has not been researched as extensively. Currently, the evidence suggest that eggs intake may be linked to increase in colon, rectal, bladder and ovarian cancer risks, putting into consideration the use of dietary alternatives to eggs (Zhang et al., 2003; Radosavljević et al., 2005; Aune et al., 2009).

Legumes are known to be beneficial in cardiovascular and type 2 diabetes risk reduction, but there is limited evidence that legumes consumption may reduce the risk of stomach, colorectal, and kidney cancer. Further investigations of these complex relations are still waited upon (Kolonel et al., 2000; Aune et al., 2009b).

Effects of nuts and seeds intake on cancer risks are limited and inconclusive (WCRF & AICR, 2007).

Aflatoxin contamination of fungus-contaminated crops and legumes remains a serious food safety problem, as aflatoxin is known to be a risk for liver cancer (Goldman & Shields, 2003; Wogan et al., 2004).

2.2.5 Table salt

Chronic intake of excessive amounts of table salt is a possible gastric cancer risk factor (WCRF & AICR, 2007; ADA, 2006a; Key et al., 2004; Béliveau et al., 2007; WHO, 2003, 2005; AICR & WCRF, 2009; Donaldson, 2004). As positive correlation between *Helicobacter pylori* infection and high salt intake has also been noted, it is possible that there is a synergy between the two factors in gastric cancer promotion. Another mechanism of stomach cancer promotion proposed is that high salt intake damages the gastric mucose, increasing the possibility of endogenous mutations, which leads to hypergastrinemia and decrease in number of gastric parietal cells, and thus to cancer promotion (Wang et al., 2009).

Processed foods are the main source of salt in the diet, and in order to reduce cancer risks in adult population, population-level strategy should start by decreasing salt intake among children, adolescents and young adults (Trajković-Pavlović et al., 2010a, 2010b).

2.2.6 Vitamins, minerals and other bioactive molecules

Micronutrients, such as vitamins and minerals, are essential nutrients in maintaining good health, while other bioactive molecules, such as phytochemicals (substances of plant origin) and zoochemicals (substances of animal origin) are non-essential, but may improve human health (Kaput, 2006). Recommendations for vitamin and mineral intake exist for different population groups (Institute of Medicine, 1998, 2000, 2001), but it is not possible to quantify the need for phytochemicals (Smolin & Grosvenor, 2010).

Many vitamins (e.g vitamin E, vitamin C), minerals (e.g selenium) and phytochemicals (e.g flavonoids) are parts of the antioxidant defense system. Substances with antioxidant properties were seen as promising in lowering risks from chronic diseases and, among them, cancer. In vitro experiments have confirmed that these molecules have antioxidant properties, but the initial hypothesis that antioxidant substances can prevent cancer (or other chronic diseases) in humans has yet to be confirmed (WCRF & AICR, 2007; Mamede et al., 2011).

The impact of calcium and vitamin D on breast and colorectal cancer is being intensively researched during the last ten years, but, up to this point, no definite answers can be given about these relations (Lin et al., 2007; Lappe et al., 2007; Manson et al., 2011).

In the complex pathways of carcinogenesis, there are numerous processes that could be targeted by phytochemicals in order to lower the risk of disease development. The interest in phytochemicals has grown substantially over the years and it has not lessen, although screening for potential chemopreventive molecules requires a systematic and wide-range approach (Tan et al., 2011; Milner, 2004). In order to reduce the risk of cancer in human population, many experiments studying herbs and spices and their effects on carcinogenesis were conducted on animals. The possibility of using herbs and spices as substitutes for unhealthy food constituents (e.g added sugars, added fat, table salt) can contribute to chemopreventive potential of herbs and spices (Tapsell et al., 2006).

If phytochemicals are added to foods, such foods become functional. Functional foods are foods that provide healthy benefits beyond basic nutrition, when consumed as part of a varied diet on a regular basis, at effective levels (ADA, 2009; Howlett, 2008). According to some authors, health effects of consuming functional foods containing bioactive substances or pharmaceuticals may be as beneficial as consumption of those substances from their natural sources (Howlett, 2008). Other authors claim that chemopreventive properties of fruits and vegetables are a result of synergistic and additive effects of phytochemicals acting together in their natural environment, and therefore, cannot be imitated by functional foods (Tapsell et al., 2006; Liu, 2003; Milner, 2006b).

Global use of dietary supplements containing vitamins, minerals and other bioactive compounds, although already enormous, is still on the rise. Dietary supplements can reduce the risk of deficiencies and promote optimal health, but should not be considered substitutes for a well-balanced, healthy diet (Mason, 2007). Evidence supporting the use of dietary supplements in cancer risk reduction are scarce, so population-based recommendation is to increase the percentage of people who are achieving optimal nutrition without the use of dietary supplements (WCRF & AICR, 2007; Myung et al., 2009). Determination of oxidative stress-based biomarkers should be regarded as "indication" for using antioxidant supplements (Ziech et al., 2010), although this is not financially viable yet.

Mediterranean diet is considered to be protective against cancers, opposite to USA and Northern Europe diet patterns. Adoption of Mediterranean eating pattern in USA and Northern Europe may help cancer risk reduction (Simopoulos, 2001; Verberne et al., 2010).

2.3 Physical activity

Regular physical activity, besides leading to fitness, provides many health benefits (Warburton et al., 2006; Miles, 2007). Physical activity increases overall well-being, and if regular, improves quality of life, helps body mass maintenance and therefore, reduces cancer risks (WCRF & AICR, 2007; WHO, 2003, 2005, 2008a, 2009b; AICR & WCRF, 2009). Cancer risks in regularly physically active are up to 40.0% lower than among physically inactive (Newton & Galvão, 2008).

Insufficient physical activity is considered to be the fourth leading risk factor in overall mortality. WHO holds insufficient physical activity responsible for 6.0% of global deaths (WHO, 2009a). Dropping levels of physical activity worldwide are in part responsible for rising prevalence of NCDs, including cardiovascular diseases, diabetes and cancer (WCRF & AICR, 2007; WHO, 2005, 2009a; Fair & Montgomery, 2009; AICR & WCRF, 2009; Newton & Galvão, 2008; Tucker et al., 2011; Hardman et al., 2011; Wannamethee et al., 2001). Insufficient physical activity accounts for 21.0-25.0% of breast and colon cancer burden (WHO, 2009a, 2010a)

Physical inactivity is a modifiable lifestyle choice and a cancer risk factor, and it is therefore of great public health significance (WCRF & AICR, 2007; WHO, 2005; AICR & WCRF, 2009; Warburton et al., 2006; Miles, 2007; Newton & Galvão, 2008; Tucker et al., 2011; Hardman, 2001; Wolin et al., 2009), but meeting physical activity recommendations has proven to be as big of a challenge on an individual level, as on the society one.

The complexity of cancer - physical activity interactions should be assessed on gene level, too. Thune & Furberg (Thune & Furberg, 2001) believe that "genetic predisposition to be physically active, combined with the knowledge that cancer is a genetic localized disease, warrants studies in general population and high-risk groups alike".

Physical activity is divided into inactivity, insufficient activity and sufficient activity. Sufficient activity is subdivided into "meeting current recommendations" (moderate physical activity) and "highly active" (WHO, 2007b, 2009a, 2009b, 2010a).

"Meeting current recommendations" is possible by 2.5 hours of moderate physical activity, or 1 hour of vigorous physical activity per week. Both are equivalent with 600 metabolic equivalents [MET] per week. Highly active individuals' energy expenditure is equivalent to 1600 MET per week. Metabolic equivalent is the ratio of energy consumption during a specific physical activity to energy consumption while sitting and resting. One MET is defined as the resting metabolic rate obtained during quiet sitting and is set by convention to 3.5 ml O_2/kg/min or 1 kcal/kg/h (WHO, 2010a). Physical activities are classified according to energy needed for their performance, using MET as a reference value. On a population level, moderate physical activity should be set as a goal for health benefits and cancer risk reduction. Indivividuals and population groups that are already moderately active, should be encouraged to become highly active.

In the "Global Recommendations on Physical Activity and Health" (WHO, 2010a), WHO aims to establish dose-response relationship between physical activity and the consequent health benefits, as well as to identify the frequency, duration, intensity, type and total amount of physical activity needed for health benefits, such as cancer or other NCDs risk reduction (WHO, 2007b, 2009b, 2010a). Currently, it is believed that diabetes, heart diseases and cancer risks, including breast and colon cancer risks, can be reduced among people who are 18 or older by 150 minutes of moderate intensity aerobic activity the least, or 60 minutes of vigorous activity weekly. At least 60 minutes of moderate to vigorous physical activity can reduce NCDs risks in 5-17 year-olds (WHO, 2009a, 2009b). For added health benefits, introduction of physical activity, with the amount, frequency, duration and intensity being gradually increased, is recommended for inactive adults, older adults and those limited in activity by their disease (WHO, 2010a).

Public health goals set by new physical activity recommendations include achieving and maintaining optimal health (WCRF & AICR, 2007; WHO, 2003, 2005, 2007, 2008a, 2009a, 2009b, 2010a; Wolin et al., 2009).

2.4 Tobacco, alcohol use and everyday drinks

Although alcoholic beverages and everyday drinks are considered foods, together with tobacco use, their consumption may pose a health risk. On the other hand, safe drinking water is not a health risk, but a prerequisite for optimal health.

2.4.1 Tobacco use

Tobacco is a plant that contains nicotine, various carcinogens and toxins, and it is considered addictive (WHO, 2011d). Around 4000 chemicals have been detected in tobacco smoke, with more than 50 of them identified as carcinogenic (WHO, 2006). Tobacco dependence is classified as a disease under the International Classification of Diseases [ICD-10] (WHO, 1999).

Tobacco use has grown into a global epidemic. The number of tobacco users is on the rise in middle and low income countries, while in decline in developed countries (Mackay et al., 2006; IARC, 2004; WHO, 2008b). Smoking is the second principal cause of global mortality participating with 8.7% (3.7% DALYs) (WHO, 2008b, 2009a; IARC, 2004). At the same time, smoking is the most modifiable single risk factor for malignant diseases and other NCDs (WHO, 2009a; Danaei et al., 2009).

Smoking causes 71.0% of lung cancer deaths (WHO, 2009a), but it is also a risk for other cancer localizations, like throat, mouth, esophagus, stomach, pancreas, kidney, bladder and cervix (WHO, 1999, 2011d). Not only smokers die of smoking-related lung cancer - 4300 secondhand smokers die from lung cancer every year in USA (IARC, 2004; WHO, 2008b, 2011e).

Tobacco use, in any form, is unhealthy. Attempts were made to create less toxic versions of tobacco products, but such products were unacceptable by consumers and consequently failed. Although not widely used, in some parts of the world smokeless tobacco represents a significant form of tobacco use (WHO, 2006; IARC, 2004, 2006, 2008).

Definitions of smoking and related terms - secondhand tobacco smoke [SHS], environmental tobacco smoke [ETS] or other people's smoke and smoking free area - are given in WHO Framework Convention on Tobacco Control [WHO FCTC] as recommended terms for smoking and secondhand smoke (WHO, 2006, 2011e).

WHO FCTC aims to protect public health policy makers from commercial interests, to provide guidance for protection against tobacco smoke, to regulate the contents of tobacco products, to implement rules for labelling, advertising and promotion of tobacco products, to educate people and communicate information about tobacco addiction. Ultimately, the goal is to decrease the number of tobacco users and increase the number of former smokers (WHO, 2011e; IARC, 2008).

There are several aspects of harmful effects of smoking. Dietary nutrient intake and plasma folate level can also be affected by smoking status. Depletion of plasma folate, an antioxidant, together with depletion of other dietary substances, might be a factor in early onset of tobacco-related morbidity and mortality in smokers. Beneficial effects of Mediterranean diet on smokers' health have been documented and they are presumably related to optimal ratio of omega-6 to omega-3 polyunsaturated fatty acids and significant amounts of bioactive molecules (Vardavas et al., 2008, 2011).

In conclusion, all tobacco products should be considered harmful and addictive, and strict regulations should be implemented in order to control the tobacco epidemic (WHO, 2011e; IARC, 2008). Public health researchers of the Oxford Vision 2020 Program, underlined not only the societal, but the individual responsibility towards health and healthy lifestyle choices. Being aware of the health risks related to tobacco use is not merely enough – motivational campaigns should be designed in order to cut down smoking prevalence by 8.0 to 10.0% per year, and achieve the resulting prevalence of less than 10.0% in all social groups (Yach et al., 2005).

2.4.2 Alcohol use

WHO has estimated that alcohol consumption causes 3.5% of global deaths (6.2% among males, and 1.1% among females) (WHO, 2011f), and it is responsible for 4.5% of DALYs (WHO, 2011f).

The link between alcohol intake and cancer is well documented. There is a positive correlation between oral, pharyngeal, laryngeal, esophageal, liver, colorectal (in men) (WCRF & AICR, 2007; WHO, 2009a, 2011f; Testino & Borro, 2010; Baan et al., 2007) and breast cancer and intake of more than 30 g of alcohol/day (3 standard drinks/day) (Allen et al., 2009; Boyle & Boffetta, 2009). Heavy drinking may correlate with higher risk of lung and pancreatic cancer, but the epidemiological evidence supporting this hypothesis is weak (WCRF & AICR, 2007; WHO, 2011f; Testino & Borro, 2010).

Heavy drinking is defined as intake of more than 80 g of alcohol per day, or more than 5 to 6 standard drinks per day (Pöschl & Seitz, 2004).

More than 30 codes of ICD-10 include the term "alcohol" in their name or definition, documenting the importance of alcohol-related health impairment (WHO, 1999).

Health effects of alcohol vary depending on the age, gender and other characteristics of consumers, but they also depend on the setting and context of drinking (Pöschl & Seitz, 2004).

International Agency for Cancer Research has stated that "acetaldehyde associated with alcoholic beverages is carcinogenic to humans (Group 1)" and confirmed the Group 1 classification of alcohol consumption and of ethanol in alcoholic beverages (Secretan et al., 2009).

Acetaldehyde is the first and the most toxic metabolite of alcohol metabolism. Alcohol dehydrogenase [ADH] oxidizes alcohol to acetaldehyde, which is then converted to acetate by aldehyde dehydrogenase [ALDH]. Ethanol also inhibits DNA methylation and interacts with retinoid metabolism. Tissue-specific levels of ethanol are in correlation with the amount of alcohol ingested, but they also depend on the genotype coding for ethanol-metabolizing enzymes, predominantly ALDH (Seitz & Stickel, 2007; Boffeta & Hashibe, 2006; Seitz & Becker, 2007).

Effects of acetaldehyde, elevated estrogen levels, production of oxygen radicals and changes in folate and vitamin B_6 metabolism, may be mechanisms responsible for the genotoxicity of alcohol (Seitz & Stickel, 2007; Boffeta & Hashibe, 2006; Seitz & Becker, 2007).

Persons with achlorhydric gastritis who consume alcohol are at greater risk of stomach cancer. Absence of hydrochloric acid creates an environment favorable for thriving of ADH-containing bacteria that can metabolize carbohydrates to ethanol and acetaldehyde (Seitz & Becker, 2007).

The WHO Global Strategy to Reduce the Harmful Use of Alcohol (WHO, 2010b) aims to raise awareness of health, social and economic aspects of alcohol abuse, and the relationship between alcohol and disease development. It points to the importance of effective stakeholders involvement in preventing harmful effects of alcohol. It also aims to provide support for national efforts to reduce the overall effects of alcohol abuse.

USDA recommendations for alcohol intake not linked to increase of cancer risks are 28 g of alcohol per day for healthy adult men, and half of that amount for healthy women (USDA & U.S. Department of Health and Human Services, 2011). The European Code Against Cancer recommends up to 20 or 30 g/day of alcohol for healthy men and, again, half of that amount for healthy women (Boyle et al., 2003). AICR made recommendations simple by advising 2 standard drinks for healthy men and 1 standard drink for healthy women (WCRF & AICR, 2007).

Tobacco and alcohol use are major risk factors for malignancies of different localizations, but mainly of the gastrointestinal tract (Testino & Borro, 2010; Pelucchi et al., 2008; Seitz & Cho, 2009) and the two also act in synergy increasing the cancer risk. Tobacco smoking combined with alcohol use increase the tissue levels of acetaldehyde, while alcohol helps in activation of different procarcinogens in tobacco smoke by induction of cytochrome-P450-2E1-dependent microsomal biotransformation system in mucose cells of the upper digestive tract and liver (IARC, 2004; Testino and Borro, 2010; Seitz & Cho, 2009). Pancreatic cancer risk is 4.3-fold higher in people who smoke more than 20 cigarettes per day and drink more than 21 standard drinks per week, than in non-smoking people who drink less than 7 standard drinks per week (Talamini et al., 2010).

2.4.3 Coffee and tea use

Coffee and tea drinking is a widespread habit. Both coffee and tea contain many bioactive substances (antioxidants, phenols) with in vitro anticarcinogenic characteristics (Ferruzzi, 2010). Consumption of 3 cups of coffee per day (equivalent to 300 mg of caffeine) is considered to be moderate (Tverdal et al., 2011).

It is still not known whether coffee consumption increases the risk of any type of cancer. Evidence concerning the link between coffee and esophageal and pancreatic cancer are inconsistent and difficult to interpret, due to the confounding effects of tobacco and alcohol use (WCRF & AICR, 2007; Ferruzzi, 2010).

Laboratory experiments and animal testing showed chemoprotective activity of tea polyphenols, but there are not enough evidence to confirm the same in human population (WCRF & AICR, 2007; Lambert & Yang, 2003).

2.4.4 Soft drinks

Soft drinks consumption shows an increase of 5.0% per year, that is an increase from 467 to 552 billion litres from 2004 to 2007 (Zenith International, 2005, 2008). Cola drinks and carbonated soft drinks reportedly accounted for 42.0% of 467 billion litres of soft drinks consumed within one year, in contrast to fruit juices, nectars and fruit drinks which accounted for 8.0% in 2004 (Zenith International, 2005).

Currently, findings on the effects of soft drinks on cancer risks are limited and inconsistent (WCRF & AICR, 2007).

Soft drinks are significant contributors to added sugar intake which leads to body mass increase, overweigh, obesity and consequently to NCDs. Eminent international organizations do not consider soft drinks to be a part of healthy and active lifestyle (WCRF & AICR, 2007; WHO, 2005; USDA & U.S. Department of Health and Human Services, 2011).

2.4.5 Water as a fluid of choice

Only air is more crucial for life than water. Access to safe drinking water is a basic human right, as well as a condition for achieving and sustaining optimal health (WHO, 2011e).

However, contaminated water is a great health risk. Inorganic arsenic from drinking water is a proven risk for lung cancer and there is limited evidence that it is also a risk factor for kidney and bladder cancer (WCRF & AICR, 2007).

Safe drinking water is a nutrient *per se*. Because it plays many important roles in the human body, water is the fluid of choice as a part of healthy lifestyle. There has been a steady growth in the sales of bottled water (6.1% in 2007) (Zenith International, 2008) which is an encouraging fact in accordance with today's active and healthy lifestyle.

Daily requirements for water depend on age, gender, pregnancy, lactation, physical activity level, diet and external conditions (Smolin & Grosvenor, 2010; ILSI, 2004).

3. Conclusion

The impact of nutrition and lifestyle on cancer development is evident. Still, there are many unanswered questions concerning the interactions among nutrition, environment and human genome. The existing and future knowledge should be used by public health professionals to promote cancer risk reduction on a population scale, especially in high risk subpopulations, as well as on the individual level. Further research and public health activities should be supported by health and government authorities.

"To eat is a necessity, to eat intelligently is an art." (François de La Rochefoucauld, French writer, 1613-1680)

"Walking is man's best medicine." (Hippocrates, ancient Greek physician, 460 BC - 377 BC)

4. References

ADA. (2006a). The Roles of Registered Dietitians and Dietetic Technicians, Registered in Health Promotion and Disease Prevention. *Journal of the American Dietetic Association*, Vol.106, No.11, (November 2006), pp. 1875-1884, ISSN 0002-8223

ADA. (2006b). Position of the American Dietetic Association: Food and Nutrition Misinformation. *Journal of the American Dietetic Association*, Vol.106, No.4, (April 2006), pp. 601-607, ISSN 0002-8223

ADA. (2008). Nutrition Care Process and Model Part I: The 2008 Update. *Journal of the American Dietetic Association*, Vol.108, No.7, (July 2008), pp. 1113-1117, ISSN 0002-8223

ADA. (2009). Position of the American Dietetic Association: Functional Foods. *Journal of the American Dietetic Association*, Vol.109, No.4, (April 2009), pp. 735-746, ISSN 0002-8223

AICR & WCRF. (2009). *Policy and Action for Cancer Prevention. Food, Nutrition, and Physical Activity: a Global Perspective*, AICR, ISBN 978-0-9722522-4-9, Washington, District of Columbia, USA

Allen, N.E., Beral, V., Casabonne, D., Kan, S.W., Reeves, G.K., Brown, A. & Green, J.; Million Women Study Collaborators. (2009). Moderate Alcohol Intake and Cancer Incidence in Women. *Journal of the National Cancer Institute*, Vol.101, No.5, (4 March 2009), pp. 296-305, ISSN 0027-8874

Allen, N.E., Sauvaget, C., Roddam, A.W., Appleby, P., Nagano, J., Suzuki, G., Key, T.J. & Koyama, K. (2004). A Prospective Study of Diet and Prostate Cancer in Japanese Men. *Cancer Causes & Control*, Vol.15, No.9, (November 2004), pp. 911-920, ISSN 0957-5243

American Cancer Society & Livestrong. (2010). *The Global Economic Cost of Cancer*, American Cancer Society, Atlanta, Georgia, USA

American Diabetic Association & ADA. (2003). *Exchange List for Meal Planning*. ADA, ISBN 978-0880913102, Alexandria, Virginia, USA

Aune, D., De Stefani, E., Ronco, A.L., Boffetta, P., Deneo-Pellegrini, H., Acosta, G. & Mendilaharsu, M. (2009a). Egg Consumption and the Risk of Cancer: a Multisite Case-control Study in Uruguay. *Asian Pacific Journal of Cancer Prevention*, Vol.10, No.5, pp. 869-876, ISSN 1513-7368

Aune, D., De Stefani, E., Ronco, A.L., Boffetta, P., Deneo-Pellegrini, H., Acosta, G. & Mendilaharsu, M. (2009b). Legume Intake and the Risk of Cancer: a Multisite Case-control Study in Uruguay. *Cancer Causes & Control*, Vol.20, No.9, (November 2009), pp. 1605-1615, ISSN 0957-5243

Aune, D., Lau, R., Chan, D.S., Vieira, R., Greenwood, D.C., Kampman, E. & Norat, T. (2011). Dairy Products and Colorectal Cancer Risk: a Systematic Review and Meta-analysis of Cohort. *Annals of Oncology*, [Epub ahead of print] 26 May 2011, ISSN 1569-8041

Baan, R., Straif, K., Grosse, Y., Secretan, B., El Ghissassi, F., Bouvard, V., Altieri, A. & Cogliano, V; WHO International Agency for Research on Cancer Monograph Working Group. (2007). Carcinogenity and Alcoholic Beverages. *Lancet Oncology*, Vol.8, No.4, (April 2007), pp. 292-293, ISSN 1470-2045

Barclay, A.W., Petocz, P., McMillan-Price, J., Flood, V.M., Prvan, T., Mitchell, P. & Brand-Miller, J.C. (2008). Glycemic Index, Glycemic Load and Chronic Disease Risk - a Meta Analysis of Observational Studies. *American Journal of Clinical Nutrition*, Vol.87, No.3, (March 2008), pp. 627-637, ISSN 0002-9165

Béliveau, R. & Gingras, D. (2007). Role of Nutrition in Preventing Cancer. *Canadian Family Physician*, Vol.53, No.11, (November 2007), pp. 1905-1911, ISSN 0008-350X

Bigaard, J., Frederiksen, K., Tjønneland, A., Thomsen, B.L., Overvad, K., Heitmann, B.L. & Sørensen, T.I.A. (2005). Waist Circumference and Body Composition in Relation to All-cause Mortality in Middle-aged Men and Women. *International Journal of Obesity*, Vol.29, (3 May 2005), pp. 778-784, ISSN 1476-5497

Boffeta, P. & Hashibe, M. (2006). Alcohol and Cancer. *Lancet Oncology*, Vol.7, No.2, (February 2006), pp. 149-156, ISSN 1470-2045

Boffetta, P., Couto, E., Wichmann, J., Ferrari, P., Trichopoulos, D., Bueno-de-Mesquita H.B., Van Duijnhoven, F.J., Büchner, F.L., Key, T., Boeing, H., Nöthlings, U., Linseisen, J., Gonzalez, C.A., Overvad, K., Nielsen, M.R., Tjønneland, A., Olsen, A., Clavel-Chapelon, F., Boutron-Ruault, M.C., Morois, S., Lagiou, P., Naska, A., Benetou, V., Kaaks, R., Rohrmann, S., Panico, S., Sieri, S., Vineis, P., Palli, D., Van Gils, C.H., Peeters, P.H., Lund, E., Brustad, M., Engeset, D., Huerta, J.M., Rodríguez, L., Sánchez, M.J., Dorronsoro, M., Barricarte, A., Hallmans, G., Johansson, I., Manjer, J., Sonestedt, E., Allen, N.E., Bingham, S., Khaw, K.T., Slimani, N., Jenab, M., Mouw, T., Norat, T., Riboli, E. & Trichopoulou, A. (2010). Fruit and Vegetable Intake and Overall Cancer Risk in the European Prospective Investigation into Cancer and Nutrition (EPIC). *Journal of the National Cancer Institute*, Vol.102, No.8, (21 April 2010), pp. 529-537, ISSN 0027-8874

Bon, G.B. (2008). Adipose Tissue: a Multifunctional Organ. *Congenital Cardiology Today*, Vol.9, No.4, (April 2008), pp. 23S-28S, ISSN 1554-7787

Bonsmann, S.S., Celemín, L.F. & Grunert, K.G. (2010). Food Labelling to Advance Better Education for Life. *European Journal of Clinical Nutrition*, Vol.64, No.3, (November 2010), pp. S14-S19, ISSN 0954-3007

Boyle, P. & Boffetta, P. (2009). Alcohol Consumption and Breast Cancer Risk. *Breast Cancer Research*, Vol.11, No.S3, pp. S3, ISSN 1465-5411

Boyle, P. & Levin, B. (Eds.) (2008). *World Cancer Report*, IARC, ISBN 9789283204237, Lyon, France

Boyle, P., Autier, P., Bartelink, H., Baselga, J., Boffetta, P., Burn, J., Burns, H.J., Christensen, L., Denis, L., Dicato, M., Diehl, V., Doll, R., Franceschi, S., Gillis, C.R., Gray, N., Griciute, L., Hackshaw, A., Kasler, M., Kogevinas, M., Kvinnsland, S., La Vecchia, C., Levi, F., McVie, J.G., Maisonneuve, P., Martin-Moreno, J.M., Bishop, J.N., Oleari, F., Perrin, P., Quinn, M., Richards, M., Ringborg, U., Scully, C., Siracka, E., Storm, H., Tubiana, M., Tursz, T., Veronesi, U., Wald, N., Weber, W., Zaridze, D.G., Zatonski, W. & Zur Hausen, H. (2003). European Code Against Cancer and Scientific Justification: Third Version (2003). *Annals of Oncology*, Vol.14, No.7, (July 2003), pp. 973-1005, ISSN 0923-7534

Brower, V. (2011). Epigenetics: Unravelling the Cancer Code. *Nature*, Vol.471, No.7339, (June 2011), pp. S12-S13, ISSN 0028-083

Butler, L.M., Sinha, R., Millikan, R.C., Martin, C.F., Newman, B., Gammon, M.D., Ammerman, A.S. & Sandler, R.S. (2003). Heterocyclic Amines, Meat Intake, and Association with Colon Cancer in a Population-based Study. *American Journal of Epidemiology*, Vol.157, No.5, (1 March 2003), pp. 434-445, ISSN 0002-9262

Buttriss, J.L. & Stokes, C.S. (2008). Dietary Fibre and Health: an Overview. *Nutrition Bulletin*, Vol.33, No.3, (September 2008), pp. 186–200, ISSN 1471-9827

Calle, E.E., Rodriguez, C., Walker-Thurmond, K., Thun, M.J. (2003). Overweight, Obesity, and Mortality from Cancer in a Prospectively Studied Cohort of U.S. Adults. *New England Journal of Medicine*, Vol.348, No.17, (24 April 2003), pp. 1625-1638, ISSN 1533-4406

Cancer Council Australia. (2007). Position Statement: Fruit, Vegetables and Cancer Prevention, 20 July 2011, Available from: http://www.cancer.org.au/File/PolicyPublications/Position_statements/PS-Fruit%20_vegetables_cancer_Aug07%20UpdatedJun09.pdf

Cani, P.D. & Delzenne, N.M. (2009). The Role of the Gut Microbiota in Energy Metabolism and Metabolic Disease. *Current Pharmaceutical Design*, Vol.15, No.13, pp. 1546-1558, ISSN 1381-6128

Cani, P.D., Amar, J., Iglesias, M.A., Poggi, M., Knauf, C., Bastelica, D., Neyrinck, A.M., Fava, F., Tuohy, K.M., Chabo, C., Waget, A., Delmée, E., Cousin, B., Sulpice, T., Chamontin, B., Ferrières, J., Tanti, J.F., Gibson, G.R., Casteilla, L., Delzenne, N.M., Alessi, M.C. & Burcelin, R. (2007a). Metabolic Endotoxemia Initiates Obesity and Insulin Resistance. *Diabetes*, Vol.56, No.7, (July 2007), pp. 1761-1772, ISSN 0012-1797

Cani, P.D., Neyrinck, A.M., Fava, F., Knauf, C., Burcelin, R.G., Tuohy, K.M., Gibson, G.R. & Delzenne, N.M. (2007b). Selective Increases of Bifidobacteria in Gut Microflora Improve High-fat-diet-induced Diabetes in Mice Through a Mechanism Associated with Endotoxaemia. *Diabetologia*, Vol.50, No.11, (November 2007), pp. 2374-2383, ISSN 0012-186X

Chan, A.T. & Giovannucci, E.L. (2010). Primary Prevention of Colorectal Cancer. *Gastroenterology*, Vol.138, No.6, (June 2010), pp. 2029-2043, ISSN 0016-5085

Chan, D.S., Lau, R., Aune, D., Vieira, R., Greenwood, D.C., Kampman, E. & Norat T. (2011). Red and Processed Meat and Colorectal Cancer Incidence: Meta-analysis of Prospective Studies. *PloS One/Public Library of Science*, Vol.6, No.6, e20456, [Epub 6 Jun 2011], ISSN 1932-6203

Colquhoun, A., Miyake, J.A. & Benadiba, M. (2009). Fatty Acids, Eicosanoids and Cancer. *Nutritional Therapy and Metabolism*, Vol.27, No.3, pp. 105-112, ISSN 1828-6232

Cross, A.J. & Sinha, R. (2004). Meat-related Mutagens/Carcinogens in the Etiology of Colorectal Cancer. *Environmental and Molecular Mutagenesis*, Vol.44, No.1, pp. 44-55, ISSN 0893-6692

Danaei, G., Ding, E.L., Mozaffarian, D., Taylor, B., Rehm, J., Murray, C.J. & Ezzati, M. (2009). The Preventable Causes of Death in the United States: Comparative Risk Assessment of Dietary, Lifestyle and Metabolic Risk Factors. *PloS One/Public Library of Science*, Vol.6, No.4, e 1000058. [Epub 28 April 2009], ISSN 1932-6203

Daniel, C.R., McCullough, M.L., Patel, R.C., Jacobs, E.J., Flanders, W.D., Thun, M.J. & Calle, E.E. (2009). Dietary Intake of Omega-6 and Omega-3 Fatty Acids and Risk of Colorectal Cancer in a Prospective Cohort of U.S. Men and Women. *Cancer Epidemiology, Biomarkers and Prevention*, Vol.18, No.2, (February 2009), pp. 516-525, ISSN 1055-9965

Donaldson, S.M. (2004). Nutrition and Cancer: a Review of the Evidence for and Anti-cancer Diet. *Nutrition Journal*, Vol.3, (20 October 2004), pp. 19, ISSN 1475-2891

Donohoe, C.L., Doyle, S.L. & Reynolds, J.V. (2011). Visceral Adiposity, Insulin Resistance and Cancer Risk. *Diabetology & Metabolic Syndrome*, Vol. 3, No.12, (22 June 2011), In press, ISSN 1758-5996

Eichholzer, M. & Gutzwiller, F. (1998). Dietary Nitrates, Nitrites, and N-nitroso Compounds and Cancer Risk: a Review of the Epidemiologic Evidence. *Nutrition Reviews*, Vol.56, No.4 Pt. 1, pp. 95-105, ISSN 0029-6643

Fair, A.M. & Montgomery, K. (2009). Energy Balance, Physical Activity and Cancer Risk. *Methods in Molecular Biology*, Vol.472, No.I , pp. 57-88, ISSN 1064-3745

FAO. (2004). *Human Energy Requirements. Report of a Joint FAO/WHO/UNU Expert Consultation*, FAO, ISBN 92-5-105212-3, Rome, Italy

FAO. (2011). FAO STAT, 22 July 2011, Available from:

http://faostat.fao.org/site/354/default.aspx

Fenech, M., El-Sohemy, A., Cahill, L., Ferguson, L.R., French, T-A.C., Tai, E.S., Milner, J.A., Koh, W.P., Xie, L., Zucker, M., Buckley, M., Cosgrove, L., Lockett, T., Fung, K.Y.C. & Head, R. (2009). Nutrigenetics and Nutrigenomics: Viewpoints on the Current Status and Applications in Nutrition Research and Practice. *Journal of Nutrigenetics and Nutrigenomics*, Vol.4, No.2, (July 2011), pp. 69-89, ISSN 1661-6499

Ferruzzi, M.G. (2010). The Influence of Beverage Composition on Delivery of Phenolic Compounds from Coffee and Tea. *Physiology and Behavior*, Vol.100, No.1, (26 April 2010), pp. 33-41, ISSN 0031-9384

Fontham, E.T.H. & Su, L.J. (2005). Prevention of Cancers of the Esophagus and Stomach, In: *Preventive Nutrition. The Comprehensive Guide for Health Professionals*, Bendich, A., Deckelbaum, R.J., (Eds.), pp. 25-54, Humana Press, ISBN 1-59259-880-3, Totowa, New Jersey, USA

Giovannuci, E., Harlan, D.M., Archer, M.C., Bergenstal, R.M., Gapstur, S.M., Habel, L.A., Pollak, M., Regensteiner, J.G. & Yee, D. (2010). Diabetes and Cancer. A Consensus Report. *Diabetes Care*, Vol.33, No.7, (July 2010), pp. 1674-1685, ISSN 0149-5992

Go, W.L.V., Butrum, R.R. & Wong, D.A. (2003). Diet, Nutrition and Cancer Prevention: The Postgenomic Era. *Journal of Nutrition*, Vol.133, No.11, (November 2003), pp. 3830S-3836S, ISSN 0022-3166

Goldman, R., Shields, P.G. (2003). Food Mutagens. *Journal of Nutrition*, Vol.133, No.3, (March 2003), pp. 965S-973S, ISSN 0022-3166

Gonzalez, C.A. (2006). Nutrition and Cancer: the Current Epidemiological Evidence. *British Journal of Nutrition*, Vol.96, No.S1, (August 2006), pp. S42-S45, ISSN 0007-1145

Goodlad, R.A., Lenton, W., Ghatei, M.A., Adrian, T.E., Bloom, S.R. & Wright, N.A. (1987). Effects of an Elemental Diet, Inert Bulk and Different Types of Dietary Fibre on the Response of the Intestinal Epithelium to Refeeding in the Rat and Relationship to Plasma Gastrin, Enteroglucagon and PYY Concentrations. *Gut*, Vol.28, No.2, (February 1987), pp. 171-180, ISSN 0017-5749

Grace, C. (2011). A Review of One-to-one Dietetic Obesity Management in Adults. *Journal of Human Nutrition & Dietetics*, Vol.24, No.1, (February 2011), pp. 13-22, ISSN 1365-277X

Gray, J. (2006). *Dietary Fibre. Definition, Analysis, Physiology and Health*. ILSI Europe, ISBN 90-78637-03-X, Brussels, Belgium

Hardman, A.E. (2011). Physical Activity and Cancer Risk. *Proceedings of the Nutrition Society*, Vol.60, pp. 107-113, ISSN 0029-6651

Havas, S., Heimendinger, J., Reynolds, K., Baranowski, T., Nicklas, T.A., Bishop, D., Buller, D., Sorensen, G., Beresford, S.A., Cowan, A. & Damron, D. (1994). 5 a Day for Better Health: a New Research Initiative. *Journal of the American Dietetic Association*, Vol.94, No.1, (January 1994), pp. 32-36, ISSN 0002-8223

Heilbronn, L.K. & Campbell, L.V. (2008). Adipose Tissue Macrophages, Low Grade Inflammation and Insulin Resistance in Human Obesity. *Current Pharmaceutical Design*, Vol.14, No.12, pp. 1225-1230, ISSN 1381-6128

Hernandez, B.Y., Park, S.Y., Wilkens, L.R., Henderson, B.E. & Kolonel, L.N. (2009). Relationship of Body Mass, Height, and Weight Gain to Prostate Cancer Risk in the Multiethnic Cohort. *Cancer Epidemiology, Biomarkers and Prevention*, Vol.18, No.9, (September 2009), pp. 2413-2421, ISSN 1055-9965

Howlett, J. (2008). *Functional Foods: From Science to Health and Claims*. ILSI Europe, ISBN 9789078637110, Brussels, Belgium

Hu, J., La Vecchia, C., De Groh, M., Negri, E., Morrison, H., Mery, L. & the Canadian Cancer Registries Epidemiology Research Group. (2011a). Dietary Cholesterol Intake and Cancer. *Annals of Oncology*, [Epub ahead of print] 4 May 2011, ISSN 1569-8041

Hu, J., La Vecchia, C.L., Groh, M.D., Negri, E., Morrison, H., Mery, L. & The Canadian Cancer Registries Epidemiology Research Group. (2011b). Dietary Transfatty Acids and Cancer Risk. *European Journal of Cancer Prevention*, [Epub ahead of print] 22 June 2011, ISSN 0959-8278

Huth, P.J., DiRienzo, D.B. & Miller, G.D. (2006). Major Scientific Advances with Dairy Foods in Nutrition and Health. *Journal of Dairy Science*, Vol.89, No.4, (April 2006), pp. 1207-1221, ISSN 0022-0302

IARC. (2004). *IARC Monographs on the Evaluation of Carcinogenic Risks to Humans, Volume 83: Tobacco smoke and involuntary smoking*, IARC, ISBN 92 832 1283 5, Lyon, France

IARC. (2006). *IARC Monographs on the Evaluation of Carcinogenic Risks to Humans, Vol. 89: Smokeless Tobacco and Some Tobacco-specific N-Nitrosamines*, IARC, ISBN 978 92 832 1289 8, Lyon, France

IARC. (2008). *IARC Handbooks of Cancer Prevention, Tobacco Control, Vol. 12: Methods for Evaluating Tobacco Control Policies*, IARC, ISBN 978-92-832-3012-0, Lyon, France

IDF. (2006). *The IDF Consensus Worldwide Definition of the Metabolic Syndrome*, IDF Communications, Brussels, Belgium

ILSI North America. (2004). Hydration: Fluids for Life, ILSI North America, ISBN 1-57881-182-1, Washington, District of Columbia, USA

ILSI. (2005). *Nutrition and Genetics. Mapping Individual Health*, ILSI Press, ISBN 1578811953, Brussells, Belgium

Institute of Medicine. (1998). *Dietary Reference Intakes for Thiamin, Riboflavin, Niacin, Vitamin B_6, Folate, Vitamin B_{12}, Pantothenic Acid, Biotin, and Choline*. National Academy Press, ISBN 978-0-309-06411-8, Washington, District of Columbia, USA

Institute of Medicine. (2000). *Dietary Reference Intakes for vitamin C, Vitamin E, Selenium and Carotenoides*. National Academy Press, ISBN 978-0-309-06935-9, Washington, District of Columbia, USA

Institute of Medicine. (2001). *Dietary Reference Intakes for Vitamin A, Vitamin K, Arsenic, Boron, Chromium, Copper, Iodine, Iron, Manganese, Molybdenum, Nickel, Silicon, Vanadium and Zinc*. National Academy Press, ISBN 978-0-309-07290-8, Washington, District of Columbia, USA

Institute of Medicine. (2005). *Dietary Reference Intakes for Energy, Carbohydrate, Fiber, Fat, Fatty Acids, Cholesterol, Protein and Amino Acids*. National Academies Press, ISBN 9780309085373, Washington, District of Columbia, USA

Jain, S., Yadav, M., Menon, S., Yadav, H. & Marotta, F. (2010). Anticarcinogenic Effects of Probiotics, Prebiotics, and Synbiotics, In: *Handbook of Prebiotics and Probiotics Ingredients*, Sungsoo, S., Finocchiaro, T.E. (Eds.), pp. 273-292, CRC Press, ISBN 9781420062137, Boca Raton, Florida, USA

Järvinen, R., Knekt, P., Hakulinen, T. & Aromaa, A. (2001). Prospective Study on Milk Products, Calcium and Cancers of the Colon and Rectum. *European Journal of Clinical Nutrition*, Vol.55, No.11, (November 2001), pp. 1000-1007, ISSN 0954-3007

Joslin Diabetes Center & Joslin Clinic. (2007). Clinical Nutrition Guideline for Overweight and Obese Adults with Type 2 Diabetes, Prediabetes or Those at High Risk for Developing Type 2 Diabetes, 21 July 2011, Available from: http://www.joslin.org/docs/Nutrition_Guideline_Graded.pdf

Jovičić, J., Novaković, B. & Torović, LJ. (2011). Health Claims Made on Foods. *Vojnosanitetski pregled*, Vol.63, No.3, (March 2011), pp. 266-269, ISSN 00428450

Kaput, J. (2006). Diet-disease Interactions at the Molecular Level: an Experimental Paradigm, In: *Phytochemicals: Nutrient-Gene Interactions*, Meskin, M.S., Bidlack, W.R. & Randolph, R.K, (Eds.)., pp. 24-39, CRC Press, ISBN 978-0849341809, Boca Raton, Florida, USA

Key, T.J., Schatzkin, A., Willett, W.C., Allen, N.E., Spencer, E.A. & Travis, R.C. (2004). Diet, Nutrition and the Prevention of Cancer. *Public Health Nutrition*, Vol.7, No.1A, (February 2004), pp. 187-200, ISSN 1368-9800

Kim, Y. (2006). Cancer, In: *Present Knowledge in Nutrition* (9th ed.), Bowman B.M., Russel R.M., (Eds.)., pp. 689-711, International Life Sciences Institute [ILSI] Press, ISBN 9781578811991, Washington, District of Columbia, USA

Kinsella, K. & He, W. (2009). *An Aging World 2008*. U.S. Government Printing Office, Washington, District of Columbia, USA, (U.S. Census Bureau, International Population Reports, P95/09-1)

Kolonel, L.N., Hankin, J.H., Whittemore, A.S., Wu, A.H., Gallagher, R.P., Wilkens, L.R., John, E.M., Howe, G.R., Dreon, D.M., West, D.W. & Paffenbarger, R.S.Jr. (2000). Vegetables, Fruits, Legumes and Prostate Cancer: a Multiethnic Case-control Study. *Cancer Epidemiology, Biomarkers and Prevention*, Vol.9, No.8, (August 2000), pp. 795-804, ISSN 1055-9965

Kryston, T.B., Georgiev, A.B., Pissis, P. & Georgakilas, A.G. (2011). Role of Oxidative Stress and DNA Damage in Human Carcinogenesis. *Mutation Research*, Vol.711, No.1-2, (3 June 2011), pp. 193-201, ISSN 0027-5107

Kushi, L.H., Byers, T., Doyle, C., Bandera, E.V., McCullough, M., McTiernan, A., Gansler, T., Andrews, K.S. & Thun, M.J. (2006). American Cancer Society Guidelines on Nutrition and Physical Activity for Cancer Prevention: Reducing the Risk of Cancer with Healthy Food Choices and Physical Activity. *CA. A Cancer Journal for Clinicians*, Vol.56, No.5, (September-October 2006), pp. 254-281, ISSN 0007-9235

Lagergren, J. (2011). Influence of Obesity on the Risk of Esophageal Disorders. *Nature Reviews Gastroenterology and Hepatology*, Vol.8, No.6, (June 2011), pp. 340-347, ISSN 1759-5045

Lambert, J.D. & Yang, C.S. (2003). Cancer Chemopreventive Activity and Bioavailability of Tea and Tea Polyphenols. *Mutation Research*, Vol.523-524, pp. 201-208, ISSN 1383-5718

Lanou, A.J. & Svenson, B. (2011). Reduced Cancer Risk in Vegetarians: an Analysis of Recent Reports. *Cancer Management and Research*, Vol.3, pp. 1-8, ISSN 1179-1322

Lappe, J.M., Travers-Gustafson, D., Davies, K.M., Recker, R.R. & Heaney, R.P. (2007). Vitamin D and Calcium Supplementation Reduces Cancer Risk: Results of a Randomized Trial. *American Journal of Clinical Nutrition*, Vol.85, No.6, (June 2007), pp. 1586-1591, ISSN 0002-9165

Lin, J., Manson, J.E., Lee, I.M., Cook, N.R., Buring, J.E. & Zhang, S.M. (2007). Intakes of Calcium and Vitamin D and Breast Cancer Risk in Women. *Archives of Internal Medicine*, Vol.167, No.10, (28 May 2007), pp. 1050-1059, ISSN 0003-9926

Liu, R.H. (2003). Health Benefits of Fruit and Vegetables are from Additive and Synergistic Combinations of Phytochemicals. *American Journal of Clinical Nutrition*, Vol.78, No.3 Suppl, (September 2003), pp. S517-S520, ISSN 0002-9165

Ma, J., Li, H., Giovannucci, E., Mucci, L., Qiu, W., Nguyen, P.L., Gaziano, J.M., Pollak, M. & Stampfer, M.J. (2008). Prediagnostic Body-mass Index, Plasma C-peptide Concentration, and Prostate Cancer-specific Mortality in Men with Prostate Cancer: a Long-term Survival Analysis. *Lancet Oncology*, Vol.9, No.11, (November 2008), pp. 1039-1047, ISSN 1470-2045

Mackay, J., Eriksen, M. & Shafey, O. (2006). *The tobacco atlas* (2nd ed.), American Cancer Society, ISBN 0-944235-58-1, Brighton, UK

Mamede, A.C., Tavares, S.D., Abrantes, A.M., Trinidade, J., Maia, J.M. & Botelho, M.F. (2011). The Role of Vitamins in Cancer: a Review. *Nutrition and Cancer*, Vol.63, No.4, (May 2011), pp. 479-494, ISSN 0163-5581

Manson, J.E., Mayne, S.T. & Clinton, S.K. (2011). Vitamin D and Prevention of Cancer: Ready for Prime Time? *New England Journal of Medicine*, Vol.364, No.15, (14 April 2011), pp. 1385-1387, ISSN 0028-4793

Mason, P. (2007). *Dietary Supplements* (3rd ed.), Pharmaceutical Press, ISBN 978-0853698838, Trowbridge, Wiltshire, UK

Miles, L. (2007). Physical Activity and Health. *Nutrition Bulletin*, Vol.32, No.4, (December 2007), pp. 314–363, ISSN 1471-9827

Milner, J.A. (2004). Molecular Targets for Bioactive Food Components. *Journal of Nutrition*, Vol.134, No.9, (September 2004), pp. 2492S-2498S, ISSN 0022-3166

Milner, J.A. (2006a). Nutrigenomics and Nutrigenetics, In: *Nutritional Oncology*, Heber, D., Blackburn, G.L, Go, V.L.W., Miler, J., (Eds.), pp. 15-24, Academic Press, ISBN 978-0-12-088393-6, Waltham, Massachusetts, USA

Milner, J.A. (2006b). Diet and Cancer: Facts and Controversies. *Nutrition and Cancer*, Vol.56, No.2, pp. 216-224, ISSN 0163-5581

Munjal, U., Glei, M., Pool-Zobel, B.L. & Scharlau, D. (2009). Fermentation Products of Inulin-type Fructans Reduce Proliferation and Induce Apoptosis in Human Colon Tumor Cells of Different Stages of Carcinogenesis. *British Journal of Nutrition*, Vol.102, No.5, (September 2009), pp. 663-671, ISSN 0007-1145

Murff, H.J., Shu, X-O., Li, H., Yang, G., Wu, X., Cai, H., Wen, W., Gao, Y-T. & Zheng, W. (2011). Dietary Polyunsaturated Fatty Acids and Breast Cancer Risk in Chinese Women: A Prospective Cohort Study. *International Journal of Cancer*, Vol.128, No.6, (15 March 2011), pp. 1434-1441, ISSN 0020-7136

Myung, S-K., Kim, Y., Ju, W., Choi, H.J. & Bae, W.K. (2009). Effects of Antioxidant Supplements on Cancer Prevention: Meta-analysis of Randomized Controlled Trials. *Annals of Oncology*, Vol.21, No.1, pp. 166-179, ISSN 0923-7534

Newton, R.U. & Galvão, D.A. (2008). Exercise in Prevention and Management of Cancer. *Current Treatment Options in Oncology*, Vol.9, No.2-3, (June 2008), ISSN 1527-2729

Novaković, B., Jovičić, J., Jusupović, F., Grujičić, M. & Đurić, D. Nutrition Care Process in Cancer. *HealthMED*, Vol.4, No.2, pp. 427-433, ISSN 1840-2291

Pelucchi, C., Gallus, S., Garavello, W., Bosetti, C. & La Vecchia, C. (2008). Alcohol and Tobacco Use, and Cancer Risk for Upper Aerodigestive Tract and Liver. *European Journal of Cancer Prevention*, Vol.17, No.4, (August 2008), pp. 340-344, ISSN 0959-8278

Popkin, B.M. (1994). The Nutrition Transition: Low-income Countries: an Emerging Crisis. Nutrition Reviews, Vol.52, No.9, (September 1994), pp. 285-298, ISSN 0029-6643

Popkin, B.M. (2001). The Nutrition Transition and Obesity in Developing World. *Journal of Nutrition*, Vol. 131, No.3, (March 2001), pp. 871S-873S, ISSN 0022-3166

Pöschl, G. & Seitz, H.K. (2004). Alcohol and Cancer. *Alcohol and Alcoholism*, Vol.39, No.3, pp. 155-165, ISSN 0735-0414

Quigley, E.M.M. (2011). Nutritional and Health Promoting Properties of Dairy Products: Colon Cancer Prevention, In: *Encyclopedia of Diary Sciences* (2nd ed.), Fuquay, J.W., Fox, P.F. & McSweeney, P.L.H. (Eds.), pp. 1016-1022, Academic Press, ISBN 978-0-12-374402-9, Waltham, Massachusetts, USA

Radosavljević, V., Janković, S., Marinković, J. & Dokić, M. (2005). Diet and Bladder Cancer: a Case-control Study. *International Urology and Nephrology*, Vol.37, No.2, pp. 283-289, ISSN 0301-1623

Redinger, R.N. (2008). The Physiology of Adiposity. *Journal of the Kentucky Medical Association*, Vol.106, No.2, (February 2008), pp. 53-62, ISSN 2155-661X

Roberfroid, M., Gibson, G.R., Hoyles, L., McCartney, A.L., Rastall, R., Rowland, I., Wolvers, D., Watzl, B., Szajewska, H., Stahl, B., Guarner, F., Respondek, F., Whelan, K., Coxam, V., Davicco, M.J., Léotoing, L., Wittrant, Y., Delzenne, N.M., Cani, P.D., Neyrinck, A.M. & Meheust, A. (2010). Prebiotic Effects: Metabolic and Health Benefits. *British Journal of Nutrition*, Vol.104, No.2, (August 2010), pp. S1-S63, ISSN 0007-1145

Schatzkin, A., Mouw, T., Park, Y., Subar, A.F., Kipnis, V., Hollenbeck, A., Leitzmann, M.F. & Thompson, F.E. (2007). Dietary Fiber and Whole-grain Consumption in Relation to Colorectal Cancer in the NIH-AARP Diet and Health Study. *American Journal of Clinical Nutrition*, Vol.85, No.2, (1 February 2007), pp. 1353-1360, ISSN 0002-9165

Secretan, B., Straif, K., Baan, R., Grosse, Y., El Ghissassi, F., Bouvard, V., Benbrahim-Tallaa, L., Guha, N., Freeman, C., Galichet, L. & Cogliano, V.; WHO International Agency for Research on Cancer Monograph Working Group. (2009). A Review of Human Carcinogens - Part E: Tobacco, Areca nut, Alcohol, Coal smoke, and Salted Fish. *Lancet Oncology*, Vol.10, No.11, (November 2009), pp. 1033-1044, ISSN 1470-2045

Seitz, H.K. & Becker, P. (2007). Alcohol Metabolism and Cancer Risk. *Alcohol Research And Health*, Vol.30, No.1, pp. 38-47, ISSN 1535-7414

Seitz, H.K. & Cho, C.H. (2009). Contribution of Alcohol and Tobacco Use in Gastrointestinal Cancer Development. *Methods in Molecular Biology*, Vol.472, pp. 217-241, ISSN 1064-3745

Seitz, H.K. & Stickel, F. (2007). Molecular Mechanisms of Alcohol-mediated Carcinogenesis. *Nature Reviews. Cancer*, Vol.7, No.8, (August 2007), pp. 599-612, ISSN 1474-175X

Simopoulos, A. & Milner, J.A. (Eds.). (2010). *Personalized Nutrition: Translating Nutrigenetic/Nutrigenomic Research into Dietary Guidelines*, S Karger Pub, ISBN 978-3805594271, Basel, Switzerland

Simopoulos, A.P. (2001). The Mediterranean Diets: What is So Special about the Diet of Greece? The Scientific Evidence. *Journal of Nutrition*, Vol.131, No.11, (1 November 2001), pp. 3065S-3073S, ISSN 0022-3166

Slimani, N. & Margetts, B. (2010). Nutrient Intakes and Patterns in the EPIC Cohorts from Ten European Countries. *European Journal of Clinical Nutrition*, Vol.63, No.S4, pp. S1-S274

Smolin, L.A. & Grosvenor, B.M. (Eds.). (2010). *Nutrition. Science and Applications* (2nd ed.), John Wiley & Sons, Inc., ISBN 9780470524749, Hoboken, New Jersey, USA

Stoll, B.A. (2002). Upper Abdominal Obesity, Insulin Resistance and Breast Cancer Risk. *International Journal of Obesity and Related Metabolic Disorders*, Vol.26, No.6, (June 2002), pp. 747-753, ISSN 1476-5497

Talamini, R., Polesel, J., Gallus, S., Dal Maso, L., Zucchetto, A., Negri, E., Bosetti, C., Lucenteforte, E., Boz, G., Franceschi, S., Serraino, D. & La Vecchia, C. (2010). Tobacco Smoking, Alcohol Consumption and Pancreatic Cancer Risk: a Case-control Study in Italy. *European Journal of Cancer*, Vol.46, No.2, (January 2010), pp. 370-376, ISSN 0959-8049

Tan, A.C., Konczak, I., Sze, D.M. & Ramzan, I. (2011). Molecular Pathways for Cancer Chemoprevention by Dietary Phytochemicals. *Nutrition and Cancer*, Vol.63, No.4, (May 2011), pp. 495-505, ISSN 0163-5581

Tapsell, L.C., Hemphill, I., Cobiac, L., Patch, C.S., Sullivan, D.R., Fenech, M., Roodenrys, S., Keogh, J.B., Clifton, P.M., Williams, P.G., Fazio, V.A. & Inge, K.E. (2006). Health Benefits of Herbs and Spices: the Past, the Present, the Future. *Medical Journal of Australia*, Vol.185, No.4 Suppl, (21 August 2006), pp. S4-S24, ISSN 0025-729X

Terry, P.D., Rohan, T.E. & Wolk, A. (2003). Intakes of Fish and Marine Fatty Acids and the Risks of Cancers of the Breast and Prostate and of Other Hormone-related Cancers: a Review of the Epidemiologic Evidence. *American Journal of Clinical Nutrition*, Vol.77, No.3, (March 2003), pp. 532-543, ISSN 0002-9165

Testino, G. & Borr, P. (2010). Alcohol and Gastrointestinal Oncology. *World Journal of Gastrointestinal Oncology*, Vol.2, No.8, (15 August 2010), pp. 322-325, ISSN 19485204

The NCD Alliance. (2011). Proposed Outcomes Document for the United Nations High-Level Summit on Non-Communicable Diseases, 15 July 2011, Available from: http://www.ncdalliance.org/sites/default/files/resource_files/NCD%20Alliance%20Proposed%20Outcomes%20Document%20for%20the%20UN%20High-Level%20Summit.pdf

Thomas, L.E., Parkinson, R.J, Frost, S.G., Goldstone, P.A. , Doré, J.C., McCarthy, P.J., Collins, L.A., Fitzpatrick, A.J., Durighel, G., Taylor-Robinson, D.S. & Bell, D.J. (2011). The Missing Risk: MRI and MRS Phenotyping of Abdominal Adiposity and Ectopic Fat. In: *Obesity*, (15 July 2011), Available from: http://www.nature.com/oby/journal/vaop/ncurrent/full/oby2011142a.html

Thune, I. & Furberg, A.S. (2001). Physical Activity and Cancer Risk: Dose-response and Cancer, All Sites and Site-specific. *Medicine and Science in Sports and Exercise*, Vol.33, No.S6, (June 2001), pp. S530-S550, ISSN 0195-9131

Trajković-Pavlović, LJ., Martinov-Cvejin, M., Novaković, B., Bijelović, S. & Torović LJ. (2010a). Analysis of Salt Content in Meals in Kindergarten Facilities in Novi Sad. *Srpski Arhiv za Celokupno Lekarstvo*, Vol.138, No.9-10, (September - October 2010), pp. 619-623, ISSN 0370-8179

Trajković-Pavlović, LJ., Novaković, B., Dragnić, N. & Torović, LJ. (2010b). Salt Content in Meals and Students' Restaurants in Novi Sad. *HealthMED*, Vol.4, No.1, pp. 45-51, ISSN 1840-2291

Tsuda, H., Sekine, K., Ushida, Y., Kuhara, T., Takasuka, N., Iigo, M., Han, B.S. & Moore, M.A. (2000). Milk and Dairy Products in Cancer Prevention: Focus on Bovine Lactoferin. *Mutation Research*, Vol.462, No.2-3, (April 2000), pp. 227-233, ISSN 0921-8262

Tucker, J.M., Welk, G.J. & Beyler, N.K. (2011). Physical Activity in U.S.: Adults Compliance with the Physical Activity Guidelines for Americans. *American Journal of Preventive Medicine*, Vol.40, No.4, (April 2011), pp. 454-461, ISSN 0749-3797

Tuohy, K.M., Rouzaud, G.C., Brück, W.M. & Gibson, G.R. (2005). Modulation of the Human Gut Microflora Towards Improved Health Using Prebiotics - Assessment of Efficacy. *Current Pharmaceutical Design*, Vol.11, No.1, pp. 75-90, ISSN 1381-6128

Tverdal, A., Hjellvik, V. & Selmer R. (2011). Coffee Intake and Oral-oesophageal Cancer: Follow-up of 389 624 Norwegian Men and Women 40-45 Years. *British Journal of Cancer*, Vol.105, No.1, (28 June 2011), pp. 157-161, ISSN 0007-0920

USDA & U.S. Department of Health and Human Services. (2011). *Dietary Guidelines for Americans 2010* (7th ed.), U.S. Government Printing Office, ISBN 978-0615449913, Washington, District of Columbia, USA

USDA. (2002). Historical Food Guides Background and Development, 17 July 2011, Available from: http://www.nal.usda.gov/fnic/history/index.html

USDA. (2011a). Food Guide Pyramid, 19 July 2011, Available from: http://www.cnpp.usda.gov/FGP.htm

USDA. (2011b). ChooseMyPlate, 19 July 2011, Available from: http://www.choosemyplate.gov/

Van der Pols, J.C., Bain, C., Gunnell, D., Smith, G.D., Frobisher, C. & Martin, R.M. (2007). Childhood Dairy Intake and Adult Cancer Risk: 65-y Follow-up of the Boyd Orr Cohort. *American Journal of Clinical Nutrition*, Vol.86, No.6, (December 2007), pp. 1722-1729, ISSN 0002-9165

Van Stuyvenberg, J.H. (1969). *Margarine: An Economic, Social and Scientific History, 1869-1969*. Liverpool University Press, ISBN 978-0853231301, Liverpool, UK

Vardavas, C.I., Flouris, A.D., Tsatsakis, A., Kafatos, A.G. & Saris, W.H. (2011). Does Adherence to the Mediterranean Diet Have a Protective Effect Against Active and Passive Smoking? *Public Health*, Vol.125, No.3, (March 2011), pp. 121-128, ISSN 0033-3506

Vardavas, C.I., Linardakis, M.K., Hatzis, C.M., Malliaraki, N., Saris, W.H. & Kafatos, A.G. (2008). Smoking Status in Relation to Serum Folate and Dietary Vitamin Intake. *Tobacco Induced Diseases*, Vol.4, No.8, (9 September 2008), ISSN 2070-7266

Verberne, L., Bach-Faig, A., Buckland, G. & Serra-Majem, L. (2010). Association Between the Mediterranean Diet and Cancer Risk: a Review of Observational Studies. *Nutrition & Cancer*, Vol.62, No.7, pp. 860-870, ISSN 0163-5581

Vinikoor, L.C., Satia, J.A., Schroeder, J.C., Millikan, R.C., Martin, C.F., Ibrahim, J.G. & Sandler, R.S. (2009). Associations Between Trans Fatty Acid Consumption and Colon Cancer Among Whites and African Americans in the North Carolina Colon Cancer Study I. *Nutrition and Cancer*, Vol.61, No.4, pp. 427-436, ISSN 0163-5581

Waldorp, M. M. (2011). The Disruptor. *Nature*, Vol.474, pp. 20-22

Wang, J. (2006). Standardization of Waist Circumference Data. *American Journal of Clinical Nutrition*, Vol.83, No.1, (January 2006), pp. 3-4, ISSN 0002-9165

Wang, X-Q., Terry, P.D. & Yan, H. (2009). Review of Salt Consumption and Stomach Cancer Risk: Epidemiological and Biological Evidence. *World Journal of Gastroenterology*, Vol.15, No.18, (14 May 2009), pp. 2204-2213, ISSN 1007-9327

Wannamethee, S.G., Shaper, A.G. & Walker, M. (2001). Physical Activity and Risk of Cancer in Middle-aged Men. *British Journal of Cancer*, Vol.85, No.2, (2 November 2001), pp. 1311-1316, ISSN 0007-0920

Warburton, D.E., Nicol, C.W. & Bredin S.S. (2006). Health Benefits of Physical Activity: the Evidence. *Canadian Medical Association Journal*, Vol.174, No.6, (14 March 2006), pp. 801-809, ISSN 1488-2329

WCRF & AICR. (2007). *Second Expert Report. Food, Nutrition, Physical Activity and the Prevention of Cancer: a Global Perspective*, American Institute for Cancer Research (AICR), ISBN 978-0972252225, Washington, USA

WHO. (1999). *International Statistical Classification of Disease and Related Heatlh Problems (ICD-10) in Occupational Health*. WHO, Geneva, Switzerland

WHO. (2003). *Diet, Nutrition and the Prevention of Chronic Diseases. Report of a Joint WHO/FAO Expert Consultation*. WHO, ISBN 92 4 120916 X, Geneva, Switzerland

WHO. (2005). *Global Strategy on Diet, Physical Activity and Health*, WHO, ISBN 92 4 159222 2, Geneva, Switzerland

WHO. (2006). Tobacco: *Deadly in any Form or Disguise*. WHO, ISBN 978 92 4 156322 2, Geneva, Switzerland

WHO. (2007a). *Protein and Amino Acid Requirements in Human Nutrition*, WHO, ISBN 92 4 120935 6, Geneva, Switzerland

WHO. (2007b). *A Guide for Population-based Approaches to Increasing Levels of Physical Activity : Implementation of the WHO Global Strategy on Diet, Physical Activity and Health*, WHO, ISBN 978 92 4 159517 9, Geneva, Switzerland

WHO. (2008a). *2008-2013 Action Plan for the Global Strategy for the Prevention and Control of Noncommunicable Diseases*, WHO, ISBN 9789241597418, Geneva, Switzerland

WHO. (2008b). *WHO Report on the Global Tobacco Epidemic, 2008: the MPOWER package*. WHO, ISBN 978 92 4 159628 2, Geneva, Switzerland

WHO. (2009a). *Global Health Risk. Mortality and Burden of Diseases Attributable to Selected Major Risks*, WHO, ISBN 978 92 4 156387 1, Geneva, Switzerland

WHO. (2009b). *Interventions on Diet and Physical Activity: What Works: summary report*, WHO, ISBN 978 92 4 159824 8, Geneva Switzerland

WHO. (2010a). *Global Recommendations on Physical Activity for Health*, WHO, ISBN 978 92 4 159 997 9, Geneva, Switzerland

WHO. (2010b). *Global Strategy to Reduce the Harmful Use of Alcohol*, WHO, ISBN 978 92 4 159993 1, Geneva, Switzerland

WHO. (2011a). *Global Status Report on Non-communicable Diseases 2010*, WHO, ISBN 978 92 4 156422 9, Geneva, Switzerland

WHO. (2011b). *Prevention and Control of Non-communicable Diseases. WHO's Role in the Preparation, Implementation and Follow-up to the High-level Meeting of the United Nations General Assembly on the Prevention and Control of Non-communicable Diseases (September 2011)*, Geneva, Switzerland

WHO. (2011c). *World Health Statistics 2011*. WHO, ISBN 978 92 4 156398 7, Geneva, Switzerland

WHO. (2011d). *WHO Report on the Global TobaccoEpidemic,2011: Warning About the Dangers of Tobacco*. WHO, ISBN 978 92 4 156426 7, Geneva, Switzerland

WHO. (2011e). *WHO Framework Convention on Tobacco Control: Guidelines for Implementation Article 5.3; Article 8; Articles 9 and 10; Article 11; Article 12; Article 13; Article 14 - 2011 Edition*. WHO, ISBN 978 92 4 150131 6, Geneva, Switzerland

WHO. (2011f). *Global Status Report on Alcohol and Health*, WHO, ISBN 978 92 4 156415 1, Geneva, Switzerland

WHO. (2011g). *Guidelines for Drinking-water Quality* (4th ed.), WHO, ISBN 978 92 4 154815 1, Geneva, Switzerland

Willet, W.C. (2010). Fruits, Vegetables and Cancer Prevention: Turmoil in the Production Section. *Journal of the National Cancer Institute*, Vol.102, No.9, (21 April 2010), pp. 510-511, ISSN 0027-8874

Wogan, G.N., Hecht, S.S., Felton, J.S., Conney, A.H. & Loeb, L.A. (2004). Environmental and Chemical Carcinogenesis. *Seminars in Cancer Biology*, Vol.14, No.6, (December 2004), pp. 473-486, ISSN 1044-579X

Wolin, K.Y., Yan, Y., Colditz, G.A. & Lee, I.M. (2009). Physical Activity and Colon Cancer Prevention: a Meta-analysis. *British Journal of Cancer*, Vol.100, No.4, (24 February 2009), pp. 611-616, ISSN 0007-0920

World Gastroenterology Organisation. (2008). *Probiotics and Prebiotics*, World Gastroenterology Organisation, Milwaukee, Visconsin, USA

Wu, S., Liang, J., Zhang, L., Zhu, X., Liu, X. & Miao, D. (2011). Fish Consumption and the Risk of Gastric Cancer: Systematic Review and Meta-analysis. *BMC Cancer*, Vol.11, [Epub ahead of print], 20 January 2011, ISSN 1471-2407

Yach, D., McKee, M., Lopez, A.D. & Novotny, T. (2005). Improving Diet and Physical Activity: 12 Lessons from Controlling Tobacco Smoking. *British Medical Journal*, Vol.330, No.7496, (16 April 2005), pp. 898-900, ISSN 0959-8138

Yan, F., Polk, D.B. (2010). Probiotics: Progress Toward Novel Therapies for Intestinal Diseases. *Current Opinion in Gastroenterology*, Vol. 26, No.2, (March 2010), pp. 95-101, ISSN 0267-1379

Zenith International. (2005). *Zenith Report on Global Soft Drinks*. Zenith International, London, UK

Zhang, J., Zhao, Z. & Berkel, H.J. (2003). Egg Consumption and Mortality from Colon and Rectal Cancers: an Ecological Study. *Nutrition and Cancer*, Vol.46, No.2, pp. 158-165, ISSN 0163-5581

Zheng, W. & Lee, S-A. (2009). Well-done Meat Intake, Heterocyclic Amine Exposure, and Cancer Risk. *Nutrition & Cancer*, Vol.61, No.4, pp. 437-446, ISSN 0163-5581

Ziech, D., Franco, R., Georgakilas, A.G., Georgakila, S., Malamou-Mitsi, V., Schoneveld, O, Pappa, A. & Panayiotidis, M.I. (2010). The Role of Reactive Oxygen Species and Oxidative Stress in Environmental Carcinogenesis and Biomarker Development. *Chemico-biological Interactions*, Vol.188, No.2, (5 November 2010), pp. 334-339, ISSN 0009-2797

Zenith International. (2008). Global Soft Drinks Report, 29 July 2011, Available from: http://www.zenithinternational.com/reports_data/117/Global+Soft+Drinks+Report

7

Risk and Protective Factors for Development of Colorectal Polyps and Cancer

Iskren Kotzev
Medical University, Varna
Bulgaria

1. Introduction

CRC is one of the most frequently diagnosed neoplastic disorders in humans worldwide. According to the National Centre for Health Information of Bulgaria the prevalence of CRC for 2005 is 304.6/100 000 cases, and the incidence - 49.2/100 000 cases (Bulletin of the National Centre for Health Information, 2005). Colorectal polyps (CRP) are established precursors of CRC. Hence, elimination of precursors is a well-known strategy for reduction of risk. In the last decade the most extensively studied etiologic factors are the risk factors for colorectal cancer development, because of its growing incidence and the possibility for its prevention. Prophylaxis of CRC we can divide in primary, secondary and tertiary. The most widely used chemopreventive drugs are: acetylsalicylic acid, polyvitamins, calcium, folic acid, selenium and NSAID.

2. Risk and protective factors for colorectal polyps and cancer

Today it is widely accepted that colorectal polyps (CRP) are preneoplastic lesions of colorectal cancer (CRC). From the 3 major groups of polyps: adenomas, hyperplastic, and serrated polyps, with the first group having the highest malignant potential. Hyperplastic polyps are the most common benign lesions, possessing very low malignant potential, and therefore do not require colonoscopic surveillance. However, recent studies prove their role in the classical model of adenoma-carcinoma sequence, and reveal common molecular features between normal mucosa, colorectal polyps, and cancer: proliferation activity, p53 overexpression, hypomethylation of c-myc, and mutations in k-ras oncogene (Hamilton, 2001). Progression of adenomas to CRC has been proven by the 'multistep model' of carcinogenesis, proposed by Fearon and Vogelstein. According to this model the stepwise progression of aberrant crypt foci, small, middle and large adenoma to carcinoma is accompanied by accumulation of mutations in the genes APC, k-ras, DCC, and p53 (Fearon, Fogelstein, 1990). Serrated polyps are histologicaly characterized by 'saw-tooth' infolding of the crypt epithelium, and are seen in 1% of the cases (Longacre & Fenoglio-Preiser, 1990). Every adenoma of the colorectum has a 5% probability for malignant transformation (Winawer et al., 1997). The growth of small adenomas is slow, requiring 10 years on average for doubling of their size (Hoff, 1987). The percentage of transformation of small adenomas into carcinomas is 0.25% (Eide, 1986). CRC is caused by complex interactions between host genetic susceptibility and certain exogenous risk factors. Geographic variation underscores the importance of environmental factors in CRC pathogenesis, since a 30-40 fold difference between regions with high and low incidence has been found (Parkin et al., 1999). It is famous that the main risk factors for CRC and CRP are obesity, high calories intake, high body mass index (BMI), and low physical activity, consumption of red meat and animal fats, and alcohol. Other risk factors include male gender, advancing age, use of laxatives, constipation, pathological gut flora, some occupations, and intake of Fe-containing supplements. There is association also between the risk of developing CRC or CRP and presence of some diseases like inflammatory bowel disease (IBD), acromegaly, diabetes mellitus, cholecystectomy, ovarian and breast cancer, history of survived cancer or availability of adenomatous polyps in the past. Many conditions increase the risk of development of CRC and the degree of their influence substantially varies, as is shown in Table 1.

Risk factor	Minimal	Moderate	Major
Dominant inheritance (FAP, HNPCC, Juvenile polyposis)			+
Diet			+
Recessive inheritance or low penetration (MAP)		+	
CRC in the past		+	
Colorectal villous adenoma in the past		+	
Low physical activity		+	
Age > 50 y.		+	
Male gender	+		
Obesity	+		
Tobacco smoking	+		
Chronic alcohol abuse	+		
Extensive IBD	+		
Acromegaly	+		
Diabetes mellitus	+		
Cholecystectomy	+		
Breast cancer, ovarian cancer, radiotherapy	+		

Table 1. Assessment of risk factors for CRC and CRP. FAP, Familial adenomatous polyposis; NHPCC, Hereditary non-polyposis colorectal cancer; MAP, MYH-associated adenomatous polyposis; IBD, inflammatory bowel disease.

3. Patients and methods (our study)

3.1 Characteristics of patients with colorectal polyps and cancer

One-hundred and sixty six patients diagnosed for large bowel polyps were included in the present study. Of the patients, 76 were female and 90 male, aged 60±13 years (range 19-86 years). Also, 107 patients with CRC (48 female and 59 male) aged 64±11 years (range 32-94 years), 3 patients with familial adenomatous polyposis (FAP), and 2 patients with

Peutz-Jeghers syndrome, aged 31±12 years were included in the study. As a control we used a group of 42 healthy individuals (18 female and 24 male), aged 55±12 years, to whom upper and lower endoscopy was performed at their will or as a screening procedure, but showed no changes. Careful personal history, including dietary habits, physical examination, and anthropometric data were taken from all patients. We studied some factors from the lifestyle and diet in our patients with CRC and CRP, and looked for any connection between these factors and the beginning of CRC and CRP. For the aim of our study, we divided food consumed from the patients into 13 groups as follows: I. Milk and dairy products; II. Eggs; III. Meat and meat products; IV. Fish and sea animals; V. Cereals and pasta; VI. Sugar and sweets; VII. Legumes; VIII. Nuts; IX. Fats; X. Vegetables; XI. Fruits; XII. Spices; XIII. Beverages. We tried to establish the preferred way of cooking and favorite drinks in the studied patients. We registered their dietary habits in qualitative and quantitative manner, until the moment of CRC or CRP occurrence. We analyzed family predisposition of the included patients and their exposition to deleterious exogenous factors. All information, including clinical data, endoscopic and histological results, surveillance, and treatment, was entered on personal cards and in a gastrointestinal register for polyps and cancer.

3.2 Statistical analysis

Logit-models were used for determining the possible risk or preventive factors, which combine regression and correlation analysis. We investigated the influence of these factors upon included patients with linear regression analysis to be able to associate the lifestyle and diet habits of population in our region. Depending on the value of the Exponent Exp(B), factors are classified in three groups: risk factors - Exp(B)>1, protective factors - Exp(B) <1 and indifferent factors - Exp(B)=1. Statistical analysis was performed using Microsoft Excel, Statistics 5. 13./W and SPSS 13.0 for Windows software programs. Values of $p<0.05$ were considered as statistically significant.

4. Risk factors for colorectal polyps according to our data

Our data find the following risk factors for colorectal polyps: consumption of red meat, meat products, sausages, fat food, high BMI, frequent use of laxatives, beer and alcohol intake, preserved foods, salty foods, grilled or barbecued meat, low physical activity, allergy, bacon, ham, margarine, fried food, preserved meat, sugar, marinated food, tobacco smoking, egg-fried food, working in heavy or petrol industry, presence of autoimmune disease, use of microwave oven, professional exposure to extremely low temperatures, passive smoking and elevated serum glucose level.

We concluded that the most important risk factors for the development of colorectal polyps are diet factors - consumption of sugar products, fried, grilled and preserved food, animal fats and margarine, egg-fried food and obesity. The most important life style and occupational risk factors for the development of colorectal polyps are: chronic alcohol intake, long lasting tobacco smoking, minimal physical activity, occupational exposure to petrol and metals. The chronic alcohol intake includes usage of beer, wine and strong drink. Substantial factors are and presence of autoimmune disease or allergy, frequent use of laxatives and elevated serum glucose level.

Factor	Intensity	Exp. (B)
Chronic alcohol abuse	+ + +	9,256
Sugar and sweets	+ + +	8,917
Fried food	+ + +	7,258
Preserved food	+ + +	5,363
Heavy industry workers	+ + +	5,259
Beer	+ + +	5,025
Meat delicacy	+ + +	4,759
Bacon	+ + +	4,582
Long lasting sausages	+ + +	4,265
Fat food	+ + +	4,023
Margarine	+ +	3,707
Exposure to petrol	+ +	3,616
Weekly consumption of grilled meal	+ +	3,093
Presence of autoimmune disease	+ +	2,958
Strong drink	+ +	2,919
Low physical activity	+ +	2,843
Wine	+ +	2,827
Salty food	+ +	2,575
Allergy	+ +	2,566
Grilled meat	+ +	2,439
Preserved meat	+ +	2,345
Ham	+ +	2,241
Smoked food	+ +	2,144
Frequent use of laxatives	+	1,796
Marinated food	+	1,658
Preserved food	+	1,511
Egg-fried food	+	1,448
Tobacco smoking	+	1,444
Frequent meat consumption	+	1,349
Elevated serum glucose level	+	1,115
Years of alcohol consumption)	+	1,074
High body mass index (BMI)	+	1,047
Years of smoking	+	1,030

Table 2. Risk factors for colorectal polyps (4,01 - 10,00 + + +), (2,01 - 4,00 + +), (1,00 - 2,00 +).

5. Protective factors for colorectal polyps according to our data

According to our results fruits (apples, plumbs, raspberries, and pears), vegetables, rye- and whole-grain bread, green tea, vegetable food consumption, yoghurt, fasting, fish, lamb, hare, garlic, legumes and mineral water have a strong protective effect against large bowel polyps.

The most significant protective factors against colorectal polyps are again diet factors - consumption of fruit, vegetables, rye- and whole-grain bread, vegetable food, green tea, yoghurt and fasting. Protective role plays and frequent consumption of fish, lamb and hare. Probably, conditions of rural life are connected with reduction of the risk factors for development of colorectal polyps.

Factor	*Intensity*	*Exp. (B)*
Fruit	+ + +	0,033
Rare consumption of grilled food	+ + +	0,094
Apples	+ + +	0,122
Vegetables	+ + +	0,126
Rye bread	+ + +	0,199
Plumbs	+ + +	0,244
Raspberries	+ + +	0,258
Pears	+ + +	0,268
Rural life	+ +	0,318
Green tea	+ +	0,325
Vegetable food	+ +	0,345
Whole-grain bread	+ +	0,352
Yoghourt	+ +	0,367
Green vegetables	+ +	0,382
Fasting	+ +	0,385
Fish	+ +	0,428
Lamb	+	0,559
Hares	+	0,588
Legumes	+	0,595
Garlic	+	0,616
Low salt diet	+	0,668
Mineral water	+	0,895

Table 3. Protective factors for colorectal polyps (0,01 - 0,3 + + +), (0,31 - 0,50 + +), (0,51 - 1,00 +).

6. Risk factors for colorectal cancer according to our data

One of the most important aims of our study was to establish the risk factors for the CRC epidemic, which is observed now and in Bulgaria. We accomplished this study considering the specific conditions in our country and made comprehensive investigation of the diet habits of all included patients with colorectal polyps and cancer. We estimated and all other possible risk factors. Detailed list of risk factors for development of colorectal cancer is presented in Table 4.

The major risk factors for CRC are dietary as well: consumption of fat food, red meat and meat diet as a whole, smoked and egg-fried food, sugar and sweets, white bread, obesity. The lifestyle has also a significant effect: long lasting alcohol intake (beer, wine, and spirits), tobacco smoking, minimal physical activity, urban life. We noticed and other risk factors for CRC development: *H. pylori* infection, presence of adenomas, diabetes mellitus, and frequent use of laxatives. Probably, urban life increases the exposition to many of the presented risk factors and therefore it is a specific risk factor for development of CRC.

7. Protective factors for colorectal cancer according to our data

According to our results consumption of dairy products, fruit, garlic, onions, fish, plant oil, boiled food, vegetables, fowls, legumes and white meat has a strong protective effect for CRC. Low salt diet, fasting, usage of acetylsalicylic acid and rural life also possess protective

Factor	Intensity	Exp. (B)
Fat food	+ + +	11,034
Adenomas with severe dysplasia	+ + +	10,784
Smoked meat	+ + +	7,282
Egg-fried food	+ + +	6,334
Long lasting alcohol intake>10y	+ + +	5,939
Sub-products	+ + +	5,625
Fried food	+ + +	5,244
Short lasting sausages	+ + +	4,646
Pork	+ + +	4,368
Sausages	+ + +	4,255
Margarine	+ + +	4,214
Beer	+ + +	4,095
Bacon	+ +	3,366
Tobacco smoking	+ +	3,622
Meat delicacy	+ +	3,546
Low gr. dysplastic adenomas	+ +	3,541
Minimal physical activity	+ +	3,446
Sugar and sweets	+ +	3,281
Urban life	+ +	3,054
Exposure to petrol	+ +	2.898
Frequent use of laxatives	+ +	2,895
Preserved food	+ +	2,339
White bread	+ +	2,248
Helicobacter pylori	+ +	2,204
Red meat	+	1,805
Meat products	+	1,508
Wine	+	1,414
Tobacco smoking >10y	+	1,058
Strong drink	+	1,054
Villous component in adenoma	+	1,052
Overweight and obesity	+	1,045
Diabetes mellitus	+	1,040
Age	+	1,036

Table 4. Risk factors for CRC (4,01 - 12,00 + + +), (2,01 - 4,00 + +), (1,00 - 2,00 +).

effect against development of CRC. Our data is similar to the findings of other authors (Zaridze, 1983). Detailed list of protective factors against development of CRC is presented in Table 5.

The most important protective factors for CRC development are: consumption of fruit, vegetables, fasting, vegetable oil, fish, poultry, white meat, legumes, boiled food, and rare consumption of grilled meat. Regular use of acetylsalicylic acid and rural life are prominent protective factors for development of CRC. Obviously, diet regime in conditions of Bulgarian rural area is much closer to the healthy Balkan diet from the first half of the 20-th century, which plays protective role in the prophylaxis of cardiovascular, metabolic and neoplastic diseases.

Factor	Intensity	Exp. (B)
Low salt diet	+ + +	0,001
Melons	+ + +	0,051
Dairy products	+ + +	0,071
Pears	+ + +	0,114
Acetylsalicylic acid	+ + +	0,119
Garlic	+ + +	0,128
Fasting	+ + +	0,133
Fish	+ + +	0,137
Poultry	+ + +	0,165
Rural life	+ + +	0,197
Water melons	+ + +	0,200
Hares	+ +	0,202
Onions	+ +	0,228
Plant oil	+ +	0,231
Grapes	+ +	0,235
Peppers	+ +	0,264
Fruit	+ +	0,294
Vegetables	+ +	0,300
Green vegetables	+ +	0,318
Boiled food	+ +	0,343
Fowls	+ +	0,367
Legumes	+	0,418
Rare use of grilled meat	+	0,430
Fasting	+	0,457
White meat	+	0,665
Peaches	+	0,668

Table 5. Protective factors for CRC (0,01 - 0,2 + + +), (0,201 - 0,40 + +), (0,41 - 1,00 +).

8. Risk and protective factors for colorectal polyps and colorectal cancer - summary

Our data show that colorectal polyps and cancer share common risk and protective factors (Kotzev et al., 2008). This finding, paired with the high frequency of existence of colorectal polyps and CRC, could serve as an evidence of the role of the colorectal polyps as CRC precursors. Common risk and protective factors for colorectal polyps and colorectal cancer are summarized in Table. 6, where factors are divided into alimentary risk factors, nonalimentary risk factors and protective factors.

9. The mode of action of risk and protective factors for colorectal polyps and cancer

The mode of action of different risk and protective factors for CRC and CRP is associated with distinct pathogenetic mechanisms, which sometimes share similar pathways.

9.1 Alimentary risk factors for colorectal polyps and cancer

9.1.1 Obesity, high BMI and high caloric intake

Obesity, high BMI and high caloric intake are associated with increased risk for cancer formation, including CRC (Giovannucci et al., 1995). These risk factors are connected with

Risk dietary factors	Risk non-dietary factors	Protective factors
Overweight	Low physical activity	Carbohydrates (long chained)
Food additives and contaminants (heterocyclic amines)	Tobacco smoking	Fish
Contaminated water	Gender	Probiotics
Fats	Age	Fibers
Red meat	Laxatives	Flavonoids
Sugar	Helicobacter pylori	Dairy products
Alcohol	Occupational risks	Calcium
Eggs	Colorectal polyps	Fluids
Way of cooking - grilled meat	IBD, diabetes. mellitus, ovarian Ca, mammary Ca	Vitt. A, B, C, D, folic acid, Selenium, Calcium
Way of cooking – fried meat	Cholecystectomy	Fruit and vegetables
Way of cooking - high t°	Radiotherapy	Cereals
Polyamines	Colorectal cancer	Bioactive components

Table 6. Summary of all protective and risk factors tor CRC and CRP.

large bowel polyp formation as well. High caloric intake in combination with low physical activity leads to hyperinsulinemia and peripheral insulin resistance, which could result in high mucosal proliferative activity, reduced apoptosis, accumulation of free radicals, and mutagenesis. Being overweight could have an inappropriate influence on the immune system, could elevate the serum level of prolactine, and raise the sensitivity of the hypothalamo-hypophyseal axis. High BMI and high caloric intake are connected with elevated risk for development of CRC and colorectal adenomas according to different experimental animal studies and epidemiological studies (Ford, S. 1999).

9.1.2 Food additives and contaminants

Food contains various food additives, contaminants, fertilizers, herbicides, food dying agents, antibiotics and antimycotics. Increased mutageneity has been observed in faeces of patients with elevated risk for CRC formation (Villa et al., 1996). Food contains a lots of carcinogens and co-carcinogens such as free radicals, N-nitrous compounds, secondary bile acids, polyamines, and heterocyclic amines (used in food processing) (Parkin et al., 1999). Co-carcinogens usually need activation in the gut. Their activation and inactivation is maintained by the gut flora, some phytochemicals and metabolites. Meat processing leads to elevated carcinogen production. Meat and fish cooking leads to formation of heterocyclic amines, especially at high temperatures or when exposed to direct fire. Our study shows that grilled, fried and egg-fried foods are associated with high CRP formation, and fried and egg-fried foods are risk factors for CRC as well. We consider preserved food as a risk factor for CRP and CRC, while marinated food is associated with CRP. Some observations propose that gut bacteria could transform bile acids into secondary bile acids (deoxycholic and litocholic) which possess high toxicity and stimulate large bowel mucosal proliferation (Burnstein, 1993). Food fatty acids also alter the composition and the quantity of bile acids. Accelerated bowel transit time could diminish exposition time of mucosa to food carcinogens, and enlarged volume could dilute them. Thus food fibers bind, inactivate and carry out the luminal carcinogens.

9.1.3 Fats

The first announcement of the relationship between high intake of fats and CRC dates from 1969 (Wynder et al., 1969). The relationship between saturated/animal fatty acids and CRC risk is tight. Saturated fats play a crucial role in the initiation, promotion and progression of CRC. Saturated fats increase the bile excretion, which is followed by toxic impact upon colon epithelium and hyperproliferation (Burnstein, 1993). The current study proved that consumption of fatty foods, bacon, and margarine is strongly associated with CRP and CRC development. The results of animal studies report that in the animals, which are on high fat diet, elevated cell proliferation and free radicals are observed. Inflammation and oxidative stress play a significant role in human carcinogenesis, besuse DNA lesions and chromosomal instability could occur (Evans et al., 2004; Kryston et al., 2011; Sedelnikova et al., 2010). On the other hand omega-3 polyunsaturated fatty acids decrease inflammation, inhibit formation and progression of preneoplastic colorectal lesions (Anti et al., 1994). The so-called "Mediterranean" diet, which is rich in fish and sea products, reduces the risk for colorectal cancer. Our study proves that regular consumption of fish and sea products (more than twice a week) strongly prevents CRP and CRC. Probably, the protective effect of omega-3 polyunsaturated fatty acids is due to stimulation of apoptotic program, decrease of inflammation, mucous prostaglandins and decrease of the secondary bile salts concentration, which are promoters for CRC. There are data that omega-3 polyunsaturated fatty acids modulate the action of COX-2 and induce the expression of 15-hydroxyprostaglandin dehydrogenase, a physiologic COX-2 antagonist (Lim et al., 2008).

9.1.4 Carbohydrates

It is believed that decreased intake of carbohydrates reduces the risk for polyp formation (Lubin et al., 1997). Complex long-chained carbohydrates are considered highly protective in contrast to saccharose (World Cancer Research Fund and American Institute for Cancer Research, Food, Nutrition and the Prevention of Cancer: A Global Perspective., 1997). Some studies confirm that persistent hyperglicaemia and the subsequent insulin release are stimuli for hyperproliferation of colon epithelium and risk factors for the development of CRC (Calle & Thun, 2004). In contrast, other studies did not observe such an association (Weijenberg et al., 2008). Complex long-chained carbohydrates must supply 46-60% of all energy intake, while refined saccharose must supply <10% according to some recommendations (World Cancer Research Fund and American Institute for Cancer Research, Food, Nutrition and the Prevention of Cancer: A Global Perspective., 1997). The results of this study support the notion that saccharose and sweets are risk factors for CRP and CRC, while complex long-chained carbohydrates have protective effect.

9.1.5 Red meat

Consumption of red meat is connected with development of CRC (Ferrucci et al., 2009). Our study also confirmed the fact that regular consumption of red meat, large amounts of meat and meat products, preserved meat, ham, long- and short lasting sausages, pork, sub-products, and meat delicacy, is strongly associated with CRP, and CRC initiation and progression. On the other hand intake of fish, hare, lamb, white meat and poultry are highly protective. The possible pro-carcinogenic effect of red meat could be explained by the elevated heme iron content which could serve as a source for production of free radicals and mucosal hyperproliferation (Nelson, 2001). The results obtained by other studies deny the role of dietary Fe and iron status for CRC development (Tseng et al., 1997). N-nitrous compounds in the red meat and produced during the food processing with high temperature polycyclic carbohydrates and heterocyclic amines are also possible reasons for the harmful effect of red meat (De Meester & Gerber, 1995) Red meat consumption in elderly individuals should be limited to 70-80g/day.

9.1.6 Alcohol

We believe that chronic alcohol abuse is a major risk factor for gastrointestinal polyps and cancer formation in esophagus, stomach, colon and rectum. High alcohol intake (>21 units/week) of beer, wine and spirits significantly increases the risk for CRP and CRC. These findings are probably due to the effect of acetaldehyde, which damages colorectal mucosa and elevates cell regeneration. Folic acid and methionine deficiency in persons who chronically abuse with alcohol are also risk factors for development of CRC (Giovannucci et al., 1995). Alcohol is an inducer of cytochrome P-405 2E1, which contributes to increased production of free radicals (Seitz & Osswald, 1992). Alcohol diminishes the transformation of retinol into retinoic acid and as result cell proliferation is upregulated (Seitz et al., 1998).

9.1.7 Food processing

We found that fried and grilled food is a risk factor for CRC and CRP. Cooking of the food at high temperatures and usage of grill induces formation of heterocyclic amines in the meat, which own mutagenic and pro-carcinogenic activity (Sigimura et al., 2004; De Meester & Gerber, 1995). Biochemical interactions between proteins, carbohydrates and fats during food processing are also of great importance for the formation of carcinogenic compounds.

9.2 Nonalimentary risk factors for colorectal polyps and cancer

9.2.1 Physical activity

Five percent of cardiovascular mortality rate is caused by low physical activity. 13% is the estimated value for CRC (Slattery & Potter, 2002). This is probably due to the combination of low physical activity, nutrition, lifestyle, and their cross-interactions. The mode of action of physical activity upon CRC is not clear, but decrease in inflammation and insulin levels is supposed. A middle intensive physical activity 3-4 times per week with 1.5 h duration is advisable. Increased physical activities, especially in men, reduce the risk for CRC with 40-50% (Scottish Intercollegiate Guidelines Network. Management of Colorectal cancer. A national clinical guideline., 2003).

9.2.2 Tobacco smoking

Many authors consider CRC as tobacco-related, taking into account the duration of smoking. It is estimated that 12% of the cases of CRC are related to smoking (Courtney et al., 2004). The present study confirmed the role of tobacco smoking as a risk factor for CRP and CRC. The risk is elevated proportionally to the years of smoking. Tobacco smoking disrupts conjugation of glutathione, cytochromes and damages DNA (Pfohl-Leskowitcz et al, 1999). Inhalation of carcinogens from tobacco smoke could trigger microsatellite instability (Yang et al., 2000).

9.2.3 Gender

The incidence of CRC is almost always higher in men (Parkin et al., 1999). Our data support these findings, as the men/women ratio was 1.2/1 in patients with CRP and 1.23/1 in patients with CRC. These differences could be explained with different life style, diet habits, physical activity, tobacco smoking, and consumption of alcohol, usage of NSAID and iron stores. There are and speculations about the protective role of female sex hormones (Crandall, 1999). Hormone replacement therapy in women is not recommended, because of the risk of vascular damages, thromboembolism and breast cancer (Scottish Intercollegiate Guidelines Network. Management of Colorectal cancer. A national clinical guideline, 2003).

9.2.4 Age

The interacting reasons for neoplastic changes in the colon are clinically manifested as a CRC during the second half of life. The mean age of our patients with CRP is 60 years and the mean age of our patients with CRC is 64 year. The mortality rate is increasing in parallel with advancing age according to reported data (Crandall, 1999).

9.2.5 Laxatives use

Frequent use of laxatives is among risk factors according to our data. This result is supported by some other studies (Van Gorkom et al., 1999). Probably, laxatives exert direct toxic effect upon colon mucosa.

9.2.6 Iron and haemochromatosis

The presumable mechanism of iron influence as a risk factor for CRC is connected with the formation of the free radicals from the unabsorbed iron, which damage colon epithelium. Heterozygotic patients who have not developed haemochromatosis are at elevated risk of developing CRC (Altes et al., 1999). The high risk of developing CRP and CRC in our patients who have regularly consumed red meat could be partially explained with the high amount of organic iron, which is available in the heme molecule.

9.2.7 Occupation

Our data show that exposure to petrol and metal is a risk factor for CRP and CRC. It is possible that petrol derivates and metals exert harmful effect upon colonic mucosa. Other exogenous risk factors are: use of anthranoid laxatives, working in petrol industry, production of synthetic materials, wood- and metal processing. Ionizing radiation increases the risk for CRC in radiation treatment of small pelvis after latent period of 15 years (Levin et al., 2002).

9.2.8 Gut flora

Pathological gut flora could produce potential carcinogens, deconjugate bile acids and impair cell DNA molecule (Aries et al., 1969). Our study ascertained the fact that *H. pylori* infection serves as a risk factor for CRC development. Similar results are reported from other authors (Zumkeller et al., 2006). However, more extensive studies are needed to prove this observation. *H. pylori* could exert negative effect not only on upper parts of gastrointestinal tract, but may be also on colorectal mucosa.

9.2.9 Association with other diseases

Chronic and extensive IBD is connected with increased cell turnover and elevated risk of developing CRC. The risk for development of CRC in patients with IBD depends on the duration (8-10 years) and the extent of disease (Ekbom et al., 1990). We observed malignant transformation in one patient with ulcer colitis and inflammatory pseudopolyposis with duration more than 10 years. Some big population based studies have found slightly elevated risk of developing CRC in right colon in women 15 years after cholecystectomy (Ekbom et al., 1993). Acromegaly is associated with elevated risk for CRC (Jenkins et al., 1997). We do not have any patient with acromegaly and CRP or CRC. We did not observe association between the patients who have undergone cholecystectomy and the frequency of CRC and CRP. The possible mechanism of this risk factor is associated with the constant free leakage of bile in the gut and with the toxic and carcinogenic effect of secondary bile salts.

9.3 The mode of action of protective factors for colorectal polyps and cancer

9.3.1 Probiotics

Our data confirm that Bulgarian yoghurt (containing *Lactobacilus acidophilus/bulgaricus* and *Streptococcus termophylus)* has a protective effect on large bowel polyp formation. Its use as a prophylactic seems perspective since it is traditionally present in Bulgarian national cuisine.

9.3.2 Fibers

According to our study the intake of large amounts of fibers is associated with reduced risk for CRP formation, although conflicting data exist. In a large prospective study, approximately 40% reduction of CRC risk in persons with high fiber consumption was reported (Bingham et al., 2003). The protective action of diet fibers is based on their capabilities to accelerate bowel transit time and enlarged volume, which could diminish exposition time of mucosa to food carcinogens and dilute them. Food fibers bind, inactivate and carry out the luminal carcinogens. Food fibers also decrease fecal pH and inhibit bacterial degradation of different alimentary compounds (Kritchevsky, 1995).

9.3.3 Flavonoids

Flavonoids are powerful antioxidants, which are found basically in fruit, vegetables, seeds, nuts, tea and wine (Middleton & Kandaswami, 1993). According to our data consumption of fruit and vegetables is protective factor for CRC and CRP, whereas regular consumption of tea is protective factor for CRP. Flavonoids inhibit cell proliferation and induce apoptosis (Wenzel et al., 2000).

9.3.4 Selenium

In supranutrtional doses selenium has protective effect against development of CRC, cancer of prostate and lung cancer (Schatzkin et al., 1996). Its mode of action is based on its antioxidant, antiproliferative, and proapoptotic properties (Zhu et al., 2000). Selenium is basic part of the selenium-dependent glutathione-reductase, which removes free radical and protects the integrity of cell membrane and DNA stability. Selenium also activates tumor-suppressor gene p53 (Seo et al., 2002). Our data in patients who use selenium as prophylaxis confirm its protective role.

9.3.5 Calcium

Our data show that consumption of milk products has protective effect against developing CRC and CRP. Calcium in milk products bind luminal bile and fat acids in insoluble soaps and inhibits proliferation of colon cells (Bostick et al., 1995). Calcium also enhances cell apoptosis in colon mucosa (Fedirko et al., 2009). Probably, calcium has a modulating role in the western diet, rather than anticarcinogenic properties. Optimal intake of calcium in >50 year old persons is 1200 mg per day (Institute of Medicine, Dietary Reference Intakes for Calcium, Phosphorus, Magnesium, Vitamin D and Fluoride. Food and Nutrition Board, Washington, DC., 1997).

9.3.6 Fluid intake

Regular intake of mineral water is protective factor for CRP according to our data. Epidemiological studies showed that protective effect of fibers depends on the volume of drank fluids (Lubin et al., 1997). This phenomenon is associated with the decreased concentration of carcinogens, accompanied with a high amount of fluid intake.

9.3.7 Vitamins

There are data that vitamin D, alone or in combination with calcium plays protective role for CRC (Hawk et al., 2004). Vitamin D induces cell differentiation and inhibits cell proliferation and metastatic potential (Giovannucci, 2006). Vitamin A has similar properties as vitamin D, but there is no clear evidence of its protective role for CRC. Significant side effects of vitamin D and vitamin A restrict their usage. No convincing data exist and for the protective role of folic acid for CRC. Combined use of some vitamins with antioxidant properties, like vitamin C and vitamin E, and minerals, like selenium could enhance their impact (Patterson et al., 2000). Our data confirm this result, because we used combination formula composed of vitamin E - 80 mg, vitamin C - 100 mg, β-caroten - 10 mg and selenium - 250 μg) as a prophylactic drug in 12 patients for period of 5 years.

9.3.8 Bioactive compounds

A lot of foods containing bioactive compounds are with protective effect for CRC and CRP according to our data - garlic, tea, fruit, vegetables, onions, grapes, vegetable food, legumes etc. Bioactive compounds include numerous chemical substances, which own anticancer properties (Greenwald, 2002). Some of the most studied bioactive compounds are found in green tea, tomatoes, and different sorts of onions, carrots, lemons and garlic. There are flavonoids and polyphenols in green tea, fruit and vegetables, which possess antioxidant properties. Bioactive compounds d-limonen and perilil alcohol are found in citrus fruit and their impact is associated with the induction of glutathione S-transferase. Red grapes have antioxidant properties, because of the bioactive compound resveratrol. In cereals and in beans are found phytoestrogens, which change the metabolism of steroid hormones. A lot of bioactive compounds present in traditional Bulgarian cuisine. Therefore, it is reasonable to keep the tradition of healthy Balkan (Bulgarian) diet from the first half of the 20-th century.

9.3.9 Cereals

Consumption of rye and whole grain bread are protective factors for CRP according to our data. Low incidence of CRC and other cancers is observed in countries with high consumption of complex long-chained carbohydrates, which is found in cereals (Gerber, 2003). This fact is based on the presumption that complex long-chained carbohydrates successfully substitute fats as a source of energy. Recommended dose of cereals is 600-800 gram per day.

9.3.10 Fruit and vegetables

Regular consumption of fruit and vegetables is a protective factor for CRC and CRP according to our data. Fruit and vegetables contain vitamins, minerals, biologically active substances and some insoluble fibers. All of them are regarded as protective. The suggested daily dose of fruit and vegetables is 400-800g/day divided in at least 5 meals. The protective role of regular consumption of fruits and vegetables is proven: the replacement of high calorie food with low calorie fruits and vegetables (cabbage and broccoli) decreases overall energy intake and reduce the risk for CRC. Compounds with hypothetical antiproliferative and anticancer action, which inactivate free radicals, are antioxidant vitamins (A, C, E), folic acid, thioethers (garlic, onions, leeks), terpens (citrus fruits), plant phenols (grapes, strawberries), carotenoids (carrots, sweet potatos, water melons), selenium, flavonoids, calcium, etc (Levin et al., 2002). With high consummation of fibres (cereals, fruits, vegetables) the risk for CRC is reduced with 40% (Guidance on Cancer Services. Improving Outcomes in Colorectal Cancers - Manual Update. National Institute for Clinical Excellence 2004). Protective effect of fibers is augmented from the fluid intake, calcium, etc. (Levin et al., 2002).

9.3.11 Dairy products

Our study confirms that dairy products and yoghourt are protective factors for CRC and CRP, but low-fat dairy products must be available, in order to prevent cardiovascular diseases. Low-fat dairy products supply calcium and vitamin D, both of which has protective effect for CRC. The contradictory data about the protective role of dairy products is associated with the quantity of the contained fat (World Cancer Research Fund and American Institute for Cancer Research, Food, Nutrition and the Prevention of Cancer, 1997).

In summary, the intake of fats cause increased influx of bile in the small intestine, whereas part of the fat and bile reaches the large bowel, where bacteria metabolize fat and bile into bile acids and fat acids. These products impair the epithelium of large bowel and stimulate cell proliferation, which is a prerequisite for carcinogenesis of large bowel. The secondary products of bile metabolism and by-products of some foods, which are cooked in certain way, could act like carcinogens, especially in persons with genetic predisposition for development of CRC. The food exerts effect upon intraluminal content and wall of the large bowel, but also part of the digested substances are absorbed and release of the local hormones and peptides, like insulin and gastrin, is induced. These hormones and peptides could also promote epithelial hyperploliferation. Apoptosis and cell differentiation are suppressed too, and DNA abnormalities could occur (Fig. 1). Adenomatous, hyperplastic or mixed colorectal polyps are morphological sign of the blended influence of genetic and exogenous factors upon the colorectal epithelium. Occurrence and progression of these polyps are evidence for the readiness of the colorectal epithelium to react in this distinct way under the influence of exogenous risk factors and inherited predisposition. Diet fibers by their volume and fluids dilute large bowel content, shorten the bowel transit time and do not permit a long contact of large bowel content with large bowel wall. As a result of bacterial fermentation of the cereal fibers, short-chain fatty acids are produced, which are very important for the metabolism and proper state of large bowel epithelium and contribute to large bowel integrity (Hague et al., 1995). Changed low pH in the large bowel inhibits dehydroxylation and dehydrogenation of bile acids. Changed low pH in the large bowel plays protective role for occurrence of CRC, because dehydroxylation and dehydrogenation of bile acids could result in formation of carcinogenic substances.

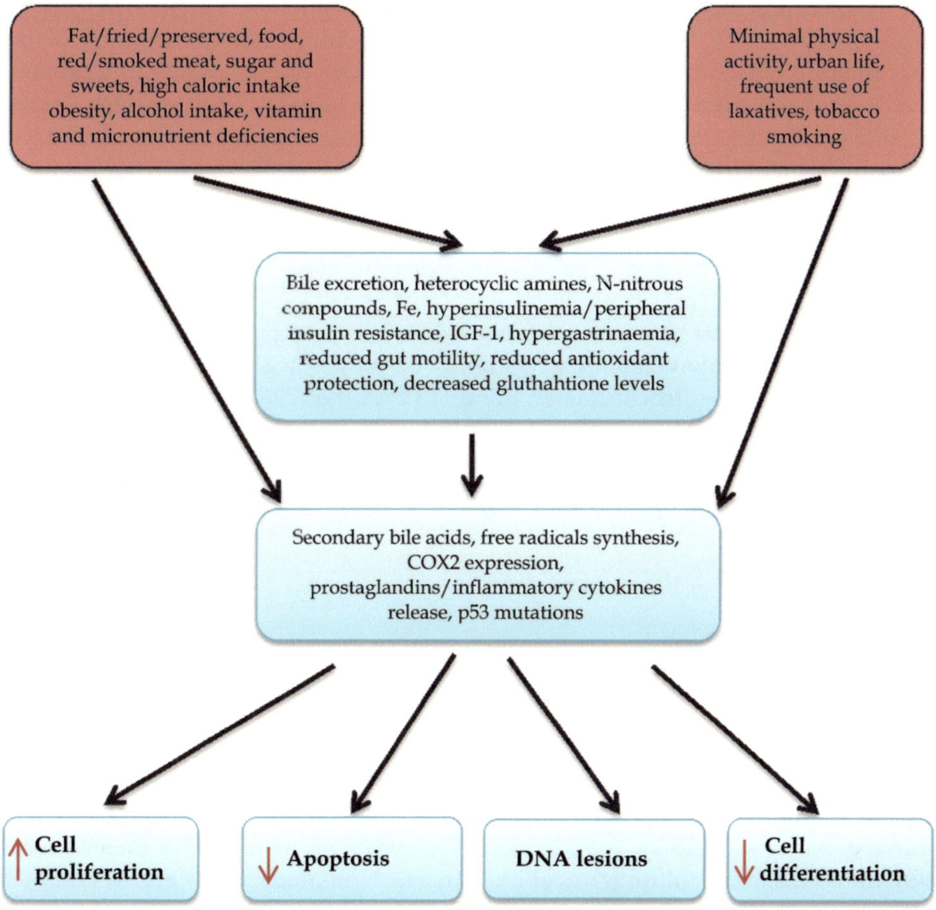

Fig. 1. Possible mechanisms of influence of diet and lifestyle upon pathogenesis of colorectal cancer. IFG-1, insulin-like growth factor-1; COX-2, cyclooxygenase-2.

Micronutrients and bioactive compounds complete their protective role by several mechanisms - in systemic way promote cell differentiation and apoptosis, and support the large bowel integrity, while intraluminally, micronutrients and bioactive compounds participate actively in detoxification of diet and metabolite carcinogens. Influence of the environmental risk factors, especially diet risk factors, could facilitate the clinic expression of recessive alleles for CRC or alleles with low penetration. Diet risk factors could also modulate the time of expression of recessive alleles for CRC. This statement could explain some of the cases of CRC in patients from a generation, which has been migrated from countries with low incidence of CRC in countries with high incidence of CRC (USA, Australia). Often, systemic genetic variations (polymorphisms) could affect the speed of detoxification or the activation of environmental carcinogens. This is happening in the process of the culinary food treatment, during tobacco smoking or from the alcohol metabolites. At the same time, shortage of anticarcinogens could be available in the regular diet.

We must not forget that from the two known etiological risk factors, the first is acquired - diet and lifestyle, and the second one is inheritable - susceptibility. Large bowel polyposis is a very good example of the interactions between exogenous and endogenous factors that take part in large bowel carcinogenesis with different rate of progression. In patients with FAP the progression from benign adenomas to cancer is rapid (2-4 years) due to inherited genetic changes; in other cases longer exposure to certain exogenous factors is needed to cause genetic changes that lead to cancer (the mean age of CRC patients in our group was 64 years); however, in certain subjects the time for neoplastic transformation exceeds life duration. Therefore a good differentiation between these groups and early prophylaxis and screening methods are needed. The most frequently used screening methods include: flexible sigmoidoscopy, fecal occult blood test, large bowel capsule endoscopy (if cheaper), double contrast barium enema, virtual colonoscopy, fibrocolonoscopy, endoscopic polypectomy, histological evaluation of all removed polyps, assessment of risk factors, and genetic testing if possible. In conclusion about 15% of the cases with CRC are hereditary, while the remaining 85% are sporadic. However, in 30% of cases a stronger correlation with dietary habits and lifestyle is suspected, while in 55% a close interaction between host susceptibility and environmental factors is more probable. The above fact leads us to the hypothesis that prevention of CRC is a possible task, which can be achieved by correction of certain exogenous factors.

10. Chemoprevention

Chemoprevention is defined as a usage of a medication or natural substances, which can prevent occurrence of benign or malignant tumor (Hakama, 1998). Chemoprevention is used in every stage of CRC prevention and includes three major groups: medications, non-medications and biologically active substances. Medications include non-steroidal anti-inflammatory drugs (NSAIDs), acetylsalicylic acid, inhibitors of cyclooxigenase-2 (COX-2), 5-aminosalicylic acid (5-ASA), folic acid, ursodeoxycholic acid, difluoromethylornithine (DFMO), dithiolethionine (oltipraz), acetilcystein, etc. Non-medications are: selenium, fibers, calcium, vit A, B, C, D, β-carotene, other retinoids, minerals, etc. Biologically active substances include: limonene and perillyl alcohol (in citruses), resveratrol (red grape), diallyl disulfide (garlic), lycopene (tomatoes), flavanols (green tea), isoflavones - genistein (soya), dithiolthiones, squalene (olive oil), ferulic and phytic acids (rice). Chemoprevention plays a substantial role in secondary and tertiary prevention of CRC. Also, it could be used for prophylaxis in patients after polypectomy of adenomas with high-grade dysplasia, polyps with invasive carcinomas, patients with familial history for cancer. Patient with IBD and inflammatory pseudopolyposis and require constant chemoprevention with 5-ASA. The most widely used medications include: acetylsalicylic acid, polyvitamins, folic acid, selenium, NSAID. So far, the most consistent data for reduction of polyp recurrence exist for acetylsalicylic acid and folic acid. Still, more large studies, examining the exact medications and possible role, are needed.

10.1 NSAIDs

Mechanisms of chemoprevention with NSAIDs include: inhibition and deactivation of possible carcinogens, inhibition of cell proliferation, promotion of cell differentiation and apoptosis, correction of genetic damages and inhibition of angiogenesis (Gustafson-Svard et al., 1996). Epidemiological studies have shown that NSAIDs and especially acetylsalicylic acid have chemopreventive properties (Lang, 2003). Regression of polyps to 28% is detected in FAP patients, who are treated in a long period with NSAIDs (Steinbach et al., 2000). The regular intake of acetylsalicylic acid and other NSAIDs reduce the incidence of CRC with 30-50% according to retrospective and prospective studies (Janne & Mayer, 2000). However, adenomas are observed in some patients, who are treated with acetylsalicylic acid, which means that chemoprevention cannot substitute completely screening colonoscopy (Sandler et al., 2003). The dose of acetylsalicylic acid is still debatable. Some studies show that reduction of the risk for colorectal polyp occurrence is achieved with lower doses of acetylsalicylic acid (Baron et al., 2003). Side effects of long intake of acetylsalicylic acid, like gastrointestinal hemorrhage and brain hemorrhage restrict the usage of acetylsalicylic acid. There is a need for development and usage of new forms of acetylsalicylic acid and NSAIDs agents, which are much safer, like NO-acetylsalicylic acid (Fiorucci & Del Soldato, 2003). Another possibility is the usage of products and substances of natural origin. For example, natural COX-2 inhibitors are yellow pigment curcumin, resveratrol (in grapes) and omega 3-fatty acids in the fish.

10.2 Folic acid

The presumable protective mechanism of folic acid is not clear, but it is supposed, that the lack of folic acid is associated with hypomethylation of DNA and oncogenic activation. Regular intake of folic acid for at least 15 years reduces the risk of development of CRC (Giovannucci et al., 1998). A study showed reduction of CRC incidence in genetically predisposed persons who use folic acid in high doses. Probably, these persons are vulnerable to methyl group deficiency, as a result of DNA aberrations with low penetration (Fuchs et al., 2002). The risk for CRC is vastly reduced if folic acid is used for a prolonged time, especially from smokers (Scottish Intercollegiate Guidelines Network. Management of Colorectal cancer. A national clinical guideline. 2003). However, there are data from animal studies that folic acid can promote the impact of some carcinogens (Kim, 2003). Moreover, no large studies are available to sustain the chemopreventive role of folic acid.

10.3 Calcium

Protective role of calcium is confirmed in different trials. A result from a study claims that regular daily intake of 3 g calcium as supplement reduce the risk of colorectal adenomas relapse 1 year after their removal. This fact is an evidence of protective action of calcium in the early stages of colorectal carcinogenesis (Baron et al., 1999). Another study reported that high calcium intake is associated with vastly lower risk of development of distal CRC, but not proximal CRC (Wu et al., 2002).

10.4 Ursodeoxycholic acid

The protective role of ursodeoxycholic acid for CRC is probably due to the reduced absorption of the secondary deoxycholic acid, which increases epithelial proliferation and promote carcinogenesis. A study proved that use of synthetic ursodeoxycholic acid is associated with reduced risk of development of CRC in patients with ulcerative colitis and primary sclerosing cholangitis (Peng et al., 1995). Other authors found that administration of ursodeoxycholic acid in patients with primary biliary cirrhosis, who have undergone polypectomy, is connected with vastly reduced risk of CRP relapse (Serfaty et al., 2003).

10.5 Selenium

Abundant data for the role of selenium as a prophylactic substance for the CRC are constantly accumulating. Epidemiological studies have shown anticancer role of selenium since 1970. In some parts of Europe there is low amount of selenium in the soil and European population show tendency of lower intake of selenium in the last 25 years (Rayman, 2000). A lower risk for CRC was detected in persons who take 200 μg selenium daily (Clark et al., 1996). Some authors found lower serum levels of selenium in patients with CRC (Scieszka et al., 1997).

We can conclude that the choice of proper chemopreventive tool is difficult. Such a tool must be effective, cheap, safe and easy to use. It is calculated, that up to 80% of the cases with CRC could be prevented by alteration of diet habits (Cummings & Bingham, 1998). These data oblige us to fully clarify the role of chemoprevention in colorectal neoplasms. Combination of chemoprevention with screening endoscopy is of great importance for reduction of the CRC mortality. The most significant chemopreventive agents are the acetylsalicylic acid and other NSAIDs, antioxidants, calcium and selenium.

10.6 Chemoprevention in our patients

The main indications for applying chemoprevention in our patients were: patients with adenomatous polyposis of large bowel; patients who have undergone endoscopic polypectomy; operated for CRC patients, IBD patients and patients with hereditary syndromes of CRC. 70 of our patients took chemopreventive agents: acetylsalicylic acid, polyvitamins, folic acid, selenium, NSAID, calcium, 5-ASA, ursodeoxycholic acid.

11. Primary prophylaxis of colorectal adenomatous polyps and CRC

Colorectal cancer prevention is divided into three groups: primary, secondary and tertiary. Diet and lifestyle are considered as targets in primary CRC prevention, which includes modification of the established risk factors for colorectal polyps. These are: limitation of certain foods, beverages and habits; improved physical activity; consumption of protective foods; eradication of *H. pylori*. Important question is whether it is possible to apply primary prophylaxis in CRC and its precursor - adenomatous colorectal polyposis and if risk factors for CRC and CRP are avoidable and at what extent? Considering the growing epidemic of CRC this issue is waiting its prompt answer. What kind of healthy style of life we can offer to threatened people, similarly to the primary prevention in other diseases like cardiovascular disease, ischaemic heart disease and arterial hypertension, and distinct type of cancers? A great part of risk factors for CRC and CRP are associated with the diet, the lifestyle, exogenous carcinogens, some diseases and disease-like conditions. However, some protective factors for CRC and CRP are famous and could be recommended. As a primary prevention in healthy persons change of diet habits, reduction of body weight, refusal of tobacco smoking and alcohol intake are recommended. Preventive role of calcium, magnesium, β-carotene, vitamins, folic acid and selenium for CRC and CRP is still disputable. Acetylsalicylic acid and other NSAIDs for this purpose are not commonly used, because of their adverse side effects (Sandler, 2004). However, if new and convincing data are available, we can try to restrict influences of known risk factors and to cure precancerous conditions and will be able to perform proper primary prevention for CRC and colorectal adenomatous polyposis.

12. Secondary prophylaxis of colorectal adenomatous polyps and CRC

Secondary CRC prevention is used for early detection of premalignant adenomas and cancer in its curative stage. It includes: screening colonoscopy; polypectomy; optimal treatment of IBD patients; chemoprevention and follow-up (Hawk, 2004; Rex, 2000). The aim of secondary prophylaxis or screening is to diminish the mortality of CRC by early detection and treatment of premalignant adenomas and cancer in its curable stage. European and national gastrointestinal and digestive endoscopy societies recommend screening to comprehend all healthy and risk groups of people. CRC screening consists of: digital rectal examination, fecal occult blood test, fecal immunochemical test for haemoglobin/haptoglobin, barium enema, sigmoidoscopy, sigmoidoscopy with fecal occult blood test, colonoscopy (with polypectomy), chromoendoscopy, NBI and high-resolution colonoscopy, virtual colonoscopy - CT or MRI, fecal DNA test (Geissler & Graeven, 2005). A useful test is invented for early detection and follow-up of CRC, similar to the noninvasive serological and fecal tests used for detection of infection with *H. Pylori*. This test is based on the idea, that proliferating cells, especially malignant cells, are expressing special isoenzyme of pyruvate kinase (PK), which plays a significant role in glycolysis. This isoenzyme consists of 4 subunits in healthy cells, while in neoplastic cells there are 2 subunits. This dimeric form M2-PK is found in gastrointestinal neoplasms. Tumor marker M2-PK is found in the blood of 47.8% of patients with CRC, while fecal test is sensible in 80% of cases with CRC (Hardt et al., 2004).

We propose stratification of healthy population in *three* groups: patients with *moderate risk* for development of colorectal polyps and cancer; patients with *elevated risk* for development of colorectal polyps and cancer; patients with *extremely high risk* for development of colorectal polyps and cancer;

The *first* group includes all patients who have no family history for cancer and no personal history for polypectomy or cancer in the past.

The *second* group includes patients with family history for CRC or related neoplasia (stomach, mammary gland, endometrium, ovary, adrenal glands), patients with polypectomy of polyps with low-grade dysplasia, patients with large bowel resection due to CRC (5 years post-surgery), male gender.

The *third* group includes patients: with familial adenomatous polyposis (FAP), with polypectomy of polyps with high-grade dysplasia, patients with large bowel resection due to CRC (up to 5 years post-surgery), with Peutz-Jeghers syndrome, juvenile polyposis, Cowden`s disease, HNPCC, IBD patients, with acromegaly and ureterosigmoidostomy.

The most appropriate follow-up method of patients, who have undergone polypectomy, is colonoscopy. The intervals according to the patients` risk and starting age are summarized in Table 7.

№	Patients	Starting age for screening colonoscopy	Interval for control colonoscopy
1	With average statistical risk for development of CRP and CRC	50 years	10 years
2	With moderately elevated risk for CRC	40 years	5 years
3	With extremely high risk for CRC	10-30 years	1-3 years

Table 7. Starting age and intervals for screening colonoscopy.

13. Tertiary prophylaxis of CRC

Follow-up, chemoprevention and polypectomy are cornerstones of tertiary CRC prvention. Tertiary prevention is performed after surgical treatment for CRC and its aim is elongation of the survival and improvement of the quality of life of patients who have been treated with resection for curable CRC. This purpose can be achieved by treatment of the patient's complaints, which are connected with the primary disease or with the systemic chemotherapy, as well and by disclosure of relapses in early and curable stage. We have not to forget, that occupational and psychosocial rehabilitation are very important in these patients. Large studies, which offer standard approach to these patients, are missing. Nevertheless, the following factors must be considered: tumor stage, general condition of the patient and life expectancy, and the patient's gain from treatment with a new, potentially curable surgeon intervention in case with proven relapse of CRC. 8,4 % of our patients develop metachronous CRC with mean age 69±11 years. The mean difference between diagnosis (CRC) of first and second localization is 6 years (2-15). This is the time for tertiary prophylaxis of CRC.

Follow-up of patients with CRC is achieved by: personal history, physical examination, carcinoembryonic antigen (CEA) test, lab tests, fecal occult blood test, chest X-ray, abdominal ultrasound, echo-endoscopy, CT, MRI, colonoscopy and PET-CT.

In conclusion, primary prophylaxis of the disease is the ultimate aim of every clinical physician. Can we apply the primary prophylaxis in colorectal adenomas and CRC?

Encouraging examples for this possibility exist. Low physical activity, high uptake of saturated fats and arterial hypertension were recognized as risk factors for cardiovascular diseases. For a few years broad public campaigns resulted in dramatic reduction of mortality from coronary heart disease. Similar results are obtained and in some countries, in which restrictive government politics for tobacco smoking exists. No single factor is responsible for CRC carcinogenesis, but combination of some important factors, which are associated with the diet and lifestyle, is crucial.

May be the true pathway is to seek some average healthy diet and lifestyle, which play preventive role for many diseases. This recommendation is especially useful for the persons who are genetically predisposed, because the environmental risk factors can promote faster carcinogenesis.

Revival of the healthy Balkan (Bulgarian) feeding habits from the first half of the 20-th century seems reasonable (Ribarova et al., 2004). More protective foods must be included in our daily meal and this task looks feasible. We have to consume regularly fruit, vegetables, cereals, low-fat dairy products, legumes, poultry, fish, sea products, fibers and to reduce the intake of animal fats, red meat and preserved food. We have to be physical active, restrict alcohol usage, and to avoid tobacco smoking and usage of grilled and fried food.

Many countries introduced a large scale programs for reduction of risk factors and promotion of protective factors for CRC. Besides that, such programs are useful and for prophylaxis of cardiovascular diseases, some other cancers and important metabolite diseases, like diabetes mellitus II type and obesity.

14. Recommendations for prophylaxis of CRC according to our data

You must follow these rules to be protected from colorectal cancer:

1. Do not eat fatty food, smoked meat, fried foods, margarine, pork, red meat and egg-fried food
2. Do not drink alcohol
3. Do not smoke
4. Sustain high physical activity and do not be obese
5. Restrict the intake of refined sugar and white flour products
6. Use plant oil, but not margarine
7. Legumes, fish, low-fat dairy products and Bulgarian yoghourt are good source of proteins
8. Consume at least 5 times per day fruits and vegetables (pears, melons, water melons, grapes, peaches, onion, garlic, pepper)
9. Prefer poultry, white meat, hares and fish from the meat
10. Healthy cooking includes decrease of the fat added in the food, reduction of the cooking temperature and refraining from the use of grilled food
11. Do not use regularly laxatives
12. Avoid contact with petrol
13. Avoid usage of preserved foods and prefer local, season`s, fresh or frozen fruits and vegetables

14. Fasting is good
15. Do endoscopic polypectomy if you have adenomatous colorectal polyps
16. Eradicate Helicobacter pylori if you are infected
17. Use daily acetylsalicylic acid if you do not have any contraindications
18. Make a screening colonoscopy after you reach 50 years, and if you are in risk group (familial predisposed to colorectal cancer or associated localization - stomach, endometrium, breast, ovary or if you have preceding polypectomy) - after you reach 40 years. Consider genetic testing if you are in risk groups

15. References

Altes, A., Gimferrer, E., Capella G., Barceló M.J. & Baiget, M. (1999). Colorectal cancer and HFE gene mutations. *Haematologica*, Vol. 84, No. 5, pp. 479-480.

Anti, M., Armelao, F., Marra, G., Percesepe, A., Bartoli, G. M., Palozza, P., Parrella, P., Canetta, C., Gentiloni, N., De Vitis, I. et al. (1994). Effects of different doses of fish oil on rectal cell proliferation in patients with sporadic colonic adenomas. *Gastroenterol*, Vol. 107, No. 6, pp. 1709-1718.

Aries, V., Crowther, S., Drasar, S., Hill, J. & Williams, E. (1969). Bacteria and the aetiology of cancer of the large bowel. *Gut*, Vol. 10, No. 5, pp. 334-335.

Baron, A., Beach, M., Mandel, J. S., van Stolk, R. U., Haile, R. W., Sandler, R. S., Rothstein, R., Summers, R. W., Snover, D. C., Beck, G. J., Bond, J. H. & Greenberg, E. R. (1999). Calcium supplements for the prevention of colorectal adenomas. Calcium polyp prevention study group. *N Engl J Med*, Vol. 340, No. 2, pp. 101-107.

Baron, J. A., Cole, B. F., Sandler, R. S., Haile, R. W., Ahnen, D., Bresalier, R., McKeown-Eyssen, G., Summers, R. W, Rothstein, R., Burke, C. A., Snover, D. C., Church, T. R., Allen, J. I., Beach, M., Beck, G. J., Bond, J. H., Byers, T., Greenberg, E. R., Mandel, J. S., Marcon, N., Mott, L. A., Pearson, L., Saibil, F. & van Stolk, R. U. (2003). A randomized trial of aspirin to prevent colorectal adenomas. *N Engl J Med*, Vol. 348, No. 10, pp. 891-899.

Bingham, S. A., Day, N. E., Luben, R., Ferrari, P., Slimani, N., Norat, T., Clavel-Chapelon, F., Kesse, E., Nieters, A., Boeing, H., Tjønneland, A., Overvad, K., Martinez, C., Dorronsoro, M., Gonzalez, C. A., Key, T. J., Trichopoulou, A., Naska, A., Vineis, P., Tumino, R., Krogh, V., Bueno-de-Mesquita, H. B., Peeters, P. H., Berglund, G., Hallmans, G., Lund, E., Skeie, G., Kaaks, R. & Riboli, E; European Prospective Investigation into Cancer and Nutrition. (2003). Dietary fibre in food and protection against colorectal cancer in the European Prospective Investigation into Cancer and Nutrition (EPIC): an observation study. *Lancet*, Vol. 361, No. 9368, pp. 1496-1501.

Bostick, R. M., Fosdick, L., Wood., J. R., Grambsch, P., Grandits, G. A., Lillemoe, T. J., Louis, T. A. & Potter, J. D. (1995). Calcium and colorectal epithelial cell proliferation in sporadic adenoma patients: a randomized, double-blinded, placebo-controlled clinical trial. *J Natl Cancer Inst*, Vol. 87, No. 17, pp. 1307-1315.

Bulletin of the National Centre for Health Information. (2005). (www.nchi.govenment.bg).

Burnstein, J. (1993). Dietary factors related to colorectal neoplasms. *Surg Clin North Am*, Vol. 73, No. 1, pp. 13-29.

Calle, E. E. & Thun, M. J. (2004) Obesity and cancer. *Oncogene*, Vol. 23, No. 38, pp. 6365-6378.

Clark, L. C., Combs, G. F., Tumbull, B. W., Slate, E. H., Chalker, D. K., Chow, J., Davis, L. S., Glover, R. A., Graham, G. F., Gross, E. G., Krongrad, A., Lesher, J. L. Jr., Park, H. K., Sanders, B. B. Jr., Smith, C. L. & Taylor, J. R. (1996). Effects of selenium supplementation for cancer prevention in patients with carcinoma of the skin. A randomized controlled trial. Nutritional Prevention of Cancer Study Group. *JAMA*, Vol. 276, No. 24, pp. 1957-1963.

Courtney, E. D., Melville, D. M. & Leicester R. J. (2004). Review article: Chemoprevention of colorectal cancer. *Aliment Pharmacol Ther,* Vol. 19, No. 1, pp. 1-24.

Crandall, C. J. (1999). Estrogen replacement therapy and colon cancer: a clinical review. *J Womens Health Gend Based Med.*, Vol. 8, No. 9, pp. 1155-1166.

Cummings, J. H. & Bingham, S. A. (1998). Diet and the prevention of cancer. *BMJ,* Vol. 317, No. 7173, pp. 1636-1640.

De Meester, C. & Gerber, G. B. (1995). The role of cooked food mutagens as possible etiological agents in human cancer: a critical appraisal of recent epidemiological investigations. *Rev Epidemiol Sante Publique,* Vol. 43, No. 2, pp. 147-161.

Eide, T. J. (1986). The age-, sex-, and site-specific occurrence of adenomas and carcinomas of the large intestine within a defined population. *Scand J Gastroenterol,* Vol. 21, No. 9, pp. 1083-1088.

Ekbom, A., Helmick, C., Zack, M. & Adami, H. O. (1990). Ulcerative colitis and colorectal cancer: a population-based study. *N Engl J Med,* Vol. 323, No. 18, pp. 1228 -1233.

Ekbom, A., Yuen, J., Adami, H. O., McLaughlin J. K., Chow, W. H., Persson, I. & Fraumeni, J. F. Jr. (1993). Cholecystectomy and colorectal cancer. *Gastroenterol,* Vol. 105, No. 1, pp. 142-147.

Evans, M. D., Dizdaroglu, M. & Cooke, M. S. (2004). Oxidative DNA damage and disease: induction, repair and significance. *Mutat. Res*, Vol. 567, No. 1, pp. 1-61.

Fearon, E. R. & Fogelstein, B. (1990). A genetic model for colorectal tumorogenesis. *Cell,* Vol. 61, No. 5. pp. 759-767.

Fedirko, V., Bostick, R. M., Flanders, W. D., Long, Q., Sidelnikov, E., Shaukat, A., Daniel, C. R., Rutherford, R. E & Woodard, J. J. Effects of Vitamin D and Calcium on proliferation and differentiation in normal colon mucosa: a randomized clinical trial. (2009). *Cancer Epidemiol Biomarkers Prev,* Vol. 18, No. 11, 2933-2941.

Ferrucci, L. M., Sinha, R., Graubard, B. I., Mayne, S. T., Ma, X., Schatzkin, A., Schoenfeld, P. S., Cash, B. D., Flood, A., & Cross, A. J. Dietary meat intake in relation to colorectal adenoma in asymptomatic women. (2009). *Am J Gastroenterol,* Vol. 104, No. 5, pp. 1231–1240.

Fiorucci, S., Del Soldato, P. (2003). NO-aspirin: mechanism of action and gastrointestinal safety. *Dig Liver Dis,* Vol. 35 (Suppl 2), pp. 9-19.

Ford, E. S. (1999). Body mass index and colon cancer in a national sample of adult US men and women. *Am J Epidemiol,* Vol. 150, No 4, pp. 390-398.

Fuchs, C. S., Willet, W. C., Colditz, G. A., Hunter, D. J., Stampfer, M. J., Speizer, F. E. & Giovannucci, E. L. (2002). The influence of folate and multivitamin use on the familial risk of colon cancer in women. *Cancer Epidemiol Biomark Pre,* Vol. 11, No. 3, pp. 227-234.

Geissler, M. & Graeven, U. (2005). Prävenzion. In: *Das kolorektale Karzinom,* pp. 27-42, Georg Thieme Verlag.

Gerber, M. (2003). Biofactors in the Mediterranean diet. *Clin Chem Lab Med,* Vol. 41, No. 8, pp. 999-1004.

Giovannucci, E., Ascherio, A., Rimm, E. B., Colditz G. A., Stampfer, M. J. & Willett, W. C. (1995). Physical activity, obesity, and risk colon cancer and adenoma in men. *Ann Intern Med,* Vol. 122, No. 5, pp. 327-334.

Giovannucci, E., Rimm, E. B., Ascherio, A, Stampfer, M. J., Colditz, G. A. & Willett, W. C. (1995). Alcohol, low methionine-low folate diets, and risk of colon cancer in men. *J Natl Cancer Inst,* Vol.v87, No. 4, pp. 265-273.

Giovannucci, E., Stampfer, M. J., Colditz, G. A., Hunter, D. J., Fuchs, C., Rosner, B. A., Speizer, F. E. & Willett, W.C. (1998). Multivitamine use, folate, and colon cancer in women in the Nurses` Health Study. *Ann Intern Med,* Vol. 129, No. 7, pp. 517-524.

Giovannucci, E. (2006). The epidemiology of vitamin D and colorectal cancer: recent findings. *Curr Opin Gastroenterol,* Vol. 22, No. 1, pp. 24-29.

Greenwald, P. (2002). Cancer chemoprevention. *BMJ,* Vol. 324, No. 7339, pp. 714-718.

Guidance on Cancer Services. (2004). Improving Outcomes in Colorectal Cancers – Manual Update. National Institute for Clinical Excellence.

Gustafson-Svärd, C., Lilja, I., Hallböök, O. & Sjödahl, R. (1996). Cyclo-oxygenase-1 and cyclooxygenase-2 gene expression in human colorectal adenocarcinomas and in azoxymethane induced colonic tumours in rats. *Gut,* Vol. 38, No. 1, pp. 79–84.

Hague, A., Elder, D. J., Hicks, D. J. & Paraskeva, C. (1995). Apoptosis in colorectal tumour cells: induction by the short chain fatty acids butyrate, propionate and acetate and by the bile salt deoxycholate. *Inl J Cancer,* Vol. 60, No.3, pp. 400-406.

Hakama, M. (1998). Chemoprevention of cancer. *Acta Oncol,* Vol, 37, No.3 , pp. 227-230.

Hamilton, S. R. (2001). Origin of colorectal cancers in hyperplastic polyps and serrated adenomas: Another truism bites the dust. *J Natl Cancer Inst,* Vol. 93, No. 17, pp. 1282-1283.

Hardt, P. D., Mazurek, S., Toepler, M., Schlierbach, P., Bretzel, R. G., Eigenbrodt, E. & Kloer H. U. (2004). Faecal tumor M2 pyruvate kinase: a new, sensitive screening tool for colorectal cancer. *Br J Cancer,* Vol. 91 No. 5, pp. 980-984.

Hawk, E. T., Umar, A. & Viner, J. L. (2004). Colorectal cancer chemoprevention-an overview of the science. *Gastroenterol,* Vol. 126, No. 5, pp. 1423-1447.

Hoff, G. (1987). Colorectal polyps. Clinical implications: Screening and cancer prevention.. *Scand J Gastroenterol,* Vol. 22, No. 7, pp. 769-775.

Institute of Medicine, Dietary Reference Intakes for Calcium, Phosphorus, Magnesium, Vitamin D and Fluoride. Food and Nutrition Board, Washington, DC. (1997) National Academy Press.

Jänne, P. A. & Mayer, R. J. (2000). Chemoprevention of colorectal cancer. *N Engl J Med,* Vol. 342, No. 26, pp. 1960-1968.

Jenkins, P. J., Fairclough, P. D., Richards, T., Lowe, D. G., Monson, J., Grossman, A., Wass, J. A. & Besser, M. (1997). Acromegaly, colon polyps carcinoma. *Clin Endocrinology,* Vol. 47, No. 1, pp. 17-22.

Kim, Y. I. (2003). Role of folate in colon cancer development and progression. *J Nutr,* Vol. 133, No. 11 (Suppl 1), pp. 3731-3739.

Kotzev, I., Mirchev, M., Manevska, B., Ivanova, I. &, Kaneva, M. (2008). Risk and protective factors for development of colorectal polyps and cancer (Bulgarian experience). Vol. 55, No. 82-83, pp. 381-387.

Kritchevsky, D. (1995). Epidemiology of fibre, resistant starch and colorectal cancer. Eur J Cancer Prev, Vol. 4, No. 5, pp. 345–352.

Kryston, T. B., Georgiev, A. B., Pissis, P. & Georgakilas, A. G. (2011). *Mutat. Res,* Vol. 711, No. 1-2, pp. 193-201.

Levin, B., Rozen, P. & Young, G. P. (2002). How should we follow up premalignant conditions?, In: *Colorectal cancer in clinical practice: prevention, early detection and management,* Paul Rozen (Ed.), pp. 67-66, Martin Dunitz, London, England.

Lim, K., Han, C., Xu, L., Isse, K., Demetris. A. J. & Wu T. (2008). Cyclooxygenase-2-derived prostaglandin E2 activates beta-catenin in human cholangiocarcinoma cells: evidence for inhibition of these signaling pathways by omega 3 polyunsaturated fatty acids. *Cancer Res,* Vol. 68, No. 2, pp. 553–560.

Longacre, T. A. & Fenoglio-Preiser, C. M. (1990). Mixed hyperplastic adenomatous polyps/serrated adenomas. A distinct form of colorectal neoplasia. *Am J Surg Pathol,* Vol. 14, No. 6, pp. 524- 537.

Lubin, F., Rozen, P., Arieli, B., Farbstein, M., Knaani, Y., Bat, L. & Farbstein, H. (1997). Nutritional and lifestyle habits and water-fiber interaction in colorectal adenoma etiology. *Cancer Epidemiol Biomarkers Prev,* Vol. 6, No. 2, pp. 79-85.

Middleton, E. & Kandaswami, C. (1993). The impact of plant flavonoids on mammalian biology: implications for immunity, inflammation and cancer. In: *The Flavonoids: Advances in Research since 1986,* J. B. Harborne (Ed.), pp. 619-652, Chapman & Hall, London.

Nelson, R. L. (2001). Iron and colorectal cancer risk: Human studies. *Nutr Rev,* Vol. 59, No. 5, pp. 140-148.

Parkin, D. M., Pisani, R. & Ferlay, J. (1999). Global cancer statistics. *CA Cancer J Clin,* Vol. 49, No. 1, pp. 33-64.

Patterson, E., Kristal, R. & Newhouser, L. (2000). Vitamin supplements and cancer risk. Epidemiologic research an recommendations, In: *Primary and Secondary Preventive Nutrition,* A. Bendich & R. J. Deckelbaum (Ed.), 21-43, Humana Press.,Totowa, NJ.

Peng, C. L., Lin, H. J., Wang, K, Lai, C. R. & Lee, S. D. (1995). Treatment of duodenal carcinoid by strip biopsy. *J Clin Gasteroenterol,* Vol. 20, No. 2, pp. 168-171.

Pfohl-Leskowitcz, A., Grosse, Y., Carrière, V., Cugnenc, P. H., Berger, A., Carnot, F., Beaune P. & de Waziers, I. (1999). High levels of DNA adducts in human colon are associated with colorectal cancer. *Cancer Res,* Vol. 55, No.23, pp. 5611-5616.

Rayman, M. P. (2000). The importance of selenium to human health. *Lancet, Vol.* 356, No. 9225, pp. 233-241.

Rex, D. K. (2000). Colonoscopy. *Gastrointest Endosc Clin N Am,* Vol. 10, No. 1, pp. 135-160.

Ribarova, F., Ilieva, Sv. & Nachev, Ch. (2004). The richness of the Balkan diet. Proceedings Varna international symposium for obesity and related diseases, pp. 62-65, Albena, Bulgaria, 30 May - 1 June, 2004.

Rustgi, A. K. (2003). Aspirin and colorectal adenoma prevention. *Gastroenterol,* Vol, 124, No. 5, p. 1176.

Sandler, R. S., Halabi, S., Baron, J. A, Budinger, S., Paskett, E., Keresztes, R., Petrelli, N., Pipas, J. M., Karp, D. D., Loprinzi, C. L, Steinbach, G. & Schilsky, R. (2003). A randomised trial of aspirin to prevent colorectal adenomas in patients with previous colorectal cancer. *N Engl J Med,* Vol. 348, No. 10, pp. 883-890.

Sandler, R. S. (2004). Aspirin prevention of colorectal cancer: more or less? *Ann Intern Med,* Vol. 140, No. 3, pp. 224-225.

Schatzkin, A., Lanza, E., Freedman, L. S., Tangrea, J., Cooper, M. R., Marshall, J. R., Murphy, P. A., Selby, J. V., Shike, M., Schade, R. R., Burt, R. W., Kikendall, J. W. & Cahill, J. (1996). The Polyp Prevention Trial I: rationale, design, recruitment, and baseline participant characteristics. *Cancer Epidemiol Biomarkers Prev,* Vol. 5, No. 5, pp. 375- 383.

Scieszka, M., Danch, A., Machalski, M. & Drózdz, M. (1997). Plasma selenium concentration in patients with stomach and colon cancer in the Upper Silesia. *Neoplasma,* Vol. 44, No. 6, pp. 395-397.

Scottish Intercollegiate Guidelines Network. Management of Colorectal cancer. A national clinical guideline. 2003.

Sedelnikova, O. A., Redon, C. E., Dickey, J. S., Nakamura, A. J., Georgakilas, A. G. & Bonner, W. M. (2010). Role of oxidatively induced DNA lesions in human pathogenesis. *Mutat. Res,* Vol. 704, No. 1-3, pp. 152-159.

Seitz, K. & Osswald, B. R. (1992). Effect of ethanol on procarcinogen activation. In: *Alcohol and cancer,* Watson R. R (Ed.), pp. 55-72, CRC Press, Boca Raton, FL.

Seitz, K., Pöchl, G. & Simanowski, U. A. (1998). Alcohol and cancer. *Recent Dev Alcohol,* Vol. 14, pp. 67-95.

Seo, Y. R., Kelley, M. R. & Smith, M. L. (2002). Selenomethionine regulation of p53 by a ref1-dependent redox mechanism. *Proc Natl Acad Sci,* Vol. 99, No. 22, pp. 14548-14553.

Serfaty, L., De Leusse, A., Rosmorduc, O., Desaint, B., Flejou, J. F., Chazouilleres, O., Poupon, R. E. & Poupon, R. (2003). Ursodesoxicholic acid therapy and the risk of colorectal adenoma in patients with primary biliary cirrhosis: an observational study. *Hepatology,* 2003, Vol. 38, No. 1, pp. 203-209.

Sigimura, T., Wakabayashi, K, Nakagama, H. & Nagao, M. (2004). Heterocyclic amines: mutagens/carcinogens produced during cooking of meat and fish. *Cancer Sci,* Vol. 94, No. 4, pp. 290-299.

Slattery, M. L. & Potter, J. D. (2002) Physical activity and colon cancer: confounding, effect modification and biological mechanism. *Med Sci Sports Exercise,* Vol. 34, No. 6, pp. 913-919.

Steinbach, G., Lynch, P. M., Philips, R. K., Wallace, M. H., Hawk, E., Gordon, G. B., Wakabayashi, N., Saunders, B., Shen, Y., Fujimura, T., Su, L. K. & Levin, B. (2000). The effect of celecoxib, a cyclooxygenase-2 inhibitor, in familial adenomatous polyposis. *N Engl J Med,* Vol. 342, No. 26 , pp. 1946-1952.

Tseng, M., Sandler, R. S., Greenberg, E. R., Mandel, J. S., Haile, R. W. & Baron, J. A. (1997). Dietary iron and recurrence of colorectal adenomas. *Cancer Epidemiol Biomarkers Prev,* Vol. 6, No. 12, pp. 1029–1032.

van Gorkom, B. A., de Vries, E. G., Karrenbeld, A. & Kleibeuker, J. H. (1999). Anthranoid laxatives and their potential carcinogenic effects. *Aliment Pharmacol Ther,* Vol. 13, No. 4, pp. 443-452.

Villa, E., Dugani, A., Rebecchi, A. M., Vignoli, A., Grottola, A., Buttafoco, P., Losi, L., Perini, M., Trande, P., Merighi, A., Lerose, R. & Manenti, F. (1996). Identification of subjects at risk for colorectal carcinoma through a test based on K-ras determination in the stool. *Gastroenterol,* Vol. 110, No. 5, pp. 1346-1353.

Weijenberg, M. P., Mullie, P. F., Brants, H. A, Heinen, M. M., Goldbohm, R. A & van den Brandt, P. A. (2008). Dietary glycemic load, glycemic index and colorectal cancer risk: results from the Netherlands Cohort Study. *Int J Cancer,* Vol. 122, No. 3, pp. 620–629.

Wenzel, U., Kuntz, S., Brendel M. D. & Daniel, H. (2000). Dietary flavone is a potent apoptosis inducer in human colon carcinoma cells. *Cancer Res,* Vol. 60, No. 14, pp. 3823-3831.

Winawer, S. J., Fletcher, R. H., Miller, L., Godlee, F., Stolar, M. H., Mulrow, C. D., Woolf, S. H., Glick, S. N., Ganiats, T. G., Bond, J. H., Rosen, L., Zapka, J. G., Olsen, S. J., Giardiello, F. M., Sisk, J. E., Van Antwerp, R., Brown-Davis, C., Marciniak, D. A. & Mayer, R. J. (1997). Colorectal cancer screening: clinical guidelines and rationale. *Gastroenterol,* Vol. 112, No. 2, pp. 594-642.

World Cancer Research Fund and American Institute for Cancer Research, Food, Nutrition and the Prevention of Cancer: A Global Perspective. (1997) Washington, DC: Banta Books.

Wu, K., Willett, W. C., Fuchs, C. S., Colditz, G. A. & Giovannucci, E. L. (2002). Calcium intake and risk of colon cancer in women and men. *J Natl Cancer Inst,* Vol. 94, No. 6, pp. 437-446.

Wynder, E. L., Kajitani, T., Ishikawa, S., Dodo, H. & Takano, A. (1969). Environmental factors of cancer of colon and rectum. II. Japanese epidemiological data. *Cancer,* Vol. 23, No. 5, pp. 1210-1220.

Yang, P., Cunningham, J. M., Halling, K. C., Lesnick, T. G., Burgart, L. J., Wiegert, E. M., Christensen, E. R., Lindor, N. M., Katzmann, J. A. & Thibodeau, S. N. (2000). Higher risk of mismatch repair-deficient colorectal cancer in α_1-antitripsin deficiency carriers and cigarette smokers. *Mol Genet Metab,* Vol. 71, No. 4 , pp.639-645.

Zaridze, D. G. (1983). Environmental etiology of large-bowel cancer. *J Natl Cancer Inst,* Vol. 70, No. 3, pp. 389-400.

Zhu, Z., Jiang, W., Ganther, H. E., Ip, C. & Thompson, H. J. (2000). In vitro effects of Se-allylselenocysteine and Se-propylselenocysteine on cell growth, DNA integrity, and apoptosis. *Biochem Pharmacol,* Vol. 60, No. 10, pp. 1467-1473.

Zumkeller, N., Brenner, H., Zwahlen, M. & Rothenbacher, D. (2006). Helicobacter pylori infection and colorectal cancer risk: a meta-analysis. *Helicobacter,* Vol. 11, No. 2, pp. 75-80.

8

Colorectal Cancer and the Preventive Effects of Food Components

Sayori Wada
Kyoto Prefectural University
Japan

1. Introduction

It has been reported that the cause of 30% of cancer is associated with eating habits (Anand et al., 2008). Colorectal cancer is one of the most common causes of death all over the world, and there is a strong association between this type of cancer and food intake. Despite this statement, the preventive effects of foods and nutrients on colorectal cancer have not completely elucidated yet.

It has been proposed that some biologically active nutrients suppress colon carcinogenesis through the mechanisms of cytostatic properties, inhibition of cell growth, induction of apoptosis, an anti-inflammation effect or modification of DNA in *in vitro* studies.

Although the positive effects of these nutrients have been shown in *in vitro* studies, it is still difficult to apply the effects of these nutrients in *in vivo* studies, due to modifications to foods during the process of absorption and delivery within the body. There might be two possible active sites, where foods and their components affect colon epithelium cells, where nutrients are distributed hematogenously after absorption, or retained in the lumen without absorption. Absorbed foods and nutrients might show the effects of anti-inflammation, anti-oxidant, and anti-proliferative par hematogenously in cancer epithelial cells and stromal cells, while on the other hand, the regulation of enterobacteria might be provided by the component in a poorly-absorbed form. Recent studies have focused on resistant carbohydrates functioning as prebiotics that prevent colorectal cancer (Davis & Milner, 2009).

The normal human intake of food has a great advantage for oral administration and safety, compared with the administration of medicine, because safety has been proven by long food experience. Thus, the prevention of colorectal cancer through the intake of specific foods and nutrients might have a great potential, however further studies are required, especially in regard to absorption and disposition. In this paper, we focused on foods, and their components, with cancer preventive aspects.

2. The preventive effects of food components against colorectal cancer

Colorectal cancer is one of the most common cancers in the world and it has been proposed that it is strongly associated with dietary habits (Anand et al., 2008; Jemal et al., 2011). Red and processed meat may convincingly increase the risk, and physical activity is only the proven method of prevention. Avoiding body fatness, especially abdominal fatness, and the consumption of an excessive amount of alcohol are also important for colorectal cancer prevention (World Cancer Research Fund, 2007b). Despite the confirmation of cancer inducing foods, foods or nutritional elements that have protective qualities against colorectal cancer have not yet been fully confirmed.

2.1 Epidemiology

Colorectal cancer is the third most commonly diagnosed cancer in males and the second in females, and it is the fourth common cause of death in males and third in females, according to a survey conducted in 2008 (Jemal et al., 2011) . The increasing rate of colorectal cancer is considered to be due to the combination of changes in dietary patterns, obesity and smoking (Jemal et al., 2011). Approximately only 5-10% of all colorectal cancers are a consequence of recognized hereditary conditions (Lynch & de la Chapelle, 2003). Since dietary habits play an important role in the incidence of colorectal cancer, this subject must be employed as one of the main strategies to investigate components derived from foods with cancer prevention properties.

It has been reported that dietary patterns are associated with the onset of colorectal cancer. The Mediterranean diet was associated with a reduced risk of recurrence of colorectal adenomas in woman. The Mediterranean diet is characterized by a high consumption of breads, vegetables, fruit, fish and olive oil (World Cancer Research Fund, 2007c, as cited in Cottet et al., 2005). The Japanese traditional diet is characterized by a high consumption of fish and seafood with a high salt content. Japanese cohort studies demonstrated that both the Japanese traditional diet and western diet were associated with an increased risk of colon cancer in women, but not in men (Kim et al., 2005). The 'Pork, processed meats and potatoes' diet was associated with an increased risk of colon cancer in women and also with rectal cancer in men. 'Pork, processed meats and potatoes' diet pattern was characterized as intakes of energy, protein carbohydrate, fat, saturated and monounsaturated fatty acids, cholesterol, B vitamins, and minerals (Dixon et al., 2004). Vegetarian diets might moderately reduce the risk of colon cancer, which is due to not only to no or low consumption of meat, but also to a high consumption of plant foods (Sanjoaquin et al., 2004; World Cancer Research Fund, 2007c), although there is a negative result of colorectal cancer prevention (Key et al., 1996).

2.2 Adenoma-to-carcinoma sequence and pathology

A genetic model for colorectal tumorigenesis has been proposed in the following procedures (Fearon & Vogelstein, 1990). 1) The mutation of APCTS gene transform normal colonic epithelia tissue to multiple polyps, 2) DNA hypomethylation is related to the onset and development of and early adenoma, 3) The K-*ras* oncogene play an important role in the progression from early to intermediate adenomas, 4) A mutation of the Thymidylate synthase gene plays an important role in the development from intermediate to late adenoma, 5) A mutation of TP53 gene is highly found in late adenomas and colorectal cancers (Tammariello & Milner, 2010) (Figure 1).

Oxidative stress, which provided by both exogenous (irradiation, chemicals, and drugs) and endogenous (O2 metabolism, immune response, and inflammation) origin, plays a critical

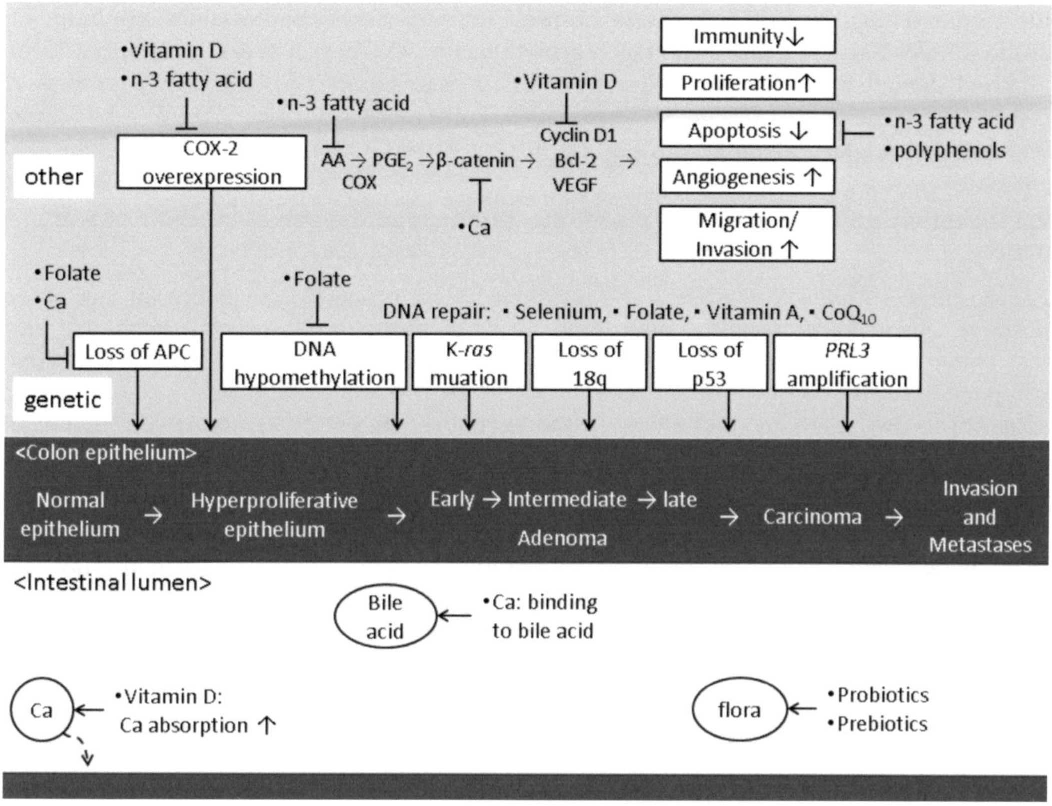

Abbreviations: COX, cyclooxygenase; AA, arachidonic acid; VEGF vascular endothelial growth factor; Ca, calcium; CoQ_{10}, coenzyme Q_{10}

Fig. 1. Proposed anticarcinogenetic effects of nutrients on colorectal cancer. Selenium, folate, vitamin A and CoQ_{10} have been reported to repair damaged DNA. Vitamin D and n-3 fatty acid may suppress the COX-2 mediated carcinogenesis. Ca plays a diverse role, including the inhibition of *APC* mutation, suppression of β-catenin and binding to bile acid. Probiotics and/or prebiotics reduce colorectal cancer to modify the proportion of gut microflora.

role in DNA damage (Kryston et al., 2011). Reactive oxygen spices (ROS) and DNA interactions induce DNA damage, which causes mutation via either double-strand break (DSB) or non-DSB lesions (Sedelnikova et al., 2010). Carcinogenesis of oxidative stress also involve immune cell activation via CCL2/MCP-1, pro-inflammatory factor (Martin et al., 2011).

The methods of accurate measurement of oxidative stress have been brought by HPLC, tandem mass spectrometry (MS/MS) electrochemical detector (Cadet et al., 2010). There are also biomarkers to assess the level of oxidative stress, such as 8-oxo-2'deoxyguanosine (8-oxo-dG) (Ziech et al., 2010). These can allow us precise studies of anti-oxidative property by food.

Cyclooxygenase (COX) also plays an important role in carcinogenesis, e.g. to induce prostaglandin E_2 (PGE_2). PGE_2 has diverse functions to promote cell proliferation, migration, invasion and angiogenesis, and also to suppress immunity and apoptosis through inducing cyclin D1, Bcl-2 and vascular endothelial growth factor (VEGF) (Chan & Giovannucci, 2010). Figure 1 demonstrates the possible anti-tumor mechanisms of nutrients in the process of colorectal carcinogenesis (Janne & Mayer, 2000; Lamprecht & Lipkin, 2003; World Cancer Research Fund, 2007a; Chan & Giovannucci, 2010; Vilar & Gruber, 2010).

2.3 Digestion, absorption, delivery and distribution, and the site of mechanisms of action

For the clinical application of foods and nutrients for the prevention of colorectal cancer, we need to elucidate thoroughly how each food is digested, absorbed, delivered, and distributed to every organ or tissue, and determine what is the biologically active component, similar to the pharmacokinetics of drugs. Food constituents showed anti-tumor properties when they are distributed hematogenously to pre-cancer or cancer epithelial cells.

We often find that there is a big gap in the effective concentration between *in vitro* and *in vivo* studies. It sometimes happens that *in vitro* studies need a much higher concentration to demonstrate significant anti-tumor effects, compared with the biological concentration. When the ingestion of a nutrient shows a cancer prevention effect in an *in vivo* study, this does not directly mean the nutrient affect will be imported into the cells, as it may change to another form after digestion and absorption. Each article of food includes a lot of constituents, so that various constituents may demonstrate additive action or synergetic effects. In addition, active constituents affect not only cancer epithelium cells, but also the cancer stromal environment, e.g. angiogenesis or the interaction between epithelial and stromal cells, since the paracrine interaction between epithelial and stroma cells affect each other for tumor progression (Ko et al., 2002; Adegboyega et al., 2004; Martinez-Outschoorn et al., 2011).

For cancer prevention of the alimentary tract, active food components can have an effect not only hematogenously, but also from the gut lumen side. This indicates that indigestible constituents, as well as easily absorbed components, can function as potent anti-cancer agents against colorectal cancer. As mentioned above, resistant starches have cancer prevention properties as prebiotics that modify intestinal microorganism (Tuohy et al., 2005). Calcium may reduce the colorectal cancer risk associated with the combination to bile acid, the risk profile in intestinal lumen (Boursi & Arber, 2007). The effective site of food components has been proposed in Figure 1 (Lamprecht & Lipkin, 2003).

Some of the blood levels of active components after the ingestion of foods have been reported, but those amounts in the gut or stool have been rarely reported. For colorectal cancer prevention in humans, we need to investigate the systemic function of food ingredients, how the food is digested, absorbed and remains in the gut, as well as the blood concentration and delivery in each organ. Further studies are necessary to illuminate the mechanisms of food components on colorectal cancer prevention.

2.4 Food, nutrition, physical activity and the prevention of cancer: a global perspective, 2007

The Food, Nutrition, Physical Activity and the Prevention of Cancer: a Global Perspective was produced by the World Cancer Research Fund and the AIRC, in order to generate a comprehensive series of recommendations on food, nutrition, and physical activity, for reducing cancer risk for all populations worldwide (World Cancer Research Fund, 2007b).

The World Cancer Research Fund and the American Institute for Cancer Research judged that the evidence that physical activity protects against colorectal cancer was convincing, and the evidence that foods containing dietary fibre, garlic, milk and calcium protect against colorectal cancer was probable. On the other hand, the evidence that red meat, processed meat, alcoholic drinks for men, body fatness, abdominal fatness and adult attained height caused colorectal cancer was convincing, and the evidence that alcoholic drinks in women caused this cancer was probable.

Table 1 shows the positive and negative results on colorectal cancer protection of foods and nutrition.

2.4.1 Foods judged to "probably" reduce the risk of colorectal cancer

The 4 foods that affected the judgement that the evidence on the reduction of the risk of colorectal cancer was probable were food containing dietary fibre, garlic, milk and calcium.

2.4.1.1 Dietary fibre

Dietary fibre was associated with a reduced risk of colon cancer (Mastromarino et al., 1976). A meta-analysis of eight studies of dietary fibre estimated that the relative risk was 0.90 (95% confidence interval (CI) 0.84-0.97) per 10 g/day increment (World Cancer Research Fund, 2007c).

A few negative results have been demonstrated. There was no association shown between dietary fibre consumption and the onset of colorectal cancer or adenoma by a 16-year follow-up prospective study (Fuchs et al., 1999). In the paper, a higher consumption of vegetable fibre was even associated with an increased risk of colorectal cancer in women. There was another negative result shown for dietary fibre, i.e., a high-fibre cereal supplement did not reduce recurrent colorectal adenomas (Alberts et al., 2000).

The mechanisms of the action of dietary fibre are not clearly elucidated yet, but it has been suggested that it dilutes faecal contents, decrease transit time, and increase stool weight (World Cancer Research Fund, 2007c, as cited in Cummings, 1981). Short-chain fatty acids, like butyrate, are produced by the gut flora from dietary carbohydrates that reach the colon, induce apoptosis and cell cycle arrest, and promote differentiation (World Cancer Research Fund, 2007c). Dietary fibre intake is important for lipid and glucose metabolism or for acting as prebiotics on microflora health in preventing colonic cancer (Donini et al., 2009). The consumption of fibre is associated to the consumption of folate (World Cancer Research Fund, 2007c), which has also been reported to be associated with a reduced risk of colorectal cancer (Sanjoaquin et al., 2005).

2.4.1.2 Garlic

In the "Global Perspective", the World Cancer Research Fund and American Institute for Cancer Research judged that garlic probably protects against colorectal cancer (World Cancer Research Fund, 2007c). Ally sulphur, which is considered to be an effective component of garlic, inhibited colon tumors in animal studies. The biologically active compounds derived from garlic have been proposed as allicin, diallyl sulphide (DAS),

Food and nutrition	Human studies	RR (95% CI) highest vs lowest exposure whcn it is not mentioned	ref.
Foods containing dietary fibre			
positive			
	Dietary fibre was associated with a reduced risk of recurrence of colorectal adenomas in woman / meta-analysis from 8 studies	0.90 (0.84-0.97) per 10g/ day increment	World Cancer Research Fund, 2007c
negative			
	Dietary fibre was not associated with colorectal cancer risk in women/ 16-year follow-up cohort study	0.95 (0.73-1.25)	Fuchs et al., 1999
	Dietary fibre from vegetable was associated with an increased risk of colorectal cancer in women/ 16-year follow-up cohort study	1.35 (1.05-1.72)	Fuchs et al., 1999
	Dietary supplement of wheat-bran fibre was not associated a reduced risk of recurrent colorectal adenomas/ randomized trial	0.88 (0.70-1.11)	Alberts et al., 2000
garlic			
positive			
	Garlic intake was probably associated with a reduced risk of colon cancer/ 2 cohort studies and 6 case-control studies	0.77 (0.51-1.16) 0.68 (0.46-1.01)	World Cancer Research Fund, 2007c
milk			
positive			
	Milk intake was associated with a reduced risk of colorectal cancer/ meta-analysis from 4 cohort studies	0.94 (0.85-1.03) per serving/ day	World Cancer Research Fund, 2007c
	Milk intake was associated with a reduced risk of colorectal cancer/ meta-analysis from 10 cohort studies	0.85 (0.78-0.94)	Cho et al., 2004
	Milk intake was associated with a reduced risk of colorectal cancer/ meta-analysis from 19 cohort studies	0.91 (0.85-0.94) per 200 g/ day of milk	Aune et al., 2011
calcium			
positive			
	Calcium supplementation was associtated with a reduced risk of adenomas/ meta-analysis from 2 cohort studies	0.95 (0.92-0.98) per 200 mg/ day	World Cancer Research Fund, 2007c
	Total calcium intake and intake of calcium from food sources was was associated with a reduced risk of colorectal cancer/ meta-analysis from 10 cohort studies	0.78 (0.69-0.88) for total calcium 0.86 (0.78-0.95) for calcium from food sources	World Cancer Research Fund, 2007c, as cited in Samad et al., 2005

Table 1.

non-starchy vegetables and fruits			
possitive			
	Conssumption of fruit was associated with a reduced risk of colorecatl cancer/meta-analysis from 8 cohort studies	0.97 (0.92-1.03) per serving/day	World Cancer Research Fund, 2007c
	Conssumption of fruit was associated with a reduced risk of colorecatl cancer in women/meta-analysis from 5 cohort studies	0.81 (0.85-0.98) per serving/day	World Cancer Research Fund, 2007c
	Consumption of fruit was associtated with a reduced risk of colorectal cancer/cohort study	0.57 (0.34-0.97)	Sanjoaquin et al., 2004
	A high consumption of vegetable and fruit was association with a reduced risk of colorectal and colon cancer/cohort study	0.86 (0.75-1.00) for colorectal cancer 0.76 (0.63-0.91) for colon cancer	van Duijnhoven et al., 2009
	There is limited evidence suggesting that non-starchy vegetables protect against colorectal cancer	1.00 (0.90–1.11) per 2 servings/day	World Cancer Research Fund, 2007c
negative			
	Vegetarians diet was not significantly associated with a reduced risk of colorectal cancer/cohort study	0.85 (0.55-1.32) vegetarians vs non-vegetarians	Sanjoaquin et al., 2004
	A high consumption of vegetable was not associated with recuded risk of rectal cancer/cohort study	0.92 (0.79-1.06)	van Duijnhoven et al., 2009
	A high consumption of fruit was not associated with recuded risk of colorectal cancer/cohort study	0.88 (0.76-1.01)	van Duijnhoven et al., 2009
Foods containing folate			
positive			
	Dietary folate intake was associated with the recuced risk of colorectal cancer/meta-analysis of 7 cohort studies	0.75 (0.64-0.89)	Sanjoaquin et al., 2005
	Total folate intake was associated with a recuced risk of colorectal cancer/metanalysis of 7 cohort studies	0.95 (0.81-1.11)	Sanjoaquin et al., 2005
Selenium and foods containing selenium			
positive			
	Dietary selenium was associated with a reduced risk of colorectal cancer/A meta-analysis from 5 case-control studies	0.86 (0.78-0.95) per 10 μg/dl serum	World Cancer Research Fund, 2007c
Fish			
positive			
	Fish consumption was associated with a reduced risk of colorectal cancer/meta-analysis from 7 cohort studies	0.96 (0.92-1.00) per serving/week	World Cancer Research Fund, 2007c
negative			

Table 1. (continued)

	Consumption of salmon or cod was not associated with local markers of inflammation, genotoxicity markers in colonocyte, and apoptotic and mitotic rate in colonic mucosa/randomized controlled study		Pot et al., 2009; Pot et al., 2010a; Pot et al., 2010b
Foods containing vitamin D			
positive			
	Food containing vitamin D was associated with a reduced risk of colorectal cancer/meta-analysis from 9 cohort studies	0.99 (0.97-1.00) per 100 IU/day	World Cancer Research Fund, 2007c
Vitamins (except vitamin D)			
positive			
	A high consumption of vitamin C and E from both food and supplements (total) was associated with a reduced risk of colon cancer risk/pooled analysis of cohort studies	0.80 (0.71-0.90) for total vitamin C 0.82 (0.74-0.91) for total vitamin E	Park et al., 2010
	Multivitamin intake was associated with a reduced risk of colon cancer/pooled analysis of cohort studies	0.88 (0.81-0.96)	Park et al., 2010
	A high intake of either dietary nutrients (vitamin C, vitamin E, β-carotene, selenium, folate, vitamin B6, and vitamin B12) was associated a reduced the risk of distal colorectal cancer in the caucasian/case-control study	0.58 (0.42-0.80) for vitamin C 0.65 (0.48-0.89) for vitamin E 0.52 (0.38-0.71) for β-carotene 0.55 (0.39-0.77) for selenium 0.50 (0.36-0.69) for folate 0.48 (0.35-0.67) for vitamin B6 0.59 (0.42-0.81) for vitamin B12	Williams et al., 2010
	A high intake of dietary selenium was associated with a reduced risk of distal coloredtal cancer in African Americans/case-control study	0.55 (0.29-1.02)	Williams et al., 2010
	β-carotene intake was associated with a reduced risk of colorectal cancer in men/cohort study	0.77 (0.763-0.95)	Park et al., 2009
negative			
	lycopene intake was associated with an increased risk of rectal cancer in men/cohort study	1.50 (1.04-2.16)	Park et al., 2009

Table 1. (continued)

Vitamin A, vitamin C, and vitamin E intake from food only were not associated with colon cancer risk /pooled analysis of cohort studies	0.92 (0.81-1.05) for vitamin A 1.06 (0.95-1.18) for vitamin C 0.99 (0.89-1.11) for vitamin E	Park et al., 2010
A high consumption of carotenoid (except for β-carotene) was not associated with a reduced resk of colorecatl cancer/cohort study	0.86 (0.71-1.04) for total carotenoids in men0.83 (0.67-1.04) for total carotenoids in men	Park et al., 2009

Abbreviations: RR, relative risk; 95% CI, 95% confidence interval

Table 1. Positive and negative result of food and nutrition on colorectal cancer protection.

diallyl disulphide (DADS), diallyl trisulfide (DATS) and ajoene. DAS, DADS and S-allylcysteie (SAC) demonstrated the inhibitory effect on colon cancer in the rat (Shukla & Kalra, 2007).

In colon tumor cells, the induction of apoptosis, cell cycle modification and inhibition of tubulin polymerisation were suggested as the mechanism of the action of DATS, and the anti-proliferative effect, G2/M cell cycle arrest, decrease of polyamine biosynthesis, inhibition of histone deacetylase activity were suggested as the mechanisms of the actions of DADS (Filomeni et al., 2003; Shukla & Kalra, 2007). It also has been reported that garlic and its constituents inhibit DNA adduct formation, scavenge free radicals and modulate P-glycoprotein-mediated multidrug resistance (Shukla & Kalra, 2007).

2.4.1.3 Milk and other dairy products

A meta-analysis of "a global perspective" produced a summary effect estimate for relative risk of 0.94 (95% CI 0.850-1.03) per serving/day (World Cancer Research Fund, 2007c). An analysis of data obtained from 10 cohort studies demonstrated that higher milk intake (≧ 250 g/day) was related to a statistically significant reduced risk of colorectal cancer with relative risk 0.85 (95% CI 0.78-0.94) compared with the lowest intake (< 70 g/day) (Cho et al., 2004). According to the latest meta-analysis study, nineteen cohort studies concluded that the summary relative risk was 0.91 (95% CI 0.85-0.94) per 200 g/day of milk, and 0.83 (95% CI 0.78-0.88) per 400 g/day of total dairy products intake. There was no significant association between the consumption of cheese and a reduced risk (Aune et al., 2011).

Dietary milk fat globule membrane reduced the incidence of aberrant crypt foci in Fisher-344 rats (Snow et al., 2010).

The cancer prevention effect of milk and dairy products is at least partly associated with the intake of calcium, which may bind to bile acids and ionized fatty acids to reduce cell proliferation and promote cell differentiation (Aune et al., 2011).

2.4.1.4 Calcium (supplemented at a dose of 1200 mg/day)

The main dietary sources of calcium in Europe and America are milk and dairy products. The meta-analysis estimate for the summary effect for colon cancer was 0.95 (95% CI 0.92-0.98) per 200 mg/day of dietary calcium (World Cancer Research Fund, 2007c). Analysis from 10 cohort studies demonstrated that the total calcium had a greater correlation (relative risk 0.78; 95% CI 0.69-0.88) to colorectal cancer than calcium from food sources (relative risk 0.86; 95% CI 0.78-0.95) (World Cancer Research Fund, 2007c, as cited in Samad et al., 2005).

On the other hand, there was a negative report regarding the chemoprevention effects of calcium, 2.5 g/kg calcium reduced the number of small intestinal tumors, but increased the number of colon tumors (Huerta et al., 2003).

Calcium binds bile acids in the bowel lumen to inhibit their proliferative and carcinogenic effects, since bile acids might promote hyper-proliferation of the colorectal epithelium and carcinogenesis. Calcium may also act directly on the colonic epithelial cells to inhibit *ras* mutation (Bautista et al., 1997; Janne & Mayer, 2000). Extracellular dietary calcium is associated with the activation of calcium-sensing receptors in intestinal epithelial cells, and then the activation of intracellular signalling pathways, including proliferation, differentiation, and apoptosis (Lamprecht & Lipkin, 2001).

2.4.2 Food judged to be "limited-suggestively" reduced cancer risk

Since there was not sufficient evidence to judge, the factors below were concluded as limited-suggestive; non-starchy vegetables (not including salted and/or pickled products), fruits, foods containing folate, foods containing selenium, fish, foods containing vitamin D, and selenium (supplements at the dose of 1200 mg/day).

2.4.2.1 Fruit and vegetable

It is quite complicated to investigate which nutrient has the most effective properties for colorectal cancer prevention, since non-starchy vegetables are a source of dietary fibre, carotenoids, folate, selenium, glucosinolates, and so on, and fruits are sources of vitamin C, carotenoids, phenols, flavonoids and other anti-oxidants. The results of the anti-cancer effects of fruit and vegetable are heterogeneous.

Dietary cruciferous vegetable intake was associated with a reduced colon risk of approximately 25% (Marshall, 2008), There was an inverse association between the consumption of fruits and the risk of colorectal cancer, although the vegetarians showed a moderate, but non-significant, decrease in the risk (Sanjoaquin et al., 2004). A high consumption of vegetable and fruit showed an inverse association with colorectal and colon cancer, but not rectal cancer in the European Prospective Investigation into Cancer and Nutrition (EPIC). There was no significant inverse association shown between vegetable consumption or fruit consumption and colorectal, colon, or rectal cancer (Key et al., 2009; van Duijnhoven et al., 2009).

Vegetable-fruit mixture intake did not decrease the number of colon polyps both in low in fat (20% of energy) and high in fat (40% of energy) in the *Apc*^{Min} mice which are genetically predisposed to intestinal polyps (van Kranen et al., 1998).

It has been reported that several fruits have a specific potency for cancer prevention. Apple is rich in quercetin (World Cancer Research Fund, 2007c). Apple juice also showed the potency of preventing colon carcinogenesis in mice, but this effect was not found under the cancer promoting conditions associated with obesity (Koch et al., 2009). On the other hand, Nandir et al. showed apple pomace increased the number and diameter of colon polyps in *Apc*^{Min} mice (Mandir et al., 2008). Citrus fruits are sources of antioxidants, such as vitamin C, phenols, flavonoid and bioactive phytochemicals. Vitamin C traps free radicals and reactive oxygen species, and protects DNA from mutagenic damage (World Cancer Research Fund, 2007c). Cruciferous vegetables, such as broccoli, cabbage and cauliflower, reduced the colorectal cancer risk (Marshall, 2008), although there was also a negative report (Graham et al., 1988).

2.4.2.2 Foods containing folate and folate

According to the meta-analysis study, there was strong association between folate consumption and colorectal cancer risk in 7 cohort studies. Dietary folate showed a stronger association (relative risk for high vs. low intake = 0.75; 95% CI 0.64-0.89) than total folate (relative risk for high vs. low =0.95; 95% CI 0.81-1.11) (Sanjoaquin et al., 2005). Folate intake was strongly correlated with dietary fibre intake (World Cancer Research Fund, 2007c).

Animal studies also supported the cancer prevention properties of folate, however, intervention with exceptionally high doses of folate (2.0-5.0 g of folic acid/kg diet) after the formation of microscopic neoplastic foci may have promoted colorectal carcinogenesis (Kim, 2003). Folate reduced the number of small intestinal tumors in mice, although the timing of folate intervention was critical in preventive properties. In contrast, this effect was not found in colon (Song et al., 2000).

Folate deficiency has the potential to modulate DNA synthesis, DNA methylation, DNA damage and impaired DNA repair, increase mutagenesis, hyperproliferation, abnormal apoptosis, and methylenetetrahydrofolate reductase (MTHFR) polymorphisms and related gene-nutrient interactions (Prinz-Langenohl et al., 2001; Kim, 2003).

Under certain conditions, folate potentialy has an inverse effect on cancer prevention. In DNA polymerase β deficiency mice, folate deficiency provided protection against tumorigenesis, the induction of apoptosis, and the suppression of cell proliferation (Ventrella-Lucente et al., 2010)

2.4.2.3 Selenium and foods containing selenium

A meta-analysis of "a global perspective" produced a summary effect estimate of 0.86 (95% CI 0.78-0.95) per 10 μg/dl serum, with high heterogeneity (World Cancer Research Fund, 2007c). Dietary selenium deficiency has been reported to cause a lack of selenoprotein expression, and some of these selenoproteins play important roles in anti-inflammatory and antioxidant properties (Ganther, 1999).

Selenium-enriched broccoli reduced the number of small intestinal tumors in multiple intestinal neoplasia mice (Davis et al., 2002). In the study, selenium-enriched diet for 10 weeks significantly increased the plasma concentration of selenium, and reduced small intestinal (46.3 ± 3.7 vs 65.6 ± 6.1) and large intestin (0.43 ± 3.7 vs 1.93 ± 6.1) tumors than control diet.

Several mechanisms have been suggested for the cancer preventiion effect of selenium, including the induction of apoptosis, cell cycle modulation (inhibition of cdk2 and protein kinase C), and the activation of thioredoxin redactase (Combs, 2004).

2.4.2.4 Fish

A meta-analysis of "a global perspective" produced a summary effect estimate of 0.96 (95% CI 0.92-1.00) per serving/week. A high consumption of fish is associated with low consumption of meat (World Cancer Research Fund, 2007c).

Increasing salmon or cod consumption for 6 months resulted in a lower concentration of the systemic inflammation marker C-reactive protein (CRP), but showed no effect on the local markers of inflammation in the colonic biopsies or feces, the genotoxicity markers in colonocyte, and apoptotic and mitotic rate in colonic mucosa (Pot et al., 2009; Pot et al., 2010a; Pot et al., 2010b).

An animal study showed that fish oil significantly reduced colon tumors (Rao et al., 2001). A diet including fish oil and pectin protects against colon cancer, compared with that of corn oil and cellulose azoxymethane, which induced colon cancer in model rats (Cho et al., 2011).

The preventive mechanisms of fish have been proposed to include the effects on gene expression, decreasing adhesion genes such as *B44galt1* at the initiation stage, lowering the expression of both cell promoters and suppressors at the aberrant crypt foci (ACF) stage, and increasing apoptosis inducing genes at the tumor stage. These modifications may be associated to the induction of apoptosis and the suppression of proliferation (Cho et al., 2011). Fish n-3 polyunsaturated fatty acids (PUFAs) may reduce eicosanoid biosynthesis derived from n-6 PUFA to protect tissue from inflammation, and inhibit COX-2 (Rao et al., 2001).

On the other hand, it has been reported that dietary fish oil containing docosahexaenoic acid (DHA) promotes inflammation through the modification of CD4+ and CD8+ T-cell populations in SMAD-/- mice and that chronic inflammation is the risk factor for colorectal cancer (Woodworth et al., 2010).

2.4.2.5 Foods containing vitamin D

A meta-analysis of "a global perspective" produced a summary effect estimate of 0.99 (95% CI 0.97-1.00) per 100 IU/day (World Cancer Research Fund, 2007c). Higher vitamin D levels are associated with a lower risk of colon cancer and overall mortality. UV exposure stimulates vitamin D production, but it may increase the risk of skin cancer. Therefore it is recommended that high-risk populations with a low level of vitamin D intake increase the consumption of fish, or take vitamin D supplements (Zeeb & Greinert, 2010).

Vitamin D induces differentiation, apoptosis and induces G1 phase arrest in intestinal cells. It also increases the absorption of calcium in the small and large intestine. Most of the pleiotropic, long-term actions of [1,25 $(OH)_2D_3$] are mediated by binding to vitamin D receptors (VDR), which are high-affinity receptors in the nucleus of cells. Activated VDR induces gene transcription, and VDR density in colonic mucosa was higher in hyperplastic polyps and in early stages of carcinogenesis, compared with normal mucosa (Lamprecht & Lipkin, 2001; Lamprecht & Lipkin, 2003; World Cancer Research Fund, 2007c).

2.4.3 Limited-non conclusive and others

There was not enough evidence for cancer prevention at the time of when "a grovel Perspective" was drawn up in 2007, so the following foods and nutrition were judged limited-non conclusive: Cereals (grains) and their products, potatoes, poultry, shellfish and other seafood, other dairy products, total fat, fatty acid, cholesterol, sugar (sucrose), coffee, tea, caffeine, total carbohydrate, starch, vitamin A, retinol, vitamin C, vitamin E, multivitamins, non-dairy sources of calcium, methionine, beta-carotene, alpha-carotene, lycopene, meal frequency, and energy intake.

Some of the latest research has demonstrated new knowledge, or confirmed the previous results.

2.4.3.1 Vitamins (except vitamin D)

A pooled analysis of cohort studies concluded that a high consumption of vitamin C and E from both food and supplements showed an inverse association with colon cancer risk, although there were some interactions with folate intake. Multivitamin intake also significantly decreases the risk of colon cancer. On the other hand, vitamin A, vitamin C, and vitamin E intake from food only were not associated with colon cancer risk (Park et al., 2010).

In the Caucasian race, a high intake of each anti-oxidant nutrient (vitamin C, vitamin E, β-carotene, selenium) and DNA methylation-related nutrients (folate, vitamin B6, vitamin B12) reduced the risk of distal colorectal cancer, and only selenium showed a lower risk in African Americans. In this study, both intake from food only and total intake (food and supplements) demonstrated cancer prevention potency (Williams et al., 2010).

In colorectal cancer patients, the level of vitamin A, vitamin C, and vitamin E were reduced, and urinary 8-oxo-dG, a biomarker of DNA oxidation, was elevated (Obtulowicz et al., 2010).

A high consumption of carotenoid did not reduce the risk of colorectal cancer, except for β-carotene intake among men, which showed an inverse association (relative risk 0.77, 95% CI 0.763-0.95). On the other hand, lycopene intake was significantly associated with an increase in the risk of rectal cancer among men (relative risk 1.50, 95% CI 1.04-2.16) (Park et al., 2009).

2.4.3.2 Other dietary factors

Avenanthraide (Avns) polyphenols from oats showed anti-proliferative effects independent of Cox-2 expression in COX-2 positive HT29, Caco-2 and LS174T cells, and COX-2 negative HCT116 cells. Avns may also reduce the colon cancer risk inhibiting PGE2 production derived from macrophage (Guo et al., 2010).

In animal studies, the oral administration of flavone (400mg/kg over 4 weeks) increased apoptosis and reduced the rate of aberrant crypt formation in mice. The down-regulation of the tricarboxylic acid cycle may be a part of the action mechanism (Winkelmann et al., 2010). In a human study, a case-control study of dietary flavonoid showed that flavonoid, especially quercetin, was significantly associated with a reduction in the colorectal cancer risk (Kyle et al., 2010).

In an SD rat study, Coenzyme Q10 reduced the number of APFs, possibly by modulating COX-2 and iNOS gene expression in colonic mucosa, and DNA damage in leukocytes (Kim & Park, 2010).

It has been reported that an increased consumption of n-3 fatty acid, Sulforaphane, Chafuroside, Curcumin and Dibenzoylmethane decreased the number of small intestinal tumors in *Apc*^{Min} mice. On the other hand, there are a few reports on colonic tumor that showed that 31 g/kg of steridonic acid or 600 ppm of sulforaphane demonstrated an inhibitory effect on colonic tumors in *Apc*^{Min} mice (Petrik et al., 2000; Shen et al., 2007).

2.5 The latest proposed action mechanisms

Various mechanisms, such as DNA repair, proapoptosis, cell cycle modification, immunity promotion, and the mediation of chemomediators, have been proposed as the effects of foods and nutrition. Recently, the focus has been on the prebiotic and probiotic effects, insulin-like growth factor (IGF) regulation, and calorie restriction.

2.5.1 Prebiotic and probiotic effects

Feeding specific food products with a prebiotic effect have been reported to reduce the incidence of tumors and cancers (Roberfroid et al., 2010). There are 100 trillion microbial organisms, called the microbiota, in human adult gut (Davis & Milner, 2009). Carbohydrate and proteolytic fermentation are the two main types of anaerobic fermentation in the gastrointestinal tract (Davis & Milner, 2009, as cited in (McIntosh et al., 1999).

Prebiotics are non-digestible food ingredients which stimulate beneficial gut microbiota (Lim et al., 2005), e.g. inulin and other oligosaccharides, lactulose and resistant starch, such as fructooligosaccharides, inulin, lactulose and galactooligosaccharides (Tuohy et al., 2005). Probiotics are live bacteria found in processed foods or in dietary supplements, e.g. yogurt, cheese, fermented milks, juices, smoothies, cereal, and nutrition bars (Penner et al., 2005; Davis & Milner, 2009). Synbiotics are a combination of a probiotic with a prebiotic. A prebiotic can support the activity of a probiotic (Gibson & Roberfroid, 1995).

Prebiotics must survive acidic conditions in the stomach and resist digestion in the small intestine. Then they need to be selectively fermented, and stimulate beneficial bacteria, usually bifidobacteria or lactobacilli, in the colon (Tuohy et al., 2005). In the randomized, double-blind, placebo-controlled trial for 12 weeks, dietary synbiotics reduced colon cancer risk, through increasing *Bifidobacterium* and *Lactobacillus*, and decreasing *Clostridium perfringens* (Rafter et al., 2007).

A 4-year supplementation regime employing *Lactobacillus casei* decreased the recurrence of atypical colonic polyps (Ishikawa et al., 2005).

Several animal studies and human trials showed that prebiotics, probiotics and synbiotics reduced toxic metabolite production, like caecal β-glucuronidase, nitrate reductase activities and caecal pH, in the gut, resulting in the prevention of colorectal cancer. On the other hand, some human studies denied the beneficial effects of prebiotics (Tuohy et al., 2005).

An increased number of bifidobacteria and/or lactobacilli may also play an important role in DNA protective modification and chemically-induced DNA damage (Tuohy et al., 2005). An increased number of biofidobacteria and/or lactobacilli in the gut may suppress the number or activity of putative enteropathogens such as *Escherichia coli* and *Clostridium perfingens* (Reddy, 1999). Prebiotics may also stimulate protective enzyme activities within the intestinal mucosa or reduce the immune inflammatory response (Burns & Rowland, 2000).

Since prebiotics are mostly oligosaccharides, it is considered that they reduce blood glucose. Increasing glycosylated hemogloin (HbA1c), which is a biomarker of glucose control for diabetes, was associated with an increased risk of colorectal cancer in women (Chan & Giovannucci, 2010). However, the consumption of short-chain fructooligosaccharides did not have a significant affect on the glucose level in blood (Luo et al., 2000).

Transplantation of the gut microflora from normal mice into germ-free recipients resulted in increasing their body fat without increasing food consumption (Bajzer & Seeley, 2006). A 1-

year low calorie diet in obese people modified the proportion of gut microbes, increasing bacteroidestes and decreasing firmicutes, while obese people had fewer bacteroidetes and firmicutes, compared with a lean control group (Ley et al., 2006).

Supplementation employing a drink fortified with short-chain fructooligosaccharides and inulin (1.5 g/day) significantly increased the absorption of calcium in adolescent girls (Griffin et al., 2002). The consumption of oligosaccharides also improved the magnesium absorption in humans and animals (Coudray et al., 2003). An optimum well-tolerated dose of prebiotics might be 10 g/day and a high dose (e.g. > 20 g/day) of some prebiotics might have a laxation effect, such as stool frequency or stool weight (Bouhnik et al., 1999).

2.5.2 IGF regulation

IGF play important roles in proliferation, differentiation and transfomation in a variety of cell types, and thus it has been suggested that dysregulation of the IGF is an important cancer risk factor (Park, 2008).

A study on colon adenocarcinoma showed that n-3 polyunsaturated fatty acids, eicosapentaenoic acid (EPA) and docosahexaenoic acid (DHA), increased IGFBP-6 in human colon adenocarcinoma Caco-2 cells, and the authors proposed that low IGF-II/IGFBP-6 ratios have resulted in less free IGF-II and a resulting slower proliferation of Caco-2 cells (Roynette et al., 2004). All-trans retinoic acid (tRA) showed an anti-proliferative effect in Caos-2 cells, and it was considered that this was due to a partly increased IGFBP-6 expression (Kim et al., 2002).

A low-calcemic vitamin D analogus decreased the secretion of IGF-II and suppressed HT-29 cell proliferation (Oh et al., 2001).

2.5.3 Calorie restriction

Calorie restriction in *Apc*^{Min} mice at the rate of 40% reduced the number of intestinal polyps by 57%, compared with mice fed ad libium. The serum levels of IGF-1 and leptin, and urinary corticosterone output were significantly reduced in the calorie restriction group, compared with that of the ad libium group. Supplementation of freeze-dried fruit and vegetable extract with a diet high in olive oil also reduced the number of polyps, even though this group had a calorie intake of about 90% of ad libium. The supplementation of fruit and vegetables significantly reduced the urinary corticosterone output levels, but did not show any effect on the serum levels of IGF-1 and leptin (Mai et al., 2003).

These results indicate that calorie restriction has a great potency for colon cancer prevention, and a diet in high fruit and vegetable without calorie restriction showed less, but still significant, intestinal tumorigenesis preventive effects.

Calorie restriction or increased exposure to n-3 fatty acid, sulforaphe, chafrroside, curcumin and dibenzoylmethane reduced the risk of colon cancer, while total fat, a diet high in calories and all-trans retinoic acid increased the risk (Tammariello & Milner, 2010).

However, even considering these interesting results, the frequency of colon polyps in the calorie restriction group and the fruit and vegetable group did not show any significant changes, compared with the ad libium group (van Kranen et al., 1998).

3. Conclusion

The contribution of diet in all cancer-related death estimates was 30-35% in the environmental factors, greater than tobacco, which was 25-30%. Colorectal cancer was strongly associated with diet, and linked to 70% of cancer related-deaths (Anand et al., 2008). Eating habits are the most important factor for colorectal cancer prevention, however, it is still difficult to specify how we should eat. It has been proposed that an increase in the consumption of fruit and vegetables and less intake of red and processed meat will comprise a better diet. However, it has not been proven yet how much of a respective increase and decrease is the best quantity, and which nutrients exactly play a key role in carcinogenesis and anti-carcinogenesis. Plenty of studies have been published on food components or nutrients to protect from carcinogenesis *in vitro*, describing the molecular action mechanisms involved. In human trials, individual nutrients, such as supplements, often showed no or less intended function, while nutrients contained in food functioned as expected. Accordingly, the judgement from a global perspective concluded that it was not appropriate to recommend the usage of supplements for cancer prevention at the present (World Cancer Research Fund, 2007d). The ideal diet for cancer prevention may be a well-balanced diet, and no one food or ingredient should be considered a miracle food. Further studies are required to elucidate precisely the disposition and safety of nutrients and the interaction of each nutrient.

4. References

Adegboyega, P.A.; Ololade, O.; Saada, J.; Mifflin, R.; Di Mari, J.F. & Powell, D.W. (2004). Subepithelial myofibroblasts express cyclooxygenase-2 in colorectal tubular adenomas. *Clin Cancer Res,* Vol. 10, No. 17, pp. 5870-5879, ISSN 1078-0432

Alberts, D.S.; Martinez, M.E.; Roe, D.J.; Guillen-Rodriguez, J.M.; Marshall, J.R.; van Leeuwen, J.B.; Reid, M.E.; Ritenbaugh, C.; Vargas, P.A.; Bhattacharyya, A.B.; Earnest, D.L. & Sampliner, R.E. (2000). Lack of effect of a high-fiber cereal supplement on the recurrence of colorectal adenomas. Phoenix Colon Cancer Prevention Physicians' Network. *N Engl J Med,* Vol. 342, No. 16, pp. 1156-1162, ISSN 0028-4793

Anand, P.; Kunnumakkara, A.B.; Sundaram, C.; Harikumar, K.B.; Tharakan, S.T.; Lai, O.S.; Sung, B. & Aggarwal, B.B. (2008). Cancer is a preventable disease that requires major lifestyle changes. *Pharm Res,* Vol. 25, No. 9, pp. 2097-2116, ISSN 0724-8741

Aune, D.; Lau, R.; Chan, D.S.; Vieira, R.; Greenwood, D.C.; Kampman, E. & Norat, T. (2011). Dairy products and colorectal cancer risk: a systematic review and meta-analysis of cohort studies. *Ann Oncol,* Vol. No., ISSN 1569-8041

Bajzer, M. & Seeley, R.J. (2006). Physiology: obesity and gut flora. *Nature,* Vol. 444, No. 7122, pp. 1009-1010, ISSN 1476-4687

Bautista, D.; Obrador, A.; Moreno, V.; Cabeza, E.; Canet, R.; Benito, E.; Bosch, X. & Costa, J. (1997). Ki-ras mutation modifies the protective effect of dietary monounsaturated fat and calcium on sporadic colorectal cancer. *Cancer Epidemiol Biomarkers Prev,* Vol. 6, No. 1, pp. 57-61, ISSN 1055-9965

Bouhnik, Y.; Vahedi, K.; Achour, L.; Attar, A.; Salfati, J.; Pochart, P.; Marteau, P.; Flourie, B.; Bornet, F. & Rambaud, J.C. (1999). Short-chain fructo-oligosaccharide administration dose-dependently increases fecal bifidobacteria in healthy humans. *J Nutr,* Vol. 129, No. 1, pp. 113-116, ISSN 0022-3166

Boursi, B. & Arber, N. (2007). Current and future clinical strategies in colon cancer prevention and the emerging role of chemoprevention. *Curr Pharm Des,* Vol. 13, No. 22, pp. 2274-2282, ISSN 1873-4286

Burns, A.J. & Rowland, I.R. (2000). Anti-carcinogenicity of probiotics and prebiotics. *Curr Issues Intest Microbiol,* Vol. 1, No. 1, pp. 13-24, ISSN 1466-531X

Cadet, J.; Douki, T. & Ravanat, J.L. (2010). Oxidatively generated base damage to cellular DNA. *Free Radic Biol Med,* Vol. 49, No. 1, pp. 9-21, ISSN 1873-4596

Chan, A.T. & Giovannucci, E.L. (2010). Primary prevention of colorectal cancer. *Gastroenterology,* Vol. 138, No. 6, pp. 2029-2043 e2010, ISSN 1528-0012

Cho, E.; Smith-Warner, S.A.; Spiegelman, D.; Beeson, W.L.; van den Brandt, P.A.; Colditz, G.A.; Folsom, A.R.; Fraser, G.E.; Freudenheim, J.L.; Giovannucci, E.; Goldbohm, R.A.; Graham, S.; Miller, A.B.; Pietinen, P.; Potter, J.D.; Rohan, T.E.; Terry, P.; Toniolo, P.; Virtanen, M.J.; Willett, W.C.; Wolk, A.; Wu, K.; Yaun, S.S.; Zeleniuch-Jacquotte, A. & Hunter, D.J. (2004). Dairy foods, calcium, and colorectal cancer: a pooled analysis of 10 cohort studies. *J Natl Cancer Inst,* Vol. 96, No. 13, pp. 1015-1022, ISSN 1460-2105

Cho, Y.; Kim, H.; Turner, N.D.; Mann, J.C.; Wei, J.; Taddeo, S.S.; Davidson, L.A.; Wang, N.; Vannucci, M.; Carroll, R.J.; Chapkin, R.S. & Lupton, J.R. (2011). A chemoprotective fish oil- and pectin-containing diet temporally alters gene expression profiles in exfoliated rat colonocytes throughout oncogenesis. *J Nutr,* Vol. 141, No. 6, pp. 1029-1035, ISSN 1541-6100

Combs, G.F., Jr. (2004). Status of selenium in prostate cancer prevention. *Br J Cancer,* Vol. 91, No. 2, pp. 195-199, ISSN 0007-0920

Cottet, V.; Bonithon-Kopp, C.; Kronborg, O.; Santos, L.; Andreatta, R.; Boutron-Ruault, M.C. & Faivre, J. (2005). Dietary patterns and the risk of colorectal adenoma recurrence in a European intervention trial. *Eur J Cancer Prev,* Vol. 14, No. 1, pp. 21-29, ISSN 0959-8278

Coudray, C.; Demigne, C. & Rayssiguier, Y. (2003). Effects of dietary fibers on magnesium absorption in animals and humans. *J Nutr,* Vol. 133, No. 1, pp. 1-4, 0022-3166

Cummings, J.H. (1981). Dietary fibre and large bowel cancer. *Proc Nutr Soc,* Vol. 40, No. 1, pp. 7-14, ISSN 0029-6651

Davis, C.D. & Milner, J.A. (2009). Gastrointestinal microflora, food components and colon cancer prevention. *J Nutr Biochem,* Vol. 20, No. 10, pp. 743-752, ISSN 1873-4847

Davis, C.D.; Zeng, H. & Finley, J.W. (2002). Selenium-enriched broccoli decreases intestinal tumorigenesis in multiple intestinal neoplasia mice. *J Nutr,* Vol. 132, No. 2, pp. 307-309, ISSN 0022-3166

Dixon, L.B.; Balder, H.F.; Virtanen, M.J.; Rashidkhani, B.; Mannisto, S.; Krogh, V.; van Den Brandt, P.A.; Hartman, A.M.; Pietinen, P.; Tan, F.; Virtamo, J.; Wolk, A. & Goldbohm, R.A. (2004). Dietary patterns associated with colon and rectal cancer: results from the Dietary Patterns and Cancer (DIETSCAN) Project. *Am J Clin Nutr,* Vol. 80, No. 4, pp. 1003-1011, ISSN 0002-9165

Donini, L.M.; Savina, C. & Cannella, C. (2009). Nutrition in the elderly: role of fiber. *Arch Gerontol Geriatr,* Vol. 49 Suppl 1, No., pp. 61-69, ISSN 1872-6976

Fearon, E.R. & Vogelstein, B. (1990). A genetic model for colorectal tumorigenesis. *Cell,* Vol. 61, No. 5, pp. 759-767, ISSN 0092-8674

Filomeni, G.; Aquilano, K.; Rotilio, G. & Ciriolo, M.R. (2003). Reactive oxygen species-dependent c-Jun NH2-terminal kinase/c-Jun signaling cascade mediates neuroblastoma cell death induced by diallyl disulfide. *Cancer Res,* Vol. 63, No. 18, pp. 5940-5949, ISSN 0008-5472

Fuchs, C.S.; Giovannucci, E.L.; Colditz, G.A.; Hunter, D.J.; Stampfer, M.J.; Rosner, B.; Speizer, F.E. & Willett, W.C. (1999). Dietary fiber and the risk of colorectal cancer and adenoma in women. *N Engl J Med,* Vol. 340, No. 3, pp. 169-176, ISSN 0028-4793

Ganther, H.E. (1999). Selenium metabolism, selenoproteins and mechanisms of cancer prevention: complexities with thioredoxin reductase. *Carcinogenesis,* Vol. 20, No. 9, pp. 1657-1666, ISSN 0143-3334

Gibson, G.R. & Roberfroid, M.B. (1995). Dietary modulation of the human colonic microbiota: introducing the concept of prebiotics. *J Nutr,* Vol. 125, No. 6, pp. 1401-1412, ISSN 0022-3166

Graham, S.; Marshall, J.; Haughey, B.; Mittelman, A.; Swanson, M.; Zielezny, M.; Byers, T.; Wilkinson, G. & West, D. (1988). Dietary epidemiology of cancer of the colon in western New York. *Am J Epidemiol,* Vol. 128, No. 3, pp. 490-503, ISSN 0002-9262

Griffin, I.J.; Davila, P.M. & Abrams, S.A. (2002). Non-digestible oligosaccharides and calcium absorption in girls with adequate calcium intakes. *Br J Nutr,* Vol. 87 Suppl 2, No., pp. S187-191, ISSN 0007-1145

Guo, W.; Nie, L.; Wu, D.; Wise, M.L.; Collins, F.W.; Meydani, S.N. & Meydani, M. (2010). Avenanthramides inhibit proliferation of human colon cancer cell lines in vitro. *Nutr Cancer,* Vol. 62, No. 8, pp. 1007-1016, ISSN 1532-7914

Huerta, S.; Irwin, R.W.; Heber, D.; Go, V.L.; Moatamed, F.; Ou, C. & Harris, D.M. (2003). Intestinal polyp formation in the Apcmin mouse: effects of levels of dietary calcium and altered vitamin D homeostasis. *Dig Dis Sci,* Vol. 48, No. 5, pp. 870-876, ISSN 0163-2116

Ishikawa, H.; Akedo, I.; Otani, T.; Suzuki, T.; Nakamura, T.; Takeyama, I.; Ishiguro, S.; Miyaoka, E.; Sobue, T. & Kakizoe, T. (2005). Randomized trial of dietary fiber and Lactobacillus casei administration for prevention of colorectal tumors. *Int J Cancer,* Vol. 116, No. 5, pp. 762-767, ISSN 0020-7136

Janne, P.A. & Mayer, R.J. (2000). Chemoprevention of colorectal cancer. *N Engl J Med,* Vol. 342, No. 26, pp. 1960-1968, ISSN 0028-4793

Jemal, A.; Bray, F.; Center, M.M.; Ferlay, J.; Ward, E. & Forman, D. (2011). Global cancer statistics. *CA Cancer J Clin,* Vol. 61, No. 2, pp. 69-90, ISSN 1542-4863

Key, T.J.; Appleby, P.N.; Spencer, E.A.; Travis, R.C.; Roddam, A.W. & Allen, N.E. (2009). Mortality in British vegetarians: results from the European Prospective Investigation into Cancer and Nutrition (EPIC-Oxford). *Am J Clin Nutr,* Vol. 89, No. 5, pp. 1613S-1619S, ISSN 1938-3207

Key, T.J.; Thorogood, M.; Appleby, P.N. & Burr, M.L. (1996). Dietary habits and mortality in 11,000 vegetarians and health conscious people: results of a 17 year follow up. *BMJ,* Vol. 313, No. 7060, pp. 775-779, ISSN 0959-8138

Kim, E.J.; Schaffer, B.S.; Kang, Y.H.; Macdonald, R.G. & Park, J.H. (2002). Decreased production of insulin-like growth factor-binding protein (IGFBP)-6 by transfection of colon cancer cells with an antisense IGFBP-6 cDNA construct leads to stimulation of cell proliferation. *J Gastroenterol Hepatol,* Vol. 17, No. 5, pp. 563-570, ISSN 0815-9319

Kim, J.M. & Park, E. (2010). Coenzyme Q10 attenuated DMH-induced precancerous lesions in SD rats. *J Nutr Sci Vitaminol (Tokyo),* Vol. 56, No. 2, pp. 139-144, ISSN 1881-7742

Kim, M.K.; Sasaki, S.; Otani, T. & Tsugane, S. (2005). Dietary patterns and subsequent colorectal cancer risk by subsite: a prospective cohort study. *Int J Cancer,* Vol. 115, No. 5, pp. 790-798, ISSN 0020-7136

Kim, Y.I. (2003). Role of folate in colon cancer development and progression. *J Nutr,* Vol. 133, No. 11 Suppl 1, pp. 3731S-3739S, ISSN 0022-3166

Ko, S.C.; Chapple, K.S.; Hawcroft, G.; Coletta, P.L.; Markham, A.F. & Hull, M.A. (2002). Paracrine cyclooxygenase-2-mediated signalling by macrophages promotes tumorigenic progression of intestinal epithelial cells. *Oncogene,* Vol. 21, No. 47, pp. 7175-7186, ISSN 0950-9232

Koch, T.C.; Briviba, K.; Watzl, B.; Fahndrich, C.; Bub, A.; Rechkemmer, G. & Barth, S.W. (2009). Prevention of colon carcinogenesis by apple juice in vivo: impact of juice constituents and obesity. *Mol Nutr Food Res,* Vol. 53, No. 10, pp. 1289-1302, ISSN 1613-4133

Kryston, T.B.; Georgiev, A.B.; Pissis, P. & Georgakilas, A.G. (2011). Role of oxidative stress and DNA damage in human carcinogenesis. *Mutat Res,* Vol. 711, No. 1-2, pp. 193-201, ISSN 0027-5107

Kyle, J.A.; Sharp, L.; Little, J.; Duthie, G.G. & McNeill, G. (2010). Dietary flavonoid intake and colorectal cancer: a case-control study. *Br J Nutr,* Vol. 103, No. 3, pp. 429-436, ISSN 1475-2662

Lamprecht, S.A. & Lipkin, M. (2001). Cellular mechanisms of calcium and vitamin D in the inhibition of colorectal carcinogenesis. *Ann N Y Acad Sci,* Vol. 952, No., pp. 73-87, ISSN 0077-8923

Lamprecht, S.A. & Lipkin, M. (2003). Chemoprevention of colon cancer by calcium, vitamin D and folate: molecular mechanisms. *Nat Rev Cancer,* Vol. 3, No. 8, pp. 601-614, ISSN 1474-175X

Ley, R.E.; Turnbaugh, P.J.; Klein, S. & Gordon, J.I. (2006). Microbial ecology: human gut microbes associated with obesity. *Nature,* Vol. 444, No. 7122, pp. 1022-1023, ISSN 1476-4687

Lim, C.C.; Ferguson, L.R. & Tannock, G.W. (2005). Dietary fibres as "prebiotics": implications for colorectal cancer. *Mol Nutr Food Res,* Vol. 49, No. 6, pp. 609-619, ISSN 1613-4125

Luo, J.; Van Yperselle, M.; Rizkalla, S.W.; Rossi, F.; Bornet, F.R. & Slama, G. (2000). Chronic consumption of short-chain fructooligosaccharides does not affect basal hepatic glucose production or insulin resistance in type 2 diabetics. *J Nutr,* Vol. 130, No. 6, pp. 1572-1577, ISSN 0022-3166

Lynch, H.T. & de la Chapelle, A. (2003). Hereditary colorectal cancer. *N Engl J Med,* Vol. 348, No. 10, pp. 919-932, ISSN 1533-4406

Mai, V.; Colbert, L.H.; Berrigan, D.; Perkins, S.N.; Pfeiffer, R.; Lavigne, J.A.; Lanza, E.; Haines, D.C.; Schatzkin, A. & Hursting, S.D. (2003). Calorie restriction and diet composition modulate spontaneous intestinal tumorigenesis in Apc(Min) mice through different mechanisms. *Cancer Res,* Vol. 63, No. 8, pp. 1752-1755, ISSN 0008-5472

Mandir, N.; Englyst, H. & Goodlad, R.A. (2008). Resistant carbohydrates stimulate cell proliferation and crypt fission in wild-type mice and in the Apc(Min/+) mouse model of intestinal cancer, association with enhanced polyp development. *Br J Nutr,* Vol. 100, No. 4, pp. 711-721, ISSN 1475-2662

Marshall, J.R. (2008). Prevention of colorectal cancer: diet, chemoprevention, and lifestyle. *Gastroenterol Clin North Am,* Vol. 37, No. 1, pp. 73-82, vi, ISSN 0889-8553

Martin, O.A.; Redon, C.E.; Nakamura, A.J.; Dickey, J.S.; Georgakilas, A.G. & Bonner, W.M. (2011). Systemic DNA damage related to cancer. *Cancer Res,* Vol. 71, No. 10, pp. 3437-3441, ISSN 1538-7445

Martinez-Outschoorn, U.E.; Pavlides, S.; Howell, A.; Pestell, R.G.; Tanowitz, H.B.; Sotgia, F. & Lisanti, M.P. (2011). Stromal-epithelial metabolic coupling in cancer: integrating autophagy and metabolism in the tumor microenvironment. *Int J Biochem Cell Biol,* Vol. 43, No. 7, pp. 1045-1051, ISSN 1878-5875

Mastromarino, A.; Reddy, B.S. & Wynder, E.L. (1976). Metabolic epidemiology of colon cancer: enzymic activity of fecal flora. *Am J Clin Nutr,* Vol. 29, No. 12, pp. 1455-1460, ISSN 0002-9165

McIntosh, G.H.; Royle, P.J. & Playne, M.J. (1999). A probiotic strain of L. acidophilus reduces DMH-induced large intestinal tumors in male Sprague-Dawley rats. *Nutr Cancer,* Vol. 35, No. 2, pp. 153-159, ISSN 0163-5581

Obtulowicz, T.; Swoboda, M.; Speina, E.; Gackowski, D.; Rozalski, R.; Siomek, A.; Janik, J.; Janowska, B.; Ciesla, J.M.; Jawien, A.; Banaszkiewicz, Z.; Guz, J.; Dziaman, T.; Szpila, A.; Olinski, R. & Tudek, B. (2010). Oxidative stress and 8-oxoguanine repair are enhanced in colon adenoma and carcinoma patients. *Mutagenesis,* Vol. 25, No. 5, pp. 463-471, ISSN 1464-3804

Oh, Y.S.; Kim, E.J.; Schaffer, B.S.; Kang, Y.H.; Binderup, L.; MacDonald, R.G. & Park, J.H. (2001). Synthetic low-calcaemic vitamin D(3) analogues inhibit secretion of insulin-like growth factor II and stimulate production of insulin-like growth factor-binding protein-6 in conjunction with growth suppression of HT-29 colon cancer cells. *Mol Cell Endocrinol,* Vol. 183, No. 1-2, pp. 141-149, ISSN 0303-7207

Park, J.H. (2008). Inhibition of colon cancer cell growth by dietary components: role of the insulin-like growth factor (IGF) system. *Asia Pac J Clin Nutr,* Vol. 17 Suppl 1, No., pp. 257-260, ISSN 0964-7058

Park, S.Y.; Nomura, A.M.; Murphy, S.P.; Wilkens, L.R.; Henderson, B.E. & Kolonel, L.N. (2009). Carotenoid intake and colorectal cancer risk: the multiethnic cohort study. *J Epidemiol,* Vol. 19, No. 2, pp. 63-71, ISSN 1349-9092

Park, Y.; Spiegelman, D.; Hunter, D.J.; Albanes, D.; Bergkvist, L.; Buring, J.E.; Freudenheim, J.L.; Giovannucci, E.; Goldbohm, R.A.; Harnack, L.; Kato, I.; Krogh, V.; Leitzmann,

M.F.; Limburg, P.J.; Marshall, J.R.; McCullough, M.L.; Miller, A.B.; Rohan, T.E.; Schatzkin, A.; Shore, R.; Sieri, S.; Stampfer, M.J.; Virtamo, J.; Weijenberg, M.; Willett, W.C.; Wolk, A.; Zhang, S.M. & Smith-Warner, S.A. (2010). Intakes of vitamins A, C, and E and use of multiple vitamin supplements and risk of colon cancer: a pooled analysis of prospective cohort studies. *Cancer Causes Control,* Vol. 21, No. 11, pp. 1745-1757, ISSN 1573-7225

Penner, R.; Fedorak, R.N. & Madsen, K.L. (2005). Probiotics and nutraceuticals: non-medicinal treatments of gastrointestinal diseases. *Curr Opin Pharmacol,* Vol. 5, No. 6, pp. 596-603, ISSN 1471-4892

Petrik, M.B.; McEntee, M.F.; Johnson, B.T.; Obukowicz, M.G. & Whelan, J. (2000). Highly unsaturated (n-3) fatty acids, but not alpha-linolenic, conjugated linoleic or gamma-linolenic acids, reduce tumorigenesis in Apc(Min/+) mice. *J Nutr,* Vol. 130, No. 10, pp. 2434-2443, ISSN 0022-3166

Pot, G.K.; Geelen, A.; Majsak-Newman, G.; Harvey, L.J.; Nagengast, F.M.; Witteman, B.J.; van de Meeberg, P.C.; Hart, A.R.; Schaafsma, G.; Lund, E.K.; Rijkers, G.T. & Kampman, E. (2010a). Increased consumption of fatty and lean fish reduces serum C-reactive protein concentrations but not inflammation markers in feces and in colonic biopsies. *J Nutr,* Vol. 140, No. 2, pp. 371-376, ISSN 1541-6100

Pot, G.K.; Habermann, N.; Majsak-Newman, G.; Harvey, L.J.; Geelen, A.; Przybylska-Philips, K.; Nagengast, F.M.; Witteman, B.J.; van de Meeberg, P.C.; Hart, A.R.; Schaafsma, G.; Hooiveld, G.; Glei, M.; Lund, E.K.; Pool-Zobel, B.L. & Kampman, E. (2010b). Increasing fish consumption does not affect genotoxicity markers in the colon in an intervention study. *Carcinogenesis,* Vol. 31, No. 6, pp. 1087-1091, ISSN 1460-2180

Pot, G.K.; Majsak-Newman, G.; Geelen, A.; Harvey, L.J.; Nagengast, F.M.; Witteman, B.J.; van de Meeberg, P.C.; Timmer, R.; Tan, A.; Wahab, P.J.; Hart, A.R.; Williams, M.P.; Przybylska-Phillips, K.; Dainty, J.R.; Schaafsma, G.; Kampman, E. & Lund, E.K. (2009). Fish consumption and markers of colorectal cancer risk: a multicenter randomized controlled trial. *Am J Clin Nutr,* Vol. 90, No. 2, pp. 354-361, ISSN 1938-3207

Prinz-Langenohl, R.; Fohr, I. & Pietrzik, K. (2001). Beneficial role for folate in the prevention of colorectal and breast cancer. *Eur J Nutr,* Vol. 40, No. 3, pp. 98-105, ISSN 1436-6207

Rafter, J.; Bennett, M.; Caderni, G.; Clune, Y.; Hughes, R.; Karlsson, P.C.; Klinder, A.; O'Riordan, M.; O'Sullivan, G.C.; Pool-Zobel, B.; Rechkemmer, G.; Roller, M.; Rowland, I.; Salvadori, M.; Thijs, H.; Van Loo, J.; Watzl, B. & Collins, J.K. (2007). Dietary synbiotics reduce cancer risk factors in polypectomized and colon cancer patients. *Am J Clin Nutr,* Vol. 85, No. 2, pp. 488-496, ISSN 0002-9165

Rao, C.V.; Hirose, Y.; Indranie, C. & Reddy, B.S. (2001). Modulation of experimental colon tumorigenesis by types and amounts of dietary fatty acids. *Cancer Res,* Vol. 61, No. 5, pp. 1927-1933, ISSN 0008-5472

Reddy, B.S. (1999). Possible mechanisms by which pro- and prebiotics influence colon carcinogenesis and tumor growth. *J Nutr,* Vol. 129, No. 7 Suppl, pp. 1478S-1482S, ISSN 0022-3166

Roberfroid, M.; Gibson, G.R.; Hoyles, L.; McCartney, A.L.; Rastall, R.; Rowland, I.; Wolvers, D.; Watzl, B.; Szajewska, H.; Stahl, B.; Guarner, F.; Respondek, F.; Whelan, K.; Coxam, V.; Davicco, M.J.; Leotoing, L.; Wittrant, Y.; Delzenne, N.M.; Cani, P.D.; Neyrinck, A.M. & Meheust, A. (2010). Prebiotic effects: metabolic and health benefits. *Br J Nutr,* Vol. 104 Suppl 2, No., pp. S1-63, ISSN 1475-2662

Roynette, C.E.; Calder, P.C.; Dupertuis, Y.M. & Pichard, C. (2004). n-3 polyunsaturated fatty acids and colon cancer prevention. *Clin Nutr,* Vol. 23, No. 2, pp. 139-151, ISSN 0261-5614

Samad, A.K.; Taylor, R.S.; Marshall, T. & Chapman, M.A. (2005). A meta-analysis of the association of physical activity with reduced risk of colorectal cancer. *Colorectal Dis,* Vol. 7, No. 3, pp. 204-213, ISSN 1462-8910

Sanjoaquin, M.A.; Allen, N.; Couto, E.; Roddam, A.W. & Key, T.J. (2005). Folate intake and colorectal cancer risk: a meta-analytical approach. *Int J Cancer,* Vol. 113, No. 5, pp. 825-828, ISSN 0020-7136

Sanjoaquin, M.A.; Appleby, P.N.; Thorogood, M.; Mann, J.I. & Key, T.J. (2004). Nutrition, lifestyle and colorectal cancer incidence: a prospective investigation of 10998 vegetarians and non-vegetarians in the United Kingdom. *Br J Cancer,* Vol. 90, No. 1, pp. 118-121, ISSN 0007-0920

Sedelnikova, O.A.; Redon, C.E.; Dickey, J.S.; Nakamura, A.J.; Georgakilas, A.G. & Bonner, W.M. (2010). Role of oxidatively induced DNA lesions in human pathogenesis. *Mutat Res,* Vol. 704, No. 1-3, pp. 152-159, ISSN 0027-5107

Shen, G.; Khor, T.O.; Hu, R.; Yu, S.; Nair, S.; Ho, C.T.; Reddy, B.S.; Huang, M.T.; Newmark, H.L. & Kong, A.N. (2007). Chemoprevention of familial adenomatous polyposis by natural dietary compounds sulforaphane and dibenzoylmethane alone and in combination in ApcMin/+ mouse. *Cancer Res,* Vol. 67, No. 20, pp. 9937-9944, ISSN 0008-5472

Shukla, Y. & Kalra, N. (2007). Cancer chemoprevention with garlic and its constituents. *Cancer Lett,* Vol. 247, No. 2, pp. 167-181, ISSN 0304-3835

Snow, D.R.; Jimenez-Flores, R.; Ward, R.E.; Cambell, J.; Young, M.J.; Nemere, I. & Hintze, K.J. (2010). Dietary milk fat globule membrane reduces the incidence of aberrant crypt foci in Fischer-344 rats. *J Agric Food Chem,* Vol. 58, No. 4, pp. 2157-2163, ISSN 1520-5118

Song, J.; Sohn, K.J.; Medline, A.; Ash, C.; Gallinger, S. & Kim, Y.I. (2000). Chemopreventive effects of dietary folate on intestinal polyps in Apc+/-Msh2-/- mice. *Cancer Res,* Vol. 60, No. 12, pp. 3191-3199, ISSN 0008-5472

Tammariello, A.E. & Milner, J.A. (2010). Mouse models for unraveling the importance of diet in colon cancer prevention. *J Nutr Biochem,* Vol. 21, No. 2, pp. 77-88, ISSN 1873-4847

Tuohy, K.M.; Rouzaud, G.C.; Bruck, W.M. & Gibson, G.R. (2005). Modulation of the human gut microflora towards improved health using prebiotics--assessment of efficacy. *Curr Pharm Des,* Vol. 11, No. 1, pp. 75-90, ISSN 1381-6128

van Duijnhoven, F.J.; Bueno-De-Mesquita, H.B.; Ferrari, P.; Jenab, M.; Boshuizen, H.C.; Ros, M.M.; Casagrande, C.; Tjonneland, A.; Olsen, A.; Overvad, K.; Thorlacius-Ussing, O.; Clavel-Chapelon, F.; Boutron-Ruault, M.C.; Morois, S.; Kaaks, R.; Linseisen, J.;

Boeing, H.; Nothlings, U.; Trichopoulou, A.; Trichopoulos, D.; Misirli, G.; Palli, D.; Sieri, S.; Panico, S.; Tumino, R.; Vineis, P.; Peeters, P.H.; van Gils, C.H.; Ocke, M.C.; Lund, E.; Engeset, D.; Skeie, G.; Suarez, L.R.; Gonzalez, C.A.; Sanchez, M.J.; Dorronsoro, M.; Navarro, C.; Barricarte, A.; Berglund, G.; Manjer, J.; Hallmans, G.; Palmqvist, R.; Bingham, S.A.; Khaw, K.T.; Key, T.J.; Allen, N.E.; Boffetta, P.; Slimani, N.; Rinaldi, S.; Gallo, V.; Norat, T. & Riboli, E. (2009). Fruit, vegetables, and colorectal cancer risk: the European Prospective Investigation into Cancer and Nutrition. *Am J Clin Nutr,* Vol. 89, No. 5, pp. 1441-1452, ISSN 1938-3207

van Kranen, H.J.; van Iersel, P.W.; Rijnkels, J.M.; Beems, D.B.; Alink, G.M. & van Kreijl, C.F. (1998). Effects of dietary fat and a vegetable-fruit mixture on the development of intestinal neoplasia in the ApcMin mouse. *Carcinogenesis,* Vol. 19, No. 9, pp. 1597-1601, ISSN 0143-3334

Ventrella-Lucente, L.F.; Unnikrishnan, A.; Pilling, A.B.; Patel, H.V.; Kushwaha, D.; Dombkowski, A.A.; Schmelz, E.M.; Cabelof, D.C. & Heydari, A.R. (2010). Folate deficiency provides protection against colon carcinogenesis in DNA polymerase beta haploinsufficient mice. *J Biol Chem,* Vol. 285, No. 25, pp. 19246-19258, ISSN 1083-351X

Vilar, E. & Gruber, S.B. (2010). Microsatellite instability in colorectal cancer-the stable evidence. *Nat Rev Clin Oncol,* Vol. 7, No. 3, pp. 153-162, ISSN 1759-4782

Williams, C.D.; Satia, J.A.; Adair, L.S.; Stevens, J.; Galanko, J.; Keku, T.O. & Sandler, R.S. (2010). Antioxidant and DNA methylation-related nutrients and risk of distal colorectal cancer. *Cancer Causes Control,* Vol. 21, No. 8, pp. 1171-1181, ISSN 1573-7225

Winkelmann, I.; Diehl, D.; Oesterle, D.; Daniel, H. & Wenzel, U. (2010). Flavone induces changes in intermediary metabolism that prevent microadenoma formation in colonic tissue of carcinogen-treated mice. *Mol Nutr Food Res,* Vol. 54 Suppl 2, No., pp. S184-195, ISSN 1613-4133

Woodworth, H.L.; McCaskey, S.J.; Duriancik, D.M.; Clinthorne, J.F.; Langohr, I.M.; Gardner, E.M. & Fenton, J.I. (2010). Dietary fish oil alters T lymphocyte cell populations and exacerbates disease in a mouse model of inflammatory colitis. *Cancer Res,* Vol. 70, No. 20, pp. 7960-7969, ISSN 1538-7445

World Cancer Research Fund & American Institute for Cancer Research (2007a). The cancer process, In: *Food, Nutrition, Physical Activity, and the Prevention of Cancer: A Global Perspective*, World Cancer Research Fund, pp. 30-46, American Institute for Cancer Research, ISBN-13: 9780972252225, Washington DC, USA

World Cancer Research Fund & American Institute for Cancer Research (2007b). Cancers; Colon and rectum, In: *Food, Nutrition, Physical Activity, and the Prevention of Cancer: A Global Perspective,* World Cancer Research Fund, pp. 280-288, American Institute for Cancer Research, ISBN-13: 9780972252225, Washington DC, USA

World Cancer Research Fund & American Institute for Cancer Research (2007c). Foods and drinks, In: *Food, Nutrition, Physical Activity, and the Prevention of Cancer: A Global Perspective,* World Cancer Research Fund, pp. 66-196, American Institute for Cancer Research, ISBN-13: 9780972252225, Washington DC, USA

World Cancer Research Fund & American Institute for Cancer Research (2007d). Summary, In: *Food, Nutrition, Physical Activity and the Prevention of Cancer: a Global Perspective*, World Cancer Research Fund, pp. xiv-xxi, American Institute for Cancer Research, ISBN-13: 9780972252225, Washington DC, USA

Zeeb, H. & Greinert, R. (2010). The role of vitamin D in cancer prevention: does UV protection conflict with the need to raise low levels of vitamin D? *Dtsch Arztebl Int*, Vol. 107, No. 37, pp. 638-643, ISSN 1866-0452

Ziech, D.; Franco, R.; Georgakilas, A.G.; Georgakila, S.; Malamou-Mitsi, V.; Schoneveld, O.; Pappa, A. & Panayiotidis, M.I. (2010). The role of reactive oxygen species and oxidative stress in environmental carcinogenesis and biomarker development. *Chem Biol Interact*, Vol. 188, No. 2, pp. 334-339, ISSN 1872-7786

9

Cervical Cancer Screening and Prevention for HIV-Infected Women in the Developing World

Jean Anderson, Enriquito Lu, Harshad Sanghvi,
Sharon Kibwana and Anjanique Lu
Jhpiego, Johns Hopkins University
USA

1. Introduction

Cervical cancer ranks as the third most common cancer in women worldwide and is the fourth leading cause of cancer deaths in women, with an estimated 270,000 deaths annually. Over 85% of both cervical cancer cases and deaths occur in developing countries with only 5% of global cancer resources (Lancet 2010). Cervical cancer is the most common cancer in women in most developing countries and most common cause of cancer deaths (Cervical Cancer Action: Report Card 2011). It is the leading cause of years of life lost to cancer in low resource settings (Yang et al. 2004). In sub-Saharan Africa cervical cancer represents 22% of all cancers in women (Parkin et al. 2003).

Currently, an estimated 33.3 million individuals worldwide are living with HIV/AIDS, approximately 68% of whom live in Sub-Saharan Africa; globally over 50% of all those living with HIV are female and in Sub-Saharan Africa, women account for 60% of HIV infections. In 2009 there were an estimated 7000 new infections per day, 51% of these among women (UNAIDS 2010). However, there have been dramatic advances in prevention, care and treatment in the areas that are hardest hit by HIV over the past 10 years, coincident with unprecedented global commitment for funding and other support. These include a global decline of 19% in number of new HIV infections and a >25% decline in HIV prevalence among young people 15–24 years of age in 15 high burden countries, a decrease in global AIDS deaths by 19% from 2004–2009, and an increase in access to antiretroviral therapy (ART) in low and middle-income (LMIC) countries from 400,000 in 2003 to 5.25 million by the end of 2009 (this however, comprises only 35% of those estimated to be in need of therapy) (WHO 2011).

The areas where cervical cancer rates are highest also often have high prevalence of HIV and the presence of HIV increases the risk of cervical precancerous and cancerous changes; furthermore there is general unavailability of effective cervical cancer screening programs in these lower resource settings. This paper will review issues related to cervical cancer screening and prevention for HIV-infected women in low resource settings, with a focus on non-cytology-based techniques.

2. Human papillomavirus infection and cervical cancer

The causal relationship between some microbial pathogens, primarily viral, and human carcinogenesis have been suspected but it has only been in the last 20 years that knowledge has accumulated to more clearly define the mechanisms and processes that chronic, persistent infections induce cancer development, see Figure 1. Replication of DNA and RNA tumor viruses involve incorporation of the viral genome into the host cell chromosomes inducing several mutations that disrupt the homeostatic balance between proliferation and cell death; in the case of oncogenic HPV, the expression of viral E2, E6, and E7 genes lead to the production of proteins that initiate cell cycle and disable control of growth, allowing the proliferation of genetic damage to accumulate in HPV infected cells. (Georgakilas et al. 2010). Oxidative stress negatively impacting genetic and cellular processes can be brought about by reactive oxygen species (ROS) or free radicals induced by chronic infection (Kryston et al. 2011; Georgakilas et al. 2010). Although additional researches are needed to accurately define the relationship, oxidative stress is linked in several studies with some tumor virus but not HPV (Kryston, et al. 2011)

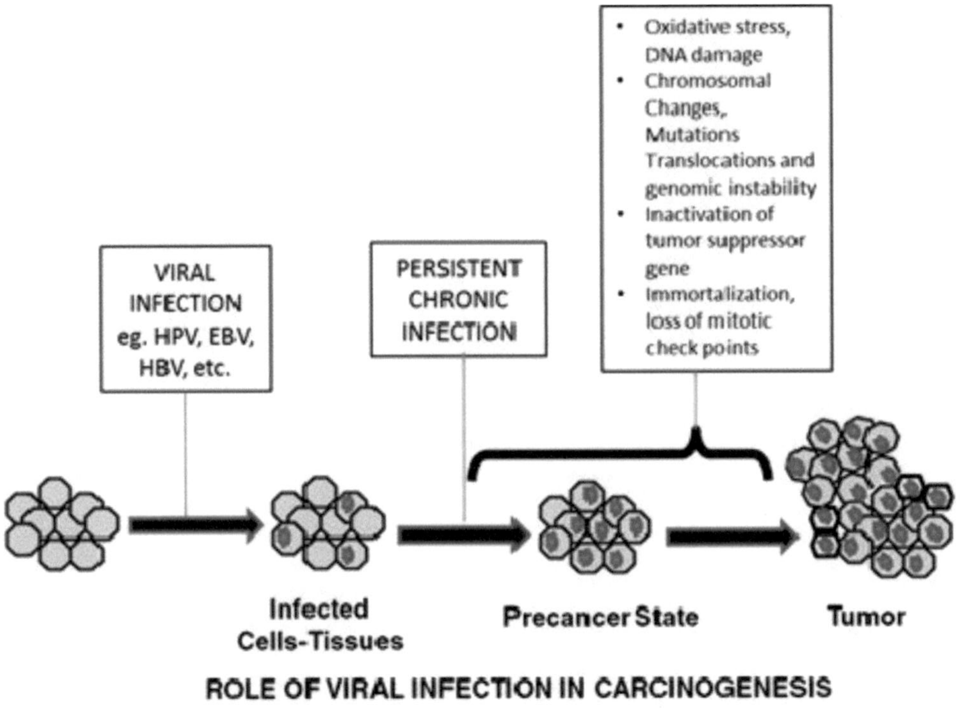

Fig. 1. Role of Viral Infection in Carcinogenesis.

Schematic pathway of viral infection leading to cancer adapted from Figure1 Viral pathogens role(s) in human carcinogenesis based on current status of knowledge and clinical evidence.

Alexandros Georgakilas, William Mosley, Stavroula Georgakila, Dominick Ziech, and Mihalis Panayiotidis. Viral-induced human carcinogenesis: an oxidative stress perspective. Molecular BioSystems Vol 6, pp 1162 – 1172, (2010).

In the 1990s a combination of large-scale epidemiologic studies and the application of new molecular techniques clearly established human papillomavirus (HPV) as the etiologic cause of cervical cancer (Clifford 2003; Walboomers 1999). Using the most sensitive assays, over

99% of invasive cervical cancers have been found to be HPV-positive (Sankaranarayanan 2008). Current evidence suggests that over 50% of sexually active adults have been infected with one or more genital HPV types (Ho 1998; Evander 1995); however, most HPV infections resolve or become latent and undetectable (Ho 1998; Moscicki 1998; Evander 1995). Furthermore, although there are well over a 100 distinct molecular subtypes of HPV, only a small subset have been associated with development of cancer and are considered "high risk" or oncogenic (Cogliano 2005). For cervical cancer to develop, persistent infection with an oncogenic HPV subtype is necessary. The oncogenic or high-risk HPV includes HPV subtypes -16, -18, -31, -33, -35, -39, -45, -51, -52, -56, -58, -59, -66, -68 which are strongly associated to cervical precancer (Schiffman 2003).

Cervical cancer is relatively unique in that there is a recognizable preinvasive phase in which progression from initial HPV infection to invasive disease evolves over several years, passing through cytologically and histologically distinct precancerous phases, known as cervical dysplasia (mild, moderate, severe, carcinoma-in-situ) or cervical intraepithelial neoplasia (CIN 1,2,3). The peak prevalence of infection with carcinogenic HPV subtypes is in the teens and twenties, following closely after the initiation of sexual activity; the majority of these infections are transient and are cleared by the body's immune system. When viral persistence and progression do occur, the median time from HPV detection to development of CIN 3 is approximately 7–8 years, with 20% progressing from CIN 1 to CIN 3 within 2 years. Progression from CIN 3 to invasive cancer occurs over an additional 5–7 years. The peak prevalence of invasive cancer occurs in the 40-50 year age range (McIndoe 1984; Kolstad 1976; Melnikow 1998; Josefsson 2000; Schiffman 2005). This prolonged natural history offers numerous opportunities to detect the presence of precancerous lesions and to prevent progression to invasive cancer.

3. HPV, cervical dysplasia and HIV

3.1 Interrelationship of HIV and Human Papillomavirus

Studies have shown that HIV-infected women have higher prevalence of HPV, higher incidence of HPV (Branca 2003; Ahdieh 2001), higher HPV viral load (Jamieson 2002), longer persistence of HPV (Ahdieh 2000; Sun 1997), higher likelihood of multiple HPV subtypes (Jamieson 2002; Firnhaber et al. 2009; Clifford et al. 2007), and greater prevalence of oncogenic subtypes (Minkoff 1998; Uberti-Foppa 1998; Acta Cytol 2009; 53: 10–17) than HIV-uninfected women. HPV viral load is independently associated with HPV persistence (Ahdieh 2001). A recent meta-analysis found that the rate of cervical HPV infection in HIV-infected women with normal cervical cytology varied from more than 55% in South and Central America and Africa to over 30% in Asia, North America, and Europe (Clifford 2006). Furthermore, in HIV-positive women the prevalence and persistence of HPV infection increases with decreasing CD4 count and increasing HIV RNA levels (Palefsky 1999; Denny 2008) and some studies show that oncogenic HPV types may be more common with lower CD4 counts and/or higher viral loads. (Luque 1999; Minkoff 1998; Clifford et al. 2007). A recent cross-sectional study of 109 HIV+ women initiating ART in South Africa (median CD4 count 125/mm3) found a high-risk HPV (HR-HPV) prevalence of 78.9% (Moodley et al. 2009). In another South African cohort of over 123 women with HIV seroconversion HR-HPV infection doubled within 36 months of seroconversion (Wang et al. 2011). Higher HPV viral loads are also associated with lower CD4 counts (Heard 2000).

3.2 HIV and cervical dysplasia

The prevalence and incidence of abnormal Pap smears are increased among HIV-infected women as compared to uninfected women, with up to 10-fold higher rates (Maiman 1998); abnormal cervical cytology is associated with the presence of HPV infection and the degree of immunosuppression. Both frequency and severity of abnormal Pap smears and histologically documented dysplasia increase with declining CD4 counts and have also been associated with higher HIV-RNA levels (Garzetti 1995; Shah 1996; Davis 2001; Ellerbrock 2000; AIDS Care 2007; 19: 1052–1057. Massad 2008; Massad 2001). Two-thirds of 109 HIV+ women initiating ART in South Africa with median CD4 125/mm3 had abnormal Pap smears (Moodley et al. 2009). Increased HPV viral load, seen in women with more advanced HIV, is also associated with increased frequency, severity, and incidence of cervical dysplasia (Heard 2000; Weissenborn 2003; Cohn 2001). HIV is also associated with more extensive/larger volume of cervical involvement, and are also more likely to involve other areas in the lower genital tract (e.g., vulva, vagina, anal regions) (Maiman 1990). Progression and regression of Pap smear abnormalities have also been associated with level of immunosuppression and plasma viremia, as reflected in CD4 count and HIV viral load (Massad 2001; Schuman 200).

The role of effective ART and immune reconstitution in reducing the incidence and progression and promoting the regression of HPV infection and cervical dysplasia remains unclear, but HPV-related lesions do not appear to respond to ART like other opportunistic illnesses. Studies examining this issue have mixed findings, which may be related to differences in study design, virologic and immunologic parameters, duration and type of ART use, length of follow-up or other factors. In one study use of ART was associated with increased likelihood of regression of cervical dysplasia after treatment for 12 months (Heard 2002). In the Women's Interagency HIV Study (WIHS), after adjustment for CD4 count and Pap status, use of ART was associated with increased regression and decreased risk of progression of cervical cytologic abnormalities (Minkoff 2001). The HIV Epidemiology Research Study (HERS), a U.S. observational, multisite cohort study, among women with preexisting abnormal cervical cytology, ART was associated with enhanced HPV clearance but not with regression of abnormal Pap results (Paramsothy et al. 2009). In a study of women initiating HAART there was a high prevalence of cervical HPV DNA at baseline, but this declined over 96 weeks of HAART (Fife et al. 2009). On the other hand, with 15 months of follow-up, persistence of high-risk HPV and progression of SIL were comparable among women without antiretroviral treatment, those treated with nucleoside analogues only, and those treated with ART (Lillo 2001). In a more recent analysis from Women's Interagency HIV Study (WIHS), the prevalence, incident detection, and clearance of HPV infection and/or SIL before versus after ART initiation were compared, using women as their own comparison group. The role of adherence, defined as use of HAART as prescribed > or = 95% of the time, and effective ART, defined as suppression of HIV replication, were also examined. ART initiation among adherent women and among women on effective ART was associated with a significant reduction in prevalence, incident detection of oncogenic HPV infection, and decreased prevalence and more rapid clearance of oncogenic HPV-positive SIL, although strength of these protective effects was only moderate. (Minkoff et al. 2010). Given these conflicting findings, HIV-positive women should continue to be followed closely for evidence of lower genital tract neoplasia, regardless of antiretroviral therapy or viral load.

3.3 Invasive Cervical Cancer (ICC) in HIV disease

In 1993, the Center for Disease Control and Prevention (CDC) expanded the case definition of AIDS to include invasive cervical cancer (ICC). As is the case with HIV- negative women, oncogenic HPV types play a central role in the relationship between HIV and cervical cancer. Recent African data found that without high-risk HPV present, the risk ratio for ICC between HIV-positive and HIV-negative women was approximately 1 (Hawes 2003). HPV types 16 and 18 were the most common HPV subtypes in a study of ICC in Kenyan HIV+ and HIV- women and were detected in 65% of ICCs in the HIV-infected patients. Almost half of the type 16 or 18 associated cancers involved multiple HPV types (De Vuyst et al. 2007).

A study matching data from AIDS registries and cancer registries in 15 US regions found that persons with AIDS (information captured 4–60 months after AIDS diagnosis) had statistically significantly elevated risk of ICC compared to the general population, with standard incidence ratios (SIR) of 68.6, 95% CI = 59.7 to 78.4 (Chaturvedi et al. 2009). During the period 1996—2004 (post-HAART introduction), ICC in women with low CD4 T-cell count was not significantly increased, possibly reflecting active screening but also not showing evidence of decline in incidence with HAART availability. There has been no evidence of increased incidence of ICC with the use of regular screening and appropriate evaluation and treatment of abnormal Paps (Massad et al. 2004; Massad et al. 2009). Case-control or cross-sectional studies in various African countries, including Cote d'Ivoire, Tanzania, South Africa, Kenya and Senegal have found that ICC was associated with HIV infection (Adjorlolo-Johnson et al. 2010; Kahesa et al. 2008; Stein et al. 2008; Hawes et al. 2003; Gichangi et al. 2003). However, studies evaluating the strength of association of HIV with cervical cancer among African women have shown conflicting results, possibly reflecting the competing risk of dying from other HIV-related conditions or other illnesses (Adjorlolo-Johnson et al. 2010; Moodley 2006). A recent mathematical modeling simulation projected that, compared with no ART and no screening, the lifetime cumulative risk of dying from ICC approximately doubled with ART and no screening; however, screening even when done once, had the potential to reduce ICC mortality (Atashili et al. 2011)

When ICC does develop in the setting of HIV, it tends to occur at younger ages and with less immunosuppression as compared with HIV-positive women with other AIDS-indicator conditions. Women with HIV and cervical cancer also tend to be 10—15 years younger than HIV-negative women with cervical cancer (Lomalisa 2000; van Bogaert 2011). HIV-positive women with invasive cervical cancer may present at more advanced stages (especially with CD4 <200/mm^3), may metastasize to unusual locations (e.g., psoas muscle, clitoris, meningeal involvement), have poorer responses to standard therapy, and have higher recurrences and death rates, as well as shorter intervals to recurrence or death, compared with HIV-negative women of similar stage (Klevens 1996; Maiman 1990).

4. Cervical cancer screening in developed countries

In the U.S. there have been marked reductions in cervical cancer incidence and mortality over the past 60 years, largely the result of the development and widespread introduction of the Papanicolau (Pap) test in 1949 (Sawaya 1999; van der Graaf et al. 1986; Eddy 1990), based on cytologic examination of cells obtained from the cervix with a simple scraping using a wooden spatula or brush. It is estimated that 60% of the women who are diagnosed with ICC have never had cervical cytology testing or have not been screened within the 5 years before diagnosis (NIH 1996). However, conventional Pap smears are not perfect: a single Pap smear is associated with false-negative rates of 10–25%, largely because of errors in sampling or interpretation. False-negative Pap smears are associated with 30% of the new cases of cervical cancer each year (NIH 1996; Shingleton et al. 1995)

Newer Pap smear screening techniques using liquid-based media appear to decrease inadequate smears and also offer the possibility of direct HPV-DNA testing on collected specimens (ACOG 2009). A recent review of over 400 HIV-infected women who underwent both conventional and liquid-based cytologic screening found a significant decrease in the proportion of smears diagnosed as ASCUS/AGUS as well as the ASCUS/SIL ratio, with liquid-based preparations (Swierczynski 2002). HPV testing for cancer-associated HPV subtypes is currently used as a triage test to stratify risk in women with a cytology diagnosis of atypical squamous cells of undetermined significance (ASC-US), in postmenopausal women with a cytology diagnosis of LSIL and is also often used as an adjunct to cytology for primary screening in women older than 30 years (ACOG 2009). The currently used classification system for Pap smear results is known as the Bethesda classification, which includes an indication of adequacy of sample, whether the result is normal and, if abnormal, degree of abnormality (Solomon 2002).

With current US-based guidelines (ACOG 2009), Pap smears are recommended beginning at age 21 and every two years until age 30 if normal. After 30, if the last 3 tests have been normal, screening interval can be increased to 3 years. Providers may consider discontinuation of screening after age 65–70; if there have been no abnormal Pap smears in 10 years and no on-going risk factors. Colposcopy with biopsy of abnormal areas for histologic confirmation is recommended with ASCUS/+HPV or greater abnormality on Pap or with repetitive ASCUS, even if HPV-. The results of both Pap smear and colposcopy/biopsy are used to determine need to treatment, follow-up or further evaluation.

Women with HIV infection are recommended to have more frequent screening with cervical cytology: twice in the first year after diagnosis of HIV and, if normal, annually thereafter (CDC 2009; ACOG 2010) More frequent Pap smears should be considered with previous abnormal Pap smears, with conservative follow-up of cervical dysplasia without treatment (after colposcopic evaluation to rule out HSIL), with other evidence of HPV infection and after treatment for cervical dysplasia (Anderson 2005).

The role of HPV-DNA testing in HIV+ women is unclear. In a WIHS substudy of HIV+ and HIV- women with normal baseline cytology, incidence of squamous intraepithelial lesions (SIL) were examined by baseline HPV DNA results and stratified by CD4 count. Through 3 year follow-up, incidence of any SIL was similar in HIV- and HIV+ with CD4>500 who had negative results for oncogenic HPV or all HPV, suggesting that similar cervical cancer screening practices may be applicable to both groups. On the other hand, after just 2 years follow-up, incidence of any SIL in HIV+ with CD4<500 was increased over HIV-, even among women with negative results for any HPV, suggesting that a closer screening strategy may be needed for women with lower CD4 counts (Harris et al. 1995). In two prospective studies of HIV-infected women with ASC-US, approximately 30% of participants had evidence of oncogenic HPV, a finding that would support the use of HPV testing in this population if HPV testing remained highly sensitive (Massad et al. 2004; Kirby et al. 2004). However, one of these studies reported a sensitivity of HPV testing for the detection of CIN 2 or higher of 100% (Kirby et al. 2004) and the other study reported a sensitivity of only 50% for detecting high-grade CIN (Massad et al. 2004). Currently CDC and ACOG do not recommend HPV testing for triage of HIV-infected women with abnormal cytology results, for follow-up after treatment for CIN, or to lengthen screening intervals (CDC 2009; ACOG 2010). A study examining HPV DNA testing as a primary screening method for cervical dysplasia in 94 HIV-positive women found that HPV DNA testing identified high-grade cervical dysplasia more accurately than Pap smear (Petry 1999).

Even in locations with high resources, screening for cervical dysplasia in the setting of HIV can be challenging. Women receiving gynecologic and primary HIV care at the same location are more likely to have had Pap smear screening within the previous year (AHRQ 2010). However, despite high rates of HPV and CIN, many women with HIV do not engage in the recommended annual Pap testing (Tello et al. 2008; Oster et al. 2009).

4.1 Cervical cancer screening in low resource countries

Cervical cancer screening is often simply not available in developing world settings. Barriers to cytology-based screening programs include poor health infrastructure, lack of trained cytology technicians and cytopathologists and cost. In addition Pap smears are not point-of-care tests; they require the ability to notify women of abnormal results and to follow-up with further evaluation or treatment. However, in low resource settings, many or most women reside at some distance from health centers, have little access to or cannot afford effective transportation, and there is a lack of effective recall mechanisms for abnormal results (Anorlu 2008). In sub-Saharan Africa there was a 60-80% default rate among those with cytologic abnormalities-(Cronje 2004).

Prevention of cervical cancer by identification and treatment of cervical cancer precursors is key, since treatment resources for invasive disease are scarce. In 2002, the survival rate for invasive cervical cancer was 21% in sub-Saharan Africa vs. 70% in US (Parkin et al. 2005). This is related to the fact that most patients present at late stages, as well as a lack of effective treatment resources, including surgical expertise and radiotherapy (Ashraf 2003). When women present with advanced cervical cancer, palliative care resources are also limited; although morphine is on the WHO list of essential medications (http://whqlibdoc.who.int/hq/2011/a95053_eng.pdf), one study of 47 African countries found that only 11 used morphine for chronic pain (Harding 2005).

Recent work has focused on service delivery models using alternatives to cytology for screening for cervical precancerous lesions in order to improve access to safe and effective treatment, minimize loss to follow-up and prioritize utilization of specialized care. Necessary programmatic components, regardless of the strategy employed, include leadership at national levels making preventing cervical cancer a priority and including development of strategies and guidelines; community awareness building; training of providers and continuing education; data collection systems and outcomes monitoring, including quality assurance measures; administrative management; patient recall and retention plans; and appropriate linkages to assure adequate supplies, timely and high quality laboratory testing, and referrals when needed for higher levels of care. In South Africa, where it is estimated that 1 in 26 women develop cervical cancer in their lifetime, a cervical screening program was initiated in 2001; it called for three free Pap smears, starting at age 30, at ten year intervals (Cronje 2003; Moodley 2006). By 2005–2006, 100% of primary health care clinics in South Africa had health professionals trained to conduct Pap smears, yet the screening rate was only 1.3% (van Schalkwyk 2008). Several studies have found a lack of awareness of cervical cancer as a disease among women, as well as stigma and cultural beliefs or perceptions related to the reproductive organs and symptoms that may delay care-seeking (Anorlu et al. 2008; Wellensiek et al. 2002; Anorlu et al. 2000); however, studies have also documented that health care workers also often have poor knowledge about cervical cancer (Tarwireyi et al. 2003; Ayinde and Omigbodun et al. 2003).

4.2 Alternatives to cervical cytology

Two primary strategies have been developed as alternatives to cytologic screening. The first technique utilizes visual inspection of the cervix without magnification after application of a dilute solution (3–5%) of acetic acid (VIA) or, less commonly, Lugol's iodine solution (VILI). Most studies report results with VIA. With visual inspection techniques, there are three possible results: negative, positive, or suspicious for cancer requiring referral and further evaluation and management. The accuracy of VIA/VILI depends on the ability to visualize the cervical transformation zone, the area where the original columnar epithelium covering the ectocervix has been replaced by squamous epithelium, and the area where oncogenesis begins. As women approach menopause and afterwards, the transformation zone recedes into the cervical canal and may no longer be visible, reducing accuracy of VIA (Cremer 2011). However, in younger women and women in whom the transformation zone is visible, the high negative predictive value of VIA (see below) suggests that significant lesions can generally reliably be excluded if VIA is negative. A major advantage of these techniques is the ability to offer treatment the same day, known as the single-visit approach (SVA).

The other major alternative to cytology is HPV testing. HPV-DNA testing, with detection of high-risk HPV subtypes, is reproducible and objective. HPV testing has been suggested as primary screening in place of cytology in the US and Europe (Kitchener et al. 2009; Cusick et al. 2006) and a negative HPV test predicts a less than 2% risk of developing cervical dysplasia (Naucler et al. 2009; Lonky et al. 2010; Mesher et al. 2010; Kitchener et al. 2009; Cusick et al. 2006). An advantage of HPV testing is that a pelvic exam is not required, but simply insertion of a swab into the vagina to obtain the sample; furthermore, studies have shown that accurate results can be obtained with self-testing, where the woman inserts the swab into her own vagina (Ogilvie et al. 2005; Balasubramanian et al. 2010), that this compares favorably to collection by clinicians (Bhatla et al. 2009; Petignat et al. 2007) and is acceptable to women (Mitchell et al. 2011; Lack et al. 2005). However, treatment of positive results clearly requires access to and good visualization of the cervix.

Sensitivity and specificity values for these screening strategies vary depending on the comparison technique used as "gold standard", as well as the detection goal, i.e., any cervical intraepithelial neoplasia (CIN) or only high grade CIN (CIN2 or CIN3) which are the immediate precursors to invasive cancer. Low-grade lesions (CIN1) may regress spontaneously up to 60% of the time (Cox et al. 2003) and are not routinely treated. Therefore, it is thought that the most appropriate detection goal is CIN 2 or higher (CIN2+), since these lesions are the ones likely to progress to cancer. Some studies have suggested that use of colposcopically-directed biopsy may overestimate sensitivity of VIA when compared to expanded biopsies, including endocervical curettage (ECC), likely due to increased detection of nonvisible lesions in the endocervical canal (Pretorius et al. 2007; Cagle et al. 2010).

In a cluster randomized trial in India, 31343 women screened with VIA were compared to 30958 controls, 30–59 years of age. Women who were VIA+ received colposcopy and biopsy with cryotherapy at the same visit for a colposcopic impression of dysplasia. With 7 years of follow-up, VIA was associated with a 24% reduction in cervical cancer incidence, stage 2 or higher, and 35% reduction in cervical cancer mortality (Sankaranarayanan 2007). In a study one year after cryotherapy, 648 women received both VIA by trained nurses and colposcopy and biopsy with VIA+ patients; 42 (6.5%) were referred for colposcopy and three of these had HSIL or cancer. Of those who were VIA-, colposcopically-based diagnosis was HSIL in only two cases (VIA sensitivity 60%, specificity 93.9%, PPV 7.1%, NPV 99.7%, comparable to Pap smear (Chumworathayi et al. 2008). A recent review of published studies of VIA accuracy with histology as the standard and CIN 2 as the outcome measure found sensitivity 79-82%, specificity 91-92% with PPV 9-10% (Sauvaget et al. 2011).

A pooled analysis of approximately 30,000 women from 17 population-based studies in China assessed the diagnostic accuracy of HPV testing for the detection of CIN 3 or greater; all positive tests were referred for colposcopy and biopsy. HPV-DNA testing had higher sensitivity of 97.5% and lower specificity of 85.1% , as compared to cytology (sensitivity 87.9%, specificity 94.7%) and VIA (sensitivity 54.6%, specificity 89.9%) (Zhao et al. 2010). HPV testing was evaluated and compared to both VIA and cytology in a cluster randomized trial in India. The trial had four arms, with >31,000 women aged 30–59 in each arm and 8 years of follow-up. In this study HPV by hybrid capture (detects 13 high risk subtypes) was compared to cytology, VIA and standard of care, which was no screening. With a positive result with any of the three screening tests, colposcopy and biopsy were performed and treatment with cryotherapy or LEEP was offered. When compared to the no screening group, HPV testing was associated with an approximately 50% reduction in detection of advanced cervical cancer and deaths from cervical cancer; neither VIA nor cytology was associated with statistically significant benefit (Sankaranarayanan et al. 2009).

In an analysis of the accuracy of five cervical cancer screening tests assessed in 11 studies in Africa and India, using colposcopically-directed biopsy as the standard and high grade CIN as the outcome, pooled sensitivity for VIA was 79.2%; for VILI 91.2%; for cytology 57% and for HPV testing (using Hybrid-Capture 2 assay) 62%(and pooled specificity for VIA was 84.7% for VILI 84.5% for cytology 93% and for HPV testing 94%). In this study pooled prevalence of CIN2+ was 2.3% and PPV was 11.6% and 12.9%, respectively for VIA and VILI and NPV >99% for both techniques. Accuracy of visual methods and cytology increased over time, while performance of the HPV test was constant (Arbyn et al. 2008).

In the setting of HIV infection, there are more limited data. In one study of 205 women correlating VIA with cytology with biopsy as the standard, VIA was more sensitive than Pap smear (76% vs. 57%, respectively) but less specific (83% vs. 95%, respectively); PPV for VIA was only 34% but was also low for cytology at 55%, but NPV for both techniques was high (97% for VIA, 95% for cytology). The prevalence for CIN in this patient population was 10.2% (Akinwuntan 2008). More recently VIA, HPV testing and cytology were compared to colposcopically-directed biopsy in 498 women in Kenya. Both HPV testing and Pap smear had higher sensitivity than VIA, with HPV showing greatest sensitivity (94%, 89% and 79%, respectively), while VIA was superior to HPV testing in terms of specificity (51% for HPV testing, 60% for cytology, 63% for VIA). PPV was low for all three methods (18% for HPV testing, 20% for Pap, 17% for VIA) and NPV was high (99% for HPV testing, 98% for PAP, 95% for VIA) (Chung CROI 2011). In a "see and treat" program in Uganda HIV-infected women had higher likelihood of inflammation, resulting in an increase in false-positive results (Mutyaba et al. 2010).A randomized clinical trial of VIA and HPV testing , with cryotherapy treatment for positive results, was performed among over 6500 women in South Africa, of whom 956 were HIV+. Women were followed for up to 36 months after randomization with colposcopy and biopsy to determine the study endpoint of CIN2+. Screen-and-treat using HPV testing significantly reduced CIN2+ in both HIV+ and HIV- women at follow-up (relative risk 0.20 [95% CI 0.06–0.69] and 0.31 [95% CI 0.20–0.50], respectively), compared to controls with sensitivity of 94% and PPV of 29.9% in HIV+ women; VIA also reduced the likelihood of CIN2+ at follow-up, but to a lesser degree and only reached statistical significance in HIV+ women (RR 0.51 [95% CI 0.29–0.89]), where sensitivity was 63.9% and PPV was (Kuhn et al. 2010). Because HIV+ women had higher rates of CIN2+, both screen-and-treat strategies had a stronger impact at the population level in HIV+ women than in HIV- women. It was estimated that for every 100 women screened HPV screen and treat could prevent 11.9 CIN2+ cases in HIV+ women and VIA screen and treat could prevent 7.4 cases of CIN2+ in HIV+ women.

A comparison of VIA and HPV testing is found in Table 1. In computer-based models, both VIA and HPV testing are cost-effective alternatives to conventional cytology-based programs, which usually require three visits, in low resource settings (Goldie et al. 2005). While HPV testing is more objective and reproducible and has higher sensitivity than VIA, it has some significant disadvantages for lower resource countries. A rapid HPV test has now been developed (Care-HPV, Qiagen Inc.) but is not yet commercially available), but costs (estimated at $5–10 US) are still largely prohibitive in areas where annual health expenditures are often under <$5 per person. Furthermore, although results can be available the same day, they are not available instantly, but are run in batches and require up to 3 hours for actual testing. VIA is inherently subjective and less reproducible, as reflected by low inter-rater agreement was seen among both midwives and gynecologists compared to lead reference physicians regarding cryotherapy treatability (Gage et al. 2009), but performance seems to improve with experience. A number of studies have shown the sensitivity of VIA to be similar to or higher than that of cytology. It is inexpensive, with low costs, including cost of supplies and cost to the patient because of the ability to treat abnormalities at the same visit. VIA can be task-shifted to lower level health workers and, most notably, allows single visit screening and treatment. Furthermore, VIA has been shown to be safe, feasible and acceptable in multiple studies (Phongsavan et al. 2011; Sankaranarayanan et al. 2007; Palanuwong 2007; Sanghvi et al. 2008). The positive predictive value of VIA is low and fairly common conditions such as cervicitis may cause false positive VIA results (Davis-Dao 2008). It remains unclear how the greater prevalence of HPV infection in HIV-infected women will affect performance characteristics of HPV testing as a primary screen in this population.

An advantage of HPV testing is that pelvic exam is not required, but simply insertion of a swab into the vagina to obtain the sample; furthermore, studies have shown that accurate results can be obtained with self-testing, where the woman insert the swab into her own vagina (Ogilvie et al. 2005; Balasubramanian et al. 2010), that this compares favorably to collection by clinicians (Bhatla et al. 2009; Petignat et al. 2007) and is acceptable to women (Mitchell et al. 2011; Lack et al. 2005). However, treatment of positive results clearly requires access to and good visualization of the cervix. On the other hand, VIA is inherently subjective and less reproducible; however a number of studies have shown its sensitivity to be similar to or higher than that of cytology, it is inexpensive, can be task-shifted to lower level health workers and, most notably allow single visit treatment. It remains unclear how the greater prevalence of HPV infection in HIV-infected women will affect performance characteristics of HPV testing as a primary screen in this population.

	Outcome	Sensitivity (%) (min-max-pooled)	Specificity (%) (min-max-pooled)
VIA	CIN 2 +	65-91-79	74-95-85
VILI	CIN 2 +	74-98-91	73-92-85
Cytology	CIN 2 +	33-82-57	87-99-93
HPV Hybrid Capture 2	CIN 2 +	48-68-62	92-95-95

Table 1. Sensitivity and specificity of 4 screening tests for CIN 2+ cervical lesion, minimum, maximum and pooled measures

Minimum, maximum and pooled measure of sensitivity and specificity adapted from Table 3.

Marc Arbyn1, Rengaswamy Sankaranarayanan, Richard Muwonge, Namory Keita, Amadou Dolo, Charles Gombe Mbalawa, Hassan Nouhou, Boblewende Sakande, Ramani Wesley, Thara Somanathan, Anjali Sharma, Surendra Shastri and Parthasarathy Basu. Pooled analysis of the accuracy of five cervical cancer screening tests assessed in eleven studies in Africa and India. Int. J. Cancer: 123, 153–160 (2008).

As yet, there has been fairly limited programmatic experience with these screening techniques in the setting of HIV. Jhpiego has introduced a VIA/SVA program in Guyana, Cote d'Ivoire and Tanzania, screening over 16,000 women from 2009–2010. Services were provided by trained nurses and midwives at HIV care and treatment sites and general health facilities. In all 3 countries HIV+ women were more likely to be VIA+ than HIV-/unknown women. In all 3 countries HIV+ women who were VIA+ were more likely to have large lesions (occupying >75% cervix) and therefore ineligible for cryotherapy. Eighty-two% of eligible women had same-day treatment with cryotherapy; of those who postponed, 44% did not return for treatment (Anderson 2011). These findings confirm cytology-based studies that HIV+ women are at greater risk for cervical dysplasia and is consistent with other studies suggesting that a larger volume of the cervix involved. It also supports the feasibility of VIA/SVA from a programmatic standpoint and suggests that this approach results in reduction of loss to follow-up as compared to screening requiring a subsequent visit.

As HPV testing becomes more affordable and accessible, and particularly if it can be done as a genuinely rapid point-of-care test, it is possible that a hybrid approach to cervical screening may maximize accuracy and minimize unnecessary treatment. In this scenario, HPV testing could be the primary screening method, with VIA performed on those who are

HPV+ to assess the presence of disease and the feasibility of treatment. Those who are HPV-negative would receive no further screening. Alternatively, VIA could be the initial screen, with those who are VIA+ having HPV testing to improve PPV.

5. Treatment

A cervical cancer screening program cannot be effective unless there is an effective intervention to prevent the development of cervical cancer. Excisional or ablative treatment is indicated for the presence of high grade lesions, which encompasses a diagnosis of moderate-severe cervical dysplasia or carcinoma-in-situ and are the immediate precursors of invasive cervical cancer (ICC). Hysterectomy should not be used as a primary treatment for high-grade cervical dysplasia without first ruling out the presence of invasive cancer with an excisional procedure. The most common procedures used for treatment are loop electrosurgical excisional procedure (LEEP), cryotherapy or cervical conization. Table 2 summarizes the key characteristics of each treatment option.

	Cervical Conization	**LEEP**	**Cryotherapy**
Anesthesia required	General or regional	Local	None
Other resources needed	Operating room supplies, instruments, personnel, anesthetics	Electrical generator, wire loops (different sizes)	Cryoprobes (different sizes), CO_2 tank
Effectiveness *	96%+	96%+	88%
Technical difficulty	Highest	Intermediate	Lowest–nurses, midwives can safely and effectively perform
Complications	Highest: bleeding, stenosis, adverse pregnancy outcomes most common	Intermediate: dependent on amount of tissue removed; excessive bleeding during or after procedure most common	Lowest: <1–2%, generally minor
Pathologic specimen	Yes	Yes	No
Cost	Highest	Intermediate	Lowest

*Effectiveness figures cited based on studies in general populations. In HIV + women, the effectiveness is expected to be lower for all techniques.

Table 2. Comparison of treatment methods for cervical dysplasia.

Cervical conization requires regional or general anesthesia and removes a larger volume of tissue. There are higher complication rates after the procedure, including postoperative bleeding (5–15%), infection (02–6.8%), cervical stenosis (approximately 8%) and increased risk of preterm delivery (Hoffman and Mann 2010; Arbyn et al. 2008). This procedure is typically used when lesions are entirely within the cervical canal (based on pathologic analysis of endocervical curettage), are thought to extend high into the cervical canal or when invasive cancer is suspected, so that accurate pathological examination can be performed and, when preinvasive, the entire lesion can be removed.

LEEP has supplanted cervical conization in many situations, including lesions that are believed to extend more superficially into the canal. LEEP utilizes a thin wire in the shape of a loop and electrosurgical generators; the loops are available in a variety of sizes and can also be passed through tissue with several passes if needed to remove the entire area of abnormality, therefore tailoring the procedure to the size of the lesion on the extocervix. The depth of excision can be fairly precisely determined and controlled. LEEP can be performed under local anesthesia and removes less tissue than conization. Complications are less common than after conization (postoperative bleeding 0–8%, infection 0–2%, cervical stenosis 4.3–7.7%; preterm delivery-no increased risk) (Hoffman and Mann 2010; Arbyn et al. 2008).

Cryotherapy uses nitrous oxide or carbon dioxide to freeze the cervix and destroy precancerous tissues and can be performed without anesthesia or electricity. Freezing is done in two cycles of three minutes with five minutes of thawing in between (Sellors 2003). Mid-level providers have been trained successfully to perform cryotherapy safely and with a high degree of acceptability (Bradley 2006; Nene et al. 2008). Carbon dioxide (CO_2) provides a less expensive alternative to nitrous oxide and produces equally low temperatures (Sirivongrangson 2007). However, some studies report that CO_2 may cause cryotherapy blockage up to 50% (Sirivongrangson 2007; Winkler 2010). The quality of cryotherapy devices rather than gas could be responsible for variant temperature (Winkler 2010). The freeze-clear-freeze technique, often employed to reduce gas blockage, may also produce temperatures not sufficiently low enough for treatment to be effective (Winkler 2010). It is important for providers to give adequate treatment by paying attention to visual cues that confirm freezing. Cryotherapy does not provide a tissue specimen. For cryotherapy to be optimally effective, the entire lesion and ideally the entire transformation zone must be visible and the lesion should occupy less than three-fourths of the transformation zone (Sankaranarayanan 2008). Adverse effects after cryotherapy are relatively uncommon and generally minor, reported in 1–2% of women (Cirisano 1999; Sankaranarayanan 2007; Nene 2008). Discomfort usually resolves within a week after treatment (Chamot 2010; Bradley 2006). Significant bleeding after cryotherapy is uncommon. After cryotherapy, watery discharge generally continues for several weeks. Post-treatment infection and pelvic inflammatory disease for LEEP and cryotherapy are both rare (Chamot 2010). The risk of cervical stenosis after cryotherapy is low (<1%) (Loobuyck and Duncan 1993) and the risk of obstetric complications, particularly preterm delivery, is lower after cryotherapy than after excisional procedures. Complications after cryotherapy do not differ among developed and developing countries.

In lower resource areas, the advantages of cryotherapy are significant: the ability to perform the procedure without anesthesia, lack of need for electricity, the lower level of technical expertise required to perform the procedure and lower costs. A significant advantage of LEEP is the ability to examine a tissue sample histologically; however, in areas with few resources, pathological evaluation is usually not available. Studies have generally found LEEP to be associated with somewhat higher cure rates (absence of persistent or recurrent disease) than cryotherapy (Melnikow et al. 2009). A randomized clinical trial of cryotherapy and LEEP for treatment of histologically confirmed high-grade cervical dysplasia found that LEEP had higher overall cure rate of 96.4% as compared to 88.3% for cryotherapy ($p=0.026$) (Chirenje et al. 2001). Treatment methods are generally consistent among high-income and low-income countries (Luciani 2008). Cryotherapy is less effective in older women, where the transformation zone and any cervical lesions are more likely to recede into the cervical canal and is less effective with large lesions. This raises potential concerns in the management of HIV+ women, who may have lesions occupying a larger volume of the cervix.

One of the treatment effects with either cryotherapy or LEEP may be stimulation of the immune response, promoting clearance of HPV after treatment, even if the entire lesion or the entire transformation zone is not excised or ablated, although one small study failed to show an effect of cryotherapy on HPV clearance one year after treatment (Taylor 2010; Chumworathayi et al. 2010).

HIV-positive women have an increased incidence of persistence or recurrence after treatment, with some studies documenting >50% recurrence rate (Tebeu et al. 2006). Recurrence rates are increased in the following situations:

- positive surgical margins with LEEP or cervical conization (present in >40% of HIV+ women) (Boardman et al. 1999; Gilles et al. 2005; Lima et al. 2009).
- glandular involvement (Lima et al. 2009).
- greater immunosuppression (Holcomb et al. 1999; Shah et al. 2008)
- lack of suppressive ART (Robinson et al. 2001).

Most recurrences in HIV+ women appear to be low-grade disease, which may be associated with new HPV infections (Massad et al. 2007) but re-excision may be necessary in some cases (Holcomb et al. 1999; Gingelmaier et al. 2007). Follow-up with cervical cytology alone or cytology and colposcopy together at 6-month intervals over the first year after treatment is recommended (CDC 2009; Wright et al. 2007).

There remain limited data on the use of LEEP and cryotherapy in the setting of HIV, especially related to efficacy. A study of HIV-infected and –uninfected women in Zimbabwe, cryotherapy had a 40.5% failure rate among HIV+ women at one year of follow-up, compared to 15.8% failure rate among HIV- women; in the same study, LEEP had 14% and 0% failure rates, respectively, among HIV+ and HIV- women (CHirenje 2003). However, over 50% of failures were low-grade lesions. LEEP was associated with higher complication rates, including excessive bleeding,and discharge, than cryotherapy. A study from Zambia of cryotherapy-ineligible women (many of whom were HIV+), referred for further management, LEEP (performed by physicians) was feasible and safe, with low levels of complications that can be managed locally (Pfaendler et al. 2008).

Abstinence should be emphasized until complete healing has occurred after treatment for cervical dysplasia, since the treatment has been shown to dramatically increase genital tract HIV shedding (Wright 2001) and may increase risk of sexual transmission of HIV. However, a recent study from Kenya found no increase in detectable cervical HIV-1 RNA among HIV-positive women (most on ART) after cryotherapy. (Chung et al. 2011).

6. Research questions and programmatic issues

There remain a number of unanswered questions and challenges regarding the implementation and integration of effective cervical cancer screening programs into HIV care and treatment. Data regarding antiretroviral treatment and CD4 counts correlated with

VIA results are important to further refine screening and treatment protocols and inform guidelines on appropriate screening strategies and intervals. Integration of cervical cancer screening for HIV+ women requires testing of different models for training, implementation and data collection. Given the information currently available of the interaction of HPV and HIV infections and the epidemiology of HIV:

- Will screening earlier in the course of HIV, when there is less immunosuppression, be associated with smaller and more treatable lesions?
- Will ART and associated immune reconstitution make a difference in rates of VIA positivity and lesion size?
- How often should screening occur in HIV+ women?
- Are HIV+ women more likely to accept SVA than HIV- women?
- What is the relative efficacy and safety of LEEP vs cryotherapy in HIV+ women?
- What are appropriate models of care and what is their feasibility?
- How will VIA and HPV testing be best integrated to enhance test performance, feasibility and scale-up?
- How will cervical cancer prevention be taken to scale in low and middle income countries?

7. Primary prevention of HPV/cervical cancer

Given the millions of new HPV infections/ year in 14-44 year olds primary prevention of HPV infections should be a priority. Consistent and correct use of condoms has been associated with reduction in risk for acquisition of genital HPV infection, including genital warts, CIN and cervical cancer (Winer et al. 2006; Vaccarella et al. 2006; Manhart and Koutsky 2002) although data are limited in the HIV setting. Male circumcision (MC) has been shown to reduce by reduce the risk of sexual HIV transmission from female to male by 60% (http://www.who.int/hiv/topics/malecircumcision/en/index.html) in randomized clinical trials. MC was also associated with a lower incidence of multiple high-risk HPV types and increased clearance of HR-HPVs as compared to controls (14.8% vs 22.3%, respectively) in Uganda (Gray et al. 2010); however, MC was not associated with decreased incidence or increased clearance of HR-HPV in the female partners of circumcised men 24 months after the procedure, as compared to partners of men in the control group (Tobian et al. 2011) However, MC has long been associated with reduced risk of cervical cancer in the wives of circumcised men; therefore further study is warranted.

Finally, two HPV preventive vaccines are now available, one quadrivalent, providing protection against HPV types 16, 18, 6, 11, and the second bivalent, protecting against HPV types 16 and 18 only. In the initial trials of these vaccines, there was >95% -100% protection against incident infection with vaccine subtypes in women not previously infected with those subtypes and in CIN2 or greater related to HPV-16 or 18 (FUTURE II Study Group, 2007; Villa et al. 2005; Paavonen et al. 2009, Garland et al. 2007) vaccine effectiveness was maintained through over 7 years of follow-up (FUTURE I/II Study Group 2010). Although there are other high risk HPV types, types 16 and 18 are responsible for approximately 70% of invasive cervical cancers worldwide (de Sanjose et al. 2010). Recent HPV seroprevalence studies in HIV+ African women found that 65% were seropositive for one of the vaccine subtypes (Firnhaber 2011), suggesting that early vaccination may provide significant protection. However, a recent review found that HIV-infected women in different geographic regions (including Zambia, Brazil, US) appear to be infected with less prevalent HR-HPV types as compared to the general population (McKenzie et al. 2010) . As yet there are limited data on safety, immune response and efficacy of the HPV vaccine in HIV+ women, although studies are on-going. Although data on the safety of the quadrivalent vaccine in HIV-infected children has been demonstrated, efficacy of the currently available HPV vaccines in women or girls with HIV has not yet been established (Levin et al. 2010).

Given the high rates of HPV and cervical cancer in countries with limited health resources, initiatives to introduce HPV vaccination for young people prior to the initiation of sexual activity in these settings are critical. The HPV vaccine is the most expensive vaccine ever developed and costs must be lowered to make this a feasible intervention in the developing world. Fortunately, groups such as GAVI and others are working with governments and other potential donors, as well as with the vaccine makers, to make these vaccines more accessible in areas where they are needed most. Given the high prevalence of both HIV and HPV in many low resource settings and the virologic synergy between these two viruses, with increased rates of HPV-related disease in HIV+ individuals, HIV+ women may be a particular target group for vaccine administration. Furthermore, with improved access to antiretroviral treatment and greater longevity, an increasing number of girls who have been perinatally infected with HIV will be living into adulthood and these girls may particularly benefit from HPV vaccination.

Mathematical models estimate that reduction in incidence and mortality of cervical cancer will be greatest in low/middle income countries with no or limited screening and that HPV vaccination may be cost-effective if cost <$10–25/vaccinated girl (Kim JJ et al. 2008). Currently, the WHO recommends including routine HPV vaccination in national immunization programs, providing prevention of cervical cancer is a public health priority, programmatically feasible, cost-effective, and has sustainable financing (WHO 2009). HIV infection is not considered a contraindication to HPV vaccination (CDC 2007; ACOG 2010; CDC 2009).

8. Conclusion

Cervical cancer is a leading cause of morbidity and mortality in countries with the fewest resources and these resources are often already over-stretched by high levels of HIV infection. Virologic synergy between HIV and HPV infections further exacerbates the problem, and HIV-infected women are at increased risk for HPV and HPV-related diseases, including cervical cancer. Furthermore, unlike other typical opportunistic infections, there is no compelling evidence that the use of effective ART reduces the burden of HPV or HPV-related complications, possibly leading to increased numbers of women at risk for cervical cancer as HIV treatment programs become more accessible and successful. Fortunately, cervical cancer is preceded by an extended precancerous period that can be detected and treated to prevent the development of invasive disease. Cervical cytology, which has revolutionized cervical cancer prevention in the U.S. and other developed countries over the past half-century, is simply not feasible for most countries with few resources. Alternatives such as VIA and HPV testing hold great promise as alternative screening strategies, coupled with the use of cryotherapy or LEEP to treat precancerous lesions. In the new WHO Global health sector strategy on HIV/AIDS an over-arching goal is to achieve universal access to comprehensive HIV prevention, treatment and care. Two of the four strategic directions noted in this strategy are to leverage broader health outcomes through HIV responses, including strengthening linkages between HIV and other related health programs, notably including cervical cancer screening and care, and to build strong and sustainable heath systems in which HIV and other essential services are available, accessible, affordable and sustainable. This renewed emphasis on comprehensiveness and integration of services is consistent with making further evaluation of the role of these screening techniques, individually or in concert, in the setting of HIV a research priority.

9. References

(2010) Moving cancer up the global health agenda. *The Lancet*, Vol. 375, No. 9371, (Jun 2010), p. 2051, ISSN 0140-6736

ACOG. Cervical cytology screening. (2009). ACOG Practice Bulletin No. 109. *Obstet Gynecol*, Vol. 114, No. 6, (Dec 2009), pp. 1409-20, ISSN 0029-7844

ACOG. Gynecologic care for women with human immunodeficiency virus. (2010). ACOG Practice Bulletin No. 117. *Obstet Gynecol*, Vol. 116, No. 6, (Dec 2010), pp. 1492–509, ISSN 0029-7844

ACOG. Human papillomavirus vaccination. (2010). ACOG Committee Opinion No. 467. *Obstet Gynecol*, Vol. 116, (Sep 2010), pp. 800–803, ISSN 1074-861X

Ahdieh L, Klein RS, Burk R, et al. (2001). Prevalence, incidence, and type-specific persistence of human papillomavirus in human immunodeficiency virus (HIV)-positive and HIV-negative women. *J Infect Dis*, Vol. 184, No. 6, (Sep 2001), pp. 682–690, ISSN 0022-1899

Ahdieh L, Munoz A, Vlahov D, Trimble C, Timpson L, Shah K. (2000). Cervical neoplasia and repeated positivity of human papillomavirus infection in human immunodeficiency virus-seropositive and -seronegative women. *Am J Epidemiol*, Vol. 151, No. 12, (Jun 2000), pp. 1148–1157, ISSN 0002-9262

AHRQ. (2010) Co-Locating Gynecologic Services Within an HIV Clinic Increases Cervical Cancer Screening Rates, Leading to Identification and Treatment of Many Cancer Cases. November 28, 2010, Available from: http://www.innovations.ahrq.gov/content.aspx?id=2393

Akinwuntan AL, Adesina OA, Okolo CA, Oluwasola OA, Oladokun A, Ifemeje AA, Adewole IF. (2008). Correlation of cervical cytology and visual inspection with acetic acid in HIV-positive women. *J Obstet Gynaecol*, Vol. 28, No. 6, (Aug 2008), pp. 638–41, ISSN 0144-3615

Anderson JR. Gynecologic problems. (2005). In: A Guide to the Clinical Care of Women with HIV (Ed. Anderson JR). U.S. Department of Health and Human Services, Health Resrources and Services Administration, HIV/AIDS Bureau. U.S. Government Printing Office, Washington, D.C. 2005

Anderson J, Lu E, Harris M, Kibwana S, Estep D, Varallo J, Coulibaly Toure K, Giattas M. (2011) Initial Results from a Multi-country Cervical Cancer Screening Program for HIV+ Women. 18th Conference on Retroviruses and Opportunistic Infections. Abstract 783. Boston, MA. Feb 27-Mar 2, 2011

Anorlu RI. (2008) Cervical cancer: the sub-Saharan African perspective. *Reprod Health Matters*, Vol. 16, No. 32, (Nov 2008), pp. 41-9, ISSN 0968-8080

Anorlu RI, Banjo AAF, Odoemhum C, et al. (2000) Cervical cancer and cervical cancer screening: level of awareness in women attending a primary health care facility in

Lagos, Nigeria. *Nigeria Postgraduate Medical Journal*, Vol. 70, (2000), pp. 25–28, ISSN: 1117-1936

Arbyn M, Sankaranarayanan R, Muwonge R, Keita N, Dolo A, Mbalawa CG, Nouhou H, Sakande B, Wesley R, Somanathan T, Sharma A, Shastri S, Basu P. (2008). Pooled analysis of the accuracy of five cervical cancer screening tests assessed in eleven studies in Africa and India. *Int. J. Cancer*, Vol. 123, No. 1, (Jul 2008), pp. 153–160, ISSN 0020-7136

Arbyn M, Kyrgiou M, Simoens C, Raifu AO, Koliopoulos G, Martin-Hirsch P, Prendiville W, Paraskevaidis E. (2008) Perinatal mortality and other severe adverse pregnancy outcomes associated with treatment of cervical intraepithelial neoplasia: meta-analysis. *BMJ*, Vol. 337:a1284, (Sep 2008), ISSN 0959-8138

Ashraf H. (2003) Poor nations need more help to slow growing cancer burden: the International Atomic Energy Agency asks donors to provide millions of dollars to buy radiotherapy equipment. *Lancet*, Vol. 361, No. 9376, (Jun 2003), p. 2209 ISSN 0140-6736

Atashili J, Smith JS, Adimora AA et al. (2011) Potential Impact of Antiretroviral Therapy and Screening on Cervical Cancer Mortality in HIV-Positive Women in Sub-Saharan Africa: A Simulation. PLoS ONE 6:4 (2011): E18527, ISSN 1932-6203

Ayinde OA, Omigbodun AO. (2003) Knowledge, attitude and practices related to prevention of cancer of the cervix among female health workers in Ibadan. *J Obstet Gynaecol*, Vol. 23, No. 1, (2003), pp. 55–58, ISSN 0144-3615

Balasubramanian A, Kulasingam SL, Baer A, Hughes JP, Myers ER, Mao C, Kiviat NB, Koutsky LA.(2010). Accuracy and cost-effectiveness of cervical cancer screening by high-risk human papillomavirus DNA testing of self-collected vaginal samples. *J Low Gen Tract Dis*, Vol. 14, No. 3, (Jul 2010), pp. 185–195, ISSN 1089-2591

Bhatla N, Dar L, Patro AR, Kumar P, Kriplani A, Gulati A, Iyer VK, Mathur SR, Sreenivas V, Shah KV, Gravitt PE. (2009) Can human papillomavirus DNA testing of self-collected vaginal samples compare with physician-collected cervical samples and cytology for cervical cancer screening in developing countries? *Cancer Epidem*, Vol. 33, No. 6, (Dec 2009), pp. 446–450, ISSN 1877-7821

Boardman LA, Peipert JF, Hogan JW, Cooper AS. (1999). Positive cone biopsy specimen margins in women infected with the human immunodeficiency virus. *Am J Obstet Gynecol*, Vol. 181, .No. 6, (Dec 1999), pp. 1395–1399, ISSN 0002-9378

Bradley J, Coffey P, Arrossi S, Agurto I, et al. (2006). Women's Perspectives on Cervical Screening and Treatment in Developing Countries: Experiences with New Technologies and Service Delivery Strategies. *Women Health*, Vol. 43, No. 3, (2006), pp. 103–121, ISSN 0363-0242

Branca M, Garbuglia AR, Benedetto A, et al. (2003). Factors predicting the persistence of genital human papillomavirus infections and Pap smear abnormality in HIV-positive and HIV-negative women during prospective follow-up. *Int J STD AIDS*, Vol. 14, No. 6, (Jun 2003), pp. 417–425, ISSN 0956-4624

Burk RD, Palefsky JM, Massad LS, Bang JY, Anastos K, et al. (1995). Incidence of Cervical Squamous Intraepithelial Lesions Associated With HIV Serostatus, CD4 Cell Counts, and Human Papillomavirus Test Results. *JAMA*, Vol. 293, No. 12, (1995), pp. 1471–1476, ISSN 0098-7484

Cagle AJ, Hu SY, Sellors JW, Bao YP, Lim JM, Li SM, et al. (2010) Use of an expanded gold standard to estimate the accuracy of colposcopy and visual inspection with acetic acid. *Int J Cancer*, Vol. 126, No. 1, (Jan 2010), pp. 156–161, ISSN 0020-7136

Castellsague X, Bosch FX, Munoz N, Meijer,C, Shah K, Sanjosé S, Eluf-Neto J, Ngelangel C, Chichareon S, Smith J, Herrero R, Moreno V, Franceschi S. (2002). Male circumcision, penile human papillomavirus infection, and cervical cancer in femal partners. *N Engl J Med*, Vol. 346, (Apr 2002), pp. 1105–1112, ISSN 0028-4793

Centers for Disease Control and Prevention. (2009). Guidelines for Prevention and Treatment of Opportunistic Infections in HIV-Infected Adults and Adolescents. *MMWR Recomm Rep*, Vol. 58(RR-4), (2009) pp. 1–207, ISSN 1057-5987

Centers for Disease Control and Prevention Advisory Committee on Immunization Practices (ACIP). (2007) Quadrivalent Human Papillomavirus Vaccine: Recommendations of the Advisory Committee on Immunization Practices (ACIP). *MMWR Recomm Rep*,Vol. 56(RR-2), (2007), pp. 1–24, ISSN 1057-5987

Cervical Cancer Action Report Card 2011. Available from http://www.cervicalcanceraction.org/pubs/CCA_reportcard_low-res.pdf

Cervical Cancer. NIH Consensus Statement. NIH, Vol. 14(1), (Apr 1996), pp. 1–38

Chamot E, Sibylle K, Stringer J SA, Mwanahamuntu MH. (2010) Are Treatments for Cervical Precancerous Lesions in Less-developed Countries Safe Enough to Promote Scaling-up of Cervical Screening Programs? A Systematic View. BMC Women's Health, 10:11, (2010), ISSN 1472-6874

Chaturvedi AK, Madeleine MM, Biggar RJ, Engels EA. (2009). Risk of human papillomavirus-associated cancers among persons with AIDS. *J Natl Cancer Inst*, Vol. 101, No. 16, (2009), pp. 1120–30, ISSN 0027-8874

Chirenje ZM, Rusakaniko S, Akino V, Mlingo M. (2001). A randomised clinical trial of loop electrosurgical excision procedure (LEEP) versus cryotherapy in the treatment of cervical intraepithelial neoplasia. *J Obstet Gynaecol*, Vol. 21, No. 6, (Nov 2001), pp. 617 -621, ISSN 0144-3615

Chirenje ZM, Rusakaniko S, Akino V, Munjoma M, Mlingo, M. (2003) Effect of HIV Disease in Treatment Outcome of Cervical Squamous Intraepithelial Lesions Among Zimbabwean Women. J Low Gen Tract Dis , Vol. 7, No. 1, (Jan 2003), pp. 16-21, ISSN 1089-2591

Chumworathayi B, Eamratsameekool W, Kularbkaew C, Chumworathayi P. (2008) Visual Inspection with Acetic Acid Test Qualities in a Secondary Setting. J. Obstet. Gynaecol Res, Vol. 34, No. 5, (Oct 2008), pp. 909-13, ISSN 1447-0756

Chumworathayi B, Thinkhamrop J, Blumenthal P, Thinkhamrop B, Pientong C, Ekalaksananan T. (2010) Cryotherapy for HPV Clearance in Women with Biopsy-confirmed Cervical Low-grade Squamous Intraepithelial Lesions. Int J Gynecol Obstet, Vol. 108, No. 2, (Feb 2010), pp. 119-22, ISSN: 0020-7292

Chung MH, McKenzie KP, Richardson BA, John-Stewart GC, Coombs RW, De Vuyst H, Njoroge JW, Nyongesa-Malava E, Sakr SR, Mugo NR. (2011) Cervical HIV-1 RNA Shedding after Cryotherapy among HIV-positive Women with Cervical Intraepithelial Neoplasia Stage 2 or 3. *AIDS*. 2011 Jun 29. [Epub ahead of print]

Chung M, McKenzie K, De Vuyst H, Pamnani R, Rana F, Njoroge J, John-Stewart G, Richardson B, Sakr S, Mugo N. (2011) Comparing Visual Inspection with Acetic Acid, High-risk HPV Testing, and Pap Smear to Colposcopic Biopsy among HIV+ Women. 18th Conference on Retroviruses and Opportunistic Infections. Abstract 41. Boston, MA. Feb 27-Mar 2, 2011.

Clifford GM, Smith JS, Aguado T, Franceschi S. (2003) Comparison of HPV type distribution in high-grade cervical lesions and cervical cancer: a meta-analysis. *Br J Cancer*, Vol. 89, No. 1, (Jul 2003),pp. 101-5, ISSN 0007-0920

Clifford GM, Goncalves MAG, Franceschi S. (2006) Human papillomavirus types among women infected with HIV: a meta-analysis. *AIDS*, Vol. 20, No. 18, (Nov 2006), pp. 2337-44, ISSN 0269-9370

Cogliano V, Baan R, Straif K, et al. (2005). Carcinogenicity of human papillomaviruses. *Lancet Oncol*, Vol. 6, No. 4, (Apr 2005), p. 204, ISSN 1470-2045

Cohn J, Gagnon S, Spence M, Harrison D, Kluzak T, Langenberg P, Brinson C, Stein A, Hellinger J. (2001) The role of human papillomavirus deoxyribonucleic acid assay and repeated cervical cytologic examination in the detection of cervical intraepithelial neoplasia among human immunodeficiency virus-infected women. Cervical Disease Study Group of the American Foundation for AIDS Research Community Based Clinical Trials Network. *Am J Obstet Gynecol*, Vol. 184, No. 3, (Feb 2001), pp. 322–330, ISSN 0002-9378

Cox J, Schiffman M, Solomon D. (2003) Prospective follow-up suggests similar risk of subsequent cervical intraepithelial neoplasia grade 2 or 3 among women with cervical intraepithelial neoplasia grade 1 or negative colposcopy and directed biopsy. ASCUS-LSIL Triage Study (ALTS) Group. *Am J Obstet Gynecol*, Vol. 188, No. 6, (Jun 2003), pp. 1406–12, ISSN 0002-9378

Cremer M, Conlisk E, Maza M, et al. (2011). Adequacy of Visual Inspection with Acetic Acid in Women of Advancing Age. *Int J Gynaecol Obstet*, Vol. 113, No. 1, (Apr 2011), pp. 68–71, ISSN 0020-7292

Cirisano FD. (1999) Management of pre-invasive disease of the cervix. *Semin Surg Oncol*, Vol. 16, No. 3, (Apr-May 1999), pp. 222-7, ISSN 8756-0437 999

Cronje H, Parham G, Cooreman B, et al. (2003). A comparison of four screening methods for cervical neoplasia in a developing country. *Am J Obstet Gynecol*, Vol. 188, No. 2, (Feb 2003), pp. 395–400, ISSN 0002-9378

Cronjé H. (2004) Screening for cervical cancer in developing countries. *Int J Gynaecol Obstet*, Vol. 84, No. 2, (Feb 2004), pp. 101-8, ISSN 0020-7292

Cusick J, Clavel C, Petry K, Meijer C, Hoyer H, Ratnam S, Szarewski A, Birembaut P, Kulasingam S, Sasieni P, Iftner T. (2006) Overview of the European and North American studies on HPV testing in primary cervical cancer screening. *Int J Cancer*, Vol. 119, No. 5, (Sep 2006), pp.1095-1101, ISSN 0020-7136

Davis AT, Chakraborty H, Flowers L, Mosunjac MB. (2001). Cervical dysplasia in women infected with the human immunodeficiency virus (HIV): a correlation with HIV viral load and CD4+ count. *Gynecol Oncol*, Vol. 80, No. 3, (Mar 2001), pp. 350–354, ISSN 0090-8258

Davis-Dao C, Cremer M, Felix J, Cortessis V. (2008). Effect of cervicitis on visual inspection with acetic acid. *J Low Genit Tract Dis*, Vol. 12, No. 4 (Oct 2008), pp. 282–286, ISSN 1089-2591

Denny L, Boa R, Williamson AL, Allan B, Hardie D, Stan R, Myer L. (2008) Human papillomavirus infection and cervical disease in human immunodeficiency virus-1-infected women. *Obstet Gynecol*, Vol. 111, No. 6, (Jun 2008), pp. 1380-7, ISSN 0029-7844

de Sanjose S, Quint WG, Alemany L, Geraets DT, Klaustermeier JE, Lloveras B et al. (2010) Human papillomavirus genotype attribution in invasive cervical cancer: a retrospective cross-sectional worldwide study. *Lancet Oncol*, Vol. 11, No 11, (Nov 2010), pp. 1048-56, ISSN 1470-2045

De Vuyst H, Gichangi P, Estambale B, Njuguna E, Franceschi S, Temmerman M. (2008) Human papillomavirus types in women with invasive cervical carcinoma by HIV status in Kenya. *Int J Cancer*, Vol. 122, No 1, (Jan 2008), pp. 244-6, ISSN 0020-7136

Eddy DM. Screening for cervical cancer. (1990) *Ann Intern Med*, Vol. 113, No. 3,(Aug 1990), pp.214-26, ISSN 0003-4819

Ellerbrock TV, Chiasson MA, Bush TJ, et al. (2000). Incidence of cervical squamous intraepithelial lesions in HIV-infected women. *JAMA*, Vol. 283, No. 8, (Feb 2000), pp. 1031–1037, ISSN 0098-7484

Evander M, Edlund K, Gustafsson A, et al. (1995). Human papillomavirus infection is transient in young women: a population-based cohort study. *J Infect Dis*, Vol. 171, No. 4, (Apr 1995), pp. 1026–1030, ISSN 0022-1899

Fang-Hui Zhao, et al. Performance of high-risk human papillomavirus DNA testing as a primary screen for cervical cancer: a pooled analysis of individual patient data from 17 population-based studies from China. (2010) *Lancet Oncol* Vol. 11, No. 12, (Dec 2010), pp. 1160-1171, ISSN 1470-2045

Fife K, W.u, J, Squires K, Watts, D, Andersen, J, Brown, D. (2009) Prevalence and Persistence of Cervical Human Papillomavirus Infection in HIV-Positive Women Initiating Highly Active Antiretroviral Therapy.*J Acquir Immune Defic Syndr*, Vol. 51, No. 3 , (Jul 2009), pp. 274-282, ISSN 0894-9255

Firnhaber C, Evans D, Khalili Friedman R, Williams S, Mallhagela K, Wester C, Grinsztejn B, Lockman S. Seroprevalence of HPV Vaccine Types 6, 11, 16 and 18 in HIV+ Women from South Africa, Brazil, and Botswana. 18th Conference on Retroviruses and Opportunistic Infections. Abstract 763. Boston, MA. Feb 27-Mar 2, 2011.

Firnhaber C, Zungu K, Levin S, Michelow P, Montaner LJ, McPhail P, Williamson AL, Allan BR, Van der Horst C, Rinas A, Sanne I. (2009) Diverse and high prevalence of human papillomavirus associated with a significant high rate of cervical dysplasia in human immunodeficiency virus-infected women in Johannesburg, South Africa. *Acta Cytol*, Vol. 53, No. 1,(Jan-Feb 2009),pp. 10-17, ISSN: 0001-5547

FUTURE II Study Group. (2007) Quadrivalent vaccine against human papillomavirus to prevent high-grade cervical lesions. *N Eng J Med*, Vol. 356, No. 19, (May 2007), pp. 1915–1927, ISSN 0028-4793

Gage JC, Rodriguez A, Schiffman M et al. (2009) An Evaluation by Midwives and Gynecologists of Treatability of Cervical Lesions by Cryotherapy Among Human Papillomavirus- Positive Women. *Int J Gynecol Cancer* Vol. 19, No. 4, (May 2009), pp. 728-33, ISSN 1048-891X

Gaffikin L, Blumenthal PD, Emerson M, Limpaphayom K; Royal Thai College of Obstetricians and Gynaecologists (RTCOG)/JHPIEGO Corporation Cervical Cancer Prevention Group. (2003). Safety, acceptability, and feasibility of a single-visit approach to cervical-cancer prevention in rural Thailand: a demonstration project. *Lancet*, Vol. 361, No. 9360, (Mar 2003), pp. 814–820, ISSN 0140-6736

Garland SM, et al. (2007). Quadrivalent vaccine against human papillomavirus to prevent anogenital diseases. *N Engl J Med*, Vol. 356, No. 19, (May 2007), pp. 1928–1943, ISSN 0028-4793

Garzetti GG, Ciavattini A, Butini L, Vecchi A, Montroni M. (1995). Cervical dysplasia in HIV-seropositive women: role of human papillomavirus infection and immune status. *Gynecol Obstet Invest*, Vol. 40, No. 1, pp. 52–56, ISSN 0378-7346

Georgakilas AG, Mosley WG, Georgakila S, Ziech D, Panayiotidis MI (2010). Viral-induced human carcinogenesis: an oxidative stress perspective. Molecular BioSystems Vol 6, pp 1162 - 1172, ISSN 1742 - 2051

Gichangi PB, Bwayo J, Estambale B, De Vuyst H, Ojwang S, Rogo K, Abwao H, Temmerman M. (2003) Impact of HIV infection on invasive cervical cancer in Kenyan women. *AIDS*, Vol. 17, No. 13,(Sep 2003),pp. 1963-8, ISSN 0269-9370

Gilles C, Manigart Y, Konopnicki D, Barlow P, Rozenberg S.(2005) Management and outcome of cervical intraepithelial neoplasia lesions: a study of matched cases according to HIV status. *Gynecol Oncol.* 2005 Jan; Vol. 96, No. 1, (Jan 2005), pp.112-8, ISSN 0090-8258

Gingelmaier A, Grubert T, Kaestner R, Mylonas I, Weissenbacher T, Bergauer F, Barthell L, Friese K. (2007) High recurrence rate of cervical dysplasia and persistence of HPV infection in HIV-1-infected women. *Anticancer Res*, Vol. 27, No. 4A, (Jul-Aug 2007), pp.1795-8,ISSN 0250-7005

Goldie S, Gaffikin L, Goldhaber-Fiebert J, Gordillo-Tobar A, Levin C, Mahe C, Wright T. (2005) Cost effectiveness of cervical screening in five developing countries. *N Engl J Med* Vol. 353, (20), (Nov 2005), pp. 2158–2168, ISSN 0028-4793

Gray RH, Serwadda D, Kong X, et al. (2010) Male circumcision decreases acquisition and increases clearance of high-risk human papillomavirus in HIV-negative men: a randomized trial in Rakai, Uganda, *J Infect Dis*, Vol. 201, No. 10, (May 2010), pp.1455–62, ISSN 0022-1899

Harding R, Higginson IJ. (2005) Palliative care in sub-Saharan Africa. *Lancet.* Vol. 365, No. 9475, (Jun 2005), pp. 1971-7, ISSN 0140-6736

Hawes SE, Critchlow CW, Faye-Niang MA, et al. (2003). Increased risk of high-grade cervical squamous intraepithelial lesions and invasive cervical cancer among African women with human immunodeficiency virus type 1 and 2 infections. *J Infect Dis*, Vol. 188, No. 4, (Aug 2003), pp. 555–563, ISSN 0022-1899

Heard I, Tassie JM, Kazatchkine MD, Orth G. (2002). Highly active antiretroviral therapy enhances regression of cervical intraepithelial neoplasia in HIV-seropositive women. *AIDS*, Vol. 16, No. 13, (Sep 2002), pp. 1799–1802, ISSN 0269-9370

Heard I, Tassie JM, Schmitz V, Mandelbrot L, Kazatchkine MD, Orth G. (2000). Increased risk of cervical disease among human immuodeficiency virus-infected women with severe immunosuppression and high human papillomavirus load. *Obstet Gynecol*, Vol. 96, No. 3, (Sep 2000), pp. 403–409, ISSN 0029-7844

Ho GY, Bierman R, Beardsley L, et al. (1998). Natural history of cervicovaginal papillomavirus infection in young women. *N Engl J Med*, Vol. 338, No. 7, (Feb 1998), pp. 423–428, ISSN 0028-4793

Hoffman MS and Man WJ. Cervical intraepithelial neoplasia: Procedures for cervical conization. Accessed on 8/19/11, Available from http://www.uptodate.com/contents/cervical-intraepithelial-neoplasia-procedures-for-cervical-conization?source=search_result&selectedTitle=1~53

Holcomb K, Matthews RP, Chapman JE, Abulafia O, Lee YC, Borges A, Buhl A. (1999) The efficacy of cervical conization in the treatment of cervical intraepithelial neoplasia in HIV-positive women. *Gynecol Oncol*, Vol. 74, No. 3, (Sep 1999), pp. 428-31, ISSN 0090-8258

International Agency for Research on Cancer. Cervical Cancer Incidence and mortality worldwide in 2008, accessed 8/15/11, Available from: http://globocan.iarc.fr/factsheets/cancer/cervix.asp

Jamieson DJ, Duerr A, Burk R, et al. (2002). HIV Epidemiology Research Study (HERS). Characterization of genital human papillomavirus infection in women who have or who are at risk of having HIV infection. *Am J Obstet Gynecol*, Vol. 186, No. 1, (Jan 2002), pp. 21–27, ISSN 0002-9378

Josefsson A, Magnusson P, Ylitalo N, Sørensen P, Qwarforth-Tubbin P, Andersen P, Melbye M, Adami H, Gyllensten U. (2000) Viral load of human papilloma virus 16 as a determinant for development of cervical carcinoma in situ: a nested case-control study. *Lancet*, Vol. 24, No. 355(9222), (Jun 2000), pp. 2189-93, ISSN 0140-6736

Kahesa C, Mwaiselage J, Wabinga HR, Ngoma T, Kalyango JN, Karamagi C. (2008) Association between invasive cancer of the cervix and HIV-1 infection in Tanzania: the need for dual screening. *BMC Public Health* 8:262, (Jul 2008), ISSN 1471-2458

Kirby T, Allen M, Alvarez R, Hoesley C, Huh W. (2004) High-risk human papillomavirus and cervical intraepithelial neoplasia at time of atypical squamous cells of undetermined significance cytologic results in a population with human immunodeficiency virus. *J Low Genit Tract Dis*, Vol. 8, No. 4, (Oct 2004), pp. 298–303 ISSN 1089-2591

Kim JJ, Brisson M, Edmunds WJ, Goldie SJ. (2008). Modelling cervical cancer prevention in developed countries. *Vaccine*, Vol. 26, Suppl. 10, (Aug 2008), pp. K76–K86, ISSN 0264-410X

Kitchener H, Almonte M, Gilham C, Dowie, R, Stoykova B, Sargent A, Roberts C, Desai M, Peto J, on behalf of the ARTISTIC Trial Study Group. (2009) ARTISTIC: a randomized trial of human papillomavirus (HPV) testing in primary cervical screening. *Health Tech Assess*, 13(51), (2009), pp. 150, ISSN 1366-5278

Klevens RM, Fleming PL, Mays MA, Frey R. (1996). Characteristics of women with AIDS and invasive cancer. *Obstet Gynecol*, Vol. 88, No. 2, (Aug 1996), pp. 269–273, ISSN 0029-7844

Kolstad P, Klem V. (1976) Long-term followup of 1121 cases of carcinoma in situ. *Obstet Gynecol*, Vol. 48, No. 2, (Aug 1976), pp. 125-9, ISSN 0029-7844

Kryston TB, Georgiev AB, Pissis P, Georgakilas AG (2011). Role of oxidative stress and DNA damage in human carcinogenesis. Mutation Research Vol. 711, pp 193 - 201, ISSN 1383-5718

Kulasingam S, Hughes J, Kiviat N, Mao C, Weiss N, Kuypers J, Koutsky L. (2002) Evaluation of human papillomavirus testing in primary screening for cervical abnormalities: Comparison of sensitivity, specificity and frequency of referral. *JAMA*, Vol. 288, No. 14, (Oct 2002), pp. 1749-1757, ISSN 0098-7484

Lack N, West B, Jeffries D, et al. (2005) Comparison of non-invasive sampling methods for detection of HPV in rural African women. *Sex Transm Infect*, Vol. 81, (2005),pp. 239 -241, ISSN 1368-4973

Kuhn L, Wang C, Tsai WY, Wright TC, Denny L. (2010) Efficacy of HPV based screen-and-treat for cervical cancer prevention among HIV-infected South African women. *AIDS*, Vol. 24, (2010), pp. 2553–2561. ISSN 0002-9378

Levin M, Moscicki A, Song L, Fenton T, Meyer W 3rd, Read J, et al. (2010) Safety and immunogenicity of a quadrivalent human papillomavirus (types 6, 11, 16, and 18) vaccine in HIV-infected children 7 to 12 years old. IMPAACT P1047 Protocol Team. *J Acquir Immune Defic Syndr*, Vol. 55, (2010), pp. 197–204, ISSN 1525-4135

Lillo FB, Ferrari D, Veglia F. (2001). Human papillomavirus infection and associated cervical disease in human immunodeficiency virus-infected women: effect of highly active antiretroviral therapy. *J Infect Dis*, Vol. 184, No. 5, (Sep 2001), pp. 547–551, ISSN 0022-1899

Lima M, Tafuri A, Araújo A, de Miranda Lima L, Melo V. (2009) Cervical intraepithelial neoplasia recurrence after conization in HIV-positive and HIV-negative women. *Int J Gynaecol Obstet*, Vol. 104, No. 2, (Feb 2009), pp. 100-4, ISSN 0020-7292

Lomalisa P, Smith T, Guidozzi F. (2000). Human immunodeficiency virus infection and invasive cervical cancer in South Africa. *Gynecol Oncol*, Vol. 77, No. 3, (Jun 2000), pp. 460–463, ISSN 0090-8258

Lonky N, Mahdavi A, Wolde-Tsadik G, Bajamundi K, Felix J. (2010) Evaluation of the clinical performance of high-risk human papillomavirus testing for primary screening: A retrospective review of the Southern California Permanente Medical Group Experience. *J Low Gen Tract Dis*, Vol. 14, No. 3, (Jul 2010), pp. 200-205. ISSN 1089-2591

Loobuyck H, Duncan I. (1993) Destruction of CIN 1 and 2 with the Semm cold coagulator: 13 years' experience with a see-and-treat policy. *Br J Obstet Gynaecol*. Vol. 100, No. 5, (1993), p. 465, ISSN 0306-5456

Luciani S, Gonzales M, Munoz S, et al. (2008). Effectiveness of Cryotherapy Treatment for Cervical Intraepithelial Neoplasia. *Int J Gynaecol Obstet*, Vol. 101, No. 2, (Nov 2008), pp. 172–177, ISSN 0020-7292

Luque A, Demeter L, Reichman R. (1999). Association of human papillomavirus infection and disease with magnitude of human immunodeficiency virus type 1 (HIV-1) RNA plasma level among women with HIV-1 infection. *J Infect Dis*, Vol. 179, No. 6, (Jun 1999), pp. 1405–1409, ISSN 0022-1899

Luque A, Hitti J, Mwachari C et al. (2010) Prevalence of Human Papillomavirus Genotypes in HIV-1-infected Women in Seattle, USA and Nairobi, Kenya: Results from the Women's HIV Interdisciplinary Network (WHIN). *IJID*, Vol. 14, No. 9, (Jul 2010), E810-814, ISSN 1201-9712

Maiman M, Fruchter RG, Serur E, Remy JC, Feuer G, Boyce J. (1990). Human immunodeficiency virus infection and cervical neoplasia. *Gynecol Oncol*, Vol. 38, No. 3, (Sep 1990), pp. 377–382, ISSN 0090-8258

Maiman M. (1998). Management of cervical neoploasia in human immunodeficiency virus-infected women. *J Natl Cancer Inst Monogr*, Vol. 23, pp. 43–49, ISSN 1052-6773

Manhart L, Koutsky L. (2002) Do condoms prevent genital HPV infection, external genital warts, or cervical neoplasia? A meta-analysis. *Sex Transm Dis*, Vol., 29, No. 11, (Nov 2002), pp. 725-35 , ISSN 0148-5717

Massad L, Ahdieh L, Benning L, et al. (2001). EVol.ution of cervical abnormalities among women with HIV-1: evidence from surveillance cytology in the women's interagency HIV study. *J Acquir Immune Defic Syndr*, Vol. 27, No. 5, (Aug 2001), pp. 432–442, ISSN 1525-4135

Massad L, Evans C, Minkoff H, Watts D, Strickler H, Darragh T,et al. (2004) Natural History of Grade 1 Cervical Intraepithelial Neoplasia in Women With Human Immunodeficiency Virus. *Obstet Gynecol* Vol. 104, (Nov 2004), pp. 1077–85 ISSN 0029-7844

Massad LS, Seaberg EC, Wright RL, Darragh T, Lee YC, Colie C, Burk R, Strickler HD, Watts DH. Squamous cervical lesions in women with human immunodeficiency virus: long-term follow-up. *Obstet Gynecol*, Vol. 111, No. 6, (Jun 2008), pp. 1388-93 ISSN 0029-7844

Massad L, Seaberg E, Watts D, Minkoff H, Levine A, Henry D, Colie C, Darragh T, Hessol N. (2009) Long-term incidence of cervical cancer in women with HIV. *Cancer*, Vol. 115, (2009), pp. 524-30, ISSN 1097-0142

Massad L, Schneider M, Watts D, Strickler H, Melnick S, Palefsky J, et al. (2004) HPV testing for triage of HIV-infected women with papanicolaou smears read as atypical squamous cells of uncertain significance. *J Womens Health*, Vol. 13, (2004), pp. 147–53, ISSN 1540-9996

Massad L, Fazzari M, Anastos K, Klein R, Minkoff H, Jamieson D, Duerr A, Celentano D, Gange S, Cu-Uvin S, Young M, Watts D, Levine A, Schuman P, Harris T, Strickler H. (2007) Outcomes after treatment of cervical intraepithelial neoplasia among women with HIV. *J Low Genit Tract Dis*, Vol. 11,(2007), pp. 90–7, ISSN 1089-2591

McIndoe W, McLean M, Jones R, Mullins P. (1984) The invasive potential of carcinoma in situ of the cervix. *Obstet Gynecol*, Vol. 64, No 4, (Oct 1984), pp. :451-8, ISSN 0029-7844

McKenzie N, Kobetz E, Hnatyszyn J, Twiggs L, Lucci J 3rd. (2010) Women with HIV are more commonly infected with non-16 and -18 high-risk HPV types. *Gynecol Oncol*, Vol. 116, No. 3, (Mar 2010), pp. 572-7, ISSN 0090-8258

Melnikow J, McGahan C, Sawaya GF, et al. (2009). Cervical intraepithelial neoplasia outcomes after treatment: long-term follow-up from the British Columbia Cohort Study. *J Natl Cancer Inst*, Vol. 101, No. 10, (May 2009), pp. 721–728, ISSN 0027-8874

Melnikow J, Nuovo J, Willan A, Chan B, Howell L. (1998) Natural history of cervical squamous intraepithelial lesions: a meta-analysis. *Obstet Gynecol*, Vol. 92, No. 4 (Pt 2), (Oct 1998), pp. 727-35, ISSN 0029-7844

Mesher D, Szarewski A, Cadman L, Cubie H, Kitchener H, Luesley D, Menon U, Hulman G, Desai M, Ho L, Terry G, Williams A, Sasieni P, Cuzick J. (2010) Long-term follow-up of cervical disease in women screened by cytology and HPV testing: Results from the HART study. *Brit J Cancer*. Vol. 102, (2010), pp. 1405-1410, ISSN 0007-0920

Minkoff H, Ahdieh L, Massad LS, et al. (2001). The effect of highly active antiretroviral therapy on cervical cytologic changes associated with oncogenic HPV among HIV-infected women. *AIDS*, Vol. 15, No. 16, pp. 2157–2164 (Nov 2001), ISSN 0269-9370

Minkoff H, Feldman J, DeHovitz J, Landesman S, Burk R. (1998). A longitudinal study of human papillomavirus carriage in human immunodeficiency virus-infected and human immunodeficiency virus-uninfected women. *Am J Obstet Gynecol*, Vol. 178, No. 5, (May 1998), pp. 982–986, ISSN 0002-9378

Minkoff H, Zhong Y, Burk R, Palefsky J, Xue X, Watts D, Levine A, Wright R, Colie C, D'Souza G, Massad L, Strickler H. (2010) Influence of adherent and effective antiretroviral therapy use on human papillomavirus infection and squamous intraepithelial lesions in human immunodeficiency virus-positive women. , Vol. 201, No 5, (Mar 2010), pp. :681-90, ISSN 0022-3476

Mitchell S, Ogilvie G, Steinberg M, Sekikubo M, Biryabarema C, Money D. (2011) Assessing women's willingness to collect their own cervical samples for HPV testing as part of the ASPIRE cervical cancer screening project in Uganda. *Int J Gynaecol Obstet*. Vol. 114, No 2, (Aug 2011), pp. 111-5, ISSN 0020-7292

Moodley J, Kawonga K, Bradley J, et al. (2006). Challenges in implementing a cervical screening program in South Africa. *Cancer Detect and Prev*, Vol. 30, No. 4, pp. 361–368, ISSN 0361-090X

Moodley J, Hoffman M, Carrara H, Allan B, Cooper D, Rosenberg L, Denny L, Shapiro S, Williamson A. (2006) HIV and pre-neoplastic and neoplastic lesions of the cervix in South Africa: a case-control study. *BMC Cancer* 23:135, (2006), ISSN 1471-2407

Moodley J, Constant D, Hoffman M, et al. (2009) Human Papillomavirus prevalence, viral load and precancerous lesions of the cervix in women initiating highly active retroviral therapy in South Africa: a cross sectional study. *BMC Cancer*, 9:275,(2009), ISSN 1471-2407

Moscicki AB, Shiboski S, Broering J, et al. (1998). The natural history of human papillomavirus infection as measured by repeated DNA testing in adolescent and young women. *J Pediatr*, Vol. 132, No. 2, (Feb 1998), pp. 277–284, ISSN 0022-3476

Mutyaba, T et al. (2010) Evaluation of 'see-see and Treat' Strategy and Role of HIV on Cervical Cancer Prevention in Uganda. *Reproductive Health* 7:4, (2010), ESSN 1742-4755

Naucler P, Ryd W, Törnberg S, Strand A, Wadell G, Elfgren K, Rådberg T, Strander B, Forslund O, Hansson B, Hagmar B, Johansson B, Rylander E, Dillner J. (2009) Efficacy of HPV DNA Testing with cytology triage and/or repeat HPV DNA testing in primary cervical cancer screening. *J Natl Cancer Inst*, Vol. 101, (2009), pp. 88-99, ISSN 0027-8874

Nene BM, Hiremath PS, Kane S, Fayette JM, Shastri SS, Sankaranarayanan R. (2008). Effectiveness, safety, and acceptability of cryotherapy by midwives for cervical intraepithelial neoplasia in Maharashtra, India. *Int J Gynaecol Obstet*, Vol. 103, No. 3, (Dec 2008), pp. 232–236, ISSN 0020-7292

Ogilvie G, Patrick DM, Schulzer M, Sellors JW, Petric M, Chambers K, White R, Fitzgerald JM. (2005). Diagnostic accuracy of self collected vaginal specimens for human papillomavirus compared to clinician collected human papillomavirus specimens: a meta-analysis. *Sex Transm Infec*, Vol. 81, No. 3, (Jun 2005), pp. 207-212, ISSN 1368-4973

Oster A, Sulllivan P, Blair J. (2009) Prevalence of cervical cancer screening of HIV-infected women in the United States. *J Acquir Immune Defic Syndr*, Vol. 51, (2009), pp. 430-436, ISSN 1525-4135

Paavonen J, Naud P, Salmerón J, Wheeler C, Chow S, Apter D et al. (2009) Efficacy of human papillomavirus (HPV)-16/18 AS04-adjuvanted vaccine against cervical infection and precancer caused by oncogenic HPV types (PATRICIA): final analysis of a double-blind, randomised study in young women. *Lancet*, Vol. 25, No. 374(9686), (Jul 2009), pp. 301-14, ISSN 0140-6736

Palanuwong B. (2007) Alternative cervical cancer prevention in low-resource settings: Experiences of visual inspection by acetic acid with single-visit approach in the first five provinces of Thailand. *Aust N Z J Obstet Gynaecol.* Vol. 47, No. 1, (feb 2007), pp. 54-60, ISSN: 0004-8666

Palefsky JM, Minkoff H, Kalish LA, et al. (1999). Cervicovaginal human papillomavirus infection in human immunodeficiency virus-1 (HIV)-positive and high risk HIV-negative women. *J Natl Cancer Inst*, Vol. 91, No. 3, (Feb 1999), pp. 226–236, ISSN 0027-8874

Paramsothy P, Jamieson D, Heilig C, Schuman P, Klein R, Shah, K, Rompalo A, Cu-Uvin S, Duerr A. (2009) The effect of highly active antiretroviral therapy on human papillomavirus clearance and cervical cytology. *Obstet Gynecol*, Vol. 113, No. 1, (2009), pp. 26-31, ISSN 0029-7844

Parkin D, Bray F, Ferlay J, et al. (2005) Global Cancer Statistics, 2002. CA: A Cancer Journal for Clinicians Vol. 55, No. 2, (Mar-Apr 2005), pp. 74–108, ISSN 0007-9235

Parkin D, Ferlay J, Hamdi-Cherif M, et al. (2003) Cancer in Africa: Epidemiology and Prevention. IARC Scientific Publications. No.153. Lyon:IARC Press, 2003.

Petignat P, Faltin D, Bruchim I, Tramèr M, Franco EL, Coutlée F. (2007) Are self-collected samples comparable to physician-collected cervical specimens for human papillomavirus DNA testing? A systematic review and meta-analysis. *Gynecol Oncol*, Vol. 105, (2007), pp. 530-535, ISSN ISSN 0090-8258

Petry KU, Bohmer G, Iftner T, Femming P, Stoll M, Schmidt RE. (1999). Human papillomavirus testing in primary screening for cervical cancer of human immunodeficiency virus-infected women, 1990-1998. *Gynecol Oncol*, Vol. 75, No. 3, (Dec 1999), pp. 427–431, ISSN 0090-8258

Phongsavan K, Phengsavanh A, Wahlström R, Marions L. (2011) Safety, feasibility, and acceptability of visual inspection with acetic acid and immediate treatment with cryotherapy in rural Laos. *Int J Gynaecol Obstet*. Vol. 114, No. 3, (Sep 2011), pp. 268-72 ISSN 0020-7292

Pretorius R, Bao Y, Belinson J, Burchette R, Smith J, Qiao Y. (2007) Inappropriate gold standard bias in cervical cancer screening studies. International *Journal of Cancer*, Vol. 121,(2007), pp. 2218–2224, ISSN: 1097-0215

Robinson W, Hamilton C, Michaels S, Kissinger P. (2001) Effect of excisional therapy and highly active antiretroviral therapy on cervical intraepithelial neoplasia in women infected with human immunodeficiency virus. *Am J Obstet Gynecol*, Vol., 184, No. 4, (mar 2001), pp. 538-43, ISSN 0002-9378

Sahasrabuddhe V, Mwanahamuntu M, Vermund S, Huh W, Lyon M, Stringer J, Parham G. (2007) Prevalence and distribution of HPV genotypes among HIV-infected women in Zambia. *Br J Cancer*. Vol. 96, No. 9, (May 2007), pp.1480-3, ISSN 0007-0920

Sanghvi H, Limpaphayom K, Plotkin M et al. (2008) Cervical Cancer Screening Using Visual Inspection with Acetic Acid: Operational Experiences from Ghana and Thailand. Reproductive Health Matters, Vol. 16, No. 32, (Nov 2008), pp. 67-77, ISSN 0968-8080

Sankaranarayanan R, Esmy PO, Rajkumar R, et al. (2007). Effect of visual screening on cervical cancer incidence and mortality in Tamil Nadu, India: a cluster randomized trial. *Lancet*, Vol. 370, No. 9585, (Aug 2007), pp. 398–406, ISSN 0140-6736

Sankaranarayanan R, Thara S, Esmy PO, Basu P. (2008) Cervical Cancer: Screening and Therapeutic Perspectives. Medicinal Principles and Practice Vol. 17, No. 5, (Aug 2008), pp. 351-64, ISSN 1011-7571

Sankaranarayanan R, Rajkumar R, Esmy PO, Fayette JM, Shanthakumary S, Frappart L, et al. (2007) Effectiveness, safety and acceptability of 'see and treat' with cryotherapy by nurses in a cervical screening study in India. *Br J Cancer* Vol. 96, No. 5, (2007), pp. 738–43, ISSN 0007-0920

Sankaranarayanan R, Nene BM, Shastri SS, Jayant K, Muwonge R, Budukh AM, Hingmire S, Malvi SG, Thorat R, Kothari A, Chinoy R, Kelkar R, Kane S, Desai S, Keskar VR, Rajeshwarkar R, Panse N, Dinshaw KA. (2009) HPV screening for cervical cancer in rural India. *N Engl J Med*. Vol. 360, No. 14, (Apr 2009), pp. 1385-94, ISSN 0028-4793

Sarkar K et al. (2011) Oncogenic HPV among HIV Infected Female Population in West Bengal, India. *BMC Infectious Diseases*, 11:72, (2011), ISSN 1471-2334

Sauvaget C, Fayette J, Muwonge R, Wasley R, Sankaranarayanan R. (2011) Accuracy of visual inspection with acetic acid for cervical cancer screening . *Int J Gynaecol Obstet* Vol. 113, No. 1, (2011), pp. 14-24, ISSN 0020-7292

Sawaya G, Grimes D. (1999) New technologies in cervical cytology screening: a word of caution. *Obstet Gynecol*. Vol. 94, No. 2, (Aug 1999), pp. 307-10, ISSN 0029-7844

Schiffman M, Castle PE. (2003). Human papillomavirus: epidemiology and public health. *Arch Pathol Lab Med*, Vol. 127, No. 8, (Aug 2003), pp. 930–934, ISSN 0003-9985

Schiffman M, Castle PE. (2005) The promise of global cervical-cancer prevention. *N Engl J Med*. Vol. 353, No. 20, Nov 2005, pp. 2101-4, ISSN 0028-4793

Schuman P, Ohmit SE, Klein RS, et al. (2003). Longitudinal study of cervical squamous intraepithelial lesions in human immunodeficiency virus (HIV)-seropositive and at risk HIV-seronegative women. *J Infect Dis*, Vol. 188, No. 1, (Jul 2003), pp. 128–136, ISSN 0022-1899

Sellors J, Sankaranarayanan R. (2003). Colposcopy and Treatment of Cervical Intraepithelial Neoplasia. Lyon: International Agency for Research on Cancer

Shah KV, Munoz A, Klein RS, et al. (1996). Prolonged persistence of genital human papillomavirus infections in HIV-infected women. *Int Conf AIDS*, Vol. 11, pp. 345 (Abst Tu.C.2466), July 7–12,1996

Shah S, Montgomery H, Crow JC, Smith CJ, Moore A, Sabin CA, Evans H, Johnson MA. (2008) Cervical intraepithelial neoplasia treatment in Human Immunodeficiency Virus-positive women. *J Obstet Gynaecol*. Vol. 28, No. 3, (Apr 2008), pp. 327-32 , ISSN 0144-3615

Sherigar B, Dalal A, Durdi et al. (2010) Cervical cancer screening by visual inspection with acetic acid - interobserver variability between nurse and physician. *Asian Pacific Journal of Cancer Prevention*, Vol. 11, (2010), pp. 323-326 ISSN 1513-7368

Shingleton H, Patrick R, Johnston W, Smith R. (1995) The current status of the Papanicolaou smear. *CA Cancer J Clin*, Vol.45,(1995)pp. 305–320, ISSN 0007-9235

Sirivongrangson P, Bollen LJ, Chaovavanich A et al. Screening HIV-infected women for cervical cancer in Thailand: findings from a demonstration project. *Sex Transm Dis*, Vol. 34, No. 2,(2007),pp. 104-7, ISSN 0148-5717

Solomon D, Davey D, Kurman R, et al. (2002). The 2001 Bethesda system. Terminology for reporting results of cervical cytology. *JAMA*, Vol. 287, No. 16, (Apr 2002), pp. 2114–2119, ISSN 0098-7484

Stein L, Urban MI, O'Connell D, Yu XQ, Beral V, Newton R, Ruff P, Donde B, Hale M, Patel M, Sitas F. (2008) The spectrum of human immunodeficiency virus-associated cancers in a South African black population: results from a case-control study, 1995-2004. *Int J Cancer*, Vol. 122, (2008), pp.2260-5, ISSN 0020-7136

Stein M, Cunningham W, Nakazono T, et al. (2001). HCSUS Consortium. Screening for cervical cancer in HIV-infected women receiving care in the United States. *J Acquir Immune Defic Syndr*, Vol. 27, No. 5 (Aug 2001), pp. 463–466, ISSN 1525-4135

Sun XW, Kuhn L, Ellerbrock TV, Chiasson MA, Bush TJ, Wright TC. (1997). Human papillomavirus infection in women infected with the human immunodeficiency virus. *N Engl J Med*, Vol. 337, No. 19, (Nov 1997), pp. 1343–1349, ISSN 0028-4793

Swierczynski SL, Lewis-Chambers S, Anderson JR, Keller JM, Hinkle DA, Ali SZ. (2004) Impact of liquid-based gynecologic cytology on an HIV-positive population. *Acta Cytol*, Vol. 48, (2004), pp. 165-72, ISSN 0001-5547

Tarwireyi F, Chirenje ZM,Rusakaniko S. (2003) Cancer of the cervix: knowledge, beliefs and screening behaviours of health workers in Mudzi District in Mashonaland East

Province, Zimbabwe. *Central African Journal of Medicine*, Vol.49, (2003), pp. 83–86, ISSN 0008-9176

Taylor, S. et al. (2010) Acquisition and Reactivation of Human Papillomavirus Infections among Older Women Treated with Cryotherapy: Results from a Randomized Trial in South Africa. *BMC Medicine* 8:40, (2010), ISSN 1741-7015

Tebeu PM, Major AL, Mhawech P, Rapiti E. (2006) The recurrence of cervical intraepithelial neoplasia in HIV-positive women: a review of the literature. *Int J STD AIDS*, Vol.17,No. 8,(Aug 2006),pp. 507-11 ,ISSN 0956-4624

Tello, M, Yeh, H, Keller, JM, Beach, MC, Anderson, JR, Moore, RD. (2008) HIV Women's health: A study of gynecologic service utilization in a U.S. urban clinic. *J Women's Health*, Vol.17, No. 10, (2008), pp. 1609-1614, ISSN 1540-9996

Tobian AA, Kong X, Wawer MJ, Kigozi G, Gravitt PE, Serwadda D et al. (2011) Circumcision of HIV-infected men and transmission of human papillomavirus to female partners: analyses of data from a randomized trial in Rakai, Uganda. *Lancet Infect Dis*, Vol. 11, No. 8, (2011), pp. 604-12, ISSN 0140-6736

Uberti-Foppa C, Origoni M, Maillard M, et al. (1998). Evaluation of the detection of human papillomavirus genotypes in cervical specimens by hybrid capture as screening for precancerous lesions in HIV-positive women. *J Med Virol*, Vol. 56, No. 2, (Oct 1998), pp. 133–137, ISSN 0146-6615

UNAIDS. (2010). Global report: UNAIDS report on the global AIDS epidemic 2010, ISBN 978-92-9173-871-7, Geneva, 2010

Van Bogaert, L. (2011) Age at diagnosis of preinvasive and invasive cervical neoplasia in South Africa: HIV-positive versus HIV-negative women. *Int J Gynecol Cancer* Vol. 21, No. 2, (Feb 2011), pp. 363-66, ISSN 1525-1438

van der Graaf Y, Klinkhamer PJJM, Vooijs GP. (1986) Effect of population screening for cancer of the uterine cervix in Nijmegen, The Netherlands. *Preventive Medicine*, Vol.15, No. 6,(1986), pp. 582-590 , ISSN 0091-7435

Van Schalkwyk SL, Maree JE, Wright SCD. (2008). Cervical cancer: the route from signs and symptoms to treatment in South Africa. *Reprod Health Matters*, Vol. 16, No. 32, pp. 9–17, ISSN 0968-8080

Vaccarella S, Franceschi S, Hererro R, et al. (2006) Sexual Behavior, Condom Use, and Human Papillomavirus: Pooled Analysis of the IARC Human Papillomavirus Prevalence Surveys. *Cancer Epidemiol Biomarkers Prev*, Vol. 15, (2006), pp. 326–33 ,ISSN 1055-9965

Villa LL, Costa RL, Petta CA, Andrade RP, Ault KA, Giuliano AR et al. (2005) Prophylactic quadrivalent human papillomavirus (types 6, 11, 16, and 18) L1 virus-like particle vaccine in young women: a randomised double-blind placebo-controlled multicentre phase II efficacy trial. *Lancet Oncol*. Vol. 6, No. 5, (May 2005), pp. 271-8. ISSN 1470-2045

Walboomers JM, Jacobs MV, Manos MM, Bosch FX, Kummer JA, Shah KV, Snijders PJ, Peto J, Meijer CJ, Muñoz N. (1999) Human papillomavirus is a necessary cause of invasive cervical cancer worldwide. *J Pathol*, Vol. 189, No. 1, (Sep 1999), pp. 12-9 ISSN 1096-0896

Wang C, Wright TC, Denny L, Kuhn L. (2011) Rapid Rise in Detection of Human Papillomavirus (HPV) Infection Soon After Incident HIV Infection Among South African Women. *Journal of Infectious Diseases*, Vol. 203, (2011): pp. 479-86 ISSN 0022-1899

Weissenborn SJ, Funke AM, Hellmich M, et al. (2003). Oncogenic human papillomavirus DNA loads in human immunodeficiency virus-positive women with high-grade cervical lesions are strongly elevated. *J Clin Microbiol*, Vol. 41, No. 6 (Jun 2003), pp. 2763–2767, ISSN 0095-1137

Wellensiek N, Moodley M, Moodley J, et al. (2002) Knowledge of cervical cancer screening and use of cervical screening facilities among women from various socioeconomic backgrounds in Durban, Kwazulu Natal, South Africa. *International Journal of Gynecological Cancer*, Vol. 12,(2002),pp. 376–82, ISSN 1525-1438

Winer RL,Hughes JP, Feng Q, O'Reilly S, Kiviat NB, Holmes KK, Koutsky LA. (2006) Condom Use and the Risk of Genital Human Papillomavirus Infection in Young *Women.N Engl J Med*, Vol. 354, (June 2006), pp. 2645-2654, ISSN 0028-4793

Winkler JL et al. (2010) Effect of the "cough Technique" on Cryotherapy Freezing Temperature.(2010) *Int J Gynecol Obstet*, Vol.108, (2010), pp.115-18 ISSN: 0020-7292

Winkler JL, Jeronimo J, Singleton J et al. (2010) Performance of Cryotherapy Devices Using Nitrous Oxide and Carbon Dioxide. *Int J Gynecol Obstet* , Vol. 111, No. 1 (2010): 73-77. ISSN: 0020-7292

World Health Organization. (2011). Global health sector strategy on HIV/AIDS 2011-2015. ISBN 978-924-1501-65-1, Geneva, 2011

World Health Organization. (2009) Human papillomavirus vaccines WHO position paper. *Weekly Epidemiological Record* Vol. 84, (Apr 2009), pp.118-130

Wright TC, Subbarao S, Ellerbrock TV, et al. (2001). Human immunodeficiency virus 1 expression in the female genital tract in association with cervical inflammation and ulceration. *Am J Obstet Gynecol*, Vol. 184, No. 3, (Feb 2001), pp. 279–285, ISSN 0002-9378

Wright TC, Massad LS, Dunton CJ, Spitzer M, Wilkiinson EJ, Solomon D for the 2006 ASCCP-sponsored consensus conference. (2007) 2006 consensus guidelines for the management of women with cervical intraepithelial neoplasia or adenocarcinoma in-situ. *Am J Obstet Gynecol*, Vol. 197, (2007), pp.340-45. , ISSN 0002-9378

Wright TC, Gagnon S, Richart RM, Ferenczy A. (1992). Treatment of cervical intraepithelial neoplasia using the loop electrosurgical excision procedure. *Obstet Gynecol*, Vol. 79, No. 2, (Feb 1992), pp. 173–178, ISSN 0029-7844

Yang BH, Bray FI, Parkin DM, Sellors JW, Zhang ZF. (2004) Cervical cancer as a priority for prevention in different world regions: an evaluation using years of life lost. *Int J Cancer*, Vol.109, No. 3, (Apr 2004), pp. 418-24. ISSN 0020-7136

Zhao FH,Lin MJ, Chen F, Hu SY, Zhang R, Belinson JL et al. (2010) Performance of high-risk human papillovirus DNA testing as a primary screen for cervical cancer: a pooled analysis of individual patient data from 17 population-based studies in China. *Lancet Oncol* Vol. 11, No. 12, (2010), pp. 1160-71. ISSN 1470-2045

10

Chemopreventive Activity of Mediterranean Medicinal Plants

A.C. Kaliora and A.M. Kountouri
Harokopio University, Department of Science of Dietetics–Nutrition, Laboratory of Chemistry–Biochemistry–Physical Chemistry of Foods, Athens, Greece

1. Introduction

Generally, the use of plants, herbs or other natural products in medicines is since humans inhabited earth. It was "since ever" when humans were trying to find out which plants might be useful to fight several pains and aches, fever, dyspepsia, or wounds. Through the ages, humans learned which plants would cure different illnesses, or might be poisonous and cause even death, and those that could be part of their diet. There are too many examples and references in the pharmaceutical, knowledge that passed from generation to generation. There is ample historical evidence for different usages of herbs by our ancestors. Herbs are the oldest drugs in the world. The initial use was primarily experimental similar to what applied to animals, e.g. against poisonous plants. The first record of the valuable properties of medicinal plants was by the Sumerians (6000 BC), followed by Chinese and Greek. The first book written about herbal plants was by Chinese (4000 BC). However, Greeks were these who spread the use of medicinal plants in West using the knowledge written down by Theophrastus (300 BC). Apollonios wrote about their uses in cosmetology and in religious ceremonies. Hippocrates recommended Pimbinella anisum, of the Umbelliferae family for sneezing and Theophrastus indicated the usefulness of 600 aromatic and medicinal plants in several pathologies. In ancient Rome, Galenus who was the personal physician to Roman emperors and is nowadays considered as "The Father of Pharmacy" was most devoted to aromatherapy. Reports about the uses of essential oils occur even in the Bible, and it was approximately during the 8th century AD when the Arabs improved the methods of extracting the essential oils from natural products and creating novel elixirs and medicines. During the Middle Ages, the essential oils producers were not affected by cholera and plague. During the Renaissance, the use of plants, essential oils, herbs and several other natural products was progressively neglected. The revolution of Chemistry and the synthesis of drugs resulted in almost complete abandonment. However, the impressive results of treating traumas with different botanical products during the two World Wars motivated scientists to further deal the potential of natural products in disease treatment. Aspirin (acetylsalicylic acid), perhaps the most popular painkiller, has a very long history and its medical use stretches back to antiquity. Medicines made from willow and other salicylate-rich plants date back at least to 400 BC. Willow bark extract became recognized for its specific effects on fever, pain and inflammation in the mid-eighteenth century. Lewis and Clark allegedly used willow bark tea in 1803-1806 as a remedy for fever for members of the famous expedition. By the nineteenth century pharmacists were experimenting with and prescribing a variety of chemicals related to salicylic acid, the active component of willow extract. Chemist Charles Frédéric Gerhardt and many other chemists established the compound's chemical structure and devised efficient methods of synthesis of acetylsalicylic acid. Aspirin's popularity grew over and it is now accepted as one of the most efficient drugs in many health problems.

The NCI (National Cancer Institute) has examined more than 30,000 plants with anticancer activity (Ipek, 2005). However, the use of plants as a means treatment is still very limited. From 250,000 to 500,000 species plants, a small percentage has been examined for its medicinal properties. The World Health Organization estimates that 80% of the inhabitants of the earth choose traditional medicine for primary health needs, much of which relies on the use of essential oils from plants. The main aromatic plants belong to the families Labiatae, Umbelliferae, Lauracae, Myrtacae and Compositae.

Today, various types of consumer products based on natural products may appear with different names, which are:

- Neutraceuticals
- Dietary supplements
- Herbal remedies
- Herbal teas and infusions

All the Mediterranean countries are extremely rich in native plants, many of which are cultivated systematically.

For several decades the majority of drug substances were either natural products or compounds. However, in the last century, synthetic chemistry and biotechnology techniques have offered alternatives to natural sources (Harvey, 2009). The past few decades have witnessed a renewed interest in the field and nowadays although to a lesser extent, the field still continues to produce new drugs; half of the drugs approved since 1994 have been based on natural products (Harvey, 2008). Contemporary Western science supports the right use of traditional medicinal plants, which have become a part of many modern therapies after thorough investigations on their quality and safety. There are of course certain steps to take before introducing medicinal plants into disease prevention or treatment. In most cases, research starts when there is knowledge of use of plants by native people for disease treatment within folk medicine. Accurate identification, phytochemical analysis, pharmacological screening, in vitro, animal model and human interventions, further identification of the most bioactive fraction or component and of the exact mechanism underlying the activity, and finally toxicity tests are steps to be taken prior consideration of the candidate medicinal plant or component to be administered in disease. To this end, collaboration among specialists in ethnobotany, ethnopharmacy, ethnopharmacology ethnomedicine, phytochemists, analytical and organic chemists is essential. Depending on the activity investigated other specialists, e.g. in microbiology or in cancer, might be required.

Ethnobotany is the study of the relationships that exist between people and plants. Ethnobotanists aim to document, describe and explain complex relationships between cultures and plants; explore how plants are used for food, medicine, clothing, hunting, and religious ceremonies.

Ethnopharmacology differs from ethnopharmacy in that it is the biological evaluation of how effective traditional medicines are, whereas ethnopharmacy deals instead with much broader considerations of drug use. These considerations are related to the perception, use, and management of pharmaceuticals within a given human society.

Ethnomedicine is the comparative study of how different cultures view disease and how they treat or prevent it; also, the medical beliefs and practices of local cultures, those that have relevant written sources, as well as knowledge and practices that have been orally transmitted over the centuries.

Phytochemistry is the study of phytochemicals that includes techniques such as extraction, isolation and structural elucidation (MS, NMR) of natural products, as well as various chromatography techniques (HPLC, LC-MS).

Although very few people nowadays would abandon the benefits of modern pharmaceutical science or the convenience of technology, a growing interest in medicinal plants and their uses occurs which began in early 1980s. It has been reported that almost 80% of the global population in developing countries use plant materials for health care (Farnsworth et al., 1985). Plants are a good source of chemical compounds many drugs originate from a natural compound isolated from a medicinal plant. Nevertheless, this extended medicinal use reported does not incorporate or result in respective drug discovery. According to estimates only 20% of all plant species have been chemically or biologically evaluated (Cordell, 2003) and therefore the evaluation of a natural product seems to be a great prospect in the seek out for new drugs. Fabricant and Farnsworth (2001) showed that 94 species of plant are utilized for the production of the 122 single agent natural products that are used as single agent drugs around the world. Of these, 72% were used clinically for the same or a related ethnomedical purpose.

This 80% of medicinal plants not yet chemically or biologically evaluated is a major challenge (Cordell & Colvard, 2005). The evidence to date with natural products is intriguing and guarantees greater attention. More research is indicated to bring about the biological effects and how susceptibility factors including nutrient–nutrient interactions and genetics influence the response. Automation, nanotechnology and proteomics, will have an increasingly important impact and thus we must be prepared to use them appropriately (Cordell & Colvard, 2005). Microarray assay systems based on the enhanced knowledge of the human genome will be brought to the level of the routine evaluation of extracts and compounds in order to assess genetic impact.

2. Mediterranean medicinal plants and cancer chemoprevention

Carcinogenesis is generally recognized as a complex and multistep process in which oxidative stress and inflammation plays a crucial role, and distinct molecular and cellular alterations occur (Franco et al., 2008; Kryston et al., 2011). Cancer chemoprevention attempts to interfere in the progress of the disease by using natural or synthetic substances. In the term of chemoprevention, many food components of the Mediterranean diet, gained the "food-borne anticarcinogens" title due to their content on components with chemopreventive properties. Those chemical compounds have proved that they may interrupt or reverse the carcinogenesis process by acting on intracellular signalling network molecules involved in the initiation and/or promotion, but also may arrest or reverse the progression stage of cancer (Ramos, 2008). Those "food-borne anticarcinogens" can be define as either "blocking agents" which act immediately before or during the initiation of carcinogenesis by chemical carcinogens, or "suppressing agents, which act after initiation during the prolonged stages of promotion and progression (I.T. Johnson, 2007). Blocking agents scavenge Reactive Oxygen Species by potentiate the antioxidant enzyme system, or prevent genotoxic carcinogens, from forming adducts with DNA, either by inhibiting their activation from carcinogens or by enhancing their detoxification and excretion (Nelson et al., 1993). Suppressing agents act after initiation, during the prolonged stages of promotion and progression. They may prevent further DNA damage, induce cell-cycle arrest or apoptosis, as well as inhibit inflammation, invasion or angiogenesis (Fig. 1).

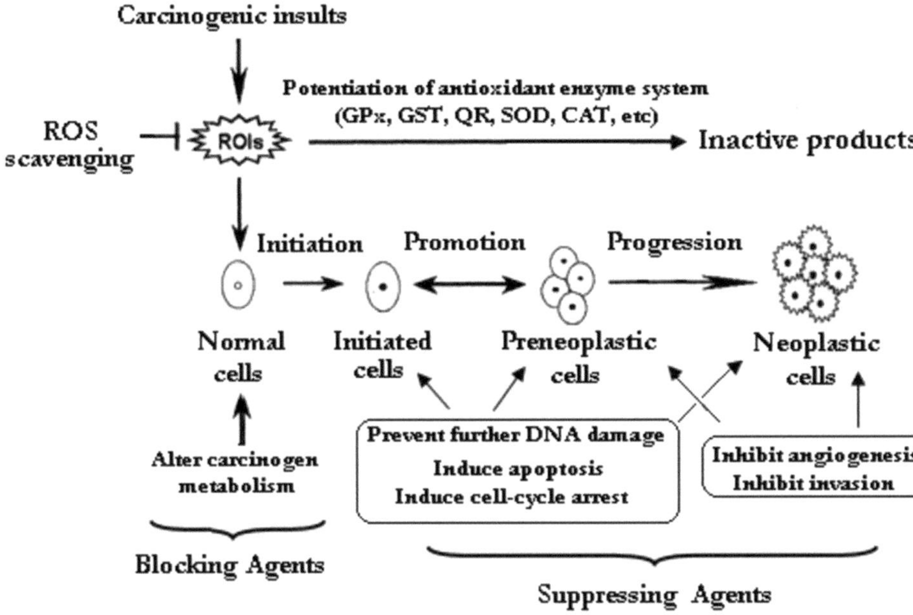

Fig. 1. Mechanism of cancer chemoprevention.

The present chapter aimed to assess the chemoprevention activity of plants derived from Mediterranean basin. Original research studies that were published in English until August 2011, were selected through a computer-assisted literature search (i.e., PubMed and Sciencedirect). We focused on the anticancer properties of phytochemicals from Chios mastic gum (Pistacia Lentiscus var. Chia) and Mediterranean herbs, derived mainly from family *Lamiaceae* (e.c. genous Origanum, Rosmarinus, Satureja, Thymus, Sideritis, Salvia, Mentha).

2.1 Chios mastic (*Pistacia lentiscus L.*) and cancer chemoprevention

Chios Mastic is the name of a resinous sap produced from the mastic tree (*Pistacia lentiscus* var. *chia*) (Fig. 2A). It is a natural, aromatic resin in teardrop shape, falling on the ground in drops from superficial scratches induced by cultivators on the tree's trunk and main branches with sharp tools (Fig. 2B). As it drips, it appears as a sticky and translucent liquid which, 15-20 days later, is solidified into irregular shapes influenced by the area's weather conditions in summertime that is intense drought and sunlight. After being solidified, it has a crystal form (Fig. 2C), while its rather bitter taste quickly subsides to leave a distinctive aroma that really makes it unique. That solid product is then harvested and washed by mastic growers, giving us finally the natural Chios mastic. Soil and climatic characteristics allow the development of mastic trees just south of the island of Chios in the Aegean Sea, Greece. Its color is initially ivory-like but as time goes by, that shade is lost and 12 to 18 months later it changes into yellowish due to oxidation. It is made of hundreds of components; such multitude probably justifies the multiple uses of Chios mastic, in the fields of food industry, health and cosmetic care, worldwide.

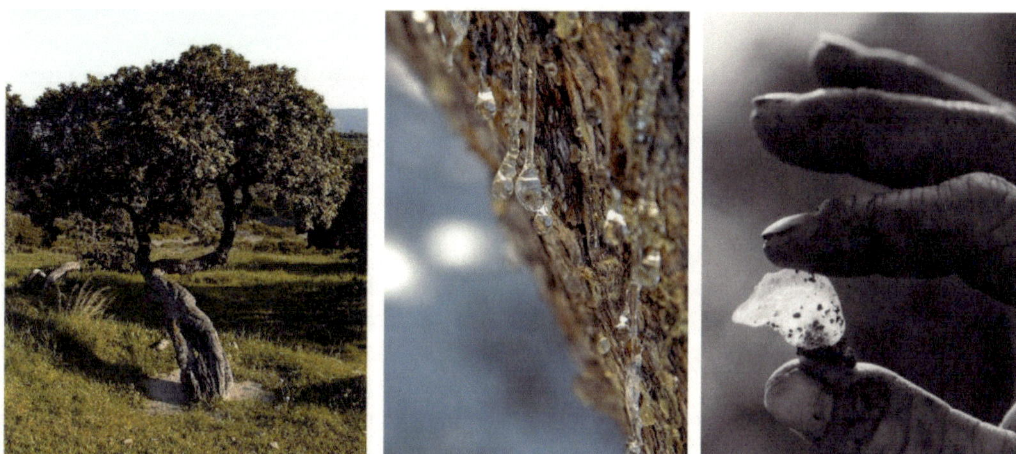
A B C

Fig. 2. **A:** Mastiha Tree, **B:** Mastiha tree trunk and **C:** Mastiha drop.

Chios mastic has been recognized since ancient times both for its distinctive aroma and its healing properties. It has been recorded as the first natural chewing gum in the ancient world. The mastic is known since antiquity for its organoleptic characteristics, but also for its beneficial properties. The first recorded promoter mastic was Dioscorides who wrote that Chios produced the best and greatest quantity of mastic, noting that it was indicated for coughing and stomach ailments, to sweeten the breath, and for facial masks. Several years later, Galen, the most important Greek physician after Hippocrates, extolled mastic's styptic and lenitive properties and recommended it for inflammations of the stomach, intestines and liver. Aretaeus, a physician from Cappadocia who lived in the second half of the 2nd century CE, left many formulas for poultices using mastic. A poultice of apple pulverized with mastic and meliloto (a species of aromatic clover) remedied delirium. A poultice of dates pulverized in wine together with mastic and aloe helped the patient regain strength after a cardiac episode. A poultice of quince, dates, nardo (valeriana) and mastic treated an upset stomach. Monk Antonio Menzani di Cuna in the pharmacy of the Franciscan Monastery of Saint Savior in Jerusalem created a most effective balsam named "The Jerusalem Balsam" using four ingredients: aloe, frankincense, myrrh, and mastic, dissolved in ethanol. The philosopher and physician al-Razi (868-932 CE) who was considered the Hippocrates of Islam, prescribed a mixture of alum and mastic to fill decayed teeth and the chewing of mastic as an appetite stimulant for pregnant women. Abu Yusuf Ya'qub ibn Ishaq al-Kindi, a physician in 9th century Baghdad, provided a medical formula "that makes those who drink happy"; it fortified the stomach, sweetened the breath, and aided the liver. It was administered before or after food and contained rose oil, clove, valeriana, cinnamon, saffron, cardamom, hazel nuts, and mastic. Abu Marwan'Abd al-Malik, born in Seville in 1091, was one of the most eminent clinicians of his time who prescribed a preparation of licorice, raisins and mastic for liver problems. The healing action of mastic was explained by the Swiss physician and alchemist Paracelsus, in his Der grossen Wundartzney (Great Surgery Book). "The biological nature of man is such that it enables him to self-heal, to re-balance and re-fill. Wounds are not healed by the balsam. Mastic, resins and other healing agents are unable to create even a fiber of flesh. They have, however, the property that enables nature to work unimpeded to heal the wound."

The first research studies on the health effects of mastic were in the mid 1980s regarding peptic ulcers (Al-Habbal et al., 1984; Al-Said et al., 1986; Huwez & Al-Habbal, 1986). Since then, more and more studies have been carried out in order to highlight the pharmaceutical effects of mastic in a number of diseases.

The research on the anticancer effects of mastic is most recent. First, Balan et al. (2005) showed that hexanoic gum extract caused apoptosis in HCT116 colon cancer cells. Although the mechanism of action was not elucidated, the resin appeared to trigger a cascade of reactions catalyzed by a family of proteases, caspases, resulting in DNA degradation and apoptosis of cancer cells. The ethanol extract of mastic gum exhibited similar properties, while the observation that cell death continued even when gum treatment stopped indicated that apoptosis was programmed (Balan et al., 2007). Also, in a study of Kaliora et al., (2010), different solvent extracts from 500 μg dried product suppressed cell proliferation, significantly ($p<0.05$) in AGS cells. In the same study, FACS indicated that extracts significantly induced cell death ($p<0.05$). All extracts statistically decreased protein and mRNA ICAM-1 levels ($p<0.05$), while IL-8 protein and mRNA levels showed no significant difference. They concluded that the ethanol-terpene-rich extract was the most effective. A similar mechanism was observed in prostate cancer cells (He et al., 2006; He et al. 2007a, 2007b).

The study of Moulos et al. (2009) was the first to investigate the effect of mastic essential oil in the expression of the whole genome (genome-wide expression analysis). This study provided novel evidence on the molecular basis of tumor growth inhibition mediated by mastic oil and set a rational basis for application of genomics and bioinformatic methodologies in the screening of natural compounds with potential cancer chemopreventive activities Microarray expression profiling was performed using Illumina mouse-6 v1 beadchips, followed by computational analysis. For a number of selected genes, RT-PCR validation was performed in Lewis lung carcinomas, cells as well as in three human cancer cell lines of different origin A549 alveolar epithelial cell, colon cancer HCT116 and K562 myelogenous leukaemic cells. DNA microarray applied in this study allows for the measurement of the expression of complete genome, including identification of functions, metabolic pathways and regulatory mechanisms in diseases such as cancer. The method of the microarray is a milestone in the science of genetics. In the study of Moulos al. the cultivation of LLC with mastic oli (0.01% v/v) resulted in regulation of the expression of 925 genes. Among them, modifications on cell cycle/proliferation, survival and NF-kappaB cascade in conjunction with concomitant regulation of genes encoding for PTEN, E2F7, HMOX1 (up-regulation) and NOD1 (down-regulation) indicated some important mechanistic links underlying the anti-proliferative, pro-apoptotic and anti-inflammatory effects of mastic oil. The expression profiles of Hmox1, Pten and E2f7 genes were similarly altered by mastic oil in the majority of test cancer cell lines. Inhibition of PTEN partially reversed mastic oil effects on tumor cell growth, indicating a multi-target mechanism of action.

A recent study in mice with colon cancer confirmed the antineoplastic role of mastic (Dimas et al., 2009). The intraperitoneal injection of hexane extract of gum at a dose equal to 200 mg/kg body weight resulted in significant suppression of tumor growth in a human colon cancer/immunodeficient mouse model. However, the schedule of administration seemed to play a key role in toxicity. When the extract given for a whole month applying 5 day administration-2 day interval, the size of tumors was significantly reduced, but none of the animals survived the intervention. Conversely, when the schedule was 4 day administration-3 day interval, tumor size was significantly decreased and all animals survived.

In none of the above studies was the bioactive compound in mastic determined. Essential oils and resins, including mastic essential oil and resin, contain a wide variety of terpenes. Specifically, essential oils consist of volatile, low molecular weight terpenes, and resins consist of a mixture of volatile and non volatile terpenes. Terpenes are hydrocarbons of plant origin with carbonate skeleton of 2-methyl-1,3-butadiene or isoprene a common organic compound with the formula $CH_2=C(CH_3)CH=CH_2$. The terpenes identified in Chios mastic are over 80 structures (Papageorgiou et al., 1997; Assimopoulou & Papagerogiou, 2005; Paraschos et al., 2007).

Numerous studies have shown the beneficial role of several terpenes known to be contained in Pistacia species against several cancers; pancreas, breast, colon, liver, and skin (Crowell, 1999). The main monoterpenes are perillyl alcohol, limonene, geraniol and α-pinene and the major triterpenes oleanolic acid and isomer ursolic acid (Fig. 3).

The chemotherapeutic action of perillyl-alcohol is established. In the study by Stark et al. (1995) Perillyl alcohol significantly reduced the growth of hamster pancreatic tumors to less than half that of controls. A percentage of 16% of perillyl alcohol-treated pancreatic tumors completely regressed whereas no control tumors regressed. Perillyl alcohol induced contact inhibition in cultured human pancreatic carcinoma cells and inhibited their anchorage-independent growth ($P<0.001$). Thus, perillyl alcohol has antitumor activity against pancreatic carcinomas at non-toxic doses, and may be an effective chemotherapeutic agent for human pancreatic cancer. As regards the mechanism of action, the perillyl alcohol has been shown to inhibit the proliferation of B12/13 adenocarcinoma pancreatic cells and also to induce apoptosis (Stayrook et al., 1997). Also, the expression of the pro-apoptotic Bak protein was multiplied up to 8 times, which was not observed in normal pancreatic D27 cells. It is rather that the antitumor activity of perillyl alcohol toward pancreatic cancers may be due to preferential stimulation of Bak-induced apoptosis in malignant versus normal cells. Bak may, therefore, be a useful biomarker for the chemopreventive and therapeutic effects of perillyl alcohol, indicative of a Bak-dependent apoptotic pathway.

In 1994, Haag and Gould examined the effect of perillyl alcohol in Wistar-Furth rats with DMBA initiated breast cancer. When tumor diameter reached 3mm, their diet was enriched with 2.5% perillyl alcohol. Three weeks later, the tumors in 22 out of 27 rats (81%) disappeared completely. This observation lead the researchers to examine the effect of different concentrations of the monoterpene in tumors already reached 10mm. After 15 weeks of 2% perillyl-alcohol intervention, 10 of the 20 animals showed complete tumor decrease and additional 5 showed some improvement. However, diet enrichment with 3% perillyl alcohol resulted to toxicity and death in some animals. On the contrary, Stark et al. (1995) have sown that 3% perillyl alcohol in the diet is absolutely secure. The results are conflicting and this is due to methodological weaknesses. Food intake depends on body weight and the number of animals present in each cell. It is noteworthy that the rats maintain a kind of hierarchy with the obvious presence of the "stronger" and more "weak". The more animals form a group, the more difficult it is to calculate food intake. In the study by Haag and Gould (1994) in each cage housed only two animals, while that of Stark et al. (1995) not listed. The choice of the strain should also be chosen with strict criteria for the purposes of the study. Thus, limonene appears to reduce the incidence of kidney cancer in F344 rats, but not in NCI-Black-Reiter rats in the absence of α2-globulin in liver cells (Dietrich & Swenberg, 1991).

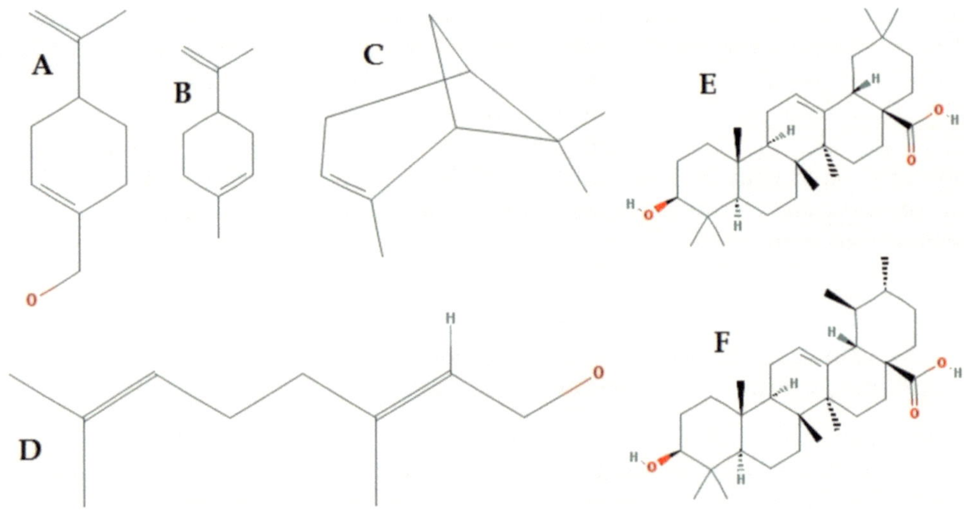

Fig. 3. Chemical structure of the main monoterpenes **A:** perillyl alcohol, **B:** limonene, **C:** geraniol and **D:** α-pinene and major triterpenes **E:** oleanolic acid and **F:** isomer ursolic acid of Chios mastic.

After 19 weeks incorporating 1% perillyl-alcohol in the diet of rats with DEN-liver cancer, the mean liver tumor weight was 10-fold less than that for the untreated animals. The monoterpene did not influence tumor cell proliferation but increased the apoptotic index approximately 10-fold. The mRNA levels for the mannose 6-phosphate/insulin-like growth factor II receptor and the transforming growth factor beta type I, II, and III receptors were also significantly increased in the liver tumors from the terpene-treated animals when compared to the corresponding receptor mRNA levels in the normal tissue surrounding the tumors and in the tumors of untreated animals. The results demonstrated that perillyl-alcohol does not promote the formation of liver tumors, but rather inhibits their growth by enhancing tumor cell loss through apoptosis (Mills et al., 1995).

Angiogenesis is essential for the progression of solid tumors and hematological malignancies. Thus, antiangiogenic therapy is one of the most promising approaches to control cancer. When Loutrari et al., (2004) examined the ability of perillyl alcohol to interfere with the process of angiogenesis, they observed prevention of new blood vessel growth in the in vivo chicken embryo chorioallantoic membrane assay and inhibition of the morphogenic differentiation of cultured endothelial cells into capillary-like networks. In addition, perillyl alcohol inhibited proliferation and induced apoptosis of endothelial cells via the caspase-3 activity and DNA fragmentation. Consistent with the observed antisurvival effect, perillyl alcohol treatment resulted in a significant inhibition of Akt phosphorylation in endothelial cells. Finally, it differentially modulated the release of two important angiogenic regulators: vascular endothelial growth factor and angiopoietin 2. A recent study in the effects of ursolic and oleanolic acid administration on the formation of 1,2-dimethyl-hydrazine (DMH)-induced aberrant crypt foci in the colon of the male Wistar rat. When either individually or as a mixturewere administered in rats, a significant reduction in the frequency of aberrant crypt foci in the group treated with the triterpenoid compounds plus DMH was recorded compared to those treated with DMH alone, suggesting that triterpenes have a protective effect against colon carcinogenesis (Furtado et al., 2008). In the study by Yamai et al. (2009) the triterpenes enhanced conventional therapy in esophageal cancer and anti-tumor activity attribted to the powerful antioxidanteffects (Ovesná et al., 2006) and their ability to block angiogenesis (Sogno et al., 2009).

Perillyl alcohol at the 1 g/kg level significantly inhibited the incidence (percentage of animals with tumors) and multiplicity (tumors/ animals) of invasive adenocarcinomas of the colon, whereas perillyl alcohol at 2 g/kg diet inhibited the incidence of total adenocarcinomas of the colon and small intestine as compared to the control diet (Reddy et al., 1997). The study indicated that the colon tumors of azoxymethane-induced colon carcinogenesis animals fed perillyl alcohol exhibited increased apoptosis as compared to those fed the control diet. These results demonstrate the potential chemopreventive activity of perillyl alcohol against colon carcinogenesis.

When investigating whether the addition of d-limonene to the diets of rats would modify the process of mammary tumor induction, diets containing 1,000 or 10,000 p.p.m. of d-limonene were fed to rats one week prior to DMBA induced tumor formation. A significant reduction in mammary carcinogenesis was observed at each level. The inhibition of carcinogenesis was mainly due to an increase in latency; however, major differences in incidence could be seen during the follow-up period. For example, rats fed 10,000 p.p.m. of d-limonene had a 72% reduction in mammary tumors when compared to controls at 18 weeks post DMBA treatment. In addition to inhibiting the appearance of mammary tumors, d-limonene was also found to cause the regression of frank mammary tumors. No toxicity was evident in these rats even at the highest d-limonene dose (Elegbede et al., 1984). Maltzman et al. (1991) observed that limonene inhibited the toxicity of DMBA, increasing the urinary excretion of DMBA and its metabolites, reducing the formation of DMBA-DNA complexes affecting the liver detoxification pathway.

Topical perillyl alcohol significantly inhibited tumor incidence and multiplicity, average tumor size, and the average tumor burden/mouse without any apparent toxicity in a nonmelanoma model of mouse skin carcinogenesis. It inhibited UVB-induced AP-1 transactivation in both cultured human keratinocytes and transgenic mice that stably express a luciferase reporter driven by AP-1 elements. The results suggested that perillyl alcohol might be used for chemoprevention of human skin cancer. (Batherlman et al., 1998).

However, clinical trials in cancer patients are intimidating. The 20 patients, of whom 15 were evaluable in the study of Bailey et al. (2008), received perillyl alcohol in doses between 1,200 and 2,000 mg/m^2 for a total of 43 courses. The most common observed toxicities were nausea, gastrointestinal distress, and fatigue. Other toxicities included diarrhea or constipation, hypokalemia, and one incidence of acute pancreatitis. Due to these toxicities, four of the patients declined further treatment either during or after the second course. While perillyl alcohol was not detected in plasma, perillic acid and dihydroperillic acid were detected in plasma, and the peak levels at 2,000 mg/m^2 per dose were approximately 600 μM perillic acid and 50 μM dihydroperillic acid. There was no evidence that levels of TGF-b plasma and the expression of Ras proteins were affected, indicative of the non significant advantages of perillyl alcohol In adults with advanced malignancies. No significant difference occurred between lesions appearing on the perillyl alcohol treated forearm vs. the placebo-treated forearm in healthy non skin cancer subjects under UV radiation (Stratton et al., 2008), indicative that most probably perillyl alcohol cream has no chemopreventive activity in skin cancer. Finally, intake of 55 mg-perillyl alcohol daily for six months, reduced 50% the size of tumors in 3.4% of adults with malignant gliomas (da Fonseca et al., 2008a, 2008b).

Conclusively, although sometimes inconsistent, the naturally occurring Chios mastic or individual terpenic components are many hoped for application as chemotherapeutic agents. The first report to display a promotion potential of Chios Mastic Gum on the formation of preneoplastic lesions comes from Doi et al., (2009). In a rat liver medium-term carcinogenesis bioassay, orally administered mastic of 1% apparently promoted GST-P foci yield after DEN-initiation but the 0.1% dose (48.3 mg/kg/day) was concluded as non-promoting dose. This 0.1% dose is almost equivalent to 2.9 g/day/person with the average human body weight regarded as 60 kg. Most Chios mastic doses previously reported in human studies were around this level, e.g. 5 g/day/person (Triantafyllou et al., 2007), 4 g/day/person (Bebb et al.,2003), 2.2 g/day/parson (Kaliora et al., 2007a, 2007b), or 1 g/day/person (Al-Habbal et al., 1984). Favorable effects of mastic such as anticarcinogenic potential could be achieved at relatively low doses without any toxicity (He et al., 2006). Further studies must elucidate the mechanisms underlying and determine safety levels in humans.

2.2 Mediterranean herbs and cancer chemoprevention

In herbal medicine the term herbs is used to refer not only to herbaceous plants but also to bark, roots, leaves, seeds, flowers and fruit of trees, shrubs, and woody vines, and extracts of the same that are valued for their savory, aromatic, or medicinal qualities. The botanical term herb refers to seed-producing plants with non-woody stems that die down at the end of the growing season (Craig, 1999).

Herbs have been grown and used for culinary and medicinal purposes since antiquity. The Mediterranean basin has been distinguished throughout the generations with a rich inventory of natural medicinal herbs and it is the place in which the sience of botany was born. Oregano (*Origanum vulgare*), Sage (*Salvia officinalis*), Thyme (*Thyumus vulgaris*), Saffron (*Crocus sativus*), Rosemary (*Rosmarinus officinalis*), Savory (*Satureja hortensis*), Bay Laurel (*Laurus nobilis*), Basil (*Ocimum basilicum L.*), Chamomile (*Marticaria chamomilla*), Dittany of Crete (*Origanum dictamnus*), Marjoram (Origanum *majorana),* Rosemary (Rosmarinus *officinalis),* Sideritis (Sideritis *syriaca),* Hypericum (*Hypericum perforatum),* Pennyroyal *(Mentha pulegium),* Olive (*Olea europaea*), Anise (*Pimpinella anisum*), Coriander (*Coriandrum sativum*), Garlic (*Allium sativum*), Fennel (*Foeniculum vulgare*), Garden cress (*Lepidium sativum*), Lavender (*Lavandula angustifolia*), Myrtle (*Myrtus communis*), Nigella (*Nigella sativa*), Sumac (*Rhus coriaria*) are some of the generally considered as native Mediterranean herbs. Herbs are used as flavorings and seasonings, for the preservation and storage of various foods and help to maintain their organoleptic properties. In most of these herbs, the flavor is provided by the aromatic ingredients in their essential oils and oleoresins (Craig, 1999). They are also used for the treatment of headaches, neuralgia, gingivitis, toothaches, tonsillitis, sore throat, common cold and against cough. Cultures throughout history have practiced the art of pain management through remedies such as oral ingestion of herbs.

Hereby are cited indicative examples of some herbs and some of the healing properties attributed to them:
Basil (*Ocimum basilicum L.*): antispasmodic, diuretic, laxative, auxiliary for memory
Bay Laurel (*Laurus nobilis*): tonic, appetizer
Rosemary (*Rosmarinus officinalis*): antiseptic, antirheumatic, tonic
Dittany (*Origanum dictamnus*): emmenagogue, tonic, healing
Thyme (*Thymus vulgaris L.*): antispasmodic, antiseptic, antirheumatic
Oregano (*Origanum vulgare)*: expectorant, antispasmodic, disinfectant
Sage (*Salvia officinalis L.*): against hypotension and anemia, antidiabetic
Chamomile (*Marticaria chamomilla*): soothing, anti-insomnia, against flu

In the past it was not known the exact way of activity of herbs and their healing properties recorded empirically. Those properties provoked the interest of researchers to conduct numerous studies in order to verify these observations and to ascertain the responsible substance for these properties. Today it is known that the properties of medicinal plants owned to chemical compounds that they contain, termed phytochemicals, with antioxidant, anti-inflammatory, anti-bacterial, anticancer and cardioprotective properties. Today much of scientific research has been focused on investigating the possible use of medicinal plants for prevention, cure and/or adjunctive treatment of chronic diseases such as cancer.

Several commonly used herbs have been identified by the National Cancer Institute as possessing cancer-preventive properties (Caragay, 1992). Many studies showed that many phytochemical compounds of herbs of the Mediterranean basin, gained the "food-borne anticarcinogens" title. These beneficial substances act as antioxidants and electrophile scavengers, stimulate the immune system, inhibit nitrosation and the formation of DNA adducts with carcinogens, induce phase I or II detoxification enzymes, act on intracellular signalling network molecules involved in the initiation and/or promotion of cancer, interrupting thus or reversing the carcinogenesis process (Bisset, 1994; Robbers et al., 1994; Cuvelier et al., 1994; Armata et al., 2008; Saddiqe et al., 2010; Lee et al., 2011).

Thyme (*Thymus vulgaris*), Rosemary (*Rosmarinus officinalis*) and Sage (*Salvia officinalis L.*) have phenolic compounds (phenolic diterpenes, flavonoids and phenolic acids) that are able to inhibit cancer, through inhibiting the initiation, as well as tumor progression (Craig 1999; Ho et al., 2000). Sideritis or "mountain tea" (*Sideritis syriaca, Sideritis clandestina*), Hypericum (*Hypericum perforatum*) and sage (*Salvia officinalis L.)* contain polyphenols (chlorogenic acid, apigenin, protocatechuic acid, caffeic acid, rosmaric acid, carnosol, qerqetin, luteolin, apigenin, p-coumaric acid, hypericine, geraniol, α-pinene, β-pinene) with anti-inflammatory and antioxidant properties (Saddiqe et al., 2010; Armata et al., 2008; Lu & Foo, 2001; Thorsen & Hildenbrandt, 2003). Carnosol has been evaluated for anti-cancer properties in prostate, breast, skin, leukemia, and colon cancer with promising results (Jonhson, 2011).

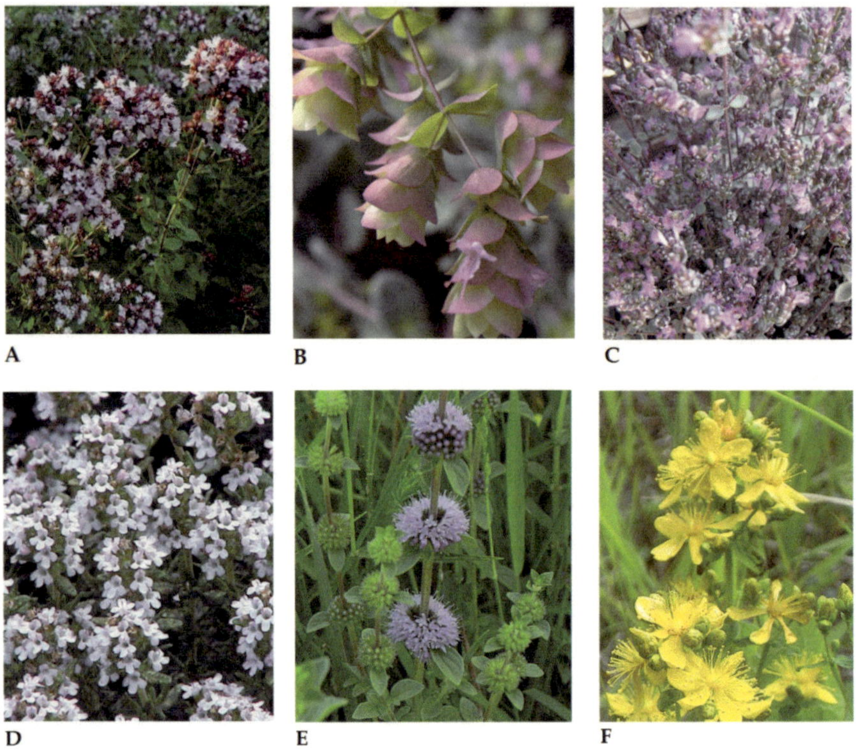

Fig. 4. **A:** Oregano (Origanum vulgare), **B:** Dittany of Crete (Origanum dictamnus), **C:** Vogel (Origanum microphilum), **D:** Thyme (Thymus vulgaris), **E:** Pennyroyal **(**Mentha pulegium), **F:** Hypericum (Hypericum perforatum).

Methanol extract of Olives (*Olea europaea*), rich in phenolic compounds, exhibits gastric cancer preventive efficacy by limiting cell proliferation, inducing cell death and suppressing inflammation in AGS cancer cells (Kountouri et al., 2009). Chamomile (*Marticaria chamomill*) and Oregano (*Origanum vulgare*) show antimicrobial activity against Helicobacter pylori, a Gram-negative bacteria that infects the stomach and strengthens the chances of stomach cancer (Stamatis et al., 2003; Bampidis et al., 2006; Couladis et al., 2003).

Many studies have been reported to that phytochemicals from herbs interfere at the initiation of cancer. In vitro studies with cancer cell lines, showed that oregano extract protect against oxidative stress and DNA damage from radiation (Rao et al., 2006; Bakkali et al., 2006). Additionally, oregano extract was found to have strong antioxidant activity, through the capture free radicals, suppression of fat oxidation, inhibition of NOS and protection of DNA from H_2O_2-induced oxidative damage (Zheng & Wang, 2001; Aherne et al., 2007; Tsai et al., 2007). The components which are responsible for this activity are carvacrol, the terpene rosmarinic acid, glycosides of protocatechuic acid and thymol (Karioti et al., 2006; Braga et al., 2006). Several phytochemicals inhibit tumor formation by stimulating the protective phase II enzyme, glutathione transferase. GT is a detoxifying enzyme that catalyzes the reaction of glutathione with electrophiles to form compounds that are less toxic, more water-soluble, and can be excreted easily. Mice fed with a diet containing thyme (*Thymus vulgaris L*, 0.5% or 2.0%) or treated orally with thymol (50-200 mg/kg) or carvacrol (50-200 mg/kg) once a day for 7 successive days, showed a significantly increased in GT protein levels (Sasaki et al., 2005). Similar results were observed when rosemary extract or carnosol alone were administered in female rats (Singletary, 1996). Limonene, geraniol, menthol, and carvone found in commonly used herbs stimulate also glutathione transferase activity (Craig, 1999).

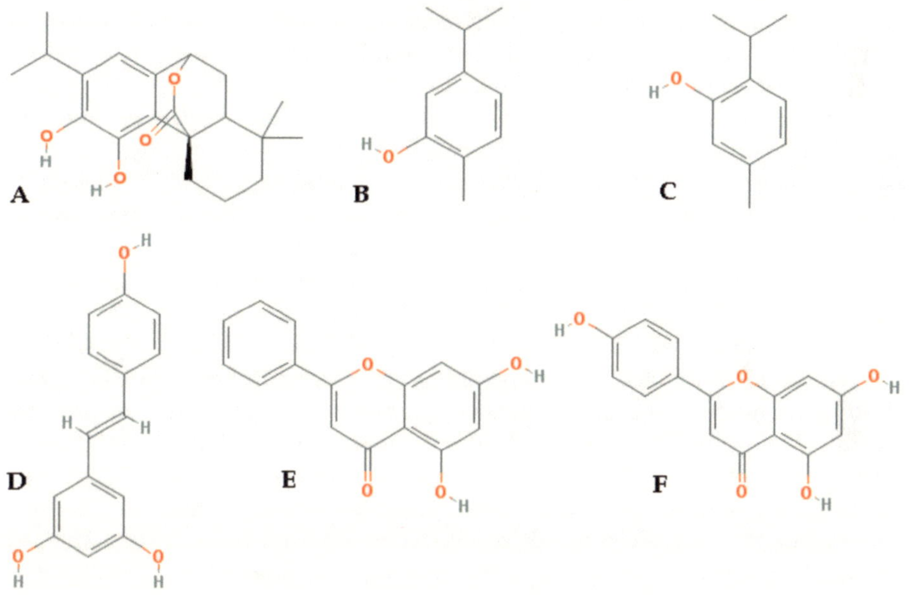

Fig. 5. Chemical structure of the terpenes **A:** carnosol, **B:** carvacrol, **C:** thymol and polyphenols **D:** resveratrol, **E:** chrysin and **F:** apigenin founds in many herbs.

Herbs phytochemicals have gained also the "suppressing agents" title. Inhibition of tumor cells proliferation has been highlighted in several studies that have been done on herbs, or on isolated components of them; nevertheless, the precise mechanism of action is not fully defined. Carnosol and thymol from oregano can inhibit the proliferation of cancerous cells or cells with active oncogenes (Sasaki et al., 2005; Slamenova et al., 2007; Mezzoug et al., 2007). Carnosol, also found in large quantities in dittany and in thyme, can inhibit the proliferation of breast cancer cells by 50% after incubation for 48h in a concentration of 100μM, by inducing apoptosis (Arunasree, 2010). An in vivo study of Moran et al. (2005) showed that dietary carnosol (0.1%) decreased APC associated adenoma formation by 46%

in the C57BL/6J/Min/+ (Min/+) mouse when compared to controls. Also, carnosol induces G2/M cell cycle arrest that targets cyclin A and cyclin B1 with an IC50 of 23 μM in Caco-2 colon adenocarcinoma cells which are representative of precancerous lesions (Visanji et al., 2006). Additional in vitro work has shown that carnosol significantly inhibited the highly metastatic mouse melanoma B16 cells through down regulation of matrix metalloproteinase 2, c-jun, as well as the redox sensitive transcription factor nuclear factor-kappa B (Nf-κB) (J.J. Johnson et al., 2008). Also, J.J. Johnson et al. (2008) shows that carnosol promoted G2 cell cycle arrest of PC3 cell line, with inhibition of cyclins A, D1, D2 and cdks 2 and 6, and targets multiple signaling pathways that include the AMPK and PI3K/Akt pathway. Resveratrol and chrysin can inhibit the proliferation of Caco-2 cells after 72h incubation when administered in combination at concentrations of 20 mM and 32 mM, respectively (Iwuchukwu et al., 2011). The effect of resveratrol to inhibit cell proliferation, has been reported previously and found to be associated with the remaining cell cycle arrest at phases S and G2/M through inhibition of Cdk7 and p34Cdc2 (Joe et al., 2002; Estrov et l., 2003; Liang et al., 2003). Similar results were reported by Jin et al. (2010) on the activity of total polyphenols from tea in cell lines of colon (IT29, LoVo, SW480, HCT116). The inhibition of cancer cell proliferation from those phytochemicals was positive correlated with the incubation time (24h-1w) and the dose administered (50-300 mg). Farnesol and geraniol, and to a lesser extent perillyl alcohol, found in spearmint (*Mentha spicata*), substantially suppressed the growth of pancreatic, colon, murine leukemia, hepatoma and melanoma tumor cells (Burke et al., 1997; Carnesecchi et al., 2001). Polyphenolics in green tea (Camellia sinensis) are known to possess antimutagenic and anticancer activity. Some evidence suggests that tea has a protective effect against stomach and colon cancers (Dreosti, 1996). The way of which tea polyphenols inhibit cell proliferation has been elucidated. More specifically, EGCG reduces cell proliferation by inhibiting enzymes that catalyze reactions of DNA replication. EGCG inhibit proteasome be forming ester bonds with it, resulting in accumulation of p27KIP1 and arrest of cell cycle in G1 phase. Additionally, EGCG induces the cyclin kinase inhibitor WAF1/p21 resulting cells arrest in phase G0/G1 (Syed et al., 2007). Also, a recent study found that genistein inhibits the proliferation of prostate cancer cells after incubation for 72h at three different concentrations (5 mg/mL, 10 mg/mL, 20 mg/mL) (Peternac et al., 2008). The essential oil of Rosemary, caused 50% inhibition of tumor cells proliferation, at breast and prostate cancer, after 24h incubation at concentrations of 190 and 180 mg/mL respectively (Hussain et al., 2010). The petroleum ether extract of Hypericum adenotrichum Spach (called "kantaron" in Turkey), a member of Hypericum perforatum genus that grows to Western Turkey, showed antiproliferative effects in HL-60 promyeloic leukaemia cells, which correlated with cyclin D1 suppression and p21 induction (Ozmen et al., 2009). Also, methanol extract of Malva Silvestris rich in phenolic compounds, inhibited cell proliferation of B16 and A375 melanoma cell lines (Danilea et al., 2007).

Many studies shows that extracts of oregano and its components have anti-inflammatory properties, as they suppress inflammation in vivo and in vitro. Braga et al. (2006) found that thymol at a concentration of 2.5-20 mg / mL inhibits the release of elastase, a marker of inflammation, by human neutrophils after stimulation with a chemotactic peptide. Resveratrol can inhibit in vitro the expression of IL-8 in monocytes stimulated with PMA (Shen et al., 2003). Additionally, resveratrol and quercetin, found that they can inhibit the secretion of IL- 8 in stimulated with IL-1 tumor cells in the liver (Gauliard et al., 2008). The apigenin, a flavone, also displays the ability to reduce secretion of IL-1b, IL-8 and TNf-α in monocytes stimulated with LPS (Nicholas et al., 2007). Zhou et al. (2004), studying the effect of hyperforins, one of the phytochemicals contained in the sedge, found that it induce gene expression of IL-8 in intestinal epithelial cells and in leukemia cells by a mechanism independent of the NF-κB. The ability of polyphenols to inhibit the secretion of IL-8 was confirmed in another study which found that ellagic acid, chrysin, genistein and EGCG can reduce significant levels of secretion of IL-8 cell line of bowel cancer (Romier et al., 2008). Carnosol can inhibit enzymes involved in the development of inflammation (5-LOX, COX-2, NOS, etc.) affecting various signaling pathways. The anticancer action has been studied in various cancers (eg prostate, breast, skin, leukemia, etc.) with encouraging results (J.J. Johnson, 2011). Apigenin, chrysin and kaempferol can suppress COX-2 transcription by mechanisms including activation of the PPARg transcription factor (Liang et al., 2001). Curcumin inhibited COX-2 activities through suppression of NF-κB activity via control of the NIK/IKK signaling complex in colon cancer cells (Plummer et al., 1999). Phenylethyl isothiocyanate in winter cress (*Barbarea vulgaris*) showed a strong anti-inflammatory activity by reducing the level of iNOS mRNA in LPS-stimulated mouse RAW264.7 macrophages (Ippoushi et al., 2003). Gingerol inhibited nitric oxide synthesis in activated J774.1 mouse macrophages and prevented peroxynitrite- induced oxidation and nitration reactions in macrophages (Chen et al., 2003). Polyphenols from green tea inhibit STAT3 expression, a transcriptional factor, and prostate cancer growth and subsequently induce apoptosis of prostate cancer cells (Siddiqui et al., 2008). Resveratrol modulates IL-6-induced intercellular adhesion molecule-1 (ICAM-1) gene expression by suppressing STAT3 phosphorylation (Wung et al., 2005). Some of the phenolic components containing herbs have been evaluated on their ability to affect the activation of NF-KB, and its commitment to the positions 'target' in DNA. More specifically, the chrysin and ellagic acid reduce the activation of NF-KB in Caco-2, which had previously stimulated with either LPS, IL-1, or with TNF-a (Romier et al., 2008). Additionally, chrysin (3 mmol/L) was found to reduce the activation of NF-KB in stimulated by TNF-a A549 human lung adenocarcinoma epithelial cell line. In contrast to the above, the chrysin caused increased binding capacity of this transcription factor to DNA, but also led to increased activation when administered to mouse macrophages that had undergone stimulation with LPS (Woo et al., 2005). Conflicting results were also studying the action of two other phenolic compounds, genistein and resveratrol. Both compounds appear to induce the activation of NF-KB in stimulated either with LPS, IL-1, or TNF- a Caco-2 colon cells (Romier et al., 2008). However, regarding genistein, Li et al. (2005) demonstrated the ability to reduce the activation of NF-KB in PC3. Also, resveratrol was found to reduce the activation of this molecule in U937, HeLa, and H4 (Holmes-McNary et al., 2000; Manna et al., 2000). Moreover, a study of the effect of resveratrol on TNF-a stimulated MCF7 cells, showed that it prevents the binding of NF-KB to DNA (Banerjee et al., 2002). Another phenolic molecule has been extensively studied is EGCG, which was found to inhibit the activation of NF-KB in cancer cell lines A431 (Gupta et al., 2004) and LNCaP (Hastak et al., 2003). One interpretation proposed to explain the contradictory results of the effect of polyphenols on levels of activation of NF-KB in cell lines of colon balances have studied is that there are probably different signaling pathways responsible for activation of NF-KB as response to various phenolic compounds. This diversity of cells in the intestinal epithelium may be associated with prolonged exposure to high concentrations of polyphenolic components in relation to blood cells and other organs are exposed to comparatively lower concentrations (Romier et al., 2008).

Historical and current studies and surveys indicate, that the region of the Mediterranean has been distinguished throughout generations with a rich inventory of natural medicinal herbs. By expanding upon the wisdom of the Greeks over the centuries, indigenous medicine has contributed greatly to the development of modern medicine in Europe and remains one of the closest forms of original European medicine. A diet in which culinary herbs are used generously to flavor food, provides a variety of active phytochemicals that promote health and protect against chronic diseases such as cancer. Charlemagne was correct when he said "a herb is a friend of physicians and the praise of cooks". Nevertheless, whereas some herbal products may be safe and may contain active constituents that have beneficial physiologic effects, others may be unsafe to use. The Food and Drug Administration has classified several herbs as unsafe, even in small amounts, and hence they should not be used in either foods or beverages (Craig, 1999). Some herbs are safe in modest amounts but they may become toxic at higher doses. Overall, when herbs are prescribed appropriately, the safety of traditional herbal medications is high. Any plant parts used or prescribed by ethnopharmacologists should be tested for safety before being recommended for human use.

3. Conclusion

Although there is a lack of definitive evidence for the association of Mediterranean diet with various types of cancer and whatever the final assessment of the overall contribution of such diets to cancer prevention turns out to be, there is no doubt that the phytochemicals they contain do exert a range of fascinating and potentially important biological effects on human health. Over the last decade, a broad spectrum of plant natural compounds, that have gained much attention for consideration as cancer chemopreventive or therapeutic agents, has been isolated from traditional herbal medicines, spices, fruits, and vegetables. These plant secondary metabolites as medicines, dietary supplements or "health food" ingredients may exhibit considerable benefits over synthetic drug approaches, as they offer an inexpensive, convenient, readily applicable and accessible health-care approach for prevention, control and management of diseases such as cancer. The continued emergence of new evidence for the multifunctional effects of these products has certainly provided much impetus for future research into their modes of action and their application in cancer prevention and treatment. Advances in cellular, biochemical and molecular biology techniques and experimental approaches using transcriptome, proteome, metabolome and bioinformatics analyses have provided useful new insights into cancer therapeutics.

One obvious weakness of the current state of research, is that much of it has been conducted in vitro, with little regard for the bioavailability of the compounds studied. In most cases the small proportion of any compound that is absorbed undergoes extensive metabolism before reaching target organs, and the products are readily excreted. In the future, long-term systematic intervention trials, that will take into consideration the bioavailability and metabolism of those phytochemicals, will be essential to gather good evidence of their anticancer potential. Such strategies will contribute to a full risk–benefit analysis, based on a thorough understanding of their overall biological effects. With the expected advances in our understanding of the specific signaling pathways, transcription factors and molecular target genes affected by chemopreventive plant compounds, these natural products will offer a great promise as anticancer therapeutics or chemopreventive agents. Moreover, further development of these potent natural products will improve the efficacy of targeted therapeutic strategies to win the long run battle against cancer.

4. References

Aherne, S.A., Kerry, J.P. & O'Brien, N.M. (2007). Effects of plant extracts on antioxidant status and oxidant-induced stress in Caco-2 cells. *British Journal of Nutrition*, Vol. 97, pp. 321-328

Al-Habbal, M.J., Al-Habbal, Z. & Huwez, F.U. (1984). A double-blind controlled clinical trial of mastic and placebo in the treatment of duodenal ulcer. *Clinical and Experimantal Pharmacology and Physiology*, Vol. 11, pp. 541-44

Al-Said, M.S., Ageel, A.M., Parmar, N.S. & Tariq, M. (1986). Evaluation of mastic, a crude drug obtained from Pistacia lentiscus for gastric and duodenal anti-ulcer activity. *Journal of Ethnopharmacology*, Vol. 15, pp. 271-78

Armata, M., Gabrieli, C., Termentzi, A., Zervou, M. & Kokkalou, M. (2008). Constituents of sideritis syriaca ssp. syriaca (Lamiaceae) and their antioxidant capacity. *Food Chemistry*, Vol. 111, pp. 179-186

Arunasree, K.M. (2010). Anti-proliferative effects of carvacrol on a human metastatic breast cancer cell line, MDA-MB 231. *Phytomedicine*, Vol. 17, pp. 581-588

Assimopoulou, A.N. & Papageorgiou, V.P. (October 2005). GC-MS analysis of penta- and tetra-cyclic triterpenes from resins of Pistacia species. Part II. Pistacia terebinthus var. Chia. *Biomedical Chromatography*, Vol. 19, pp. 586-605

Bailey, H.H., Attia, S., Love, R.R., Fass, T., Chappell, R., Tutsch, K., Harris, L., Jumonville, A., Hansen, R., Shapiro, G.R. & Stewartm, J.A. (2008). Phase II trial of daily oral perillyl alcohol (NSC 641066) in treatment-refractory metastatic breast cancer. *Chemotherapy and Pharmacology*, Vol. 62, pp. 149-57

Bailey, H.H., Wilding, G., Tutsch, K.D., Arzoomanian, R.Z., Alberti, D., Feierabend, C., Simon, K., Marnocha, R., Holstein, S.A., Stewart, J., Lewis, K.A. & Hohl, R.J. (2004). A phase I trial of perillyl alcohol administered four times daily for 14 days out of 28 days. *Cancer Chemotherapy and Pharmacology*, Vol. 54, pp. 368-76

Bakkali, F., Averbeck, S., Averbeck, D., Zhiri, A., Baudoux, D. & Idaomar, M. (2006). Antigenotoxic effects of three essential oils in diploid yeast (S. cerevisiae) after treatments with UV radiation, 8-MPO plus UVA, and MMS. *Mutation Research*, Vol. 606, pp. 27-38

Balan, K.V., Demetzos, C., Prince J., Dimas, K., Cladaras, M., Han, Z., Wyche, J.H. & Pantazis, P. (2005). Induction of apoptosis in human colon cancer HCT116 cells treated with an extract of the plant product, Chios mastic gum. *In Vivo*, Vol. 19, pp. 93-102

Balan, K.V., Prince, J., Han, Z., Dimas, K., Cladaras, M., Wyche, J.H., Sitaras, N.M. & Pantazis, P. (2007). Antiproliferative activity and induction of apoptosis in human colon cancer cells treated in vitro with constituents of a product derived from Pistacia lentiscus L. var. chia. *Phytomedicine*, Vol. 14, pp. 263-72

Bampidis, V.A., Christodoulou, V., Florou-Paneri, P. & Christaki, E. (2006). Effect of dried oregano leaves versus neomycin in treating newborn calves with colibacillosis. *Journal of Veterinary Medicine A-Physiology Pathology Clinical Medicine*, Vol. 53, pp. 154-156

Banerjee, S., Bueso-Ramos, C. & Aggarwal, B.B. (2002). Suppression of 7, 12-dimethylbenz (α)anthracene-induced mammary carcinogenesis in rats by resveratrol: role of nuclear NFκB, cyclooxygenase 2 and matrix metalloprotease 9. *Cancer Research*, Vol. 62, pp. 4949-4954

Barthelman M., Chen W., Gensler H.L., Huang, C., Dong, Z. & Bowden, G.T. (1998). Inhibitory effects of perillyl alcohol on UVB-induced murine skin cancer and AP-1 transactivation. *Cancer Research*, Vol. 58, pp. 711-16

Bebb, J.R., Bailey-Flitter, N., Ala'Aldeen, D. & Atherton, J.C. (2003). Mastic gum has no effect on Helicobacter pylori load in vivo. *Journal of Antimicrobial Chemotherapy*, Vol. 52, pp. 522-23

Bisset NG, ed. (1994). *Herbal drugs and phytopharmaceuticals. A handbook for practice on a scientific basis*. Medpharm Scientific Publishers, ISBN 3-88763-100-5, Stuttgart, Germany

Braga, P., DalSasso, M., Culici, M., Bianchi, T., Bordoni, L. & Marabini, L. (2006). Anti-inflammatory activity of thymol: inhibitory effect on the release of human neutrophil elastase. *Pharmacology*, Vol. 77, pp. 130-136

Burke, Y.D., Stark, M.J., Roach, S.L., Sen, S.E. & Crowell, P.L. (1997). Inhibition of pancreatic cancer growth by the dietary isoprenoids farnesol and geraniol. *Lipids*, Vol. 32, pp.151–5

Caragay AB. (1992). Cancer-preventative foods and ingredients. *Food Technology*, Vol. 46, pp. 65–68

Carnesecchi, S., Schneider, Y., Ceraline, J., Duranton, B., Gosse, F., Seiler, N., & Raulf, F. (2001). Geraniol, a Component of Plant Essential Oils, Inhibits Growth and Polyamine Biosynthesis in Human Colon Cancer Cells. *Journal of Pharmacology and Experimental Therapeutics*, Vol. 298, pp. 197–200

Chen, Y.H., Dai, H.J. & Chang, H.P. (2003). Suppression of inducible nitric oxide production by indole and isothiocyanate derivatives from Brassica plants in stimulated macrophages. *Planta Medica*, Vol. 69, pp. 696–700

Cordell, G.A., (2003). Discovering our gifts from nature, now and in the future. Part II. *Revista de Quimica*, Vol. 17, pp. 3–15

Cordell, G.A., & Colvard, M.D. (2005). Some thoughts on the future of ethnopharmacology. *Journal of Ethnopharmacology*, Vol. 100, pp. 5–14

Couladis, M., Tzakou, O., Verykokidou, E. & Harvala, C. (2003). Screening of some Greek aromatic plants for antioxidant activity. *Phytotherapy Research*, Vol. 17, pp. 194-195

Craig, J.W. (1999). Health-promoting properties of common herbs. *American Journal of Clinical Nutrition*, 70 (suppl), pp. 491S–9S

Crowell, P.L. (1999). Symposium on phytochemicals: biochemistry and physiology. Prevention and therapy of cancer by dietary monoterpenes. *Journal of Nutrition*, Vol. 129, pp. 775-78

Cuvelier, M.E., Berset, C. & Richard, H. (1994). Antioxidant constituents in sage (Salvia officinalis). *Journal of Agricultural and Food Chemistry*, Vol. 42, pp. 665–669

Da Fonseca, C.O., Linden, R., Futuro D., Gattass, C.R. & Quirico-Santos, T. (2008a). Ras pathway activation in gliomas: a strategic target for intranasal administration of perillyl alcohol. *Archivum Immunologiae et Therapia Experimentalis*, Vol. 56(4), pp. 267-76

Da Fonseca, C.O., Schwartzmann, G., Fisher, J., Nagel, J., Futuro, D., Quirico-Santos, T. & Gattass, C.R. (2008b). Preliminary results from a phase I/II study of perillyl alcohol intranasal administration in adults with recurrent malignant gliomas. *Surgical Neurology*, Vol. 70, pp. 259-67

Daniela, A., Pichichero1, E., Canuti, L., Cicconi, R., Karou, D., D'Arcangelo, G., & Canini, A. (2007). Identification of phenolic compounds from medicinal and melliferous plants and their cytotoxic activity in cancer cells. *Caryologia*, Vol. 60, pp. 90-95

Dietrich, D.R. & Swenberg, J.A. (1991). The presence of a2u-globulin is necessary for d-limonene promotion of male rat kidney tumors. *Cancer Research*, Vol. 51, pp. 3512-17

Dimas K., Hatziantoniou S., Wyche J.H. & Pantazis, P. (2009). A mastic gum extract induces suppression of growth of human colorectal tumor xenografts in immunodeficient mice. *In Vivo.*, Vol. 23, pp. 63-68

Doi, K., Wei, M., Kitano, M., Uematsu, N., Inoue, M. & Wanibuchi, H. (2009). Enhancement of preneoplastic lesion yield by Chios Mastic Gum in a rat liver medium-term carcinogenesis bioassay. *Toxicology and Applied Pharmacology*, Vol. 234, pp. 135-42

Dreosti, IE. (1996). Bioactive ingredients: antioxidants and polyphenols in tea. *Nutrition Reviews*, Vol. 54, pp. S51–58

Elegbede, J.A., Elson, C.E., Qureshi, A., Tanner, M.A. & Gould, M.N. (1984). Inhibition of DMBA-induced mammary cancer by the monoterpene d-limonene. *Carcinogenesis*, Vol. 5, pp. 661-65

Estrov, Z., Shishodia, S., Faderl, S., Harris, D., Van, Q., Kantarjian, H.M., Talpaz, M. & Aggarwal, B.B. (2003). Resveratrol blocks interleukin-1beta-induced activation of the nuclear transcription factor NF-kappaB, inhibits proliferation, causes S-phase arrest, and induces apoptosis of acute myeloid leukemia cells. *Blood*, Vol. 102, pp. 987-995

Fabricant, D.S. & Farnsworth, N.R. (2001). The value of plants used in traditional medicine for drug discovery. *Environmental Health Perspectives*, Vol. 109, pp. 69–75

Farnsworth, N.R., Akerele, O., Bingel, A.S., Soejarto, D.D. & Guo, Z., (1985). Medicinal Plants in therapy. *Bulletin of the World Health Organization*, Vol. 63, pp. 965–981, ISSN

Franco, R., Schoneveld, O., Georgakilas, G.A., Panayiotidis, I.M. (2008) Oxidative stress, DNA methylation and carcinogenesis. *Cancer Letters*, Vol. 266, pp. 6–11

Furtado, R.A., Rodrigues, E.P., Araújo, F.R., Oliveira, W.L., Furtado, M.A., Castro, M.B., Cunha, W.R. & Tavares, D.C. (2008). Ursolic acid and oleanolic acid suppress preneoplastic lesions induced by 1,2-dimethylhydrazine in rat colon. *Toxicologic Pathology*, Vol. 36, pp. 576-80, ISSN: 1533-1601

Gupta, S., Hastak, K., Afaq, F., Ahmad, N. & Mukhtar, H. (2004). Essential role of caspases in EGCG-mediated inhibition of nuclear factor kappa B and induction of apoptosis. *Oncogene*, Vol. 14, pp. 2507-2522

Haag, J.D. & Gould, M.N. (1994). Mammary carcinoma regression induced by perillyl alcohol, a hydroxylated analog of limonene. *Cancer Chemotherapy and Pharmacology*, Vol. 34, pp. 477-83

Harvey, A.L. (2008). Natural products in drug discovery. *Drug Discovery Today*, Vol. 13, pp. 894–901

Harvey, A.L. (2009). Bridging the Gap: using natural products in drug discovery research in academia and industry. In: *M.C. Novel Therapeutic Agents from Plants,* Carpinella and M. Rai (eds.). pp. 167–175. Science Publishers, ISBN: 978-1578085460, Enfield, NH, USA.

Hastak, K., Gupta, S., Ahmad, N., Agarwal, M.K., Agarwal, M.L. & Mukhtar, H. (2003). Role of p53 and NF-κB in epigallocatechingallate- induced apoptosis of LNCap cells. *Oncogene,* Vol. 22, pp. 4851-4859

He, M.L., Yuan, H.Q., Jiang, A.L., Gong, A.Y., Chen, W.W., Zhang, P.J., Young, C.Y. & Zhang, J.Y. (2006). Gum mastic inhibits the expression and function of the androgen receptor in prostate cancer cells. *Cancer,* Vol. 106, pp. 2547-55

He, M.L., Li, A., Xu, C.S., Wang, S.L., Zhang, M.J., Gu, H., Yang, Y.Q. & Tao, H.H. (2007a). Mechanisms of antiprostate cancer by gum mastic: NF-kappaB signal as target. *Acta Pharmacologica Sinica,* Vol. 28, pp. 446-52

He, M.L., Chen, W.W., Zhang, P.J., Jiang, A.L., Fan, W., Yuan, H.Q., Liu, W.W. & Zhang, J.Y. (2007b). Gum mastic increases maspin expression in prostate cancer cells. *Acta Pharmacologica Sinica,* Vol. 28, pp. 567-72

Ho, C.T., Wang, M., Huang, G.J. & Huang, M.T. (2000). Chemistry and antioxidative factors in rosemary and sage. *Biofactors,* Vol. 13, pp. 161-166, ISSN: 1872-8081

Holmes-McNary, M. & Baldwin, A.S. (2000). Chemopreventive properties of trans-resveratrol are associated with inhibition of activation of the IkB kinase. *Cancer Research,* Vol. 60, pp. 3477-3483

Hussain, I.V., Anwar, F., Chatha, S.A., Jabbar, A., Mahboob, S. & Nigam, S.P. (2010). Rosmarinus officinalis essential oil: Antiproliferative, antioxidant and antibacterial activities., *Brazilian Journal of Microbiology,* Vol. 41, pp. 1070-1078, ISSN 1517-8382

Huwez, F.U. & Al-Habbal, M.J. (1986). Mastic in treatment of benign gastric ulcers. *Gastroenterologia Japonica,* Vol. 21, pp. 273-74

Ipek, E., Zeytinoglu, H., Okay, S., Tuylu, B., Kurkouglu, M., Hisnu, C. & Baser, K. (2005). Genotoxicity and antigenotoxicity of Origanumoil and carvacrol evaluated by Ames Salmonella/microsomal test. *Food Chemistry,* Vol. 93, pp. 551-556

Ippoushi, K., Azuma, K., Ito, H., Horie, H. & Higashio, H. (2003). [6]-Gingerol inhibits nitric oxide synthesis in activated J774.1 mouse macrophages and prevents peroxynitrite-induced oxidation and nitration reactions. *Life Science,* Vol. 73, pp. 3427–3437 |

Iwuchukwu, O.F., Tallarida, R.J., & Nagar, S. (2011). Resveratrol in combination with other dietary polyphenols concomitantly enhances antiproliferation and UGT1A1 induction in Caco-2 cells. *Life Science,* Vol. 88, pp. 1047-1054

Jin, H., Tan, X., Liu, X. & Ding, Y. (2010). The study of effect of tea polyphenols on microsatellite instability colorectal cancer and its molecular mechanism. *International Journal of Colorectal Disease,* Vol. 25, pp. 1407-1415

Joe, A.K., Liu, H., Suzui, M., Vural, M.E., Xiao, D. & Weinstein, I.B. (2002). Resveratrol induces growth inhibition, S-phase arrest, apoptosis, and changes in biomarker expression in several human cancer cell lines. *Clinical Cancer Research,* Vol. 8, pp. 893-903

Johnson, I.T. (2007). Phytochemicals and cancer. *Proceedings of the Nutrition Society,* Vol. 66, pp. 207-215

Johnson, J.J., Syed, N.D., Heren, R.C., Suh, Y., Adhami, M.V. & Mukhtar, H. (September 2008). Carnosol, a dietary diterpene, displays growth inhibitory effects in human prostate cancer PC3 cells leading to G2-phase cell cycle arrest and targets the 5'-AMP-activated protein kinase (AMPK) pathway. *Pharmacological Research*, Vol. 25, pp. 2125–2134

Johnson, J.J. (June 2011). Carnosol: a promising anti-cancer and anti-inflammatory agent. *Cancer Letters*, Vol. 305, pp. 1-7

Kaliora, A.C., Stathopoulou, M.G., Triantafillidis, J.K., Dedoussis, G.V. & Andrikopoulos, N.K. (2007a). Chios mastic treatment of patients with active Crohn's disease. *World Journal of Gastroenterology*, Vol. 13, pp. 748-53, ISSN: 1007-9327

Kaliora, A.C., Stathopoulou, M.G., Triantafillidis, J.K., Dedoussis, G.V. & Andrikopoulos, N.K. (2007b). Alternations in the function of circulating mononuclear cells derived from patients with Crohn's disease treated with mastic. *World Journal of Gastroenterology*, Vol. 13, pp. 6031-36, ISSN: 1007-9327

Kaliora, A.C., Kountouri, A.M., Stathopoulou, G.M., & Andrikopoulos, N.K. (2010). Antioxidant and Anti-inflammatory properties of Mastic Terpenes: A natural product of the Mediterranean. Book of abstract of *Terpenes: Application, Activity, Analysis* (abstact no.P47), Istanbul, Turkey, 26-29 September, 2010

Karioti, A., Vrahimi-Hadjilouca, T., Droushiotis, D., Rancic A., Hadjipavlou-Litina, D. & Skaltsa, H. (2006). Analysis of the essential oils of Origanum dubium growing wild in Cyprus: investigation of its antioxidant capacity and antimicrobial activity. *Planta Medica*, Vol. 72, pp. 1330-1334

Kountouri, A.M., Kaliora, A.C., Koumbi, L. & Andrikopoulos, N.K. (2009). In-vitro gastric cancer prevention by a polyphenol-rich extract from olives through induction of apoptosis. *European Journal of Cancer Prevention*. Vol. 18, pp. 33-39

Kryston, B.T., Georgiev, B.A., Pissis, P. & Georgakilas, G.A. (2011). Role of oxidative stress and DNA damage in human carcinogenesis. *Mutation Research*, Vol. 711, pp. 193–201Lee, K.W., Bode, A.M. & Dong, Z. (2011). Molecular targets of phytochemicals for cancer prevention. *Nature Reviews Cancer*, Vol. 11, pp. 211-218

Li, Y., Ahmed, F., Ali, S., Philip, P.A., Kucuk, O. & Sarkar, F.H. (2005). Inactivation of nuclear factor kB by soy isoflavone genistein contributes to increased apoptosis induced by chemotherapeutic agents in human cancer cells. *Cancer Research*, Vol. 65, pp. 6934-6942

Liang, Y.C., Tsai, S.H., Tsai, D.C., Lin-Shiau, S.Y. & Lin, J.K. (2001). Suppression of inducible cyclooxygenase and nitric oxide synthase through activation of peroxisome proliferatoractivated receptor-gamma by flavonoids in mouse macrophages. *FEBS Letters*, Vol. 496, pp. 12–18

Liang, Y.C., Tsai, S.H., Chen, L., Lin-Shiau, S.Y. & Lin, J.K. (2003). Resveratrol-induced G2 arrest through the inhibition of CDK7 and p34CDC2 kinases in colon carcinoma HT29 cells. *Biochemical Pharmacology*, Vol. 65, pp. 1053-1060

Loutrari, H., Hatziapostolou, M., Skouridou, V., Papadimitriou, E., Roussos, C., Kolisis, F.N. & Papapetropoulos, A. (2004). Perillyl alcohol is an angiogenesis inhibitor. *Journal of Pharmacology and Experimental Therapeutics*, Vol. 311, pp. 568-75

Lu, Y. & Foo, L.Y. (2001). Antioxidant activities of polyphenols from sage (Salvia officinalis). *Food Chemistry*, Vol. 75, pp. 197-202

Maltzman, T.H., Christou, M., Gould, M.N. & Jefcoate, C.R. (1991). Effects of monoterpenoids on in vivo DMBA-DNA adduct formation and on phase I hepatic metabolizing enzymes. *Carcinogenesis*, Vol. 12, pp. 2081-90

Manna, S.K., Mukhopadhyay, A.A. & Aggarwal, B.B. (2000). Resveratrol suppresses TNF-induced activation of nuclear transcription factors NF-kappa B, activator protein-1, and apoptosis: potential role of reactive oxygen intermediates and lipid peroxidation. *Journal of Immunology*, Vol. 164, pp. 6509-6519, ISSN: 1550-6606

Mills, J.J., Chari, R.S., Boyer, I.J., Gould, M.N. & Jirtle, R.L. (1995). Induction of apoptosis in liver tumors by the monoterpene perillyl alcohol. *Cancer Research*, Vol. 55, pp. 979-83

Mezzoug, N., Elhadri, A., Dallouh, A., Amkiss, S., Skali, N.S., Abrini, J., Zhiri, A., Baudoux, D., Diallo, B., El Jaziri, M. & Idaomar, M. (2007). Investigation of the mutagenic and antimutagenic effects of Origanum compactum essential oil and some of its constituents. *Mutation Research*, Vol. 629, pp. 100-110

Moran, A.E., Carothers, A.M., Weyant, M.J., Redston, M., & Bertagnolli, M.M. (2005). Carnosol inhibits betacatenin tyrosine phosphorylation and prevents adenoma formation in the C57BL/6J/Min/+ (Min/+) mouse. *Cancer Research*, Vol. 65, pp. 1097–1104

Moulos, P., Papadodima, O., Chatziioannou, A., Loutrari, H., Roussos, C. & Kolisis, F.N. (2009). A transcriptomic computational analysis of mastic oil-treated Lewis lung carcinomas reveals molecular mechanisms targeting tumor cell growth and survival. *BMC Medical Genomics*, Vol. 2, pp. 1-15

Nelson, D.R., Kamataki, T., Waxman, D.J., Guengerich, F.P., Estabrook, R.W., Feyereisen, R Gonzalez FJ, Coon MJ, Gunsalus IC, Gotoh O, et al. (1993) The P450 superfamily: update on new sequences, gene mapping, accession numbers, early trivial names of enzymes, and nomenclature. *DNA and Cell Biology* 12, 1–51

Nicholas, C., Batra, S., Vargo, M.A., Voss, O.H., Gavrilin, M.A., Wewers, M.D., Guttridge, D.C., Grotewold, E. & Doseff, A.I. (2007). Apigenin blocks lipopolysaccharide-induced lethality in vivo and proinflammatory cytokines expression by inactivating NF-kappaB through the suppression of p65 phosphorylation. *Journal of Immunology*, 1Vol. 79, pp. 7121-7127

Ovesná, Z., Kozics, K. & Slamenová, D. (2006). Protective effects of ursolic acid and oleanolic acid in leukemic cells. *Mutation Research*, Vol. 600, pp. 131-137

Özmen, A., Bauer, S., Gridling, M., Singhuber, J., Krasteva, S., Madlener, S., Nha Vo, T.P., Stark, N., Saiko, P., Fritzer-Szekers, M., Szekeres, T., Askin-Celik, T., Krenn, L., & Krupitza, G. (2009). In vitro anti-neoplastic activity of the ethno-pharmaceutical plant Hypericum adenotrichum Spach endemic to Western Turkey. *Oncology Reports*, Vol. 22, pp. 845-852

Papageorgiou, V.P., Bakola-Christianopoulou, M.N., Apazidou, K.K. & Psarros, E.E. (1997). Gas chromatographic-mass spectroscopic analysis of the acidic triterpenic fraction of mastic gum. *Journal of Chromatography A*, Vol. 769, pp. 263-73

Paraschos, S., Magiatis, P., Mitakou, S., Petraki, K., Kalliaropoulos, A., Maragkoudakis, P., Mentis, A., Sgouras, D. & Skaltsounis, A.L. (2007). In vitro and in vivo activities of Chios mastic gum extracts and constituents against Helicobacter pylori. *Antimicrobial Agents and Chemotherapy*, Vol. 51, pp. 551-59

Peternac, D., Klima, I., Cecchini, M.G., Schwaninger, R., Studer, U.E. & Thalmann, G.N. (2008). Agents used for chemoprevention of prostate cancer may influence PSA secretion independently of cell growth in the LNCaP model of human prostate cancer progression., *Prostate*, Vol. 68, pp. 1307-1318

Plummer, S.M., Holloway, K.A., Manson, M.M., Munks, R.J., Kaptein, A., Farrow, S. & Howells, L. (1999). Inhibition of cyclo-oxygenase 2 expression in colon cells by the chemopreventive agent curcumin involves inhibition of NFkappaB activation via the NIK/IKK signaling complex. *Oncogene*, Vol. 18, pp. 6013–6020, ISSN 0950-9232

Rao, B.S., Shanbhoge, R., Upadhya, D., Jagetia, G.C., Adiga, S.K., Kumar, P., Guruprasad, K. & Gayathri, P. (2006). Antioxidant, anticlastogenic and radioprotective effect of Coleus aromaticus on Chinese hamster fibroblast cells (V79) exposed to gamma radiation. *Mutagenesis*, Vol. 21, pp. 237-242

Ramos, S. (2007) Effects of dietary flavonoids on apoptotic pathways related to cancer chemoprevention. *Journal of Nutritional Biochemistry*, Vol. 18, pp. 427–442

Ramos, S. (2008) Cancer chemoprevention and chemotherapy: Dietary polyphenols and signalling pathways. *Molecular Nutrition and Food Research*, Vol. 52, pp. 507 - 526

Reddy, B.S., Wang, C.X., Samaha, H., Lubet, R., Steele, V.E., Kelloff, G.J. & Rao, C.V. (1997). Chemoprevention of colon carcinogenesis by dietary perillyl alcohol. *Cancer Research*, Vol. 57, pp. 420-425

Robbers, J.E., Speedie, M.K., & Tyler, V.E. (1994). *Pharmacognosy and pharmacobiotechnology*. Williams & Wilkins. Baltimore

Romier, B., Van De Walle, J., During, A., Larondelle, Y. & Schneider, Y.J. Modulation of signalling nuclear factor-kB activation pathway by polyphenols in human intestinal Caco-2 cells. 2008, *British Journal of Nutrition*, Vol. 100, pp. 542-551

Saddiqe, Z., Naeem, I. & Maimoona, A. (2010). A review of the antibacterial activity of Hypericum perforatum L. *Journal of Ethnopharmacology*, Vol. 131, pp. 511-521

Sasaki, K., Wada, K., Tanaka, Y., Yoshimura, T., Matuoka, K. & Anno, T. (2005). Thyme (Thymus vulgaris L.) leaves and its constituents increase the activities of xenobiotic-metabolizing enzymes in mouse liver. *Journal of Medicinal Food, Vol.* 8, pp. 184-189

Shen, F., Chen, S.J., Dong, X.J., Zhong, H., Li, Y.T. & Cheng, G.F. (2003). Suppression of IL-8 gene transcription by resveratrol in phorbol ester treated human monocytic cells. *Journal of Asian Natural Products Research*, Vol. 5, pp. 151-157

Siddiqui, I.A., Shukla, Y., Adhami, V.M., Sarfaraz, S., Asim, M., Hafeez, B.B. & Mukhtar, H. (2008). Suppression of NFkappaB and its regulated gene products by oral administration of green tea polyphenols in an autochthonous mouse prostate cancer model. *Pharmaceutical Research*, Vol. 25, pp. 2135–2142

Singletary, K.W. (1996). Rosemary extract and carnosol stimulate rat liver glutathione-S-transferase and quinone reductase activities. *Cancer Letters*. Vol. 10, pp. 139-44

Slamenova, D., Horvathova, E., Sramkova, M. & Marsalkova, L. (2007). DNA-protective effects of two components of essential plant oils carvacrol and thymol on mammalian cells cultured in vitro. *Neoplasma*, Vol. 54, pp. 108-112, ISSN 1337-9569

Sogno, I., Vannini, N., Lorusso, G., Cammarota, R., Noonan, D.M., Generoso, L., Sporn, M.B. & Albini, A. (2009). Anti-angiogenic activity of a novel class of chemopreventive compounds: oleanic acid terpenoids. *Recent Results in Cancer Research*, Vol. 181, pp. 209-212

Stamatis, G., Kyriazopoulos, P., Golegou, S., Basayiannis, A., Skaltsas, S. & Skaltsa, H. (2003). In vitro anti-Helicobacter pylori activity of Greek herbal medicines. *Journal of Ethnopharmacology*, Vol. 88, pp. 175-179

Stark, M.J., Burke, Y.D., McKinzie, J.H., Ayoubi, A.S. & Crowell, P.L. (1995). Chemotherapy of pancreatic cancer with the monoterpene perillyl alcohol. *Cancer Letters*, Vol. 96, pp. 15–21

Stayrook, K.R., McKinzie, J.H., Burke, Y.D., Burke, Y.A. & Crowell, P.L. (1997). Induction of the apoptosis-promoting protein Bak by perillyl alcohol in pancreatic ductal adenocarcinoma relative to untransformed ductal epithelial cells. *Carcinogenesis*, Vol. 18, pp. 1655-58

Stratton, S.P., Saboda, K.L., Myrdal, P.B., Gupta, A., McKenzie, N.E., Brooks, C., Salasche, S.J., Warneke, J.A., Ranger-Moore, J., Bozzo, P.D., Blanchard, J., Einspahr, J.G., Dorr, R.T., Levine, N. & Alberts, D.S. (2008). Phase 1 study of topical perillyl alcohol cream for chemoprevention of skin cancer. *Nutrion and Cancer*, Vol. 60, pp. 325-330

Syed, D.N., Khan, N., Afaq, F. & Mukhtar, H. (2007). Chemoprevention of Prostate Cancer through Dietary Agents: Progress and Promise. *Cancer Epidemiology, Biomarkers and Prevention*, Vol. 16, pp. 2193-2203

Thorsen, M.A. & Hildebrandt, K.S. (2003). Quantitative determination of phenolic diterpenes in rosemary extracts. Aspects of accurate quantification. *Journal of Chromatography A*, Vol. 995, pp. 119-125

Triantafyllou, A., Chaviaras, N., Sergentanis, T.N., Protopapa, E. & Tsaknis, J. (2007). Chios mastic gum modulates serum biochemical parameters in a human population. *Journal of Ethnopharmacology*, Vol. 111, pp. 43-9

Tsai, P.J., Tsai, T.H., Yu, C.H., and Ho, S.C. (2007). Evaluation of NO-suppressing activity of several Mediterranean culinary spices. *Food and Chemical Toxicology*, Vol. 45, pp. 440-447

Visanji, J.M., Thompson, D.G. & Padfield, P.J. (2006). Induction of G2/M phase cell cycle arrest by carnosol and carnosic acid is associated with alteration of cyclin A and cyclin B1 levels. *Cancer Letters*, Vol. 237, pp. 130–136

Woo KJ, Jeong YJ, Inoue H, Park, J.W. & Kwon, T.K. (2005). Chrysin suppresses lipopolysaccharide-induced cyclooxygenase- 2 expression through the inhibition of nuclear factor for IL-6 (NF-IL6) DNA-binding activity., *FEBS Letters*, Vol. 579, pp. 705-711

Wung, B.S., Hsu, M.C., Wu, C.C. & Hsieh, C.W. (2005). Resveratrol suppresses IL-6 induced ICAM-1 gene expression in endothelial cells: effects on the inhibition of STAT3 phosphorylation. *Life Science*, Vol. 78, pp. 389–397

Yamai, H., Sawada, N., Yoshida, T., Seike, J., Takizawa, H., Kenzaki, K., Miyoshi, T., Kondo, K., Bando, Y., Ohnishi, Y. & Tangoku, A. (2009). Triterpenes augment the inhibitory effects of anticancer drugs on growth of human esophageal carcinoma cells in vitro and supress experimental metastasis in vivo. *International Journal of Cancer*, vol. 125, pp. 952-960

Zheng, W. & Wang, S.Y. (2001). Antioxidant activity and phenolic compounds in selected herbs. *Journal of Agriculture and Food Chemistry*, Vol. 49, pp. 5165-5170

Zhou, C., Tabb, M.M., Sadatrafiei, A., Grün, F., Sun, A. & Blumberg, B. (2004). Hyperforin, the active component of St. John's wort, induces IL-8 expression in human intestinal epithelial cells via a MAPK-dependent, NF-kappaB-independent pathway. *Journal of Clinical Immunology*, Vol. 24, pp. 623-636

11

Dietary Manipulation for Therapeutic Effect in Prostate Cancer

Carol A Gano[1], Kieran Scott[2], Joseph Bucci[2], Heather Greenfield[3], Qihan Dong[4,5] and Paul L de Souza[1*]

[1]*University of Western Sydney School of Medicine and Ingham Institute, Liverpool Hospital, Campbelltown and Liverpool, NSW*
[2]*St. George Hospital Clinical School, UNSW, Kogarah, NSW*
[3]*Adjunct Professor, University of Sydney and University of NSW, Randwick, NSW*
[4]*University of Western Sydney School of Health Science, Campbelltown, NSW*
[5]*University of Sydney Central Clinical School, Sydney, NSW*
Australia

1. Introduction

Given that there is a wealth of literature on the potential effect of a wide variety of phytochemicals on the growth of prostate cancer cells, we have limited our discussion to arguably four of the most important: isoflavones, lycopene, resveratrol, and curcumin. The focus of this review is on the clinical pharmacology of these compounds, as there are already an extensive number of reviews in the literature on all of these compounds for various cancers, including our previous review of isoflavones in prostate cancer (de Souza et al., 2009). Here, we use the loose term "phytochemicals" to describe this group of plant-based compounds with biological activity *in vitro,* for simplicity. Like other phytochemicals, isoflavones, lycopene, resveratrol and curcumin have a wide variety of potential mechanisms of action in many different cancer cell lines. Many of these biological effects involve key components of signal transduction pathways within cancer cells, but in this review, we will be focusing on studies specifically in prostate cancer.

Reactive oxidative species (ROS) may have an overall contribution to the development of cancer (Kryston et al., 2011; Benhar et al., 2002), but the mechanism is far from clear, though the general thrust of the argument is that DNA damage wrought by ROS may be left unchecked or uncorrected by mismatch repair enzymes, thereby contributing to carcinogenesis (Benhar et al., 2002, Ziech et al., 2010, Kryston et al., 2011). However, it is also apparent that higher levels of ROS can activate intrinsic apoptosis (Benhar et al., 2002), which would imply that antioxidants should not be used indiscriminately as it could prevent a desirable outcome in cancer cells. The biological mechanisms underpinning some of the potential anti-oxidant mechanisms of phytochemicals are complex and as yet speculative, and will not be discussed here. Instead, readers are referred to recent reviews (Ziech et al., 2010; Kryston et al., 2011).

---

* Corresponding author

Table 1 lists the major sources of our selected phytochemicals (Holden et al., 1999; Neveu et al., 2010; Nutrient Data, L. & Knovel, 2008; Tayyem et al., 2009), though we acknowledge that many other foods contain smaller amounts as well, though they are not reviewed here.

Food	Curcumin mg/100g	Lycopene mg/100g	Isoflavones mg/100g	Resveratrol mg/100g
Apricots, tinned		0.065		
Bilberry				0.67
Chocolate, dark				0.04
Cranberries, European				1.92
Curry	50-580			
Grape, black				0.15
Grapefruit, pink		1.3-1.5		
Guava, fresh		5.4		
Guava, juice		3.3		
Lingonberry				3.00
Peanut			0.02	0.08
Peanut butter			0.01	0.04
Pistachio			3.6	0.11
Red currant				1.57
Soy paste, miso			41.4	
Soybean, tofu,firm			22.5	
Soybean,tofu, silken			30.0	
Strawberry				0.35
Tomato, raw		3.0		
Tomato, boiled		4.4		
Tomato juice		9.3		
Tomato paste		6.5-29.3		
Tomato, sauce (ketsup)		17.0		
Tomato, tinned		9.7		
Turmeric powder	580-3,140			
Wine, Red				0.27
Wine, Rose				0.12
Wine, White				0.04

Table 1. Dietary sources of selected phytochemicals.

2. Isoflavones

Soy and soy products, rye bread, and red clover, are good sources of flavonoids (Adlercreutz, 2002). Flavonoids, in turn, are made up of isoflavones, flavonones, flavones, flavonols, catechins, anthocyanins, and chalcones, of which the isoflavones are but a small part, though disproportionately studied. Isoflavone intake is approximately 50mg daily in Asia, about ten times more than in Western countries (Messina et al., 2006).

2.1 Pharmacology

There are many intermediates and metabolites of isoflavones produced in humans, but the majority have not been studied. Genistin, daidzin and glycitin are thought to be the predominant isoflavones found in soy foods, of which the glycoside moiety is the major form with anticancer activity. Through the action of α - glucosidase provided by gut bacteria, and hydrolysis, the conversion of glycosides to aglycones (Setchell et al., 2002; Yuan et al., 2007; Zubik & Meydani, 2003) allows absorption into the blood. One hypothesis for the variable absorption values obtained from studies is the variability of the gut microbacterial environment amongst humans. Some support for this concept was provided by Rufer et al., (2008), who gave pure daidzein in both its aglycone and glycoside forms to seven volunteer men in a randomized, double - blind study, at a dose of 1mg/kg. Bioavailability of the glycoside form was found to be 3-6 times higher than that of the aglycone form, with half - life measured at 6.4h for the glycoside and 8.9h for the aglycone. Given the differences recorded for maximum concentration (Cmax) and urinary excretion, it is not unreasonable to speculate that this observation could be explained by the time taken by gut microflora to generate metabolites. Inter - individual variability in pharmacokinetic parameters was very high for these metabolites, which clearly could not be explained by differences in pharmacogenomic factors, due to the randomized crossover design.

There are few other pharmacokinetic reports of isoflavones and data are derived largely from single dose administration studies. In general, aglycones appear in the blood within two hours of ingestion (Atkinson et al., 2005; Franke et al., 1995; Richelle et al., 2002; Setchell et al., 2001). Peak plasma concentrations (Cmax) for aglycones occur at 4-7h, whereas the corresponding time for glycosides is 8-11h, implying that the rate limiting step for absorption is initial hydrolysis of the isoflavone (Setchell et al., 2001; Zubik & Meydani, 2003). After about 48hrs, plasma concentrations are no longer detectable. In a study reported by Setchell et al., (2003), higher doses of isoflavones did not produce linear pharmacokinetic parameters, suggesting that uptake was rate - limiting and saturable. Administration of approximately 80mg isoflavones a day is thought to give concentrations of genistein and daidzein consistent with that found in patients on a high isoflavone diet (Howes et al., 2002).

2.2 *In vitro* data

The literature attests to a large array of potential biological effects of isoflavones, despite their similarity in chemical structure: genistein binds estrogen receptor better than daidzein (Kuiper et al., 1998) for example, and equol is more potent than daidzein in inhibiting prostate cancer cell growth (Hedlund et al., 2003). Genistein produces apoptosis in prostate cancer cells (Kyle et al., 1997), but it is also possible that low doses promote cancer cell growth while higher doses inhibit growth (Bergan et al., 1996). This apparently conflicting data is not limited to isoflavones, and if the potential biphasic effects of phytochemicals are true, the underlying mechanisms for this observation could represent an important area of future research.

Tyrosine kinase phosphorylation appears to be a key event influencing the fate of many cancer cells, and inhibition may increase apoptosis or inhibit prostate cancer cell growth. Some isoflavones appear to have this ability; for example, genistein has been shown to reduce FAK (focal adhesion kinase) activity just prior to apoptosis (Kyle et al., 1997). It can also transiently activate the FAK : beta - 1 - integrin complex (Bergan et al., 1996; Liu et al., 2000), which could theoretically help explain its ability to reduce metastases. Further, isoflavones may reduce activity of ERK1/2 and various cyclin dependent kinases (Agarwal et al., 2000). A range of other potential mechanisms for the growth inhibiting effects of isoflavones have been described (see Table 2).

2.3 *In vivo* data

Soy protein or biochanin A (another isoflavone) inhibits growth and increases apoptosis in the LNCaP prostate cancer xenograft model (Bylund et al., 2000; Rice et al., 2002). Dietary genistein supplementation can reduce the incidence of poorly differentiated adenocarcinoma in a transgenic strain of mice (Mentor-Marcel et al., 2001), and can improve survival. In a model where prostate cancer is induced by chemical carcinogens methyl nitrosourea (NMU) or 3,2-dimethyl-4-aminobiphenyl (DMAB) (Kato et al., 2000), soy protein or genistein can prevent growth (McCormick et al., 2007; Wang et al., 2002). Dose - response studies involving subcutaneously and orthotopically implanted tumours (Zhou et al., 1999; 2002) demonstrated clear reduction of tumor growth with a variety of isoflavone preparations, though changes in a variety of biomarkers were not consistent, and depended on the type of isoflavone preparation.

2.4 Clinical studies in prostate cancer

An interesting study of 40 men randomized post-prostatectomy to a low fat / high isoflavone diet (Li et al., 2008) or a control diet showed lower 6 month IGF-1 concentrations in the treatment group. Sera collected from treated patients were able to reduce *in vitro* growth of LNCaP cancer cells by 20%, suggesting biologically relevant concentrations were achieved. Soy has been shown to suppress growth of localized, but not for advanced disease (Kurahashi et al., 2007), perhaps not surprisingly, since prostate cancer is a heterogenous disease, and more advanced disease may have different underlying biology. Pharmacogenomic work suggests that the reduction in risk of prostate cancer may be positively associated with a greater ability to produce equol from other isoflavones (Akaza et al., 2002, 2004). "Nutrigenomic" factors may therefore play an important part in predicting those who might benefit from phytoestrogen supplementation (Steiner et al, 2008).

Many studies do not show evidence of benefit for isoflavones. One randomized, placebo-controlled trial of 12 weeks treatment with genistein in men with early prostate cancer found no significant difference in PSA levels between the treatment and placebo groups (Kumar et al., 2004), although the authors suggested that surrogate measures were being affected by treatment. Other trials support the idea that isoflavones, even given over relatively short periods of time, can possibly slow the rate of rise of PSA, though no statistically significant conclusions can be drawn (Dalais et al., 2004; Hussain et al., 2003; Maskarinec et al., 2006; Pendleton et al., 2008). Even by administering high doses, up to 600mg genistein daily, no statistically significant PSA changes were noted in a Phase I and

	Action	References
Androgen related functions		
5α reductase	a. Inhibited by genistein	a. (Evans et al., 1995)
PART-1	a. Prostate androgen regulated transcript 1 inhibited by genistein and daidzein	a. (Yu et al., 2003)
AR	a. Transcriptionally downregulated by genistein b. In LNCaP cells, Lycopene inhibited AR gene element in a dose response manner c. Resveratrol inhibits AR transcription activity in LNCaP d. Curcumin downregulates AR gene expression in androgen dependent and castration resistant prostate cancer cells	a. (Davis et al., 2000; Takahashi et al., 2006; Tepper et al., 2007) b. (Zhang et al., 2010) c. (Wang et al, 2010) d. (Nakamura et al, 2002; Tsui et al., 2008)
PSA	a. mRNA expression and secretion reduced by genistein b. PSA mRNA not downregulated by lycopene in LNCaP c. Resveratrol downregulates expression in LNCaP cells d. Curcumin inhibits PSA expression	a. (Davis et al., 2000; Rice et al., 2007) b. (Peternac et al., 2008) c. (Hsieh & Wu, 2000; Mitchell et al., 1999) d. (Tsui et al., 2008)
Cell survival and proliferation		
DNA synthesis	b. Lycopene reduces DNA synthesis in primary cultures of prostate epithelia	b. (Barber et al, 2006)
Cyclins	a. Cyclin B downregulated by genistein b. Lycopene downregulates cyclin D1 c. C1/Cdk4 kinase and D1, E, B and cdk1 all downregulated by resveratrol in LNCaP lines; resveratrol increases cyclin A and cyclin E in LNCaP cells d. Curcumin downregulates cyclin expression	a. (Davis et al., 1998) b. (Palozza et al., 2010) c. (Benitez et al., 2007; Kuwajerwala et al., 2002) d. (Aggarwal et al., 2009)
Myt-1	a. Upregulated by genistein	a. (Touny & Banerjee, 2006)
Wee-1	a. Phosphorylation reduced by genistein	a. (Touny & Banerjee, 2006)
$p21^{WAF1}$	a. Upregulated by genistein c. Decreased by resveratrol in LNCaP d. Upregulated by curcumin	a. (Davis et al., 1998; Lian et al., 1998) c. (Benitez et al., 2007; Kuwajerwala et al., 2002; Mitchell et al., 1999) d. (Aggarwal et al., 2007)

p27^{Kip1}	a. Increased by genistein c. Upregulated by resveratrol in LNCaP only, not in PC-3 cells; repressed by resveratrol in LNCaP cells d. Upregulated by curcumin	a. (Bhatia & Agarwal, 2001; Kazi et al., 2003; Rice et al., 2007) c. (Benitez et al., 2007; Kuwajerwala et al., 2002) d. (Aggarwal et al., 2007)
Protein tyrosine kinase	a. Inhibition of EGF tyrosine kinase activation by genistein c. Resveratrol inhibits tyrosine kinase d. Curcumin inhibits EGF-R signaling	a. (Akiyama et al., 1987) c. (Sallman et al., 2007) d. (Dorai et al., 2000)
PTEN	a.Expression is induced by genistein and daidzein in PC3 and LNCaP	a. (Cao et al., 2006)
Akt	a. Inhibited by genistein b. Lycopene decreases AKT activation, leading to apoptosis in both androgen-responsive and independent PCa cells c. Inhibited by resveratrol d. Inhibited by curcumin; PI3K inhibited by curcumin	a. (Bemis et al., 2004; Li & Sarkar, 2002; El Touny & Banerjee, 2007; Park et al., 2005) b. (Ivanov et al., 2007) c. (Aziz et al., 2006; Chen et al., 2010) d. (Yu et al., 2008; Shankar & Srivastava, 2007)
mTOR	a. Inhibited by genistein c. Resveratrol inhibits mTOR d. Inhibited by curcumin in PC-3 cells,	a. (Rice et al., 2007) c. (Brito et al, 2009; Chen et al., 2010) d. (Yu et al., 2008)
MAPK	a. MAPK inhibited by genistein b. Lycopene, at least partially inhibits MAPK c. MAPK is inhibited by resveratrol d. P38 is activated by curcumin in PC3 cells	a. (Huang et al., 2005; Xu & Bergan, 2006) b. (Palozza et al., 2010) c. (Nguyen et al., 2008) d. (Hilchie et al., 2010)
ERK1/2	a. Inhibited by genistein; induced by isoflavones	a. (Agarwal, 2000; Bhatia & Agarwal, 2001; Wang et al., 2006; Wang et al., 2004)
JNK	a. Activation by genistein d. Activated by curcumin	a. (Lazarevic et al., 2008) d. (Hilchie et al., 2010)
NFκB	a. Inhibited by genistein and soy isoflavones b. Downregulated by resveratrol	a. (Davis et al., 1999; Li & Sarkar, 2002; Raffoul et al., 2007; Singh-Gupta et al., 2009) b. (Benitez et al., 2009)
IGF-1/R	a. Inhibition by genistein b. Lycopene decreases IGF-1R expression in PC-3 cells	a. (Takahashi et al., 2006, Wang et al., 2003) b. (Kanagaraj et al., 2007)

STAT	a. Activated by genistein c. Resveratrol inhibits Src and Jak kinases d. STAT 3 is inhibited by curcumin, but even more so by synthetic analogues of curcumin	a. (Pinski et al., 2006) c. (Sallman et al., 2007) d. (Lin et al., 2009)
TGFβ	a. TGFβ inhibited by genistein d. IL6 induction via TGFβ inhibited via curcumin	a. (Xu & Bergan, 2006) d. (Park et al., 2003)
Apoptosis		
Mdm2	a. Downregulated by genistein d. mRNA reduced by Curcumin in a dose dependent manner	a. (Li et al., 2005) d. (Li et al., 2007)
Bax	a. Increased by genistein b. Lycopene upregulates Bax in LNCaP c. Increased due to resveratrol in LNCaP d. Curcumin upregulates	a. (Kazi et al., 2003) b. (Palozza et al., 2010) c. (Benitez et al., 2007) d. (Shankar & Srivastava, 2007)
Bcl-XL	a. Downregulated by genistein d. Down regulated by curcumin	a. (Li et al., 2001) d. (Shankar & Srivastava, 2007)
XIAP	a. Inhibited by phenoxodiol in ovarian cancer cells and melanoma cells c. Resveratrol promotes interaction of XIAP with Bax to cause apoptosis d. Inhibited by curcumin	a. (Alvero et al., 2006; Herst et al., 2007; Kamsteeg et al., 2003, Kluger et al., 2007; Sapi et al., 2004) c. (Gogada et al., 2011) d. (Deeb et al., 2007)
Caspases	a. Activated and caspase inhibition overcome by phenoxodiol in HN12 cells; Caspase mediation by genistein induced apoptosis c. Resveratrol activates caspase: 9,6,7 and 3 leading to apoptosis d. In PC-3 cells, apoptosis caused by curcumin is independent of caspases; In LNCaP curcumin initiates caspase-dependent mitochondrial death	a. (Aguero et al., 2005; Choueiri et al., 2006; Kumi-Diaka et al., 2000; Kumi-Diaka & Butler, 2000) c. (Benitez et al., 2007) d. (Hilchie et al., 2010) PC-3 results, (Shankar & Srivastava, 2007) LNCaP results
Other targets		
HIF1α	a. Inhibition by genistein in PC3 cancer cells d. Curcumin inhibits gene transcription of HIF 1 alpha	a. (Singh-Gupta, 2009) d. (Thomas et al, 2008)

VEGF	a. Downregulated by genistein b. Inhibited by lycopene in xenografts c. Suppressed by resveratrol d. Inhibited by curcumin in LNCaP xenografts	a. (Cao et al., 2006; Guo et al., 2007; Li & Sarkar, 2002) b. (Yang, 2011) c. (Ganapathy et al., 2010) d. (Shankar et al., 2007)
ERβ	a. Antagonist and partial agonist by genistein; expression reduced by genistein d. Estradiol binding inhibited by > 85% in PC-3 cells	a. (Booth et al., 2006; Cao et al., 2006; Kuiper et al., 1998; Pike et al., 1999; Wang et al., 2006) d. (Shenouda, et al., 2004)
COX-2	a. mRNA and protein expression reduced by genistein in LNCaP and PC3	a. (Swami et al., 2009)
Sphingosine Kinase	a. Inhibited by phenoxodiol in endothelial cells c. Inhibited by resveratrol	a. (Gamble et al., 2006) c. (Brizuela, 2010)
TNOX	a. Inhibited by phenoxodiol	a. (Davies & Bozzo, 2006; DeLuca et al., 2005)
Focal adhesion kinase	a. Activity reduced by genistein	a. (Kyle et al., 1997)
Hypermethylation	a. Reversal of DNA methyltransferase activity by genistein	a. (Fang et al., 2007; Skogseth et al., 2005)
MMP	a. MMP2 and 9 downregulated by genistein; MMP2 expression inhibited by phenoxodiol c. MMP3 and MMP9 suppressed by resveratrol d. Curcumin inhibited expression of MMP2 and MMP9	a. (Gamble et al., 2006; Huang et al., 2005; Kumi-Diaka, 2006; Li & Sarkar, 2002 ; Xu & Bergan, 2006) c. (Ganapathy et al., 2010) d. (Hong et al., 2006)
Urokinase plasminogen activator	a. Inhibited by genistein b. Lycopene upregulates UPA receptor	a. (Jarred et al., 2002) b. (Forbes et al., 2003)

Table 2. Selected molecular targets of phytochemicals in prostate cancer cells: (a), (b), (c), (d) refer to isoflavone, lycopene, resveratrol, and curcumin related literature, respectively. While many of these targets have been shown to be relevant in other cancer cell lines, here we have focused on publications on prostate cancer cell lines.

pharmacokinetic study (Fischer et al., 2004), though serum dehydroepiandrosterone was reduced by 31.7% (P = 0.0004) at the end of the study, and estrogenic side effects were encountered. Biologically relevant concentrations of genistein, commensurate with *in vitro* activity, can be achieved with high doses of genistein - enriched isoflavone extracts (Takimoto et al., 2003). Peak plasma concentrations reached between 4.3 and 16.3uM at doses up to 8mg/kg orally (equivalent to 560mg for a 70kg person) in this study.

3. Lycopene

Once water is reduced, the lycopene content of tomato products surpasses all other foods, weight for weight. Although lycopene melts at 172-173 degrees Celsius (Zapalis & Beck, 1985), processing and cooking improves availability of tomato-sourced lycopene. Being fat soluble, tomato sources of lycopene are best absorbed when cooked or consumed with a fat, such as with olive oil in Mediterranean cooking (Itsiopoulos et al., 2009). As lycopene synthesis correlates with tomato ripening, it is older, vine ripened-in-the sun tomatoes that offer the highest lycopene content (Ronen et al., 1999). Other sources of lycopene, in descending order of content are: guava, watermelon, pink grapefruit (Mangels et al., 1993), apricots (Curl, 1960) and rosehips (Böhm et al., 2003).

3.1 Pharmacology

Lycopene is a non-provitamin A carotenoid. The frequency of light absorption, due to its alternating double bond system, defines visual color ranging from pink through to deep red. Once consumed, lycopene micelles are believed to be formed by bile salts and along with fat, pass from the mucosa and into general circulation via low-density lipoproteins (Sharma & Goswami, 2011). It is the only carotenoid associated with plasma cholesterol level (Campbell et al., 1994). Within the body, lycopene is preferentially stored in the liver, seminal vesicles and the prostate tissue. In particular it becomes localized to the nuclear membrane and the nuclear matrix, suggesting that it may have a receptor or transporter role. In Western populations, blood lycopene concentrations range from 0.29-0.60 uM, with a half-life of 2-3 days (Schwedhelm et al., 2003).

A Phase I single-dose study on lycopene pharmacokinetics using increasing doses from 10 to 120 mg found dose dependent half-lives between 28 and 62 hours. Lycopene peaks between 16 and 33 hours after dosing levels of 0.075 to 0.21 uM (Gustin et al., 2004).

3.2 *In vitro* data

Like other phytochemicals, many potential mechanisms of action have been put forward to explain the anticancer properties of lycopene. Of relevance to prostate cancer, lycopene has been shown to inhibit DNA synthesis (Barber et al., 2006). Lycopene also inhibits growth of hormone-dependent LNCaP and C4-2 prostate cancer cell lines without affecting PSA mRNA expression (Peternac et al., 2008), and increases expression of PPARgamma and LXRalpha in LNCaP cells (Yang et al., 2011). It also inactivates Ras and reduces NFkappaB, as well as inducing apoptosis in LNCaP cells (Palozza et al., 2010). While it can reduce Akt activation (Ivanov et al., 2007), its ability to induce apoptosis may be cell line-dependent. Other potential mechanisms of action by lycopene in prostate cancer are listed in Table 2.

In combination with docetaxel, lycopene inhibits growth of hormone independent prostate cancer DU145 cells through insulin-like growth factor 1 receptors leading to downstream inhibition of survivin expression and subsequent apoptosis (Tang et al., 2011).

Almost certainly, variations in experimental conditions, doses and techniques could contribute to these apparent biological effects. At physiological concentrations, however, lycopene may not have growth inhibitory effects on a variety of cell lines (Burgess et al., 2008). This was confirmed recently in experiments where supraphysiological concentrations were required to reduce growth, possibly through alterations in the cell cycle (Ford et al., 2011).

3.3 *In vivo* data

Athymic mice models used by Yang et al., (2011) show strong inhibition of PC3 xenograft growth by high doses of lycopene (16 mg/kg), possibly via increased levels of insulin-like growth factor-binding protein 3, or a reduction in plasma vascular endothelial growth factor (VEGF) levels. In a provocative study of androgen expressing prostate cancer cell lines treated with serum from rats fed a control diet, or diets supplemented with red, or yellow tomato (containing no lycopene), connexin43 (a protein regulating cell growth) was upregulated by both the red and yellow tomato supplemented diet (Gitenay et al., 2007). This suggests tomato compounds other than lycopene may have a role in reducing prostate cancer cell growth; one such candidate might be FruHis, a carbohydrate derivative found in tomato products (Mossine et al., 2008). However, in humans at least, dietary lycopene has been shown to affect gene expression, regardless of whether it is included in its food matrix (Talvas et al., 2010)

In a transgenic mouse model, early intervention with selenium, vitamin E and lycopene supplements was able to significantly reduce prostate cancer and liver metastases (Venkateswaran et al, 2009). Limpens et al., (2006) had earlier reached the same conclusion, but they did not see any activity from the single agents. Naturally, it is difficult to know how much the additional supplements contributed to prostate cancer control, though both groups suggest the combination was important. Not all data are supportive of the growth inhibitory effect of lycopene however, possibly because of differences in the rat model used by Imaida et al., (2001).

3.4 Clinical studies in prostate cancer

Mills et al., (1989), through the Seventh Day Adventist men study, showed a link between low prostate cancer risk and frequent tomato consumption, along with beans, lentils and peas, raisins, dates, and other dried fruit. Giovannucci et al., (2007) performed an analysis on data from the Health Professionals study and found that higher tomato sauce (assumed to be lycopene) intake correlated inversely with prostate cancer incidence; indeed, this was only one of four factors (in addition to African American race, positive family history, and alpha-linolenic acid intake) that predicted for incidence and advanced prostate cancer.

In a small, randomized trial of 30mg lycopene supplementation over 3 weeks prior to prostatectomy, margin positivity at surgery was reduced by lycopene, though no other endpoints were affected (Kucuk et al., 2001). The study was extremely small, and no conclusions can be drawn.

Zhang et al., (2010) recently reported a study in 41 men with localized prostate cancer given 10mg lycopene once a day. Seventy percent of men had a reduced slope of PSA rise, and 21% had a decrease in their PSA levels. However, scant details were available for the study, and we do not know whether there were confounding variables; further, this would appear to be the same patient population as in a previous publication (Barber et al., 2006). In a study of 41 men with localised prostate cancer (Barber et al., 2006) given 20 mg lycopene daily, nearly 70% of patients had a slower rate of PSA rise post-treatment. A study in 20 consecutive men with hormone refractory prostate cancer treated with lycopene 10mg daily had shown a response rate (complete and partial) of 35% (Ansari et al., 2004). However, this phenomenal response rate has not been able to be repeated. Indeed, Vaishampayan et al., (2007) reported a study in 38 men with hormone sensitive and resistant cancer randomized to the lycopene alone arm and found only PSA stabilization, without any patient qualifying for a partial response. Adding soy isoflavones (to men randomized to the other arm) did not appear to improve outcome. Another study in 46 patients with androgen-independent prostate cancer prescribed 15mg lycopene daily found only one patient with a PSA response; toxicity included mainly grade 1-2 diarrhea, nausea, flatulence, and abdominal distension (Jatoi et al., 2007).

4. Resveratrol

Resveratrol is a phytoalexin found in the skins and seeds of red grapes *Vitaceaea vinifera*. Therefore, red wines are especially rich in resveratrol, as is grape juice (Romero-Perez, 1999). Other sources include lentils (as resveratrol-3-O-glucoside), peanuts, dark chocolate and berries (Neveu, 2010).

4.1 Pharmacology

Resveratrol is well-absorbed, but has poor bioavailability due to extensive first pass metabolism by the liver.

A pharmacokinetic study of trans-resveratrol (25, 50, 100 or 150mg single doses, repeated over 13 dosings) showed Cmax detected 48 to 90 minutes post-dosing (Almeida et al., 2009), but there was wide interindividual variability reported, also noted in another pharmacokinetic study (Nunes et al., 2009). In another study in 40 healthy volunteers given a single dose ten times the quantities used in the previous study (500, 1000, 2,500 or 5,000mg), peak plasma concentrations were achieved in 90 minutes, and were associated with a range of plasma resveratrol concentrations between 73 and 539 ng/mL (Boocock et al., 2007). Absorption may be faster after oral dosing (Goldberg et al., 2003), possibly due to delayed absorption by food (Vaz-da-Silva et al., 2008).

Resveratrol is rapidly metabolized. Radioactively labeled carbon-14 distribution studies (Vitrac et al., 2003) have been performed in mice with trans-resveratrol; it distributes to the stomach, intestines, liver and kidney, regions of highest uptakes. Mice, like men (de Santi et al., 2000 a,b,c) also form both sulfur and glucuronide conjugates, but a proportion remains unchanged as trans-resveratrol. A toxicological study with trans-resveratrol (as resVida®) in rats over 4 weeks has tested up to 300 mg/kg/d, with no observed serious adverse events (Edwards et al., 2011).

A phase I trial and repeated dose study to determine safety, pharmacokinetics and the effect on insulin-like growth factor (IGF) axis by resveratrol was recently reported (Brown et al., 2010). Doses of 0.5, 2.5 or 5.0 g per day over 29 days was given to forty volunteers. Levels of resveratrol metabolites in plasma were about 20 times higher than that of free resveratrol, and a reduction of circulating plasma IGF-1 and IGFBP-3 was noted ($P < 0.04$ in both). It is not clear to what extent the metabolites contributed to the fall in plasma IGF-1 and IGFBP-3 levels.

4.2 *In vitro* data

Resveratrol results in dose-dependent inhibition of PI3K and pAkt in LNCaP cells that in turn modulates anti-apoptotic bcl2 family proteins (Aziz et al., 2006). Resveratrol reduces ERK 1/2 activation in PC3 cells (Stewart & O'Brian, 2004) amongst many other targets; some of these are listed in Table 2. For example, resveratrol also reduces the activity of clusterin by functioning as a tyrosine kinase inhibitor (Sallman et al., 2007), phosphoAkt and mTOR (Chen et al., 2010), and NFkB (Benitez et al., 2009). Resveratrol causes growth inhibition in typical prostate cancer cell lines: PC-3, DU145, and LNCaP (Hsieh & Wu, 1999), but interestingly, whole cranberry extract (containing resveratrol) was also effective in inducing apoptosis (Maclean et al., 2011). As in all whole-food extract studies, however, there is no certainty that the molecule of interest is responsible for the effect seen.

4.3 *In vivo* data

In a PC3 xenograft study, resveratrol alone inhibited tumour growth, enhanced TRAIL induced apoptosis, and inhibited angiogenenesis (Ganapathy et al., 2010). Resveratrol is also able to reduce or delay prostate cancer in the TRAMP mouse model (Slusarz et al., 2010), possibly via inhibition of HedgeHog signaling. Conflicting evidence was provided by Wang et al., (2008), who found that resveratrol increased angiogenesis and inhibited apoptosis, at least in LNCaP xenografts.

4.4 Clinical studies in prostate cancer

A review on clinical trials of resveratrol has already been recently published (Patel et al., 2011), and will not be discussed in detail here. Selected prostate cancer trials are listed in Table 3.

Resveratrol dosing studies have been performed at up to 5 grams per day. However, mild gastrointestinal side effects (abdominal pain, nausea, diarrhea) were common in subjects administered resveratrol at a dose 1g daily (Brown et al., 2010; Elliott et al., 2009; la Porte et al, 2010). A Phase I study of resveratrol in 10 volunteers demonstrated that even at the highest 5 g per day cohort, saturation kinetics were not observed (Boocock et al., 2007) and that plasma concentrations remained quite low, 500 ng/mL. This possibly is considerably less that the 5uM concentration required for *in vitro* activity, but six plasma and urine metabolites were identified; whether these compounds contribute to the anticancer activity of resveratrol remains unknown. Two monoglucuronide metabolites of resveratrol area under the curve concentrations were 23-fold hold higher than that of cis-resveratrol (Boocock et al., 2007). Inter-individual pharmacokinetic variability has been found to be high (Almeida et al., 2009). Complicating the picture is that other phytochemicals ingested in the diet, such as quercetin and to a lesser degree, kaempferol, fisetin, apigenin and myricetin, may inhibit phenol sulfotransferase and in doing so, increase resveratrol absorption (de Santi et al., 2000 a, b).

As the studies in Table 3 have noted, data for resveratrol are not all favourable or particularly convincing. The reasons are not well understood, but could include ineffective plasma concentrations derived from inadequate doses, inter-individual pharmacokinetic

Intervention / Diet	Design	Outcome	Reference
Isoflavones			
	N=34. Randomized crossover trial. 6 week intervention	Reduced cholesterol but no change in PSA	(Urban et al., 2001)
Single dose formulations of genistein, daidzein, glycitein	Pharmacokinetic study	Mean elimination half - lives of genistein was 3.2h and daidzein was 4.2h	(Busby et al., 2002)
160mg daily of red clover isoflavone preparation (genistein, daidzein, formonetin, biochanin A)	N=38, pilot study of treatment prior to prostatectomy. 18 treated vs 18 untreated patients. Non - randomized and non - blinded study	Apoptosis in treated patient specimens significantly higher than controls. No changes in PSA, testosterone.	(Jarred, 2002)
Soy isoflavone preparation for 3 - 6 months	N=41, Pilot study in 3 groups (watchful waiting, rising PSA after local therapy, hormone insensitive)	Reduction of rate of rise of PSA in whole group. Serum genistein concentrations increased from 0.11 to 0.65μM and daidzein from 0.11 to 0.51μM. PSA stabilization in 83% of hormone sensitive group and 35% hormone insensitive patients	(Hussain et al., 2003)
Single doses of two soy isoflavone preparations	N=13. Phase I dose escalation with genistein at 2, 4, 8mg/kg.	Cmax between 4.3 and 16.3μM, half - life between 15 and 22h.	(Takimoto et al., 2003)
Approximately 300mg or 600mg genistein and daidzein in soy formulation	N=20. Phase I multiple dose, orally over 84 days	31% reduction in dehydroepiandrosterone. Possibly slowing of PSA rise (non - significant)	(Fischer et al., 2004)
Soy vs Soy + linseed vs wheat in bread diet	N=29, Pilot study. randomized comparison prior to prostatectomy	-12% and 24% change in PSA and free/total ratio respectively. In favour of phytoestrogen activity.	(Dalais et al., 2004)
Genistein - rich extract for 6 months	N=62, range of rising PSA states including post - prostatectomy, off cycle during intermittent hormones, surveillance.	One patient had PSA decline >50% and 8 patients had PSA decline <50%.	(de Vere White et al., 2004)
60mg soy isoflavone preparation	N=59 evaluable patients who completed 12 weeks treatment. Gleason grade 6 or less.	Reduction of testosterone in 61% of treatment group vs 33% of controls. PSA stabilization in 69% of treatment group vs 55% controls.	(Kumar et al., 2004)
Supplement of soy, isoflavones, lycopene, silymarin, antioxidants	N=46 (intent to treat). Randomized, double blind, crossover analysis. 10 week treatment periods separated by 4 week washout	Statistically significant reduction in slope of PSA induced by treatment. Increase in PSA doubling time from 445 to 1150 days (2.6 fold) with supplement	(Schroder et al., 2005)

Intervention / Diet	Design	Outcome	Reference
240mg clover phytoestrogens daily for 2 weeks prior to prostatectomy	N=20, pilot study, placebo controlled.	Non - significant decline in testosterone levels, but compensated rise in LH levels	(Rannikko et al., 2006)
High or low soy diet for 3 months	N=24, randomized crossover to alternative diet after 1 month washout	Decline of PSA (not significant) of 14% while on high soy diet	(Maskarinec et al., 2006)
Lycopene with or without soy isoflavones for 6 months	N=71, includes hormone sensitive and resistant patients. Randomized trial.	95% of patients in lycopene group and 67% of patients in the combined group achieved PSA stabilization.	(Vaishampayan et al., 2007)
80mg daily, purified isoflavones	N=50 men with prostate cancer Gleason grad 6 or less completed treatment. Randomized, placebo controlled, double blind	No changes in sex hormones or PSA over 12 weeks	(Kumar et al., 2007)
Soy milk 3 times daily for 12 months	N=20, open label study observing rate of PSA rise after local therapy	Regression modeling showed slowing of the rate of PSA rise, from 56% per year to 20% per year while on study	(Pendleton et al., 2008)
Soy isoflavone supplement for 2 -4 weeks prior to prostatectomy	N=25 (12 placebo, 13 soy). Randomized, double blind, placebo controlled	Tissue COX-2 mRNA expression were reduced by soy isoflavones. Statistically significant correlation between isoflavone levels and p21 mRNA expression in the treatment group.	(Swami et al., 2009)
Soy vs Soy + linseed vs wheat in bread diet	N=29, Pilot study. randomized comparison prior to prostatectomy	-12% and 24% change in PSA and free/total ratio respectively. In favour of phytoestrogen activity.	(Dalais et al., 2004)
Lycopene			
15 mg Lycopene daily for 6 months	N=18, Phase II pilot study in men with advanced hormone refractory disease. 29% withdrew from the study before the end of the 6 month observation period.	Endpoints included PSA progression rate, QOL, analgesic use. Stable PSA noted in 29%, but otherwise no benefit.	(Schwenke, et al., 2009)
30 mg/d lycopene supplement tomato oleoresin (LycoRed®)	N=105. Randomized Phase II, placebo controlled, double blind study in African Americans. 21 day treatment prior to prostate biopsy.	Mean Plasma lycopene concentration 0.74 to 1.43 µmol/L ($P<0.0001$), Mean Prostate tissue lycopene 0.45 to 0.59 pmol/mg. No significant changes in 8-oxo-deoxyguanosine or malondialdehyde was seen.	(van Breemen et al., 2011)

Intervention / Diet	Design	Outcome	Reference
3 months of 30mg lycopne per day, 3g fish oil per day, or placebo	N = 69 (22 on lycopene, 21 on fish oil, 26 placebo). Randomized, Phase II double-blind trial.	IGF-1 and COX-2 gene expression did not change compared to placebo in men with early stage, low grade prostate cancer.	(Chan et al., 2011)
10mg daily for 3 months	N=20, metastatic hormone refractory prostate cancer	One patient (5%) with complete response, 6 with partial response (30%)	(Ansari & Gupta,2004)
10mg daily	N=41, localized prostate cancer on surveillance	Regression slopes of (log) PSA vs time decreased in 26/37 (70%, 95% CI: 53–84%) of the patients after supplementation and in eight cases (21%) the post-treatment slope was negative	(Barber et al., 2006)
15mg, 30mg, or 45mg for 30 days	N=45, randomized to one of 3 doses of lycopene prior to prostatectomy	No toxicity, but reduced serum free testosterone and increased total estradiol was noted.	(Kumar et al., 2008)
Resveratrol			
Trans-resveratrol at: 0, 25,50,100 and 150 mg, 6 times/d for 13 doses-	Double blind, randomized, placebo controlled Healthy volunteers, N=40, as 4 x 10 per group 5 males Phase I	Mean plasma concentration was 3.9, 7.4, 23.1 and 63.8 ng/mL and peaked in 0.8-1.5 hours post dose: Mean area under curve for plasma, post the 13th dose was 3.1, 11.2, 33.0 and 78.9 ng/mL; coefficients of variation >40% Adverse events were mild and similar between groups, but low plasma concentrations achieved	(Almeida, et al., 2009)
2 g resveratrol BID over 8 days	N=8 Healthy subjects Steady state and pharmacokinetics study Tolerability with food, quercetin and alcohol Phase I	6/8 has loose stool or mild diarrhea at the start of the study 1 subject developed rash and headache	(la Porte et al., 2010)
Up to 975 mg/d as: 25,50,100,150 mg given 6 times per day over 2 days	N=8 Healthy volunteers Double blind Randomized Placebo-controlled Phase I 4 men, one per dosing level	Mild adverse events experience d; low plasma concentrations achieved	(Almeida , 2009)
28 day x 36 μg resveratrol per day- as Chardonnay cava wine containing *trans*-resveratrol, *cis*-resveratrol, and *cis*-piceid	Healthy volunteers Phase I	Decrease in inflammatory markers: IL-6, high sensitivity CRP, intercellular adhesion molecule-1 (ICAM-1), monocyte chemo attractant protein 1 (MCP-1)	(Soleas et al., 2002)
270 mg/d resveratrol over 7 days	N=19 Phase I	"did not cause discomfort"	(Wong et al., 2010)

Intervention / Diet	Design	Outcome	Reference
2.5 versus 5 g per day for 28 days	N = Healthy volunteers Phase I	Mild and reversible AEs	(Elliott et al., 2009)
Single resveratrol doses of 0.5, 1, 2.5 and 5 g using 500 mg capsules	Healthy volunteers 10/level = 40 Pharmacokinetic study and metabolite	6 metabolites found in urine and plasma No serious adverse events Peak Plasma 539 ng/mL 1.5 hour post dose, peak AUC for metabolites were up to 23 time that of resveratrol, rapid urinary excretion.	(Boocock et al., 2007)
25mg to 5 g resveratrol	Dose escalation Phase I 40 Healthy volunteers	No evidence of saturation with a continuing linear response- very limited plasma concentrations, at high 5 g intake only 500 ng/mL levels achieved	(Boocock et al., 2007a,b)
500 mg caps resveratrol At 0.5, 1, 1.25 or 5.0 g once daily over 29 days	Healthy adults 22 Males, 18 Females Safety, Pharmacokinetics Phase I	Lower IGF-1 and IGFBP-3 in plasma.In all ,28/40 healthy adults had at least one adverse event,: nausea, diarrhea or abdominal pain, all above 1 g daily	(Brown et al., 2010)
Curcumin			
Soy isoflavones (40mg) + Curcumin (100mg) or placebo for 6 months	Randomised trial, N=85 men who had previous prostate biopsies but were negative for cancer and PIN.	PSA reduction was greater in subgroup of men who had higher baseline PSA value, but overall, there was no statistical difference between those who had supplements and those on placebo	(Ide et al., 2010)

Table 3. Selected clinical trials of phytochemicals in prostate cancer.

and pharmacodynamic variability, and other factors such as drug interaction. For example, resveratrol has been shown to inhibit cytochrome P 450; 3A4, 2D6, 2C9 and alternately induce 1A2 (Chow et al., 2010), a key factor that has not been taken into account in many clinical studies. Theoretically, interactions with concomitant medications whilst on trial may therefore result in either unwanted toxicity or reduced concentrations of resveratrol.

5. Curcumin

Curcumin is only found as an active component of whole or ground turmeric, within the rhizome or root nodule, specifically of two branches of the ginger family, Zingiberaceas, of the species, *Curcuma longa* Linneas, *Curcuma aromatica* or *Curcuma zantorrhiza* and in tropical ginger, *Zingiber cassumaunar*. In India, turmeric in dried curry powders range considerably from 10 to 32% (Govindarajan, 1980).

5.1 Pharmacology

Structurally, curcumin (diferuloylmethane, a polyphenolic molecule) is a diketone and can also be classified as a phenylpropanoid. It is known to have poor solubility and poor bioavailability (Anand et al., 2007). Absorption and transformation occurs at the intestinal wall, where enzymes such as sulfotransferases, UDP-glucoronyltransferase, and P450 ensure its rapid breakdown (Ireson et al., 2002). Pharmacokinetic studies, including Phase I and other trials confirm the poor bioavailability of the compound (Cheng et al, 2001; Sharma et al., 2004; Garcea et al., 2005; Garcea et al., 2004). Data from these studies show that curcumin seems to be absorbed from the gut within 1-2hrs, and doses up to 8000mg have produced minimal toxicity. Nausea and diarrhea have been the principal toxicities encountered. Vareed et al (2008) studied doses of either 10g or 12g in volunteers, and found Cmax to be around 1.7-2.3 ug/mL, with time taken to reach maximum concentration (Tmax) and half-life estimated to be 3.3h and 6.8h, respectively. Sharma et al., (2004) studied escalating doses in a Phase I trial up to 3.6g daily and found no dose-limiting toxicity. Mild nausea and diarrhea was encountered, but plasma concentrations of only around 10nM could be elicited in this study; nevertheless, inducible PGE2 production was reduced by about 50-60% at that dose level.

5.2 *In vitro* data

There is a wealth of literature on the potential mechanism of action of curcumin *in vitro* (see Table 2), but it is not clear which is the predominant mode of action. It is highly likely that different mechanisms of action exist for different cell lines. Curcumin can inhibit Akt and mTOR in PC3 cell lines (Yu et al., 2008), and enhance Apo2L/TRAIL induced apoptosis, at least in ovarian cancer cells (Wahl et al., 2007). EF24, a curcumin analogue, and curcumin itself can inhibit HIF1alpha gene transcription in PC3 prostate cancer cells (Thomas et al., 2008). Teiten et al., (2011) showed that curcumin induced cell cycle arrest in G2 phase and could modulate Wnt signaling in androgen-dependent prostate cancer cells, but not in androgen-independent cells.

Apoptotic and growth inhibitory pathways are affected by curcumin in numerous ways (Ravindran et al., 2009). One example is its ability to abrogate survival mechanisms via suppression of constitutive and inducible NF-kappaB activation (Mukhopadhyay et al., 2001). It can also induce apoptosis of DU145 and LNCaP, associated with reduction of expression of Bcl2 and bcl-xL (Mukhopadhyay et al., 2001).

5.3 *In vivo* data

Curcumin inhibits LNCaP xenograft growth, induces apoptosis, and sensitizes tumours to TRAIL induced apoptosis (Shankar et al., 2007). Others have also demonstrated the growth inhibitory properties of curcumin *in vivo* (Barve et al., 2008; Khor et al., 2006), possibly via antiangiogenic mechanisms such as reduction of MMP-2 and MMP-9 expression (Hong et al., 2006). Liposomal encapsulation of curcumin, particularly in combination with resveratrol, significantly reduces prostate cancer tumours *in vivo* (Narayanan et al., 2009).

5.4 Clinical studies

Despite the intense interest in curcumin as a possible cancer prevention agent, there is a surprising lack of clinical data in prostate cancer. Efforts have focused on improving bioavailability by incorporating curcumin in nanoparticles, or developing more potent analogues. Whilst ongoing trials in prostate cancer are yet to be reported, the only trial we could find described a randomized study of the combination of soy isoflavone and curcumin compared to placebo in men who did not have prostate cancer after undergoing prostate biopsy (Ide et al., 2010); its relevance for prostate cancer can therefore be questioned.

6. Studies on the the combination of phytochemicals and androgen ablation

Even though androgen suppression for metastatic disease is effective treatment, invariably, castrate resistance develops. However the recent development of new drugs that act on the androgen receptor (AR) suggest that there is still a role for androgen manipulation beyond the point traditionally defined as "castration resistance". As a result, there is renewed interest in whether phytochemicals modulate androgen receptor function in prostate cancer. It appears each phytochemical discussed in this review accomplishes androgen receptor inhibition, but all may use different mechanisms. For example, isoflavones have been shown to reduce androgen receptor transcription (Gao et al., 2004), and down regulate prostate androgen-regulated transcript-1 gene expression (Yu et al, 2003), whereas androgen receptor gene element is inhibited by lycopene in a dose-dependent manner in studies with LNCaP cells (Zhang et al., 2010). Lycopene appears to interact with AR by affecting β-catenin nuclear localization and inhibiting IGF-1 stimulated prostate cancer growth (Kucuk et al., 2002; Liu et al 2008). Resveratrol functions include the inhibition of androgen receptor transcription activity (Wang et al., 2010; Shi et al 2009) and down regulation of PSA expression (Mitchell at al, 1999; Hsieh & Wu, 2000) as tested in LNCaP cell lines. Others have shown that it also inhibits DNA binding of androgen receptor (Harada et al., 2011). Finally, androgen receptor function is inhibited by curcumin in LNCaP (Tsui et al., 2008) and in PC3 (Nakamura et al., 2002) cell lines. Curcumin appears to down regulate transactivation and expression of AR and AR-related cofactors, including activator protein-1 (AP-1), NF-kB, and cAMP response element binding protein (CREB) (Nakamura et al., 2002).

Burich et al., (2008), showed that the combination of genistein combined polysaccharide (GCP) and bicalutamide had enhanced activity against LNCaP and LNCaPR237H cell lines. Presumably, the basis of synergistic activity observed was the ability of GCP to downregulate AR and suppress mTOR (Tepper et al., 2007).

7. Studies on the combination of phytochemicals and chemotherapy

In many clinical studies, the possibility that something other than the phytochemical of interest, obtained from the diet, may influence outcome has probably not been given sufficient weight in the literature. Given that foods contain many phytochemicals other than those proposed to have anti-cancer activity, it is surprising to find little work on the potential synergistic or antagonistic interactions between different phytochemicals on cancer cell lines. Further, since many experiments involve unspecified doses, sources and contents of phytochemicals, it is not possible to conclude whether true synergistic growth inhibition occurs when these agents are used in combination.

Synergy or enhanced activity has been reported in prostate cancer cell lines using isoflavones in combination with paclitaxel (Ping et al., 2010), radiation (Raffoul et al., 2007), and docetaxel (Burich et al., 2008). Phenoxodiol, a novel isoflavone, in combination with cisplatin has been shown to be synergistic against DU145 cells and probably additive in PC3 cells (McPherson et al., 2009). *In vivo* combination therapy of soy isoflavones and radiation for prostate cancer has also been investigated, with favorable effects on the control of the disease (Raffoul et al., 2007; Wang et al., 2006).

Docetaxel effect in castration-resistant prostate cancer patients was improved by lycopene via insulin-like growth factor 1 receptor perturbation (Tang et al., 2011). Using an animal model to confirm these findings, a 38% improvement over docetaxel was found (P=0.047). Lycopene appeared to work by inhibiting IGF-1 stimulation and increasing expression and secretion of IGF-BP3. Downstream effects included reduced AKT kinase activity and survivin production and increased apoptosis.

Resveratrol enhances ionizing radiation - induced cell death in DU145 cells, which are thought to be relatively radiation-resistant (Scarlatti et al., 2007), and as previously noted, enhances TRAIL-induced apoptosis *in vivo* (Ganapathy et al., 2010). Radiosensitisation properties, at least in PC3 cells, also appear to belong to curcumin (Chendil et al., 2004; Li et al., 2007), and like resveratrol, curcumin also enhances TRAIL-induced apoptosis in prostate cancer cells (Deeb et al., 2005). Synergy between curcumin and a number of cytotoxic agents including doxorubicin, 5FU and paclitaxel occurs in PC3 and DU145 cells (Hour et al., 2002), as well as gemcitabine in PC3 (Li et al., 2007).

The advantage of finding synergy lies in an increased benefit: risk ratio if compounds being combined are more effective (synergistic) without necessarily being more toxic, particularly if they are known to be well-tolerated as single agents. Further, because some phytochemicals have poor bioavailability, the discovery of synergistic interactions with other phytochemicals in prostate cancer gives rise to the hypothesis that therapeutic effects may be obtained from a variety of combinations, even though individual phytochemicals may have questionable clinical effect.

8. Conclusions

The literature surrounding the idea of using phytochemicals for the prevention of prostate cancer is considerable, yet there are disproportionately few clinical studies, and just about none that show a convincing effect for biological outcomes in a clinical setting. Showing meaningful outcomes in a prostate cancer prevention trial with phytochemicals would ideally involve a prospective, randomized, placebo controlled trial that would require large numbers of patients to provide statistical power. Given that prostate cancer patients can live for many years, long-term follow up, is also required. Both of these requirements make such studies extremely difficult to mount. Nevertheless, many have investigated the effect of phytochemical administration in men with established prostate cancer (see Table 3). The lack of standardization in endpoints (eg. PSA, sex hormone changes) means that drawing systematic conclusions from such data is problematic, if not impossible. Other flaws in these studies include short-term administration of the phytochemical in question, highly variable sources, preparations and combinations, underpowered studies, and almost certainly inadequate dosing and scheduling of these compounds. However, the wealth of preclinical literature concerning the potential use and mechanisms of action of phytochemicals for prostate cancer will no doubt continue to provide impetus for therapeutic trials for some time to come. There are some serious pharmacological challenges in simply administering a single agent though, and it remains to be seen whether new approaches such as developing analogues of phytochemicals, or improving their bioavailability through better formulations will ultimately prove successful.

9. Acknowledgements and statement of conflict of interest

Carol Gano is funded by an Australian Postgraduate scholarship. Prof. de Souza is a holder of a project grant from the Prostate Cancer Foundation of Australia, and a Translational Cancer Research Grant from the NSW Cancer Institute. Prof. de Souza was a consultant in 2002 for Novogen Pty Ltd, the manufacturer of phenoxodiol.

10. References

Adlercreutz, H. "Phyto-Oestrogens and Cancer." *Lancet Oncol* 3, no. 6 (2002): 364-73.

Agarwal, C., Y. Sharma & R. Agarwal. "Anticarcinogenic Effect of a Polyphenolic Fraction Isolated from Grape Seeds in Human Prostate Carcinoma Du145 Cells: Modulation of Mitogenic Signaling and Cell-Cycle Regulators and Induction of G1 Arrest and Apoptosis." *Mol Carcinog* 28, no. 3 (2000): 129-38.

Aggarwal, B. B., S. Banerjee, U. Bharadwaj, B. Sung, S. Shishodia & G. Sethi. "Curcumin Induces the Degradation of Cyclin E Expression through Ubiquitin-Dependent Pathway and up-Regulates Cyclin-Dependent Kinase Inhibitors P21 and P27 in Multiple Human Tumor Cell Lines." *Biochem Pharmacol* 73, no. 7 (2007): 1024-32.

Aggarwal, B. B. & B. Sung. "Pharmacological Basis for the Role of Curcumin in Chronic Diseases: An Age-Old Spice with Modern Targets." *Trends Pharmacol Sci* 30, no. 2 (2009): 85-94.

Aguero, M. F., M. M. Facchinetti, Z. Sheleg & A. M. Senderowicz. "Phenoxodiol, a Novel Isoflavone, Induces G1 Arrest by Specific Loss in Cyclin-Dependent Kinase 2 Activity by P53-Independent Induction of P21waf1/Cip1." *Cancer Res* 65, no. 8 (2005): 3364-73.

Akaza, H., N. Miyanaga, N. Takashima, S. Naito, Y. Hirao, T. Tsukamoto, T. Fujioka, M. Mori, W. J. Kim, J. M. Song & A. J. Pantuck. "Comparisons of Percent Equol Producers between Prostate Cancer Patients and Controls: Case-Controlled Studies of Isoflavones in Japanese, Korean and American Residents." *Jpn J Clin Oncol* 34, no. 2 (2004): 86-9.

Akaza, H., N. Miyanaga, N. Takashima, S. Naito, Y. Hirao, T. Tsukamoto & M. Mori. "Is Daidzein Non-Metabolizer a High Risk for Prostate Cancer? A Case-Controlled Study of Serum Soybean Isoflavone Concentration." *Jpn J Clin Oncol* 32, no. 8 (2002): 296-300.

Akiyama, T., J. Ishida, S. Nakagawa, H. Ogawara, S. Watanabe, N. Itoh, M. Shibuya & Y. Fukami. "Genistein, a Specific Inhibitor of Tyrosine-Specific Protein Kinases." *J Biol Chem* 262, no. 12 (1987): 5592-5.

Almeida, L., M. Vaz-da-Silva, A. Falcao, E. Soares, R. Costa, A. I. Loureiro, C. Fernandes-Lopes, J. F. Rocha, T. Nunes, L. Wright & P. Soares-da-Silva. "Pharmacokinetic and Safety Profile of Trans-Resveratrol in a Rising Multiple-Dose Study in Healthy Volunteers." *Mol Nutr Food Res* 53 Suppl 1 (2009): S7-15.

Alvero, A. B., D. O'Malley, D. Brown, G. Kelly, M. Garg, W. Chen, T. Rutherford & G. Mor. "Molecular Mechanism of Phenoxodiol-Induced Apoptosis in Ovarian Carcinoma Cells." *Cancer* 106, no. 3 (2006): 599-608.

Anand, P., A. B. Kunnumakkara, R. A. Newman & B. B. Aggarwal. "Bioavailability of Curcumin: Problems and Promises." *Mol Pharm* 4, no. 6 (2007): 807-18.

Ansari, M. S. & N. P. Gupta. "Lycopene: A Novel Drug Therapy in Hormone Refractory Metastatic Prostate Cancer." *Urol Oncol* 22, no. 5 (2004): 415-20.

Atkinson, C., C. L. Frankenfeld & J. W. Lampe. "Gut Bacterial Metabolism of the Soy Isoflavone Daidzein: Exploring the Relevance to Human Health." *Exp Biol Med (Maywood)* 230, no. 3 (2005): 155-70.

Aziz, M. H., M. Nihal, V. X. Fu, D. F. Jarrard & N. Ahmad. "Resveratrol-Caused Apoptosis of Human Prostate Carcinoma LNCaP Cells Is Mediated Via Modulation of Phosphatidylinositol 3'-Kinase/Akt Pathway and Bcl-2 Family Proteins." *Molecular Cancer Therapeutics* 5, no. 5 (2006): 1335-41.

Barber, N. J., X. Zhang, G. Zhu, R. Pramanik, J. A. Barber, F. L. Martin, J. D. H. Morris & G. H. Muir. "Lycopene Inhibits DNA Synthesis in Primary Prostate Epithelial Cells *in Vitro* and Its Administration Is Associated with a Reduced Prostate-Specific Antigen Velocity in a Phase Ii Clinical Study." *Prostate Cancer Prostatic Dis* 9, no. 4 (2006): 407-13.

Barve, A., T. O. Khor, X. Hao, Y. S. Keum, C. S. Yang, B. Reddy & A. N. Kong. "Murine Prostate Cancer Inhibition by Dietary Phytochemicals--Curcumin and Phenyethylisothiocyanate." *Pharm Res* 25, no. 9 (2008): 2181-9.

Bemis, D. L., J. L. Capodice, M. Desai, R. Buttyan & A. E. Katz. "A Concentrated Aglycone Isoflavone Preparation (Gcp) That Demonstrates Potent Anti-Prostate Cancer Activity *in Vitro* and *in Vivo*." *Clin Cancer Res* 10, no. 15 (2004): 5282-92.

Benhar, M., D. Engelberg & A. Levitzki. "Ros, Stress-Activated Kinases and Stress Signaling in Cancer." *EMBO Rep* 3, no. 5 (2002): 420-5.

Benitez, D. A., M. A. Hermoso, E. Pozo-Guisado, P. M. Fernandez-Salguero & E. A. Castellon. "Regulation of Cell Survival by Resveratrol Involves Inhibition of Nf Kappa B-Regulated Gene Expression in Prostate Cancer Cells." *Prostate* 69, no. 10 (2009): 1045-54.

Benitez, D. A., E. Pozo-Guisado, A. Alvarez-Barrientos, P. M. Fernandez-Salguero & E. A. Castellon. "Mechanisms Involved in Resveratrol-Induced Apoptosis and Cell Cycle Arrest in Prostate Cancer-Derived Cell Lines." *J Androl* 28, no. 2 (2007): 282-93.

Bergan, R., E. Kyle, P. Nguyen, J. Trepel, C. Ingui & L. Neckers. "Genistein-Stimulated Adherence of Prostate Cancer Cells Is Associated with the Binding of Focal Adhesion Kinase to Beta-1-Integrin." *Clin Exp Metastasis* 14, no. 4 (1996): 389-98.

Bhatia, N. & R. Agarwal. "Detrimental Effect of Cancer Preventive Phytochemicals Silymarin, Genistein and Epigallocatechin 3-Gallate on Epigenetic Events in Human Prostate Carcinoma Du145 Cells." *Prostate* 46, no. 2 (2001): 98-107.

Böhm, V., K. Fröhlich & R. Bitsch. "Rosehip -- a "New" Source of Lycopene?" *Molecular Aspects of Medicine* 24, no. 6 (2003): 385-89.

Boocock, D. J., G. E. Faust, K. R. Patel, A. M. Schinas, V. A. Brown, M. P. Ducharme, T. D. Booth, J. A. Crowell, M. Perloff, A. J. Gescher, W. P. Steward & D. E. Brenner. "Phase I Dose Escalation Pharmacokinetic Study in Healthy Volunteers of Resveratrol, a Potential Cancer Chemopreventive Agent." *Cancer Epidemiol Biomarkers Prev* 16, no. 6 (2007): 1246-52.

Boocock, D. J., K. R. Patel, G. E. Faust, D. P. Normolle, T. H. Marczylo, J. A. Crowell, D. E. Brenner, T. D. Booth, A. Gescher & W. P. Steward. "Quantitation of Trans-Resveratrol and Detection of Its Metabolites in Human Plasma and Urine by High Performance Liquid Chromatography." *J Chromatogr B Analyt Technol Biomed Life Sci* 848, no. 2 (2007): 182-7.

Booth, N.L., C.R. Overk, P. Yao, J.E. Burdette, D. Nikolic, S. Chen, J.L. Bolton, R.B. van Breemen,G.F. Pauli and N.R. Farnsworth. "The Chemical and Biologic Profile of a Red Clover(*Trifolium pratense* L.) Phase II Clinical Extract" *The Journal of Alternative and Complementary Medicine* no.12 (2006): 133-139.

Brito, P. M., R. Devillard, A. Negre-Salvayre, L. M. Almeida, T. C. Dinis, R. Salvayre & N. Auge. "Resveratrol Inhibits the Mtor Mitogenic Signaling Evoked by Oxidized Ldl in Smooth Muscle Cells." *Atherosclerosis* 205, no. 1 (2009): 126-34.

Brizuela, L., A. Dayon, N. Doumerc, I. Ader, M. Golzio, J. C. Izard, Y. Hara, B. Malavaud & O. Cuvillier. "The Sphingosine Kinase-1 Survival Pathway Is a Molecular Target for the Tumor-Suppressive Tea and Wine Polyphenols in Prostate Cancer." *FASEB J* 24, no. 10 (2010): 3882-94.

Brown, V. A., K. R. Patel, M. Viskaduraki, J. A. Crowell, M. Perloff, T. D. Booth, G. Vasilinin, A. Sen, A. M. Schinas, G. Piccirilli, K. Brown, W. P. Steward, A. J. Gescher & D. E. Brenner. "Repeat Dose Study of the Cancer Chemopreventive Agent Resveratrol in Healthy Volunteers: Safety, Pharmacokinetics, and Effect on the Insulin-Like Growth Factor Axis." *Cancer Res* 70, no. 22 (2010): 9003-11.

Burgess, L.C., E. Rice, T. Fischer, J.R. Seekins, T.P. Burgess, S.J. Sticka & K. Klatt. "Lycopene Has Limited Effect on Cell Proliferation in Only Two of Seven Human Cell Lines (Both Cancerous and Noncancerous) in an *in Vitro* System with Doses across the Physiological Range." *Toxicology in Vitro* 22, no. 5 (2008): 1297-300.

Burich, R.A., W.S. Holland, R.L. Vinall, C. Tepper, R.W. DeVere White & P.C. Mack. "Genistein Combined Polysaccharide Enhances Activity of Docetaxel, Bicalutamide and Src Kinase Inhibition in Androgen-Dependent and Independent Prostate Cancer Cell Lines." *BJU International* 102, no. 10 (2008): 1458-66.

Busby, M. G., A. R. Jeffcoat, L. T. Bloedon, M. A. Koch, T. Black, K. J. Dix, W. D. Heizer, B. F. Thomas, J. M. Hill, J. A. Crowell & S. H. Zeisel. "Clinical Characteristics and Pharmacokinetics of Purified Soy Isoflavones: Single-Dose Administration to Healthy Men." *American Journal of Clinical Nutrition* 75, no. 1 (2002): 126-36.

Bylund, A., J. X. Zhang, A. Bergh, J. E. Damber, A. Widmark, A. Johansson, H. Adlercreutz, P. Aman, M. J. Shepherd & G. Hallmans. "Rye Bran and Soy Protein Delay Growth and Increase Apoptosis of Human LNCaP Prostate Adenocarcinoma in Nude Mice." *Prostate* 42, no. 4 (2000): 304-14.

Campbell, D. R., M. D. Gross, M. C. Martini, G. A. Grandits, J. L. Slavin & J. D. Potter. "Plasma Carotenoids as Biomarkers of Vegetable and Fruit Intake." *Cancer Epidemiol Biomarkers Prev* 3, no. 6 (1994): 493-500.

Cao, F., T. Y. Jin & Y. F. Zhou. "Inhibitory Effect of Isoflavones on Prostate Cancer Cells and Pten Gene." *Biomed Environ Sci* 19, no. 1 (2006): 35-41.

Chan, J. M., V. Weinberg, M. J. Magbanua, E. Sosa, J. Simko, K. Shinohara, S. Federman, M. Mattie, M. Hughes-Fulford, C. Haqq & P. R. Carroll. "Nutritional Supplements, Cox-2 and Igf-1 Expression in Men on Active Surveillance for Prostate Cancer." *Cancer Causes & Control* 22, no. 1 (2011): 141-50.

Chen, Q., S. Ganapathy, K. P. Singh, S. Shankar & R. K. Srivastava. "Resveratrol Induces Growth Arrest and Apoptosis through Activation of Foxo Transcription Factors in Prostate Cancer Cells." *PLoS One* 5, no. 12 (2010): e15288.

Chendil, D., R. S. Ranga, D. Meigooni, S. Sathishkumar & M. M. Ahmed. "Curcumin Confers Radiosensitizing Effect in Prostate Cancer Cell Line Pc-3." *Oncogene* 23, no. 8 (2004): 1599-607.

Cheng, A. L., C. H. Hsu, J. K. Lin, M. M. Hsu, Y. F. Ho, T. S. Shen, J. Y. Ko, J. T. Lin, B. R. Lin, W. Ming-Shiang, H. S. Yu, S. H. Jee, G. S. Chen, T. M. Chen, C. A. Chen, M. K. Lai, Y. S. Pu, M. H. Pan, Y. J. Wang, C. C. Tsai & C. Y. Hsieh. "Phase I Clinical Trial of Curcumin, a Chemopreventive Agent, in Patients with High-Risk or Pre-Malignant Lesions." *Anticancer Res* 21, no. 4B (2001): 2895-900.

Choueiri, T. K., R. Wesolowski & T. M. Mekhail. "Phenoxodiol: Isoflavone Analog with Antineoplastic Activity." *Curr Oncol Rep* 8, no. 2 (2006): 104-7.

Chow, H. H., L. L. Garland, C. H. Hsu, D. R. Vining, W. M. Chew, J. A. Miller, M. Perloff, J. A. Crowell & D. S. Alberts. "Resveratrol Modulates Drug- and Carcinogen-Metabolizing Enzymes in a Healthy Volunteer Study." *Cancer Prev Res (Phila)* 3, no. 9 (2010): 1168-75.

Curl, A.L.. "The Carotenoids of Apricots." *Journal of Food Science* 25, no. 2 (1960): 190-96.

Dalais, F. S., A. Meliala, N. Wattanapenpaiboon, M. Frydenberg, D. A. Suter, W. K. Thomson & M. L. Wahlqvist. "Effects of a Diet Rich in Phytoestrogens on Prostate-Specific Antigen and Sex Hormones in Men Diagnosed with Prostate Cancer." *Urology* 64, no. 3 (2004): 510-5.

Davies, S. L. & J. Bozzo. "Spotlight on Tnox: A Tumor-Selective Target for Cancer Therapies." *Drug News Perspect* 19, no. 4 (2006): 223-5.

Davis, J. N., O. Kucuk & F. H. Sarkar. "Genistein Inhibits Nf-Kappa B Activation in Prostate Cancer Cells." *Nutr Cancer* 35, no. 2 (1999): 167-74.

Davis, J. N., N. Muqim, M. Bhuiyan, O. Kucuk, K. J. Pienta & F. H. Sarkar. "Inhibition of Prostate Specific Antigen Expression by Genistein in Prostate Cancer Cells." *International Journal of Oncology* 16, no. 6 (2000): 1091-7.

Davis, J. N., B. Singh, M. Bhuiyan & F. H. Sarkar. "Genistein-Induced Upregulation of P21waf1, Downregulation of Cyclin B, and Induction of Apoptosis in Prostate Cancer Cells." *Nutr Cancer* 32, no. 3 (1998): 123-31.

De Luca, T., D. M. Morre, H. Zhao & D. J. Morre. "Nad+/Nadh and/or Coq/Coqh2 Ratios from Plasma Membrane Electron Transport May Determine Ceramide and Sphingosine-1-Phosphate Levels Accompanying G1 Arrest and Apoptosis." *BioFactors* 25, no. 1-4 (2005): 43-60.

de Santi, C., A. Pietrabissa, F. Mosca & G. M. Pacifici. "Glucuronidation of Resveratrol, a Natural Product Present in Grape and Wine, in the Human Liver." *Xenobiotica* 30, no. 11 (2000): 1047-54.

de Santi, C., A. Pietrabissa, R. Spisni, F. Mosca & G. M. Pacifici. "Sulphation of Resveratrol, a Natural Compound Present in Wine, and Its Inhibition by Natural Flavonoids." *Xenobiotica* 30, no. 9 (2000): 857-66.

———. "Sulphation of Resveratrol, a Natural Product Present in Grapes and Wine, in the Human Liver and Duodenum." *Xenobiotica* 30, no. 6 (2000): 609-17.

de Souza P., Russell, P. J., Kearsley, J.H., Howes, L.G. "Clinical pharmacology of isoflavones and its relevance for potential prevention of prostate cancer" *Nutrition Reviews* 68 no. 9 (2010): 542-555.

Deeb, D., H. Jiang, X. Gao, S. Al-Holou, A. L. Danyluk, S. A. Dulchavsky & S. C. Gautam. "Curcumin [1,7-Bis(4-Hydroxy-3-Methoxyphenyl)-1-6-Heptadine-3,5-Dione; C21h20o6] Sensitizes Human Prostate Cancer Cells to Tumor Necrosis Factor-Related Apoptosis-Inducing Ligand/Apo2l-Induced Apoptosis by Suppressing Nuclear Factor-Kappab Via Inhibition of the Prosurvival Akt Signaling Pathway." *Journal of Pharmacology and Experimental Therapeutics* 321, no. 2 (2007): 616-25.

Deeb, D. D., H. Jiang, X. Gao, G. Divine, S. A. Dulchavsky & S. C. Gautam. "Chemosensitization of Hormone-Refractory Prostate Cancer Cells by Curcumin to Trail-Induced Apoptosis." *J Exp Ther Oncol* 5, no. 2 (2005): 81-91.

deVere White, R. W., R. M. Hackman, S. E. Soares, L. A. Beckett, Y. Li & B. Sun. "Effects of a Genistein-Rich Extract on PSA Levels in Men with a History of Prostate Cancer." *Urology* 63, no. 2 (2004): 259-63.

Dorai, T., N. Gehani & A. Katz. "Therapeutic Potential of Curcumin in Human Prostate Cancer. Ii. Curcumin Inhibits Tyrosine Kinase Activity of Epidermal Growth Factor Receptor and Depletes the Protein." *Molecular Urology* 4, no. 1 (2000): 1-6.

Edwards, J. A., M. Beck, C. Riegger & J. Bausch. "Safety of Resveratrol with Examples for High Purity, Trans-Resveratrol, Resvida." *Annals of the New York Academy of Sciences* 1215, no. 1 (2011): 131-37.

El Touny, L. H. & P. P. Banerjee. "Akt Gsk-3 Pathway as a Target in Genistein-Induced Inhibition of Tramp Prostate Cancer Progression toward a Poorly Differentiated Phenotype." *Carcinogenesis* 28, no. 8 (2007): 1710-7.

Elliott, P. J., S. M. Walpole, L. Morelli, P. D. Lambert, W. Lunsmann, C. H. Westphal & S. Lavu. "Resveratrol/Srt501 Sirtuin Sirt1 Activator Treatment of Type 2 Diabetes." *Drugs of the Future* 34, no. 4 (2009): 291-95.

Evans, B. A., K. Griffiths & M. S. Morton. "Inhibition of 5 Alpha-Reductase in Genital Skin Fibroblasts and Prostate Tissue by Dietary Lignans and Isoflavonoids." *J Endocrinol* 147, no. 2 (1995): 295-302.

Fang, M., D. Chen & C. S. Yang. "Dietary Polyphenols May Affect DNA Methylation." *Journal of Nutrition* 137, no. 1 Suppl (2007): 223S-28S.

Fischer, L., C. Mahoney, A. R. Jeffcoat, M. A. Koch, B. E. Thomas, J. L. Valentine, T. Stinchcombe, J. Boan, J. A. Crowell & S. H. Zeisel. "Clinical Characteristics and Pharmacokinetics of Purified Soy Isoflavones: Multiple-Dose Administration to Men with Prostate Neoplasia." *Nutr Cancer* 48, no. 2 (2004): 160-70.

Forbes, K., K. Gillette & I. Sehgal. "Lycopene Increases Urokinase Receptor and Fails to Inhibit Growth or Connexin Expression in a Metastatically Passaged Prostate Cancer Cell Line: A Brief Communication." *Exp Biol Med (Maywood)* 228, no. 8 (2003): 967-71.

Ford, N. A., A. C. Elsen, K. Zuniga, B. L. Lindshield & J. W. Erdman, Jr. "Lycopene and Apo-12'-Lycopenal Reduce Cell Proliferation and Alter Cell Cycle Progression in Human Prostate Cancer Cells." *Nutr Cancer* 63, no. 2 (2011): 256-63.

Franke, A. A., L. J. Custer, C. M. Cerna & K. Narala. "Rapid Hplc Analysis of Dietary Phytoestrogens from Legumes and from Human Urine." *Proc Soc Exp Biol Med* 208, no. 1 (1995): 18-26.

Gamble, J. R., P. Xia, C. N. Hahn, J. J. Drew, C. J. Drogemuller, D. Brown & M. A. Vadas. "Phenoxodiol, an Experimental Anticancer Drug, Shows Potent Antiangiogenic Properties in Addition to Its Antitumour Effects." *Int J Cancer* 118, no. 10 (2006): 2412-20.

Ganapathy, S., Q. Chen, K.P. Singh, S. Shankar & R.K. Srivastava. "Resveratrol Enhances Antitumor Activity of Trail in Prostate Cancer Xenografts through Activation of Foxo Transcription Factor." *PLoS One* 5, no. 12 (2010): e15627.

Gao, S., G. Z. Liu & Z. Wang. "Modulation of Androgen Receptor-Dependent Transcription by Resveratrol and Genistein in Prostate Cancer Cells." *Prostate* 59, no. 2 (2004): 214-25.

Garcea, G., D. P. Berry, D. J. Jones, R. Singh, A. R. Dennison, P. B. Farmer, R. A. Sharma, W. P. Steward & A. J. Gescher. "Consumption of the Putative Chemopreventive Agent Curcumin by Cancer Patients: Assessment of Curcumin Levels in the Colorectum and Their Pharmacodynamic Consequences." *Cancer Epidemiol Biomarkers Prev* 14, no. 1 (2005): 120-5.

Garcea, G., D. J. Jones, R. Singh, A. R. Dennison, P. B. Farmer, R. A. Sharma, W. P. Steward, A. J. Gescher & D. P. Berry. "Detection of Curcumin and Its Metabolites in Hepatic Tissue and Portal Blood of Patients Following Oral Administration." *Br J Cancer* 90, no. 5 (2004): 1011-5.

Giovannucci, E. "Does Prostate-Specific Antigen Screening Influence the Results of Studies of Tomatoes, Lycopene, and Prostate Cancer Risk?" *J Natl Cancer Inst* 99, no. 14 (2007): 1060-2.

Gitenay, D., B. Lyan, J. Talvas, A. Mazur, S. George, C. Caris-Veyrat & E. Rock. "Serum from Rats Fed Red or Yellow Tomatoes Induces Connexin43 Expression Independently from Lycopene in a Prostate Cancer Cell Line." *Biochem Biophys Res Commun* 364, no. 3 (2007): 578-82.

Gogada, R., V. Prabhu, M. Amadori, R. Scott, S. Hashmi & D. Chandra. "Resveratrol Induces P53-Independent, X-Linked Inhibitor of Apoptosis Protein (Xiap)-Mediated Bax Protein Oligomerization on Mitochondria to Initiate Cytochrome C Release and Caspase Activation." *J Biol Chem* 286, no. 33 (2011): 28749-60.

Goldberg, D. M., J. Yan & G. J. Soleas. "Absorption of Three Wine-Related Polyphenols in Three Different Matrices by Healthy Subjects." *Clin Biochem* 36, no. 1 (2003): 79-87.

Govindarajan, V. S. "Turmeric--Chemistry, Technology, and Quality." *Crit Rev Food Sci Nutr* 12, no. 3 (1980): 199-301.

Guo, Y., S. Wang, D. R. Hoot & S. K. Clinton. "Suppression of Vegf-Mediated Autocrine and Paracrine Interactions between Prostate Cancer Cells and Vascular Endothelial Cells by Soy Isoflavones." *J Nutr Biochem* 18, no. 6 (2007): 408-17.

Gustin, D. M., K. A. Rodvold, J. A. Sosman, V. Diwadkar-Navsariwala, M. Stacewicz-Sapuntzakis, M. Viana, J. A. Crowell, J. Murray, P. Tiller & P. E. Bowen. "Single-Dose Pharmacokinetic Study of Lycopene Delivered in a Well-Defined Food-Based Lycopene Delivery System (Tomato Paste-Oil Mixture) in Healthy Adult Male Subjects." *Cancer Epidemiol Biomarkers Prev* 13, no. 5 (2004): 850-60.

Harada, N., K. Atarashi, Y. Murata, R. Yamaji, Y. Nakano & H. Inui. "Inhibitory Mechanisms of the Transcriptional Activity of Androgen Receptor by Resveratrol: Implication of DNA Binding and Acetylation of the Receptor." *J Steroid Biochem Mol Biol* 123, no. 1-2 (2011): 65-70.

Hedlund, T. E., W. U. Johannes & G. J. Miller. "Soy Isoflavonoid Equol Modulates the Growth of Benign and Malignant Prostatic Epithelial Cells *in Vitro*." *Prostate* 54, no. 1 (2003): 68-78.

Herst, P. M., T. Petersen, P. Jerram, J. Baty & M. V. Berridge. "The Antiproliferative Effects of Phenoxodiol Are Associated with Inhibition of Plasma Membrane Electron

Transport in Tumour Cell Lines and Primary Immune Cells." *Biochem Pharmacol* 74, no. 11 (2007): 1587-95.

Hilchie, A. L., S. J. Furlong, K. Sutton, A. Richardson, M. R. Robichaud, C. A. Giacomantonio, N. D. Ridgway & D. W. Hoskin. "Curcumin-Induced Apoptosis in Pc3 Prostate Carcinoma Cells Is Caspase-Independent and Involves Cellular Ceramide Accumulation and Damage to Mitochondria." *Nutr Cancer* 62, no. 3 (2010): 379-89.

Holden, J.M., A.L. Eldridge, G.R. Beecher, I. M. Buzzard, S. Bhagwat, C.S. Davis, L.W. Douglass, S. Gebhardt, D. Haytowitz & S. Schakel. "Carotenoid Content of U.S. Foods: An Update of the Database." *Journal of Food Composition and Analysis* 12, no. 3 (1999): 169-96.

Hong, S. I., H. J. Kwak, M. J. Park, H. Cho, C. M. Park, S. I. Moon, H. C. Lee, I. C. Park, M. S. Kim & C. H. Rhee. "Transforming Growth Factor-Beta 1 Induces Tissue Inhibitor of Metalloproteinase-1 Expression Via Activation of Extracellular Signal-Regulated Kinase and Sp1 in Human Fibrosarcoma Cells." *Molecular Cancer Research* 4, no. 3 (2006): 209-20.

Hour, T. C., J. Chen, C. Y. Huang, J. Y. Guan, S. H. Lu & Y. S. Pu. "Curcumin Enhances Cytotoxicity of Chemotherapeutic Agents in Prostate Cancer Cells by Inducing P21(Waf1/Cip1) and C/Ebpbeta Expressions and Suppressing Nf-Kappab Activation." *Prostate* 51, no. 3 (2002): 211-8.

Howes, J., M. Waring, L. Huang & L. G. Howes. "Long-Term Pharmacokinetics of an Extract of Isoflavones from Red Clover (Trifolium Pratense)." *J Altern Complement Med* 8, no. 2 (2002): 135-42.

Hsieh, T. C. & J. M. Wu. "Differential Effects on Growth, Cell Cycle Arrest, and Induction of Apoptosis by Resveratrol in Human Prostate Cancer Cell Lines." *Exp Cell Res* 249, no. 1 (1999): 109-15.

———. "Grape-Derived Chemopreventive Agent Resveratrol Decreases Prostate-Specific Antigen (PSA) Expression in LNCaP Cells by an Androgen Receptor (Ar)-Independent Mechanism." *Anticancer Res* 20, no. 1A (2000): 225-8.

Huang, X., S. Chen, L. Xu, Y. Liu, D. K. Deb, L. C. Platanias & R. C. Bergan. "Genistein Inhibits P38 Map Kinase Activation, Matrix Metalloproteinase Type 2, and Cell Invasion in Human Prostate Epithelial Cells." *Cancer Res* 65, no. 8 (2005): 3470-8.

Hussain, M., M. Banerjee, F. H. Sarkar, Z. Djuric, M. N. Pollak, D. Doerge, J. Fontana, S. Chinni, J. Davis, J. Forman, D. P. Wood & O. Kucuk. "Soy Isoflavones in the Treatment of Prostate Cancer." *Nutr Cancer* 47, no. 2 (2003): 111-7.

Ide, H., S. Tokiwa, K. Sakamaki, K. Nishio, S. Isotani, S. Muto, T. Hama, H. Masuda & S. Horie. "Combined Inhibitory Effects of Soy Isoflavones and Curcumin on the Production of Prostate-Specific Antigen." *Prostate* 70, no. 10 (2010): 1127-33.

Ireson C.R., DJL Jones, S. Orr, MWH Coughtrie, DJ Boocock, ML Williams, PB Farmer, WP Steward & A J Gescher. "Metablisim of the Cancer Chemoprevetive Agent Curcumin in Human and Rat Intestine." Ca Epi Bio & Prev 11 (2002) :105- 111.

Imaida, K., S. Tamano, K. Kato, Y. Ikeda, M. Asamoto, S. Takahashi, Z. Nir, M. Murakoshi, H. Nishino & T. Shirai. "Lack of Chemopreventive Effects of Lycopene and Curcumin on Experimental Rat Prostate Carcinogenesis." *Carcinogenesis* 22, no. 3 (2001): 467-72.

Itsiopoulos, C., A. Hodge & M. Kaimakamis. "Can the Mediterranean Diet Prevent Prostate Cancer?" *Molecular Nutrition & Food Research* 53, no. 2 (2009): 227-39.

Ivanov, N. I., S. P. Cowell, P. Brown, P. S. Rennie, E. S. Guns & M. E. Cox. "Lycopene Differentially Induces Quiescence and Apoptosis in Androgen-Responsive and -Independent Prostate Cancer Cell Lines." *Clin Nutr* 26, no. 2 (2007): 252-63.

Jarred, R. A., M. Keikha, C. Dowling, S. J. McPherson, A. M. Clare, A. J. Husband, J. S. Pedersen, M. Frydenberg & G. P. Risbridger. "Induction of Apoptosis in Low to Moderate-Grade Human Prostate Carcinoma by Red Clover-Derived Dietary Isoflavones." *Cancer Epidemiol Biomarkers Prev* 11, no. 12 (2002): 1689-96.

Jatoi, A., P. Burch, D. Hillman, J. M. Vanyo, S. Dakhil, D. Nikcevich, K. Rowland, R. Morton, P. J. Flynn, C. Young & W. Tan. "A Tomato-Based, Lycopene-Containing Intervention for Androgen-Independent Prostate Cancer: Results of a Phase Ii Study from the North Central Cancer Treatment Group." *Urology* 69, no. 2 (2007): 289-94.

Kamsteeg, M., T. Rutherford, E. Sapi, B. Hanczaruk, S. Shahabi, M. Flick, D. Brown & G. Mor. "Phenoxodiol--an Isoflavone Analog--Induces Apoptosis in Chemoresistant Ovarian Cancer Cells." *Oncogene* 22, no. 17 (2003): 2611-20.

Kanagaraj, P., M. Vijayababu, B. Ravisankar, J. Anbalagan, M. Aruldhas & J. Arunakaran. "Effect of Lycopene on Insulin-Like Growth Factor-I, Igf Binding Protein-3 and Igf Type-I Receptor in Prostate Cancer Cells." *Journal of Cancer Research and Clinical Oncology* 133, no. 6 (2007): 351-59.

Kato, K., S. Takahashi, L. Cui, T. Toda, S. Suzuki, M. Futakuchi, S. Sugiura & T. Shirai. "Suppressive Effects of Dietary Genistin and Daidzin on Rat Prostate Carcinogenesis." *Jpn J Cancer Res* 91, no. 8 (2000): 786-91.

Kazi, A., K. G. Daniel, D. M. Smith, N. B. Kumar & Q. P. Dou. "Inhibition of the Proteasome Activity, a Novel Mechanism Associated with the Tumor Cell Apoptosis-Inducing Ability of Genistein." *Biochem Pharmacol* 66, no. 6 (2003): 965-76.

Khor, T.O., Y.-S. Keum, W. Lin, J.-H. Kim, R. Hu, G. Shen, C. Xu, A. Gopalakrishnan, B. Reddy, X. Zheng, A.H. Conney & A.-N. T. Kong. "Combined Inhibitory Effects of Curcumin and Phenethyl Isothiocyanate on the Growth of Human Pc-3 Prostate Xenografts in Immunodeficient Mice." *Cancer Research* 66, no. 2 (2006): 613-21.

Kluger, H. M., M. M. McCarthy, A. B. Alvero, M. Sznol, S. Ariyan, R. L. Camp, D. L. Rimm & G. Mor. "The X-Linked Inhibitor of Apoptosis Protein (Xiap) Is up-Regulated in Metastatic Melanoma, and Xiap Cleavage by Phenoxodiol Is Associated with Carboplatin Sensitization." *J Transl Med* 5 (2007): 6.

Kryston, T. B., A.B. Georgiev, P. Pissis, and A.G. Georgakilas. "Role of Oxidative Stress and DNA Damage in Human Carcinogenesis." *Mutation Research/Fundamental and Molecular Mechanisms of Mutagenesis* 711, no. 1-2 (2011): 193-201.

Kucuk, O., F. H. Sarkar, Z. Djuric, W. Sakr, M. N. Pollak, F. Khachik, M. Banerjee, J. S. Bertram & D. P. Wood, Jr. "Effects of Lycopene Supplementation in Patients with Localized Prostate Cancer." *Exp Biol Med (Maywood)* 227, no. 10 (2002): 881-5.

Kucuk, O., F. H. Sarkar, W. Sakr, Z. Djuric, M. N. Pollak, F. Khachik, Y. W. Li, M. Banerjee, D. Grignon, J. S. Bertram, J. D. Crissman, E. J. Pontes & D. P. Wood, Jr. "Phase Ii Randomized Clinical Trial of Lycopene Supplementation before Radical Prostatectomy." *Cancer Epidemiol Biomarkers Prev* 10, no. 8 (2001): 861-8.

Kuiper, G. G., J. G. Lemmen, B. Carlsson, J. C. Corton, S. H. Safe, P. T. van der Saag, B. van der Burg & J. A. Gustafsson. "Interaction of Estrogenic Chemicals and Phytoestrogens with Estrogen Receptor Beta." *Endocrinology* 139, no. 10 (1998): 4252-63.

Kumar, N. B., K. Besterman-Dahan, L. Kang, J. Pow-Sang, P. Xu, K. Allen, D. Riccardi & J. P. Krischer. "Results of a Randomized Clinical Trial of the Action of Several Doses of Lycopene in Localized Prostate Cancer: Administration Prior to Radical Prostatectomy." *Clin Med Urol* 1 (2008): 1-14.

Kumar, N. B., A. Cantor, K. Allen, D. Riccardi, K. Besterman-Dahan, J. Seigne, M. Helal, R. Salup & J. Pow-Sang. "The Specific Role of Isoflavones in Reducing Prostate Cancer Risk." *Prostate* 59, no. 2 (2004): 141-7.

Kumar, N. B., J. P. Krischer, K. Allen, D. Riccardi, K. Besterman-Dahan, R. Salup, L. Kang, P. Xu & J. Pow-Sang. "A Phase Ii Randomized, Placebo-Controlled Clinical Trial of Purified Isoflavones in Modulating Steroid Hormones in Men Diagnosed with Localized Prostate Cancer." *Nutr Cancer* 59, no. 2 (2007): 163-8.

Kumi-Diaka, J. & A. Butler. "Caspase-3 Protease Activation During the Process of Genistein-Induced Apoptosis in Tm4 Testicular Cells." *Biol Cell* 92, no. 2 (2000): 115-24.

Kumi-Diaka, J., N. A. Sanderson & A. Hall. "The Mediating Role of Caspase-3 Protease in the Intracellular Mechanism of Genistein-Induced Apoptosis in Human Prostatic Carcinoma Cell Lines, Du145 and LNCaP." *Biol Cell* 92, no. 8-9 (2000): 595-604.

Kumi-Diaka, J. K., M. Hassanhi, K. Merchant & V. Horman. "Influence of Genistein Isoflavone on Matrix Metalloproteinase-2 Expression in Prostate Cancer Cells." *J Med Food* 9, no. 4 (2006): 491-7.

Kurahashi, N., M. Iwasaki, S. Sasazuki, T. Otani, M. Inoue & S. Tsugane. "Soy Product and Isoflavone Consumption in Relation to Prostate Cancer in Japanese Men." *Cancer Epidemiol Biomarkers Prev* 16, no. 3 (2007): 538-45.

Kuwajerwala, N., E. Cifuentes, S. Gautam, M. Menon, E. R. Barrack & G.P.V. Reddy. "Resveratrol Induces Prostate Cancer Cell Entry into S Phase and Inhibits DNA Synthesis." *Cancer Research* 62, no. 9 (2002): 2488-92.

Kyle, E., L. Neckers, C. Takimoto, G. Curt & R. Bergan. "Genistein-Induced Apoptosis of Prostate Cancer Cells Is Preceded by a Specific Decrease in Focal Adhesion Kinase Activity." *Molecular Pharmacology* 51, no. 2 (1997): 193-200.

la Porte, C., N. Voduc, G. Zhang, I. Seguin, D. Tardiff, N. Singhal & D. W. Cameron. "Steady-State Pharmacokinetics and Tolerability of Trans-Resveratrol 2000 Mg Twice Daily with Food, Quercetin and Alcohol (Ethanol) in Healthy Human Subjects." *Clin Pharmacokinet* 49, no. 7 (2010): 449-54.

Lazarevic, B., S. J. Karlsen & F. Saatcioglu. "Genistein Differentially Modulates Androgen-Responsive Gene Expression and Activates Jnk in LNCaP Cells." *Oncol Rep* 19, no. 5 (2008): 1231-5.

Li, M., Z. Zhang, D. L. Hill, X. Chen, H. Wang & R. Zhang. "Genistein, a Dietary Isoflavone, Down-Regulates the Mdm2 Oncogene at Both Transcriptional and Posttranslational Levels." *Cancer Res* 65, no. 18 (2005): 8200-8.

Li, M., Z. Zhang, D.L. Hill, H. Wang & R. Zhang. "Curcumin, a Dietary Component, Has Anticancer, Chemosensitization, and Radiosensitization Effects by Down-Regulating the Mdm2 Oncogene through the Pi3k/Mtor/Ets2 Pathway." *Cancer Research* 67, no. 5 (2007): 1988-96.

Li, X., M. Marani, R. Mannucci, B. Kinsey, F. Andriani, I. Nicoletti, L. Denner & M. Marcelli. "Overexpression of Bcl-X(L) Underlies the Molecular Basis for Resistance to Staurosporine-Induced Apoptosis in Pc-3 Cells." *Cancer Res* 61, no. 4 (2001): 1699-706.

Li, Y. & F. H. Sarkar. "Down-Regulation of Invasion and Angiogenesis-Related Genes Identified by Cdna Microarray Analysis of Pc3 Prostate Cancer Cells Treated with Genistein." *Cancer Lett* 186, no. 2 (2002): 157-64.

Li, Z., W. J. Aronson, J. R. Arteaga, K. Hong, G. Thames, S. M. Henning, W. Liu, R. Elashoff, J. M. Ashley & D. Heber. "Feasibility of a Low-Fat/High-Fiber Diet Intervention with Soy Supplementation in Prostate Cancer Patients after Prostatectomy." *Eur J Clin Nutr* 62, no. 4 (2008): 526-36.

Lian, F., M. Bhuiyan, Y. W. Li, N. Wall, M. Kraut & F. H. Sarkar. "Genistein-Induced G2-M Arrest, P21waf1 Upregulation, and Apoptosis in a Non-Small-Cell Lung Cancer Cell Line." *Nutr Cancer* 31, no. 3 (1998): 184-91.

Limpens, J., F. H. Schroder, C. M. de Ridder, C. A. Bolder, M. F. Wildhagen, U. C. Obermuller-Jevic, K. Kramer & W. M. van Weerden. "Combined Lycopene and Vitamin E Treatment Suppresses the Growth of Pc-346c Human Prostate Cancer Cells in Nude Mice." *Journal of Nutrition* 136, no. 5 (2006): 1287-93.

Lin, L., B. Hutzen, S. Ball, E. Foust, M. Sobo, S. Deangelis, B. Pandit, L. Friedman, C. Li, P.-K. Li, J. Fuchs & J. Lin. "New Curcumin Analogues Exhibit Enhanced Growth-Suppressive Activity and Inhibit Akt and Signal Transducer and Activator of Transcription 3 Phosphorylation in Breast and Prostate Cancer Cells." *Cancer Science* 100, no. 9 (2009): 1719-27.

Liu, X., J. D. Allen, J. T. Arnold & M. R. Blackman. "Lycopene Inhibits Igf-I Signal Transduction and Growth in Normal Prostate Epithelial Cells by Decreasing Dht-Modulated Igf-I Production in Co-Cultured Reactive Stromal Cells." *Carcinogenesis* 29, no. 4 (2008): 816-23.

Liu, Y., E. Kyle, R. Lieberman, J. Crowell, G. Kellof & R. C. Bergan. "Focal Adhesion Kinase (Fak) Phosphorylation Is Not Required for Genistein-Induced Fak-Beta-1-Integrin Complex Formation." *Clin Exp Metastasis* 18, no. 3 (2000): 203-12.

MacLean, M. A., B. E. Scott, B. A. Deziel, M. C. Nunnelley, A. M. Liberty, K. T. Gottschall-Pass, C. C. Neto & R. A. Hurta. "North American Cranberry (Vaccinium Macrocarpon) Stimulates Apoptotic Pathways in Du145 Human Prostate Cancer Cells *in Vitro*." *Nutr Cancer* 63, no. 1 (2011): 109-20.

Mangels, A. R., J. M. Holden, G. R. Beecher, M. R. Forman & E. Lanza. "Carotenoid Content of Fruits and Vegetables: An Evaluation of Analytic Data." *J Am Diet Assoc* 93, no. 3 (1993): 284-96.

Maskarinec, G., Y. Morimoto, S. Hebshi, S. Sharma, A. A. Franke & F. Z. Stanczyk. "Serum Prostate-Specific Antigen but Not Testosterone Levels Decrease in a Randomized Soy Intervention among Men." *Eur J Clin Nutr* 60, no. 12 (2006): 1423-9.

McCormick, D. L., W. D. Johnson, M. C. Bosland, R. A. Lubet & V. E. Steele. "Chemoprevention of Rat Prostate Carcinogenesis by Soy Isoflavones and by Bowman-Birk Inhibitor." *Nutr Cancer* 57, no. 2 (2007): 184-93.

McPherson, R. A., P. T. Galettis & P. L. de Souza. "Enhancement of the Activity of Phenoxodiol by Cisplatin in Prostate Cancer Cells." *Br J Cancer* 100, no. 4 (2009): 649-55.

Mentor-Marcel, R., C. A. Lamartiniere, I. E. Eltoum, N. M. Greenberg & A. Elgavish. "Genistein in the Diet Reduces the Incidence of Poorly Differentiated Prostatic Adenocarcinoma in Transgenic Mice (Tramp)." *Cancer Res* 61, no. 18 (2001): 6777-82.

Messina, M., C. Nagata & A. H. Wu. "Estimated Asian Adult Soy Protein and Isoflavone Intakes." *Nutr Cancer* 55, no. 1 (2006): 1-12.

Mills, P. K., W. L. Beeson, R. L. Phillips & G. E. Fraser. "Cohort Study of Diet, Lifestyle, and Prostate Cancer in Adventist Men." *Cancer* 64, no. 3 (1989): 598-604.

Mitchell, S. H., W. Zhu & C. Y. Young. "Resveratrol Inhibits the Expression and Function of the Androgen Receptor in LNCaP Prostate Cancer Cells." *Cancer Res* 59, no. 23 (1999): 5892-5.

Mossine, V. V., P. Chopra & T. P. Mawhinney. "Interaction of Tomato Lycopene and Ketosamine against Rat Prostate Tumorigenesis." *Cancer Res* 68, no. 11 (2008): 4384-91.

Mukhopadhyay, A., C. Bueso-Ramos, D. Chatterjee, P. Pantazis & B. B. Aggarwal. "Curcumin Downregulates Cell Survival Mechanisms in Human Prostate Cancer Cell Lines." *Oncogene* 20, no. 52 (2001): 7597-609.

Nakamura, K., Y. Yasunaga, T. Segawa, D. Ko, J. W. Moul, S. Srivastava & J. S. Rhim. "Curcumin Down-Regulates Ar Gene Expression and Activation in Prostate Cancer Cell Lines." *International Journal of Oncology* 21, no. 4 (2002): 825-30.

Narayanan, N. K., D. Nargi, C. Randolph & B. A. Narayanan. "Liposome Encapsulation of Curcumin and Resveratrol in Combination Reduces Prostate Cancer Incidence in Pten Knockout Mice." *Int J Cancer* 125, no. 1 (2009): 1-8.

Neveu, V., Perez-Jiménez J., Vos F., Crespy V., du Chaffaut L., Mennen L., Knox C., Eisner R., Cruz J., Wishart D., Scalbert A. (2010) "Phenol-Explorer: an online comprehensive database on polyphenol contents in foods." *Database*, doi: 10.1093/ database/ bap024.

Neveu, V., J. Perez-Jimenez, F. Vos, V. Crespy, L. du Chaffaut, L. Mennen, C. Knox, R. Eisner, J. Cruz, D. Wishart & A. Scalbert. "Phenol-Explorer: An Online Comprehensive Database on Polyphenol Contents in Foods." *Database (Oxford)* 2010 (2010): bap024.

Nguyen, T. H., F. B. Mustafa, S. Pervaiz, F. S. Ng & L. H. Lim. "Erk1/2 Activation Is Required for Resveratrol-Induced Apoptosis in Mda-Mb-231 Cells." *International Journal of Oncology* 33, no. 1 (2008): 81-92.

Nunes, T., L. Almeida, J. F. Rocha, A. Falcao, C. Fernandes-Lopes, A. I. Loureiro, L. Wright, M. Vaz-da-Silva & P. Soares-da-Silva. "Pharmacokinetics of Trans-Resveratrol Following Repeated Administration in Healthy Elderly and Young Subjects." *Journal of Clinical Pharmacology* 49, no. 12 (2009): 1477-82.

Nutrient Data, Laboratory, and Knovel. "USDA Database for the Isoflavone Content of Selected Foods." U.S. Dept. of Agriculture; http://ezproxy.uws.edu.au/ login?url=http://www.knovel.com/web/portal/browse/display?_EXT_KNOVEL _DISPLAY_bookid=3708.

Palozza, P., M. Colangelo, R. Simone, A. Catalano, A. Boninsegna, P. Lanza, G. Monego & F. O. Ranelletti. "Lycopene Induces Cell Growth Inhibition by Altering Mevalonate Pathway and Ras Signaling in Cancer Cell Lines." *Carcinogenesis* 31, no. 10 (2010): 1813-21.

Park, J. I., M. G. Lee, K. Cho, B. J. Park, K. S. Chae, D. S. Byun, B. K. Ryu, Y. K. Park & S. G. Chi. "Transforming Growth Factor-Beta1 Activates Interleukin-6 Expression in Prostate Cancer Cells through the Synergistic Collaboration of the Smad2, P38-Nf-Kappab, Jnk, and Ras Signaling Pathways." *Oncogene* 22, no. 28 (2003): 4314-32.

Park, S.-S., Y.-N. Kim, Y.K. Jeon, Y.A. Kim, J.E. Kim, H. Kim & C.W. Kim. "Genistein-Induced Apoptosis Via Akt Signaling Pathway in Anaplastic Large-Cell Lymphoma." *Cancer Chemotherapy and Pharmacology* 56, no. 3 (2005): 271-78.

Patel, K. R., E. Scott, V. A. Brown, A. J. Gescher, W. P. Steward & K. Brown. "Clinical Trials of Resveratrol." *Ann N Y Acad Sci* 1215 (2011): 161-9.

Pendleton, J. M., W. W. Tan, S. Anai, M. Chang, W. Hou, K. T. Shiverick & C. J. Rosser. "Phase Ii Trial of Isoflavone in Prostate-Specific Antigen Recurrent Prostate Cancer after Previous Local Therapy." *BMC Cancer* 8 (2008): 132.

Peternac, D., I. Klima, M. G. Cecchini, R. Schwaninger, U. E. Studer & G. N. Thalmann. "Agents Used for Chemoprevention of Prostate Cancer May Influence PSA Secretion Independently of Cell Growth in the LNCaP Model of Human Prostate Cancer Progression." *Prostate* 68, no. 12 (2008): 1307-18.

Pike, A. C., A. M. Brzozowski, R. E. Hubbard, T. Bonn, A. G. Thorsell, O. Engstrom, J. Ljunggren, J. A. Gustafsson & M. Carlquist. "Structure of the Ligand-Binding Domain of Oestrogen Receptor Beta in the Presence of a Partial Agonist and a Full Antagonist." *EMBO J* 18, no. 17 (1999): 4608-18.

Ping, S. Y., T. C. Hour, S. R. Lin & D. S. Yu. "Taxol Synergizes with Antioxidants in Inhibiting Hormal Refractory Prostate Cancer Cell Growth." *Urol Oncol* 28, no. 2 (2010): 170-9.

Pinski, J., Q. Wang, M. L. Quek, A. Cole, J. Cooc, K. Danenberg & P. V. Danenberg. "Genistein-Induced Neuroendocrine Differentiation of Prostate Cancer Cells." *Prostate* 66, no. 11 (2006): 1136-43.

Raffoul, J. J., S. Banerjee, M. Che, Z. E. Knoll, D. R. Doerge, J. Abrams, O. Kucuk, F. H. Sarkar & G. G. Hillman. "Soy Isoflavones Enhance Radiotherapy in a Metastatic Prostate Cancer Model." *Int J Cancer* 120, no. 11 (2007): 2491-8.

Rannikko, A., A. Petas, T. Raivio, O. A. Janne, S. Rannikko & H. Adlercreutz. "The Effects of Short-Term Oral Phytoestrogen Supplementation on the Hypothalamic-Pituitary-Testicular Axis in Prostate Cancer Patients." *Prostate* 66, no. 10 (2006): 1086-91.

Ravindran, J., S. Prasad & B. B. Aggarwal. "Curcumin and Cancer Cells: How Many Ways Can Curry Kill Tumor Cells Selectively?" *AAPS J* 11, no. 3 (2009): 495-510.

Rice, L., R. Handayani, Y. Cui, T. Medrano, V. Samedi, H. Baker, N. J. Szabo, C. J. Rosser, S. Goodison & K. T. Shiverick. "Soy Isoflavones Exert Differential Effects on Androgen Responsive Genes in LNCaP Human Prostate Cancer Cells." *Journal of Nutrition* 137, no. 4 (2007): 964-72.

Rice, L., V. G. Samedi, T. A. Medrano, C. A. Sweeney, H. V. Baker, A. Stenstrom, J. Furman & K. T. Shiverick. "Mechanisms of the Growth Inhibitory Effects of the Isoflavonoid Biochanin a on LNCaP Cells and Xenografts." *Prostate* 52, no. 3 (2002): 201-12.

Richelle, M., S. Pridmore-Merten, S. Bodenstab, M. Enslen & E. A. Offord. "Hydrolysis of Isoflavone Glycosides to Aglycones by Beta-Glycosidase Does Not Alter Plasma and Urine Isoflavone Pharmacokinetics in Postmenopausal Women." *Journal of Nutrition* 132, no. 9 (2002): 2587-92.

Romero-Perez, A. I., M. Ibern-Gomez, R. M. Lamuela-Raventos & M. C. de La Torre-Boronat. "Piceid, the Major Resveratrol Derivative in Grape Juices." *J Agric Food Chem* 47, no. 4 (1999): 1533-6.

Ronen, G., M. Cohen, D. Zamir & J. Hirschberg. "Regulation of Carotenoid Biosynthesis During Tomato Fruit Development: Expression of the Gene for Lycopene Epsilon-Cyclase Is Down-Regulated During Ripening and Is Elevated in the Mutant Delta." *Plant J* 17, no. 4 (1999): 341-51.

Rufer, C. E., A. Bub, J. Moseneder, P. Winterhalter, M. Sturtz & S. E. Kulling. "Pharmacokinetics of the Soybean Isoflavone Daidzein in Its Aglycone and

Glucoside Form: A Randomized, Double-Blind, Crossover Study." *American Journal of Clinical Nutrition* 87, no. 5 (2008): 1314-23.

Sallman, D. A., X. Chen, B. Zhong, D. L. Gilvary, J. Zhou, S. Wei & J. Y. Djeu. "Clusterin Mediates Trail Resistance in Prostate Tumor Cells." *Mol Cancer Ther* 6, no. 11 (2007): 2938-47.

Sapi, E., A. B. Alvero, W. Chen, D. O'Malley, X. Y. Hao, B. Dwipoyono, M. Garg, M. Kamsteeg, T. Rutherford & G. Mor. "Resistance of Ovarian Carcinoma Cells to Docetaxel Is Xiap Dependent and Reversible by Phenoxodiol." *Oncol Res* 14, no. 11-12 (2004): 567-78.

Scarlatti, F., G. Sala, C. Ricci, C. Maioli, F. Milani, M. Minella, M. Botturi & R. Ghidoni. "Resveratrol Sensitization of Du145 Prostate Cancer Cells to Ionizing Radiation Is Associated to Ceramide Increase." *Cancer Lett* 253, no. 1 (2007): 124-30.

Schroder, F. H., M. J. Roobol, E. R. Boeve, R. de Mutsert, S. D. Zuijdgeest-van Leeuwen, I. Kersten, M. F. Wildhagen & A. van Helvoort. "Randomized, Double-Blind, Placebo-Controlled Crossover Study in Men with Prostate Cancer and Rising PSA: Effectiveness of a Dietary Supplement." *Eur Urol* 48, no. 6 (2005): 922-30; discussion 30-1.

Schwedhelm, E., R. Maas, R. Troost & R. H. Boger. "Clinical Pharmacokinetics of Antioxidants and Their Impact on Systemic Oxidative Stress." *Clin Pharmacokinet* 42, no. 5 (2003): 437-59.

Schwenke, C., B. Ubrig, P. Thurmann, C. Eggersmann & S. Roth. "Lycopene for Advanced Hormone Refractory Prostate Cancer: A Prospective, Open Phase Ii Pilot Study." *Journal of Urology* 181, no. 3 (2009): 1098-103.

Setchell, K. D., N. M. Brown, P. Desai, L. Zimmer-Nechemias, B. E. Wolfe, W. T. Brashear, A. S. Kirschner, A. Cassidy & J. E. Heubi. "Bioavailability of Pure Isoflavones in Healthy Humans and Analysis of Commercial Soy Isoflavone Supplements." *Journal of Nutrition* 131, no. 4 Suppl (2001): 1362S-75S.

Setchell, K. D., N. M. Brown, L. Zimmer-Nechemias, W. T. Brashear, B. E. Wolfe, A. S. Kirschner & J. E. Heubi. "Evidence for Lack of Absorption of Soy Isoflavone Glycosides in Humans, Supporting the Crucial Role of Intestinal Metabolism for Bioavailability." *American Journal of Clinical Nutrition* 76, no. 2 (2002): 447-53.

Setchell, K. D., M. S. Faughnan, T. Avades, L. Zimmer-Nechemias, N. M. Brown, B. E. Wolfe, W. T. Brashear, P. Desai, M. F. Oldfield, N. P. Botting & A. Cassidy. "Comparing the Pharmacokinetics of Daidzein and Genistein with the Use of 13c-Labeled Tracers in Premenopausal Women." *American Journal of Clinical Nutrition* 77, no. 2 (2003): 411-9.

Shankar, S., Q. Chen, I. Siddiqui, K. Sarva & R. K. Srivastava. "Sensitization of Trail-Resistant LNCaP Cells by Resveratrol (3, 4', 5 Tri-Hydroxystilbene): Molecular Mechanisms and Therapeutic Potential." *J Mol Signal* 2 (2007): 7.

Shankar, S. & R. K. Srivastava. "Involvement of Bcl-2 Family Members, Phosphatidylinositol 3'-Kinase/Akt and Mitochondrial P53 in Curcumin (Diferulolylmethane)-Induced Apoptosis in Prostate Cancer." *International Journal of Oncology* 30, no. 4 (2007): 905-18.

Sharma, N. & U. Goswami. "Functioning of Lycopene in Mammalian System: A Review." *Proceedings of the Zoological Society* 64, no. 1 (2011): 1-7.

Sharma, R. A., S. A. Euden, S. L. Platton, D. N. Cooke, A. Shafayat, H. R. Hewitt, T. H. Marczylo, B. Morgan, D. Hemingway, S. M. Plummer, M. Pirmohamed, A. J.

Gescher & W. P. Steward. "Phase I Clinical Trial of Oral Curcumin: Biomarkers of Systemic Activity and Compliance." *Clin Cancer Res* 10, no. 20 (2004): 6847-54.

Shenouda, N. S., C. Zhou, J. D. Browning, P. J. Ansell, M. S. Sakla, D. B. Lubahn & R. S. Macdonald. "Phytoestrogens in Common Herbs Regulate Prostate Cancer Cell Growth *in Vitro*." *Nutr Cancer* 49, no. 2 (2004): 200-8.

Shi, W. F., M. Leong, E. Cho, J. Farrell, H. C. Chen, J. Tian & D. Zhang. "Repressive Effects of Resveratrol on Androgen Receptor Transcriptional Activity." *PLoS One* 4, no. 10 (2009): e7398.

Singh-Gupta, V., H. Zhang, S. Banerjee, D. Kong, J. J. Raffoul, F. H. Sarkar & G. G. Hillman. "Radiation-Induced Hif-1alpha Cell Survival Pathway Is Inhibited by Soy Isoflavones in Prostate Cancer Cells." *Int J Cancer* 124, no. 7 (2009): 1675-84.

Skogseth, H., E. Larsson & J. Halgunset. "Inhibitors of Tyrosine Kinase Inhibit the Producion of Urokinase Plasminogen Activator Human Prostatic Cancer Cells." *Apmis* 113, no. 5 (2005): 332-39.

Slusarz, A., N. S. Shenouda, M. S. Sakla, S. K. Drenkhahn, A. S. Narula, R. S. MacDonald, C. L. Besch-Williford & D. B. Lubahn. "Common Botanical Compounds Inhibit the Hedgehog Signaling Pathway in Prostate Cancer." *Cancer Res* 70, no. 8 (2010): 3382-90.

Soleas, G.J., L. Grass, P.D. Josephy, D.M. Goldberg & E.P. Diamandis. "A Comparison of the Anticarcinogenic Properties of Four Red Wine Polyphenols." *Clinical Biochemistry* 35, no. 2 (2002): 119-24.

Steiner, C., S. Arnould, A. Scalbert & C. Manach. "Isoflavones and the Prevention of Breast and Prostate Cancer: New Perspectives Opened by Nutrigenomics." *Br J Nutr* 99 E Suppl 1 (2008): ES78-108.

Stewart, J. R. & C. A. O'Brian. "Resveratrol Antagonizes Egfr-Dependent Erk1/2 Activation in Human Androgen-Independent Prostate Cancer Cells with Associated Isozyme-Selective Pkc Alpha Inhibition." *Invest New Drugs* 22, no. 2 (2004): 107-17.

Swami, S., A.V. Krishnan, J. Moreno, R.S. Bhattacharyya, C. Gardner, J.D. Brooks, D.M. Peehl & D. Feldman. "Inhibition of Prostaglandin Synthesis and Actions by Genistein in Human Prostate Cancer Cells and by Soy Isoflavones in Prostate Cancer Patients." *International Journal of Cancer* 124, no. 9 (2009): 2050-59.

Takahashi, Y., S. D. Hursting, S. N. Perkins, T. C. Wang & T. T. Wang. "Genistein Affects Androgen-Responsive Genes through Both Androgen- and Estrogen-Induced Signaling Pathways." *Mol Carcinog* 45, no. 1 (2006): 18-25.

Takimoto, C. H., K. Glover, X. Huang, S. A. Hayes, L. Gallot, M. Quinn, B. D. Jovanovic, A. Shapiro, L. Hernandez, A. Goetz, V. Llorens, R. Lieberman, J. A. Crowell, B. A. Poisson & R. C. Bergan. "Phase I Pharmacokinetic and Pharmacodynamic Analysis of Unconjugated Soy Isoflavones Administered to Individuals with Cancer." *Cancer Epidemiol Biomarkers Prev* 12, no. 11 Pt 1 (2003): 1213-21.

Talvas, J., C. Caris-Veyrat, L. Guy, M. Rambeau, B. Lyan, R. Minet-Quinard, J. M. Lobaccaro, M. P. Vasson, S. George, A. Mazur & E. Rock. "Differential Effects of Lycopene Consumed in Tomato Paste and Lycopene in the Form of a Purified Extract on Target Genes of Cancer Prostatic Cells." *American Journal of Clinical Nutrition* 91, no. 6 (2010): 1716-24.

Tayyem, R. F., D.D. Heath, W.K. Al-Delaimy, C.L. Rock. " Curcumin Content of Turmeric and Curry Powders" *Nutrition and Cancer* Vol. 55,no. 2, (2009) : 126-131.

Tang, Y., B. Parmakhtiar, A. R. Simoneau, J. Xie, J. Fruehauf, M. Lilly & X. Zi. "Lycopene Enhances Docetaxel's Effect in Castration-Resistant Prostate Cancer Associated with Insulin-Like Growth Factor I Receptor Levels." *Neoplasia* 13, no. 2 (2011): 108-19.

Teiten, M. H., F. Gaascht, M. Cronauer, E. Henry, M. Dicato & M. Diederich. "Anti-Proliferative Potential of Curcumin in Androgen-Dependent Prostate Cancer Cells Occurs through Modulation of the Wingless Signaling Pathway." *International Journal of Oncology* 38, no. 3 (2011): 603-11.

Tepper, C.G., R.L. Vinall, C.B. Wee, L. Xue, X.-B. Shi, R. Burich, P.C. Mack & R.W. de Vere White. "Gcp-Mediated Growth Inhibition and Apoptosis of Prostate Cancer Cells Via Androgen Receptor-Dependent and -Independent Mechanisms." *The Prostate* 67, no. 5 (2007): 521-35.

Thomas, S. L., D. Zhong, W. Zhou, S. Malik, D. Liotta, J. P. Snyder, E. Hamel & P. Giannakakou. "Ef24, a Novel Curcumin Analog, Disrupts the Microtubule Cytoskeleton and Inhibits Hif-1." *Cell Cycle* 7, no. 15 (2008): 2409-17.

Touny, L. H. & P. P. Banerjee. "Identification of Both Myt-1 and Wee-1 as Necessary Mediators of the P21-Independent Inactivation of the Cdc-2/Cyclin B1 Complex and Growth Inhibition of Tramp Cancer Cells by Genistein." *Prostate* 66, no. 14 (2006): 1542-55.

Tsui, K. H., T. H. Feng, C. M. Lin, P. L. Chang & H. H. Juang. "Curcumin Blocks the Activation of Androgen and Interlukin-6 on Prostate-Specific Antigen Expression in Human Prostatic Carcinoma Cells." *J Androl* 29, no. 6 (2008): 661-8.

Urban, D., W. Irwin, M. Kirk, M. A. Markiewicz, R. Myers, M. Smith, H. Weiss, W. E. Grizzle & S. Barnes. "The Effect of Isolated Soy Protein on Plasma Biomarkers in Elderly Men with Elevated Serum Prostate Specific Antigen." *J Urol* 165, no. 1 (2001): 294-300.

Vaishampayan, U., M. Hussain, M. Banerjee, S. Seren, F. H. Sarkar, J. Fontana, J. D. Forman, M. L. Cher, I. Powell, J. E. Pontes & O. Kucuk. "Lycopene and Soy Isoflavones in the Treatment of Prostate Cancer." *Nutr Cancer* 59, no. 1 (2007): 1-7.

van Breemen, R. B., R. Sharifi, M. Viana, N. Pajkovic, D. Zhu, L. Yuan, Y. Yang, P. E. Bowen & M. Stacewicz-Sapuntzakis. "Antioxidant Effects of Lycopene in African American Men with Prostate Cancer or Benign Prostate Hyperplasia: A Randomized, Controlled Trial." *Cancer Prev Res (Phila)* 4, no. 5 (2011): 711-8.

Vareed, S. K., M. Kakarala, M. T. Ruffin, J. A. Crowell, D. P. Normolle, Z. Djuric & D. E. Brenner. "Pharmacokinetics of Curcumin Conjugate Metabolites in Healthy Human Subjects." *Cancer Epidemiol Biomarkers Prev* 17, no. 6 (2008): 1411-7.

Vaz-da-Silva, M., A. I. Loureiro, A. Falcao, T. Nunes, J. F. Rocha, C. Fernandes-Lopes, E. Soares, L. Wright, L. Almeida & P. Soares-da-Silva. "Effect of Food on the Pharmacokinetic Profile of Trans-Resveratrol." *Int J Clin Pharmacol Ther* 46, no. 11 (2008): 564-70.

Venkateswaran, V., L. H. Klotz, M. Ramani, L. M. Sugar, L. E. Jacob, R. K. Nam & N. E. Fleshner. "A Combination of Micronutrients Is Beneficial in Reducing the Incidence of Prostate Cancer and Increasing Survival in the Lady Transgenic Model." *Cancer Prev Res (Phila)* 2, no. 5 (2009): 473-83.

Vitrac, X., A. Desmouliere, B. Brouillaud, S. Krisa, G. Deffieux, N. Barthe, J. Rosenbaum & J. M. Merillon. "Distribution of [14c]-Trans-Resveratrol, a Cancer Chemopreventive

Polyphenol, in Mouse Tissues after Oral Administration." *Life Sci* 72, no. 20 (2003): 2219-33.

Wahl, H., L. Tan, K. Griffith, M. Choi & J. R. Liu. "Curcumin Enhances Apo2l/Trail-Induced Apoptosis in Chemoresistant Ovarian Cancer Cells." *Gynecol Oncol* 105, no. 1 (2007): 104-12.

Wang, J., I. E. Eltoum & C. A. Lamartiniere. "Genistein Alters Growth Factor Signaling in Transgenic Prostate Model (Tramp)." *Molecular and Cellular Endocrinology* 219, no. 1-2 (2004): 171-80.

Wang, J., I.-E. Eltoum & C.A. Lamartiniere. "Dietary Genistein Suppresses Chemically Induced Prostate Cancer in Lobund–Wistar Rats." *Cancer Letters* 186, no. 1 (2002): 11-18.

Wang, S., V. L. DeGroff & S. K. Clinton. "Tomato and Soy Polyphenols Reduce Insulin-Like Growth Factor-I-Stimulated Rat Prostate Cancer Cell Proliferation and Apoptotic Resistance *in Vitro* Via Inhibition of Intracellular Signaling Pathways Involving Tyrosine Kinase." *Journal of Nutrition* 133, no. 7 (2003): 2367-76.

Wang, T. T., T. S. Hudson, T. C. Wang, C. M. Remsberg, N. M. Davies, Y. Takahashi, Y. S. Kim, H. Seifried, B. T. Vinyard, S. N. Perkins & S. D. Hursting. "Differential Effects of Resveratrol on Androgen-Responsive LNCaP Human Prostate Cancer Cells *in Vitro* and *in Vivo*." *Carcinogenesis* 29, no. 10 (2008): 2001-10.

Wang, T. T., N. W. Schoene, Y. S. Kim, C. S. Mizuno & A. M. Rimando. "Differential Effects of Resveratrol and Its Naturally Occurring Methylether Analogs on Cell Cycle and Apoptosis in Human Androgen-Responsive LNCaP Cancer Cells." *Mol Nutr Food Res* 54, no. 3 (2010): 335-44.

Wang, Y., J. J. Raffoul, M. Che, D. R. Doerge, M. C. Joiner, O. Kucuk, F. H. Sarkar & G. G. Hillman. "Prostate Cancer Treatment Is Enhanced by Genistein *in Vitro* and *in Vivo* in a Syngeneic Orthotopic Tumor Model." *Radiat Res* 166, no. 1 Pt 1 (2006): 73-80.

Wong, Y., G. Osmond, K. I. Brewer, D. S. Tyler & M. B. Andrus. "Synthesis of 4'-Ester Analogs of Resveratrol and Their Evaluation in Malignant Melanoma and Pancreatic Cell Lines." *Bioorganic & Medicinal Chemistry Letters* 20, no. 3 (2010): 1198-201.

Xu, L. & R. C. Bergan. "Genistein Inhibits Matrix Metalloproteinase Type 2 Activation and Prostate Cancer Cell Invasion by Blocking the Transforming Growth Factor Beta-Mediated Activation of Mitogen-Activated Protein Kinase-Activated Protein Kinase 2-27-Kda Heat Shock Protein Pathway." *Molecular Pharmacology* 70, no. 3 (2006): 869-77.

Yang, C. M., I. H. Lu, H. Y. Chen & M. L. Hu. "Lycopene Inhibits the Proliferation of Androgen-Dependent Human Prostate Tumor Cells through Activation of Ppargamma-Lxralpha-Abca1 Pathway." *J Nutr Biochem* (2011).

Yang, C. M., Y. T. Yen, C. S. Huang & M. L. Hu. "Growth Inhibitory Efficacy of Lycopene and Beta-Carotene against Androgen-Independent Prostate Tumor Cells Xenografted in Nude Mice." *Mol Nutr Food Res* 55, no. 4 (2011): 606-12.

Yu, L., G. L. Blackburn & J. R. Zhou. "Genistein and Daidzein Downregulate Prostate Androgen-Regulated Transcript-1 (Part-1) Gene Expression Induced by Dihydrotestosterone in Human Prostate LNCaP Cancer Cells." *Journal of Nutrition* 133, no. 2 (2003): 389-92.

Yu, S., G. Shen, T. O. Khor, J. H. Kim & A. N. Kong. "Curcumin Inhibits Akt/Mammalian Target of Rapamycin Signaling through Protein Phosphatase-Dependent Mechanism." *Mol Cancer Ther* 7, no. 9 (2008): 2609-20.

Yuan, J. P., J. H. Wang & X. Liu. "Metabolism of Dietary Soy Isoflavones to Equol by Human Intestinal Microflora--Implications for Health." *Mol Nutr Food Res* 51, no. 7 (2007): 765-81.

Zapalis, Charles. *Food Chemistry and Nutritional Biochemistry / Charles Zapalis, R. Anderle Beck.* Edited by R. Anderle Beck. New York :: Wiley, 1985.

Zhang, X., Q. Wang, B. Neil & X. Chen. "Effect of Lycopene on Androgen Receptor and Prostate-Specific Antigen Velocity." *Chin Med J (Engl)* 123, no. 16 (2010): 2231-6.

Zhou, J. R., E. T. Gugger, T. Tanaka, Y. Guo, G. L. Blackburn & S. K. Clinton. "Soybean Phytochemicals Inhibit the Growth of Transplantable Human Prostate Carcinoma and Tumor Angiogenesis in Mice." *Journal of Nutrition* 129, no. 9 (1999): 1628-35.

Zhou, J. R., L. Yu, Y. Zhong, R. L. Nassr, A. A. Franke, S. M. Gaston & G. L. Blackburn. "Inhibition of Orthotopic Growth and Metastasis of Androgen-Sensitive Human Prostate Tumors in Mice by Bioactive Soybean Components." *Prostate* 53, no. 2 (2002): 143-53.

Ziech, D., R. Franco, A.G. Georgakilas, S. Georgakila, V. Malamou-Mitsi, O. Schoneveld, A. Pappa & M.I. Panayiotidis. "The Role of Reactive Oxygen Species and Oxidative Stress in Environmental Carcinogenesis and Biomarker Development." *Chemico-Biological Interactions* 188, no. 2 (2010): 334-39.

Zubik, L. & M. Meydani. "Bioavailability of Soybean Isoflavones from Aglycone and Glucoside Forms in American Women." *American Journal of Clinical Nutrition* 77, no. 6 (2003): 1459-65.

12

Phytoestrogens as Nutritional Modulators in Colon Cancer Prevention

Michele Barone, Raffaele Licinio and Alfredo Di Leo
Gastroenterology Unit, Department of Emergency and Organ Transplantation (D.E.T.O.), University of Bari "A. Moro", Bari, Italy

1. Introduction

Intestinal carcinogenesis is the final outcome of a multi-step process resulting from genetic alterations that are influenced by two categories of factors: environmental factors and host-related factors such as cytokines and hormones (including sex steroid hormones). One of the most important environmental factors involved in the development of colon cancer is dietary components. However, variations in cancer incidence among and within populations with similar dietary patterns suggest that the predominant pathogenetic factor is the individual response, through the expression of different protein and metabolite patterns (1). Among host-related factors particular attention is paid in this work to the relationship between estrogens, as well as their agonists (phytoestrogens), and colon cancer, and the possible role of these latter substances in the prevention of colon cancer.

2. APC gene in colorectal cancer

Colorectal cancer (CRC) is the final outcome of a multi-step process that, in most cases, proceeds down the adenoma–carcinoma sequence pathway (2).

The tumor suppressor gene mutation involving the *Adenomatous Polyposis Coli* (APC) gene is present in 80% of sporadic CRCs and 100% of cases of *Familial Adenomatous Polyposis* (FAP). In humans, the APC mutation provides the genetic background to the onset of the tumor process, making intestinal cells susceptible to tumor progression and promotion through the accumulation of further mutations as a result of epigenetic phenomena largely influenced by environmental factors (3).

FAP offers an ideal model for the study of CRC since in these patients "normal" mucosa coexists with low and high-grade dysplastic lesions as well adenocarcinoma, i.e. all the stages of the carcinogenetic process. For this reason the modifications occurring during the carcinogenetic process are easily comparable and free from individual variations (4).

3. Estrogens in colorectal cancer

Phytoestrogens (heterocyclic non steroid phenols) are plant-derived compounds with a structural and functional action as estrogen agonists in mammals. To understand their biological activities and the possible interactions between phytoestrogens and colorectal cancer, a knowledge of some fundamental data on estrogens is essential.

Estrogen biological activities are mainly mediated by their binding with two specific receptors: estrogen receptor alpha (ER-α) and estrogen receptor beta (ER-β). Both of these estrogen receptors (ERs) belong to the steroid/thyroid hormone receptor superfamily of nuclear receptors, which are activated upon binding of the ligand. After binding, activated ERs are able to interact directly with cis-regulatory elements of target genes by binding to estrogen-response elements (EREs), or indirectly through interaction with another DNA-bound transcription factor, such as activator protein 1 (AP-1), thus facilitating the assembly of basal transcription factors into a stable pre-initiation complex, followed by increased transcription rates for target mRNAs (5).

Both ERs consist of three main regions: 1) a hypervariable N-terminal, that contributes to the transactivation function, 2) a highly conserved DNA-binding domain, responsible for specific DNA-binding and dimerization and 3) a C-terminal domain, involved in ligand-binding (LBD) and nuclear localization, as well as ligand-dependent transactivation functions. ER-α and ER-β are produced by different genes located on different chromosomes (6).

In mammals, both ER-α and ER-β have conserved DNA binding domains (96%) but they have different LBD showing only 58% homology. ER-α has two distinct transcriptional activation functions (AF): AF-1 and AF-2. AF-1, located at the N-terminal, is ligand-independent, constitutively active and contributes to the transcriptional activity of the receptor by recruiting co-activator proteins such as GRIP1 and SRC-1 and the histone acetyltransferases (HAT) p300/CBP and pCAF. The AF-2 domain is under the control of ligands in both ER-α and ER-β.

Variations observed in the phenotypes of knock-out mice lacking ER-α or ER-β suggest that these two proteins have different biological activities. This view has been further supported by in vitro and in vivo studies in ER-β knock-out mice, indicating that ER-β is a modulator of ER-α activity as it is able to reverse the effects of ER-α and to inhibit estradiol (E_2)-dependent proliferation (7). In addition, it is known that ER-α and ER-β have a different distribution in the various organs and apparatuses. ER-α is essentially expressed in the breast, bone, cardiovascular tissue, urogenital tract and central nervous system, while ER-β is the prevalent form in the gut. Both receptors bind E_2 but they activate promoters in different ways. Studies on breast and prostate carcinogenesis suggest an opposite role of ER-α and ER-β in the proliferation and differentiation of target tissues, a hypothesis described as the ying/yang relationship (8).

Estrogens regulate cellular function also through non-genomic pathways. In fact, after palmitoylation ERs can localize at the plasma membrane, associate to caveolin-1 and, upon estrogens stimulation, activate rapid signals. In the case of ER-α, palmitoylation stimulates proliferation, while ER-β localization at the plasma membrane and its association with caveolin-1 activates p38 (a member of the MAPK family), that promotes apoptosis (9). This finding is confirmed by the observation, in the tumor tissue, of a reduction of ER-β and an increased alpha/beta ratio, that is related to a reduction of apoptosis and an increased rate of proliferation.

In the last few years, numerous epidemiological, clinical and experimental studies have explored the role of estrogens in intestinal carcinogenesis, suggesting their protective role and potential use in CRC prevention (10-14). In particular, estrogen protective activities are thought to be related to their receptor subtype beta (ER-β), suggesting the use of selective ER-β agonists in primary CRC prevention .

Since the early 80s, the role of a progressive silencing of Estrogen Receptor beta (ERβ) expression in intestinal cells, as a pathogenetic factor involved in intestinal tumorigenesis and its progression to an overt cancerous phenotype, has been studied in both animal models and clinical settings (11-14).

There is some evidence supporting ER-β as a prognostic factor in sporadic adenocarcinoma, and suggesting its role as a relevant surrogate biomarker in the follow-up of intestinal neoplasia development and dysplastic severity (15-18).

In the $Apc^{Min/+}$ mouse, that represents the animal model equivalent to FAP in humans, the loss of apoptotic control also occurs in non adenomatous (normal) mucosa, again depending upon a decreased ER-β expression and related decreased TUNEL and caspase-3 expression. In intact male $Apc^{Min/+}$ mice it has been demonstrated that supplementing the diet with selected, weak but specific ER-β agonists reversed the hyperproliferative behavior in non adenomatous mucosa, and reduced the number and the degree of polyp dysplasia in adenomatous mucosa (19).

In human sporadic polyps, a progressive, significant decrease of ER-β expression has been demonstrated, a finding confirmed in subjects affected by Familial Adenomatous Polyposis (FAP) (4). In these patients, in fact, a progressive, significant decrease of ER-β expression was observed in the different stages of the disease, correlated with apoptosis ($r=0.76$, $p< 0.001$), and inversely correlated with cell proliferation.

4. Phytoestrogens and CRC

Phytoestrogens are heterocyclic, non steroid phenols extracted from plants. These compounds are structurally similar and have a functional action as estrogen-agonists in mammals. Four classes of phytoestrogens can be distinguished, on the basis of their different molecular structure and different biological activities, namely isoflavones, lignans, coumestans and lactones (20-21).

Isoflavones, including genistein and quercitin, are the most known phytoestrogens. They are primarily found in the Fabaceae family, which includes legumes, soybean, peanut and clover.

Lignans were first identified in plants and later in biological fluids of mammals. These compounds are found in whole grain, seeds, fruits and vegetables but also in beverages such as coffee and tea (22). The cyclic urinary excretion of these phenolic compounds during the menstrual cycle led to investigations of their biological role, and they are now considered as a new hormone class (23).

Coumestans are less common in the human diet than isoflavones; they are extracted from fodder, clover, legumes and soybean.

Lactones are the least common phytoestrogens in the human diet.

Natural phytoestrogens undergo glycosidic binding to carbohydrates to produce complex molecules that are hard for the intestinal tract to absorb. For this reason, after ingestion, this glycosidic binding is broken up by glycosidases, enzymes produced by intestinal microflora. This enzymatic digestion generates "aglycone", a compound that is quickly absorbed and can bind ERs (24).

Phytoestrogens are characterized by a higher binding affinity to ER-β as compared to the other estrogen receptor subtype, alpha (ER-α). This biological characteristic explains why the administration of phytoestrogens does not produce the classic side effects associated to estrogen administration (cerebro- and cardiovascular attacks, a higher incidence of endometrial and breast cancer) (25-27), making these substances ideal candidates for CRC prevention.

As proposed for estrogens, genomic and non-genomic mechanisms have been also suggested for phytoestrogens to explain their biological activities (20; 28-32).

One of the most interesting compounds is Silymarin, initially extracted from Silybum marianum. It is a mixture of four flavolignans (silibinin, isosilibinin, silydianin and silychristin) and the isoflavone taxifolin. It is already used in the treatment of alcoholic liver disease and as an anti-fibrotic agent (33).

Extensive research within the last decade has shown that silymarin can suppress the proliferation of a variety of tumor cells (e.g., prostate, breast, ovary, colon, lung, bladder); this is accomplished through cell cycle arrest at the G1/S-phase, induction of cyclin-dependent kinase inhibitors (such as p15, p21 and p27), down-regulation of anti-apoptotic gene products (e.g., Bcl-2 and Bcl-xL), inhibition of cell-survival kinases (AKT, PKC and MAPK) and inhibition of inflammatory transcription factors (e.g., NF-kappaB). Silymarin can also down-regulate gene products involved in the proliferation of tumor cells (cyclin D1, EGFR, COX-2, TGF-beta, IGF-IR), invasion (MMP-9), angiogenesis (VEGF) and metastasis (adhesion molecules). The antiinflammatory effects of silymarin are mediated through suppression of NF-kappaB-regulated gene products, including COX-2, LOX, inducible iNOS, TNF and IL-1 (35).

Silymarin has also been shown to sensitize tumors to chemotherapeutic agents through down-regulation of the MDR protein and other mechanisms. It binds to both estrogen and androgen receptors, and down-regulates PSA. In addition to its chemopreventive effects, silymarin exhibits antitumor activity against human tumors (e.g., prostate and ovary) in rodents (35)

Seidlova-Wuttke et al. (34) have demonstrated the selective binding of silymarin to ER-β and no binding to ER-α, but, how mentioned above, beyond its specific ER-β agonism silymarin, exerts an anti 5-lipoxygenase (LOX) and anti-COX_2 effect (35-36).

There is strong positive correlation has been recently established between 5-LOX overexpression and the appearance of typical high-risk factors for malignant transformation of polyps, such as histological epithelial localization, increased polyp size, villous and tubulovillous adenomas, high grade of intraepithelial neoplasia, and patient age because both inflammatory enzymes are up-regulated in colon carcinogenesis and involved in silencing apoptosis (37).

Finally have been demonstrated that, without any apparent toxicity, the feeding of polyphenols from silymarin suppressed the tumor growth of the human SW480 CRC, implanted in *nu/nu* mice. The inhibitory activity was associated with strong anti-proliferative (β-catenin, c-Myc and cyclin D1 suppression) and pro-apoptotic effects. (36).

Even lignans exert similar activity in several human cancers. For example Touillaud et al. examined associations between the risk of postmenopausal invasive breast cancer and dietary intakes of four plant lignans (pinoresinol, lariciresinol, secoisolariciresinol, and matairesinol) and estimated exposure to two enterolignans (enterodiol and enterolactone), as measured with a self-administered diet history questionnaire, among postmenopausal French women who were not taking soy isoflavone supplements. They demonstrate that high dietary intakes of plant lignans and high exposure to enterolignans were associated with reduced risks of Estrogen receptor negative and Progesteron receptor positive postmenopausal breast cancer in a Western population that does not consume a diet rich in soy (56). On the other hand Kuiisten et al. studied the associations between plasma enterolignans and the risk of colorectal adenomas in a Dutch case-control study . Colorectal adenomas are considered to be precursors of colorectal cancer. Cases with at least one histologically confirmed colorectal adenoma and controls with no history of any type of adenoma were included. Plasma enterodiol and enterolactone concentrations were measured by liquid chromatography with tandem mass spectrometry and they observed a substantial reduction in colorectal adenoma risk among subjects with high plasma concentrations of enterolignans, in particular, enterodiol (42).

Lignans exert a similar activity in several human colon cancer cells and are easily metabolized and absorbed in the colon (38-41). Lignin is a documented absorbant of carcinogens in the intestinal lumen. Its degradation to enterolignans by human intestinal microbiota could delay lignan release (42).

5. Phytoestrogens in experimental CRC

Mice with the Apc gene ($Apc^{Min/+}$) mutation are highly susceptible to spontaneous intestinal adenoma formation and are therefore considered the most suitable model for experimental CRC studies (43). A recent experimental study demonstrated that in ovariectomized $Apc^{Min/+}$ female mice, the administration of a diet enriched with the phytoestrogen cumestrol induced a reduction of the number of polyps and an increased enterocyte migration as compared to control animals. Cumestrol was chosen in this study because it is a potent ER-β agonist, with a 200-fold higher affinity than estradiol (44).

Seidlova-Wuttke et al. (34) compared the effect of silymarin and estradiol in ovariectomized female mice and confirmed the selective binding of silymarin to ER-β by in vitro experiments. In another study, conducted by Khono et al., a silymarin-enriched diet significantly reduced azoxymethane-induced intestinal carcinogenesis in male mice. This effect was dose-dependent and determined a reduction of the number of cryptic adenomas, that are known to precede the development of colic adenocarcinoma (45).

The effect of a 0.02% silymarin-enriched diet on tumor development was also tested in intact $Apc^{Min/+}$ male mice, i.e. in physiological conditions. Intestinal polyp development was evaluated together with ER-β expression, as well as other biological parameters influencing tumor growth (epithelial cell proliferation, apoptosis and migration), following the addition of a combination of the ER-β-selective agonist silymarin and/or lignin to a high-fat/low-fiber diet, which has been shown to foster tumor growth. The addition of silymarin or lignin to the diet and, to an even greater extent, the specific combination of the two, significantly counteracted intestinal tumorigenesis and increased ER-β mRNA and protein levels. Cell proliferation and apoptosis were rebalanced and cell migration accelerated, restoring values similar to those observed in wild type animals. These results further support a protective effect of ER-β in CRC, suggesting that dietary supplementation with the combination of silymarin and lignin could be a potential approach to CRC prevention (46).

6. Phytoestrogens in human CRC

Several studies have reported a reduction of the CRC risk associated with the consumption of soy foods (the main source of isoflavones) and non-fermented soy foods (e.g. tofu) (47-52). The main limitations of these studies are that they all assessed only specific soy foods intake rather than total phytoestrogen intake: none of the studies was designed to evaluate phytoestrogen intake.

Another study investigated the association between colorectal cancer and lignans commonly present in Western diets. Dietary lignan intake produced a significant reduction in colorectal cancer risk (53).

Few epidemiologic studies have been conducted on the relationship between phytoestrogens and colorectal polyps formation. A case-control study on the role of lignans (54) suggests that these compounds may be protective against cardiovascular diseases and polyps (55).

Our research group aimed to assess whether a specifically ERβ-targeted dietary management of human, recurrent sporadic adenopolyposis could have any impact on ERβ-controlled apoptosis and/or proliferative behavior. As a preliminary step, we assessed whether non adenomatous (normal) mucosa of patients affected by sporadic adenopolyposis displayed an impaired apoptotic control of cell proliferation, dependent upon a reduced ER-β expression similar to that observed in the $Apc^{Min/+}$ mouse. We designed a randomized, double blind placebo-controlled study to further assess whether a proprietary blend of ER-β agonists (a mixture of silymarin, 30% of which as silibinin) could positively affect the ERβ-dependent apoptotic control of cell proliferation, in the normal mucosa of patients affected by sporadic adenopolyposis, prone to polyp recurrence, and enrolled in a surveillance program for the follow-up of polyp recurrence by screening colonoscopy every 3-5 years.

We also assessed urinary phytoestrogens to check for compliance to sylimarin supplementation, and to see whether biomarkers expression was differently related to the phytoestrogens from the regular diet as opposed to the supplements given during the study period, in the two study groups. All patients were instructed to maintain their regular diet over the study period. Urinary phytoestrogens (ng/mL), namely the active lignans: enterodiol (ED) and enterolactone (EL), were measured on spot urinary samples.

In this clinical trial, we similarly hypothesized a ERβ down-modulation, paving the way for an altered apoptotic control of cell proliferation, in the non adenomatous colon mucosa of patients affected by sporadic adenopolyposis, presenting with a similar cell proliferation rate. We found that the normal mucosa of an APC-mutated intestinal environment is prone to polyp development and recurrence because of an altered proliferation-apoptosis ratio, related to a decreased ER-β expression. Moreover, we demonstrated that ER-β dependent apoptosis can be restored by administering specific phytoestrogens supplements with a selective action on ERβ, in a similar manner to what we had previously observed in $Apc^{Min/+}$ mice. This randomized, double-blind placebo-controlled study showed that sylimarin, lignans and lignin can positively affect the ERβ-driven apoptotic control of colon epithelial turnover, by increasing ER-β expression in the normal mucosa of sporadic adenopolyposis patients prone to polyp recurrence. This is achieved via an increased ERβ content and was demonstrated in all patients, regardless of whether they were free from polyps or not, at screening colonoscopy.

7. References

[1] Van Engeland M, Derks S, Smits KM, Meijer GA, Herman JG (2011) Colorectal cancer epigenetics: complex simplicity. J Clin Oncol. 2011 29(10):1382-91

[2] Vogelstein, B. et al. (1988). N. Engl. J. Med., 319, 525–532.. (1988) Genetic alteration during colorectal-tumor development.

[3] Yang, K. et al. (1998) Dietary modulation in a mouse model for human familial adenomatous polyposis. Cancer Res., 58, 5713–5717.

[4] Barone M, Scavo MP, Papagni S, Piscitelli D, Guido R, Di Lena M, Comelli MC, Di Leo A. 2010 ERβ expression in normal, adenomatous and carcinomatous tissues of patients with familial adenomatous polyposis.Scand J Gastroenterol. Nov;45(11):1320-8. Epub

[5] Pettersson, K et al. 2000 Estrogen receptor beta acts as a dominant regulator of estrogen signaling Oncogene 19(8):4970–497). 19(8):4970–4978

[6] Menasce LP et al. (1993) Localization of the estrogen receptor locus (ESR) to chromosome 6q25.1 by FISH and a simple post-FISH banding technique.Genomics 17(1):263–265

[7] Weihua Z et al. (2000) Estrogen receptor (ER) beta, a modulator of ERalpha in the uterus. Proc Natl Acad Sci USA 97(11):5936–5941.

[8] Nelson LR et. al. Bulun SE (2001) Estrogen production and action. J Am Acad Dermatol 45(1):S116–S124

[9] Galluzzo P. et al. (2007) 07) Role of ERbeta palmitoylation in the inhibition of human colon cancer cell proliferation. Endocr Relat Cancer 14(1):153–167

[10] Di Leo, A. et al. (1994). Prognostic value of cytosolic estrogen receptors in human colorectal carcinoma and surrounding mucosa. Preliminary results. Dig. Dis. Sci., 39, 2038–2042.

[11] Fernandez, E. et al. 1998 Hormone replacement therapy and risk of colon and rectal cancer. Cancer Epidemiol. Biomarkers Prev., 7, 329–333.

[12] Notarnicola, M. et al. (2001) Oestrogen receptors and microsatellite instability in colorectal cancer patients. Cancer Lett., 168, 65–70.

[13] Woodson, K. et al. (2001 Hormone replacement therapy and colorectal adenoma recurrence among women in the Polyp Prevention Trial. Report J. Natl Cancer Inst., 93, 1799–1805.

[14] Newcomb, P.A. et al. (2002). Postmenopausal hormone replacement therapy: scientific review. JAMA, 110, 219–227.

[15] Lindberg, M.K. et al. 2003 Estrogenreceptor(ER)-betareduces ERalpharegulated gene transcription, supporting a "ying yang" relationship between ERalpha and ERbeta in mice. Mol. Endocrinol., 17, 203–208.

[16] Gustafsson, J.A. (1999) Estrogen receptor b: a new dimension in estrogen mechanism of action. J. Endocrinol., 163, 379–383.

[17] Giroux,V. et al. (2008) Estrogen receptor beta/deficiency enhances small intestinal tumorigenesis in ApcMin/þ mice. Int. J. Cancer, 123,303–311.

[18] Kronenberg F, Fugh-Berman A (2002). Complementary and alternative medicine for menopausal symptoms. A review of randomized, controlled trials. Ann Intern Med 137(7):805–813

[19] Barone M, Tanzi S, Lofano K, et al. Dietary-induced ERβ upregulation counteracts intestinal neoplasia development in intact male $Apc^{Min/+}$ mice. Carcinogenesis 2010;31:269-274

[20] Matsuda H, et al. 2001 Phytoestrogens from the roots of Polygonum cuspidatum:structure requirement of hydroxyanthraquinones for estrogenic activity. Bioorg Mol Chem Lett 11(14):1839–184

[21] Whitten PL, Naftolin F (1998) Reproductive actions of phytoestrogens.Baillieres Clin Endocrinol Metab 12(4):667–690

[22] Adlercreutz H, Fotsis T, Heikkinen R, Dwyer JT, Goldin BR, Gorbach SL, Lawson AM, Setchell KD (1981) Diet and urinary excretion of lignans in female subjects. Med Biol 59(4):259–261

[23] Adlercreutz H, Höckerstedt K, Bannwart C, Bloigu S, Ha¨ma¨la¨inen E, Fotsis T, Ollus A (1987) Effect of dietary components, including lignans and phytoestrogens, on enterohepatic circulation and liver metabolism of estrogens and on sex hormone binding globulin (SHBG). J Steroid Biochem 27(4–6):1135–1344

[24] Otieno DO, Shah NP (2007) Endogenous beta-glucosidase and beta-galactosidase activities from selected probiotic microorganisms and their role in isoflavone biotransformation in soymilk.J Appl Microbiol 103(4):910–91

[25] Kronenberg F, Fugh-Berman A (2002) Complementary and alternative medicine for menopausal symptoms. A review of randomized, controlled trials. Ann Intern Med 137(7):805–813

[26] Setchell KD (1998) Phytoestrogens: the biochemistry, physiology and implications for human health of soy isoflavones. Am J Clin Nutr 68(6 Suppl):1333s–1146s

[27] Kuiper GGJM et al Lemmen JG, Carlsson B et al (1996) Interaction of estrogenic chemicals and phytoestrogens with estrogen receptor beta. Endocrinology 139(10):4252–4263

[28] Anderson JJB, Anthony M, Messina M, Garner SC (1999) Effect of phytoestrogens on tissues. Nutr Res Rev 12(3):75–116

[29] Adlercreutz H et al (2000) Food containing phytoestrogens, and breast cancer. Biofactors 12(1–4):89–93

[30] Santti R, Makela S, Strauss L, Korkman J, Kostian ML (1998) Phytoestrogens: potential endocrine disruptors in males. Toxicol Ind Health 14(1–2):223–237

[31] Messina MJ, Loprizi CL (2001) Soy for breast cancer survivors: a critical review of the literature. J Nutr 131(11 Suppl):3095s–3108s

[32] Kurzer MS (2002) Hormonal effects of soy in premenopausal women and men. J Nutr 132(3):570s–573s

[33] Polyak,S.J. et al. (2007) Inhibition of T-cell inflammatory cytokines, hepatocyte NF-kappaB signaling, and HCVinfection by standardized Silymarin.Gastroenterology, 132, 1925–1936.

[34] Wuttke-Seidlova D, Becker T, Cristoffel V, Jarry H, Wuttke W (2003) Silymarin is a selective estrogen receptor beta (ER beta) agonist and has estrogenic effects in the metaphysis of the femur but no antiestrogenic effects in the uterus of ovariectomized rats.J Steroid Biochem Mol Biol 86(1):179–188

[35] Agarwal R, Agarwal C, Ichikawa H, et al. 2006 Anticancer potential of silymarin: from bench to bed side. Anticancer Res;26:4457-98.

[36] Velmuragan B. et al. 2010 Silibinin exerts sustained growth suppressive effect against human colon carcinoma SW480 xenograft by targeting multiple signaling molecules. Pharm Res;27:2085-2097.

[37] Wasilewiwicz M et al. 2010 Overexpression of 5-lipoxygenase in sporadic adenomas and a possible new aspect of colon carcinogenesis. Int J Colorectal Dis;25:1079-1085.

[38] Begum A et al. 2004 Dietary lignins are precursors of mammalian lignans in rats. J Nutr;134:120-12.

[39] Rajamanickam S, Agarwal R. 2008 Natural products and colon cancer: current status and future prospects. Drug Dev Res;69:460-471.

[40] Kuijsten A, et al. 2006 Plasma enterolignans are associated with lower colorectal adenoma risk. Cancer Epidemiol Biomarkers Prev;15:1132-1136.

[41] Touré A, Xueming X. 2010 Flaxseed lignans: source, biosynthesis, metabolism, antioxidant, bio-active components, and health benefits. Compreh Rev Food Sci Food Safety;9:261-269

[42] Mueller S, Simon S, Chae K, et al. 2004 Phytoestrogens and their human metabolites show distinct agonistic and antagonistic properties on Estrogen Receptor α (ERα) and ERβ in Human Cells. Toxicol Sci;80: 14-25

[43] Moser, A.R. et al. (1990) A dominant mutation that predisposes to multiple intestinal neoplasia in the mouse. Science, 247, 322–324.

[44] Javid, S.H. et al. (2005) Modulation of tumor formation and intestinal cell migration by estrogens in the ApcMin/þ mouse model of colorectal cancer. Carcinogenesis, 26, 587–595.

[45] Khono H et al. 2002 Silymarin, a naturally occurring polyphenolic antioxidant flavonoid, inhibits azoxymethane-induced colon carcinogenesis in male F344 rats. Int J Cancer 101(5):461–468

[46] Michele Barone et al. (2010). Dietary-induced ERb upregulation counteracts intestinal neoplasia development in intact male ApcMin/1 mice. Carcinogenesis vol.31 no.2 pp.269–274

[47] Grodstein F et al. 1998. Postmenopausal hormone use and risk for colorectal cancer and adenoma. Ann Intern Med 128(9):705–712

[48] Hoshiyama Y et al. (1993) A case-control study of colorectal cancer and its relation to diet, cigarettes, and alcohol consumption in Saitama Prefecture, Japan. Tohoku J Exp Med 171(2):153–165

[49] Jacobson JS et al. 1996. Hormone replacement therapy is associated with lower risk of adenomatous polyps of the large bowel: the Minnesota cancer prevention research unit case control study.Cancer Epidemiol Biomarkers Prev 5(10):779–784

[50] Peipins A, Newman B, Sandler RS (1997) Use of exogenous hormones and risk of colorectal adenomas. Cancer Epidemiol Biomarkers Prev 6(4):671–675

[51] Weyant MJ, Carothers AM, Mahmoud NN et al (2001) Reciprocal expression of ERalpha and ERb is associated with estrogen-mediated modulation of intestinal tumorigenesis. Cancer Res 6(1):2547–2551

[52] Theodoratou E. et al. (2007) Dietary flavonoids and the risk of colorectal cancer. Cancer Epidemiol Biomarkers Prev 16(4):684–693

[53] Cotterchio M et al. (2006) Dietary phytoestrogen intake is associated with reduced colorectal cancer risk. J Nutr 136(12):3046–3053

[54] Axelson M, Sjo¨vall J, Gustafsson BE, Setchell KD (1982) Origin of lignans in mammals and identification of a precursor from plants. Nature 298(5875):659–660

[55] Kuijsten A, Arts ICW, Holmann PCH, van't Veer P, Kampman E (2006) Plasma enterolignans are associated with lower colorectaladenoma risk. Cancer Epidemiol Biomarkers Prev 15(6):1132–1136

[56] Touillaud, M.S. et al. (2007) Dietary lignan intake and postmenopausal breast cancer risk by estrogen and progesterone receptor status. J. NatlCancer Inst., 99, 475–486

[57] Di Leo Alfredo et al. (2011) Human sporadic adenocarcinoma and dietary management of Estrogen Receptors (ERs)-driven biomarkers of proliferation and apoptosis (Ki-67; caspase 3, TUNEL) in the colorectal mucosa of patients undergoing screening colonoscopy. Submitted to GASTROENTEROLOGY.

13

The Therapeutic Potential of Pomegranate and Its Products for Prevention of Cancer

Arzu Akpinar-Bayizit, Tulay Ozcan and Lutfiye Yilmaz-Ersan
Uludag University
Turkey

1. Introduction

Pomegranate (*Punica granatum* L.) is considered one of the oldest known edible fruits and is the symbolic of abundance and prosperity. For thousand of years, many cultures have believed that pomegranate have beneficiary effects on health, fertility, longevity and rebirth. The recent interest for this fruit is not only because of the pleasant taste, but also due to the scientific evidences that suggest therapeutic activity such as anti-atherogenic, antiparasitic, antimicrobial, antioxidant, anticarcinogenic and antiinflammatory effects. These beneficial effects were attributed to the antioxidative properties of pomegranate phenolic compounds, tannins and anthocyanins as well as other phytochemicals. The constituents of pomegranate have been thoroughly investigated, however, clinical trials are in progress to explore the therapeutic potential of pomegranate products, particularly determining preventive efficacy of pomegranate extracts in cancer, cardiovascular diseases, inflammation, diabetes and ultraviolet radiation-induced skin damage. In order to facilitate the further investigations the information contained in this work is based upon the immense work on impact of administration of pomegranate extracts, particularly in cancer prevention such as skin, prostate, breast, and colon.

2. The constituents of pomegranate and derived products

Along with olives, figs and grapes, pomegranates are among the first plants to have been cultivated by man. Pomegranate (*Punica granatum* L.) is considered one of the oldest known edible fruit that is mentioned in the Koran, the Bible, the Jewish Torah, and the Babylonian Talmud as 'Food of Gods' that is symbolic of plentyness, fertility and prosperity (Madihassan, 1984; Aviram et al., 2000; Seeram et al., 2006). The pomegranate, a mystical and highly distinctive fruit, is the predominant member of two species comprising the *Punicaceae* family. The genus name Punica, was the Roman name for Carthage, where the best pomegranates were known to grow. Pomegranate is known by the French as grenade, the Spanish as granada (derived from the ancient city of Granada), and literally translates to seeded ("granatus") apple ("ponium") (Jurenka, 2008).

In ancient Greek mythology, the edible part of pomegranate known as the "fruit of the dead", containing considerable amounts of saccharides, polyphenol, and available in Hades for its residents. Hades benefitted amorously when six pomegranate seeds from his kingdom sealed for him the betrothal of the daughter of Zeus and Demeter. The

Babylonians regarded the seeds as an agent of resurrection, the Persians as conferring invincibility on the battle field and for ancient Chinese alchemical adepts; the bright red juice was mythopoetically regarded as a "soul concentrate", a synonym to human blood, conferring to longevity and immortality (Dahham et al., 2010). Since ancient times, the pomegranate has been used extensively in the folk medicine of many cultures as a "healing food" in order to eliminate parasites, as an antihelmintic and vermifuge, antipyretic, and to treat and cure aphtae, ulcers, diarrhea, acidosis, dysentery, hemorrhage, microbial infections, and respiratory pathologies. It also features prominently in the ceremonies, art, and mythology of the Egyptians and Greeks, and was the personal emblem of Maximilian, the Holy Roman Emperor (Longtin, 2003; Larrosa et al., 2010; Lee et al., 2010).

The pomegranate fruit is round, with leathery skin or rind, typically yellow, overlaid with light or deep pink or rich red. The edible part of the fruit, the arils can be preserved as syrup or used for juice, jam, jelly, wine, vinegar, and fruit leather production, and can be an alternative to flavoring and coloring used in beverages (Maestre et al., 2000; Fadavi et al., 2005; Ozgen et al., 2008; Al-Said et al., 2009; Mousavinejad et al., 2009; Akbarpour et al., 2010).

2.1 Chemical composition of pomegranates

The pomegranate tree can be divided into several anatomical compartments: seed, juice, peel, leaf, flower and root bark, each of which is widely used in therapeutic and food formulas, and cosmetics due in large part to the scientifically supported health benefits on arteriosclerosis, cholesterol levels and cancer prevention.The other parts are good source of tannins, dyes, and alkaloids (Khan, 2009; Viuda-Martos et al., 2010; Wang et al., 2010). The chemical composition of the pomegranate and its products depends on the cultivar, growing region, and climate, the fruit's stage of maturity, cultural practices and manufacturing systems (Badenes et al., 1998; Dumas et al., 2003; Toor et al., 2006; Raffo et al., 2006, Borochov-Neori et al., 2009; Zarei et al., 2011). Tables 1 & 2 show the chemical composition of pomegranate fruit and phytochemicals in pomegranate and its parts.

Constituent	
Moisture	72.6-86.4%
Protein	0.05-1.6%
Fat	0.01-0.9%
Mineral elements	0.36-0.73%
Fibre	3.4-5.0%
Carbohydrates	15.4-19.6%
Calcium	3.0-12.0 mg
Phosphorus	8.0-37.0 mg
Iron	0.3-1.2 mg
Sodium	3.0 mg
Magnesium	9.0 mg
Ascorbic acid (Vitamin C)	4.0-14.0 mg
Thiamine (Vitamin B_1)	0.01 mg
Riboflavine (Vitamin B_2)	0.012-0.03 mg
Niacine	0.18-0.3 mg

*Values per 100 g of edible portions

Table 1. Chemical Composition of Pomegranate* (Yilmaz, 2007).

Plant Component	Constituents
Pomegranate juice	Anthocyanins; glucose; ascorbic acid; phenolics such as ellagic acid, gallic acid, caffeic acid, catechin, epigallocatechin gallate (EGCG), quercetin, rutin; mineral elements; aminoacids
Pomegranate seed oil	Punicic acid; ellagic acid; fatty acids; sterols
Pomegranate pericarp (peel, rind)	Phenolic compounds like punicalagins, gallic acid, catechin, EGCG, quercetin, rutin, anthocyanidins, other flavonoids
Pomegranate leaves	Ellagitannins (punicalin and punicafolin); flavonols such as luteolin and apgenin
Pomegranate flower	Gallic acid, triterpenoids such as ursolic,maslinic and asiatic acid
Pomegranate roots and bark	Ellagitannins; piperidine alkaloids

Table 2. Phytochemicals of Pomegranate (Jurenka, 2008).

About 50% of the total fruit weight corresponds to the peel, which is an important source of bioactive compounds such as phenolics, flavonoids, ellagitannins (ETs), and proanthocyanidin compounds (Li et al., 2006), minerals (Mirdehghan & Rahemi, 2007), and complex polysaccharides (Jahfar et al., 2003). Significant variations in organic acids, phenolic compounds, sugars, water-soluble vitamins, and minerals of pomegranates have been reported by various researchers (Davidson et al., 2009; Tezcan et al., 2009).

The edible part of the pomegranate fruit consists of 40% arils and 10% seeds. The arils are comprised of approximately 80% juice and 20% seed. The juice of arils contain 85% water, 10% total sugars (glucose, sucrose, and fructose) (Melgarejo & Artes, 2000), and 1.5% pectin, organic acids (citric, malic, tartaric, succinic, fumaric, ascorbic acid) (Tezcan et al., 2009), fatty acids (i.e. conjugated linoleic acid, linoleic acid, punicic acid and eleostearic acid) (Fadavi et al., 2006) and amino acids (i.e. proline, valin, and methionine) (Seppi & Franciosi, 1980), and bioactive compounds (phenolics and flavonoids) (Dahham et al., 2010). Pomegranate fruit is a rich source of two types of polyphenolic compounds: anthocyanins and hydrolyzable tannins, which account for 92% of the antioxidant activity of the whole fruit (Gil et al., 2000). The soluble polyphenol content in pomegranate juice varies between 0.2 and 1.0% depending on variety (Narr Ben et al., 1996). The seeds are a rich source of lipids; of which comprised to 12% to 20% of total seed weight and characterized by a high content of polyunsaturated (*n*-3) fatty acids such as linolenic, linoleic, and other lipids such as punicic acid, oleic acid, stearic acid, and palmitic acid (Ozgul-Yucel, 2005). The seeds also contain protein, crude fibers, vitamins, minerals, pectin, sugars, polyphenols, isoflavones (mainly genistein), the phytoestrogen coumestrol, and the sex steroid, estrone (Singh et al., 1990; Singh & Sethi, 2003; El-Nemr et al., 2006; Syed et al., 2007).

Pomegranate flowers (*gulnar*) contain a variety of secondary metabolites: i) polyphenols, including gallic acid (Huang et al., 2005b), ellagic acid and ethyl brevifolin-carboxylate (Wang et al., 2006), and ii) triterpene acids consisting of oleanolic, ursolic (Huang et al., 2005a), maslinic and asiatic (Batta & Rangaswami, 1973). In folk medicine the decoction of flowers is used to stop bleeding and purging (Sivarajan & Balachandran, 1994; Jafri et al.,

2000). The polyphenols in pomegranate flowers have strong antioxidant activity (Oswa et al., 1987); ellagic acid had a marked inhibitory effect on the occurrence and development of tumours in mice (Boukharta et al., 1992), triterpenes show antimutagenic and anticarcinogenic effects (Ovesná et al., 2004); and oleanolic acid significantly enhanced acute glucose-stimulated insulin secretion at basal and stimulatory glucose concentrations in pancreatic b-cell , and such effects may contribute to the antidiabetic properties (Teodoro et al., 2008).

Pomegranate fruit extracts/constituents possesses immense biological activities such as anticarcinogenic (Whitley et al., 2003; Afaq et al., 2005), antibacterial (Akiyama et al., 2001; Prashanth et al., 2001; Duman et al., 2009), antidiarrhoeal (Das et al., 1999), antifungal (Dutta et al., 1998), antiulcer (Gharzouli et al., 1999), antioxidant activity and free radical scavenging capability (Schubert et al., 1999; Aviram et al., 2000; Festa et al., 2001), strengthening of the immune system (Lee et al., 2008), prevention of heart disease (Johanningsmeier & Harris, 2011) and liver fibrosis (Thresiamma & Kuttan, 1996), and inhibition of lipid peroxidation even at lower concentrations than vitamin E (Rosenblat et al., 2003). All these therapeutical activities are related to the presence of diverse *'phenolic compounds'*, including gallic acid, protocatechinunic acid, chlorogenic acid, caffeic acid, ferulic acid, coumaric acid, and catechin and hydrolysable tannins (such as punicalin, pedunculagin, punicalagin, corilagin, casuarinin, punicacortein, granatin and ellagic acid), and anthocyanins (delphinidin, cyanidin and pelargonidin 3-glucosides and 3,5-diglucosides) (Amakura et al., 2000; Noda et al., 2002; Poyrazoglu et al., 2002; Kulkarni & Aradya, 2005; Viuda-Martos et al., 2010).

The bright colour of pomegranate flowers and arils is due to anthocyanins (Afaq et al., 2005); however, only one anthocyanin compound (i.e. pelargonidin-3,5-diglucoside) has yet been identified in pomegranate flowers using HPLC (Miguel et al., 2009), whereas in pomegranate juice, principally cyanidin-3-*O*-glucoside, cyanidin-3,5-di-*O*-glucoside, delphinidin-3-*O*-glucoside, delphinidin-3,5-di-*O*glucoside, pelargonidin-3-*O*-glucoside, and pelargonidin-3,5-di- *O*-glucoside, have been reported (Lansky & Newman 2007; Jaiswal et al., 2010).

Tannins, high-molecular-weight plant polyphenols, are divided into 3 chemically and biologically distinct groups: condensed tannins or proanthocyanidins, hydrolyzable tannins or elagitannins (ETs), and gallotannins (GTs) (Seeram et al., 2005). Pomegranate leaves contain unique tannins such as punicalin and punicafolin, and also have glycosides of apigenin, a flavone with progestinic (Zand et al., 2000) and anxiolytic (Paladini et al., 1999) properties. Pomegranate peel are rich in hydrolyzable tannins, mainly punicalin, pedunculagin, and punicalagin (Seeram et al., 2006), which differ from proanthocyanidins in their chemical structures. In addition to ETs, pomegranate peel contains hydroxybenzoic acids such as gallagic, ergot alkaloid (EA), and EA glycosides (Amakura et al., 2000); anthocyanidins are principally cyanidin, pelargonidin, and delphinidin (Noda et al., 2002) and flavonoids such as kaempferol, luteolin, and quercetin (Van Elswijk et al., 2004).

Al-Maiman & Ahmad (2002) showed the amounts of potassium, calcium and sodium were highest in both juice and seeds followed by magnesium, phosphorous, zinc, iron and copper. The authors stated that pomegranate can be a good source of nutrients and variation could originate from the pomegranate cultivar, and agro-climatic. Akpinar-Bayizit (2010) reported that although processing steps include clarification and filtration, the pomegranate juices in Turkish market were a good source for minerals such as potassium (1283.30 mg/L), calcium (107.53 mg/L), sodium (96.02 mg/L), phosphorus (76.54 mg/L) and magnesium (67.22 mg/L). The high mineral content of pomegranate juices could contribute to the daily intake of these constituents in the human diet.

2.2 Pomegranate fruit derived products

Pomegranate can be consumed as fresh, fruit juice, fermented fruit juice, dried aril, frozen aril, minimally-processed aril, canned aril, jam, jelly, wine, vinegar, paste, fruit leather and in flavoring products.

Pomegranate arils can either be consumed fresh or procesed (dried, frozen, canned and minimally-processed). The conventional utilization of wild pomegranate fruit lies in the drying seeds along with pulp (arils), which constitute a traditional product called as '*Anardana*' (Pruthi & Saxena, 1984). The dehydrated arils are acidic (7.8–15.4%), help in improving mouth-feel and digestion, and are widely used as acidulent in culinary preparations. The dried anardana contains acid (5.8-15.4%), total sugars (9.3-17.5%) and crude fiber as compared to fresh fruit. To obtain frozen arils the arils are put into polyethylene bags either with syrup of 15° Brix or coated with solid sugar and frozen in a chest freezer. For canned arils, used generally as an appartiser, the arils were put into metal tins with syrup of 15° Brix and sterilised for 10 minutes. In the production of minimally-processed pomegranate aril pomegranates are chilled to 0°C, selected, washed and dried with a current of air at room temperature. They are conditioned in polyethylene bags that were heat-sealed and conserved in a chamber at 0°C for 10-15 days. These arils are used as a garnish for desserts and salad (Al-Maiman & Ahmad, 2002).

Pomegranate juice can be extracted by using a spiral-type screw press without crushing the seeds. The juice is clarified by heating in a flash pasteurizer at 79-82°C cooling, settled for 24 hours and filtered. The clear juice can be preserved by heat treatment or by using chemicals. The use of sulphur dioxide is banned for pomegranate due to loss of colour by bleaching action of SO_2. Pomegranate juice represents one of the foods recently promoted for its health benefits since a glass of pomegranate juice contains about 40% of the Recommended Daily Allowance (RDA) of Vitamin C (Singh & Singh, 2004).

Pomegrenate syrup of 60° Brix with an added acidity of 1.5% as citric acid has a bright purplish-red colour and a delightful taste and flavour. It was preserved by pasteurization. Preparation of jelly on a small-scale from sweet-sour pomegranates is described by Adsule et al. (1992) and Singh & Singh (2004). When making the jellies, approximately 50% of the total anthocyanins present in the juice of are lost. During storage at 5°C, certain colour differences were observed, which indicates that the pH was not the only parameter responsible for this characteristic.

For preparation of wine, the whole furits are pressed without crushing or juice may be extracted from pomegranate grains, which gives a yield of 76 to 85% (Adsule & Patil, 1995). Sugar is added to the juice to obtain 22-23° Brix. The juice is fermented as in the same manner of red grape wine. The wine is flash pasteurized at 60°C and bottled hot (Singh & Singh, 2004).

Pomegranate seed is a residue obtained from pomegranate juice production, ranging between 40 and 100 g/kg of fruit weight (Fadavi et al., 2006; Lansky & Newman, 2007). The seeds are rich source of lipids, and the fatty acid component of pomegranate seed oil comprises over 95% of the oil, of which 99% is triacylglycerols. Minor components of the oil include vitamin E, sterols, steroids, and a key component of mammalian myelin sheaths, cerebroside (Tsuyuki et al., 1981).

'*Pekmez*', a concentrated and shelf-life extended Turkish product, is generally produced from fruits containing high amounts of sugar such as grape, mulberry, carnob, apple, pomegranate, plum and apricot (Alparslan & Hayta, 2002; Demirozu et al., 2002). The first steps in pomegranate pekmez production is washing, granulating and crushing of the pomegranates. The pomegranate juice, obtained by pressing the crushed pomegranates by a pneumatical or mechanical press, is boiled with a calcareous substance called '*pekmez earth*', white soil containing 70.40% $CaCO_3$ or technical $CaCO_3$, for deacidification and neutralization. The juice is clarified and concentrated usually in open vessels, and rarely under vacuum at 565 mm Hg and 66°C, up to 65–68° Brix; this product is called '*liquid pekmez*'. The liquid pekmez can be consumed either as liquid or solidified at 6°C for 2-3 days via addition of hydrocolloids, to produce '*solid pekmez*', which has a pasty form that is easily spread on a slice of bread.

The '*pomegranate leather (pestil)*' is another Turkish pomegranate derived product that can be stored for a long time without deterioration. Pomegranates are washed, granulated, crushed, pressed and filtered to separate the seeds and skin. Pekmez earth is added to neutralize and clarify the fresh pomegranate juice. Clarified juice is filtered and is mixed with the wheat starch. Nuts such as walnut or hazelnut can be added in small pieces if desired. The juice and starch mixture is concentrated upto 40° Brix by boiling and continuous stirring. The puree is spread on cloths of 0.5–2.00 mm thickness and sun-dried until a mild, tasty, light and chewable leathery product is obtained. The dried pestil is folded, cut and stored in dry conditions (Maskan et al., 2002).

The '*pomegranate molasses (sour pomegranate pekmez, nar eksisi, pomegranate sauce)*', a traditional seasoning commonly used in salads and many dishes to improve the taste and aroma characteristics in Turkey, is a concentrated product produced simply by boiling, without the addition of further sugar or other additives (Poyrazoglu et al., 2002; Incedayi et al., 2010). Pomegranate molasses is a highly nutritive product since it is more concentrate and the have a high mineral content. Traditional methods are still being used to produce pomegranate molasses, of which requires cleaning, crushing, extraction, filtration, and evaporation (upto 35-65° Brix) in an open vessel or under vacuum. Clarification is not recommended in pomegranate molasses since customers prefer bitterness and sourness that comes from phenolic substances and acidity (Vardin & Abbasoglu, 2004; Kaya & Sozer, 2005).

3. The biochemistry and pharmokinetics of pomegranate

There is little knowledge about the absorption, bioavailability, biodistribution, and metabolism of the bioactive compounds present in pomegranate and in other fruits, although they probably have a similar pathway (Petti & Scully, 2009). The bioavailability of polyphenols varies according to the structure, glycosylation and solubility of the molecules which defined their extractability (Lecerf, 2006; Ozcan et al., 2011). In view of limited human studies, it appears that the bioavailability determinations of pomegranate polyphenols is affected by individual variability, differential processing of pomegranate juice, and the analytical techniques used, which need to be sensitive enough to detect low postprandial concentrations of these metabolites (Basu & Penugonda, 2009). An *in vitro* study of pomegranate juice showed that phenolic compounds are available during the digestion in a quite high amount (29%), however, due to pH, anthocyanins are in large transformed into non-red forms and/or degraded and similar results are obtained for vitamin C (Pérez-Vicente et al., 2002).

The recent interest in pomegranate products is due to the fruit's beneficial role in the prevention of prostate cancer, the prevention of the oxidation of both low density lipoprotein (LDL), high density lipoprotein (HDL), and cholesterol, reductions in blood pressure, arthritis, anemia, diarrhea, inflammation, gynecological diseases, atherosclerosis development, the stimulation of T-cell functions and production of cytokines, Alzheimer's disease, and improvoment of sperm quality (Figure 1). These beneficial effects were attributed to the wide range of phytochemicals found in pomegranate. These phytochemicals are predominantly phenolic compounds as well as to those of sugar-containing polyphenolic tannins and anthocyanins, including primarily hydrolysable ellagitannins, anthocyanins and other polyphenols. Gil et al. (2000) have demonstrated that one of the ellagitannins, punicalagins, is responsible for over 50% of the antioxidant activity of the pomegranate juice. The same reserachers indicated that as being water-soluble, commercial pomegranate juice obtained by pressing the fruit contain significant amounts of punicalagins, depending on the cultivar. Seeram et al. (2005) proposed punicalagin as a proper chemical marker for the authentication, quality control and standardization of pomegranate products.

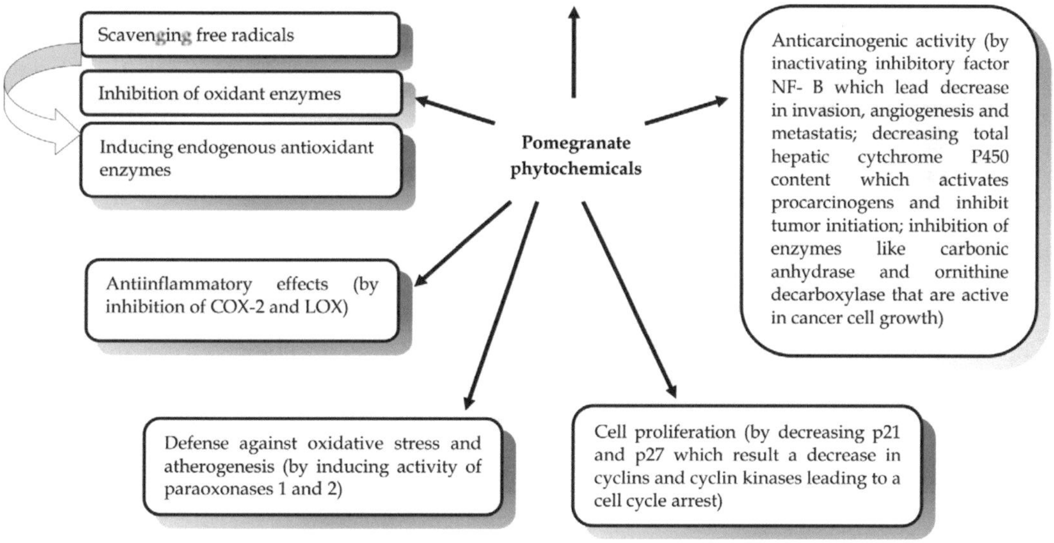

Fig. 1. Bioactive effects of pomegranate constituents.

4. The health benefits of pomegranate derived products

In recent years, the focus is on understanding the mechanisms of nutraceutic and health promoting potentials of the foods nutrients. Cancer, in terms of morbidity and mortality, is a major health issue, eventhough there are advances in early detection and in treatment options. Cancer is an aggressive disease, which if not detected at an early stage can metastasize to other organs of the body. *Carcinogenesis* (cancer development) is a multistage process, influenced by mainly age, dietary habits and hormonal balance. There are three stages of cancer: *initiation*, *promotion* and *progression* (Surh, 2003). The hypothesis of alternative methods to prevent cancer seems to be practical and promising strategy to reduce cancer incidinces since treatment options for metastasized cancers remain inadequate. Chemoprevention focuses on cancer prevention by the administration of one or more synthetic or naturally occurring agents to suppress reverse or prolong the process of carcinogenesis (Mukhtar & Ahmad, 1999).

It is clear that bioactive compounds present in daily diet, mainly in fruits and vegetables, have prevention potential in cancer by inhibiting carcinogenesis through cell-defensive and cell-death mechanism regulation. These chemopreventive effects may be attributed to a complex effect of various phenolic substances of antioxidant capacity (Khan et al., 2008).

Pomegranate is rich in anthocyanins, 3-glucosides, 3,5-diglucosides of delphinidin, cyanidin and pelargonidin, ellagitannins and other phenolic compounds, which are known bioactive compounds with antioxidant and antitumoral activity (Ozgen et al., 2008; Chaturvedula et al., 2011; Zhang et al., 2011). Major hydrolysable tannins in pomegranates are gallotannins, ellagic acid tannins and gallagyl tannins, generally termed as *punicalagins*, and they have been shown to inhibit the proliferation of human cancer cells and modulate inflammatory subcellular signaling pathways due to a high antioxidant activity (Seeram et al., 2005).

There are several studies conducted to evaluate the efficacy of pomegranate and its products as an anti-proliferative, anti-invasive, and pro-apoptotic agent in various cancer cell lines such as skin, prostate, breast, column, and blood cancer. Adams et al. (2006) revealed that pomegranate juice suppresses cancer activity through the combined antioxidant and anti-inflammatory effects by modulating inflammatory cell signaling in colon cancer cells. Malik et al. (2005) suggested that pomegranate juice may have cancer chemopreventive as well as cancer-chemotherapeutic effects against prostate cancer in humans. Pomegranate fruit extract possesses remarkable antitumor-promoting effects in mouse skin.

Researchers found that daily consumption of pomegranate juice may improve stress-induced myocardial ischemia in patients who have coronary heart disease (CHD) and the pomegranate juice not only prevented hardening of the arteries by reducing blood vessel damage, but also reversed the progression of CHD (Sumner et al., 2005). Hartman et al. (2006) reported that pomegranate juice had beneficial effect on animal model of Alzheimer's disease since polyphenols are responsible for neural protection.

4.1 Antioxidant activity

Over the past few years, consumer demand-based research on functional foods gave a basis for traditional using of pomegranate, which lead to an increase in number of scientific papers concerning pomegranate and its products with health-improving effects (Mehta & Lansky, 2004; Rettig et al., 2008; Turk et al., 2008; Alam et al., 2010; Dai et al., 2010; Jadeja et al., 2010; Park et al., 2010). The reports have focused on *in vitro, ex vivo,* and *in vivo* antioxidant actions, of pomegranate and its products, which are attributed to the chemical composition. However, many other cellular processes are likely to be involved along with bioactive compounds to enhance reactive oxygen species (ROS) elimination and inhibit ROS generation. Oxidative stress, refers to a cell state characterized by excessive production of ROS, has been given growing attention, as the generation of ROS, thus improved oxidative stress, can induce DNA damage and trigger redox-dependent transcription factors which lead to cancer, inflammatory, cardiovascular and neurodegenerative diseases, and aging (Evans et al., 2004; Franco et al., 2008; Ziech et al., 2010; Sedelnikova et al., 2010; Kryston et al., 2011; Martin et al., 2011). Nishikawa (2008) mentioned that sublethal levels of ROS can induce additional changes in DNA of tumor cells to make those cells malignant, stimulate the proliferation of cancer cells, and activate the expression of various molecules, some of which assist cancer cells to form metastatic colonies.

The effect of pomegranate cultivars on antioxidant activity was target of study by some authors (Borochov-Neori et al., 2009; Mousavinejad et al., 2009; Pande & Akoh, 2009; Sadeghi et al. 2009). All authors reported considerable variation in some of the chemical composition profile (lipids, phenols, organic acids, vitamins, sugars) and antioxidant properties of pomegranate samples, independent on the antioxidant method performed. The antioxidant activity of pomegranate and its products was almost determined via *in vitro* trials and several methods could be used for its determination, however, pomegranate showed an antioxidant activity, independent on the antioxidant test assayed and generally with significant linear correlation between phenolic content and antioxidant capacity (Elfalleh et al., 2009). Seeram et al. (2005) stated that the antioxidant level in pomegranate juice was higher than found in other fruit juices, such as blueberry, cranberry, and orange. Schubert et al. (1999) and Gil et al. (2000) demonstrated that pomegranate juice and seed extracts have 2-3 times the *in vitro* antioxidant capacity of either red wine or green tea.

Rosenblat et al. (2006) have shown that pomegranate extracts scavenge free radicals, and decrease macrophage oxidative stress and lipid peroxidation in animals. Studies in rats and mice confirmed the antioxidant properties of a pomegranate by-product extract made from whole fruit minus the juice, showing a 19% reduction in oxidative stress in mouse peritoneal macrophages (MPMs), a 42% decrease in cellular lipid peroxide content, and a 53% increase in reduced glutathione levels. A study in rats with chemically induced liver damage demonstrated that pretreatment with a methanolic extract of pomegranate peel enhanced or maintained the free-radical scavenging activity of the hepatic enzymes such as catalase, peroxidase, and superoxide dismutase to values comparable with control values, whereas resulted in 54% reduction of lipid peroxidation values compared to controls (Chidambara Murthy et al., 2002).

Using the FRAP (ferric reducing/antioxidant power) assay, Guo et al. (2008) found that consumption of 250 mL pomegranate pulp juice daily for four weeks by healthy elderly subjects resulted in increased plasma antioxidant capacity, while subjects consuming apple juice experienced no significant increase. In addition, subjects consuming the pomegranate pulp juice exhibited significantly decreased plasma carbonyl content, a biomarker for oxidant/antioxidant barrier impairment in various inflammatory diseases.

Several works have demonstrated that peel, seeds, arils have antioxidant activity, nevertheless, after ingestion those antioxidant compounds, mainly tannin components, are metabolized by gut bacteria into urolithins, which readily enter systemic circulation. Bialonska et al. (2009a) studied the antioxidant activities of seven urolithins derivatives in a cell-based assay in order to reflect bioavailability of the test compound to the cells, and the antioxidant activity is evaluated in the cellular environment and in terms of inhibition of intracellular generation of reactive oxygen species. They found that urolithins exhibited a significant antioxidant activity correlated with the number of hydroxyl groups as well as lipophilicity of the molecules.

4.2 Anticarcinogenic/antitumoral activity

The critical success factor in cancer chemoprevention is the capacity of the agent to selectively inhibit proliferation and/or induce apoptosis in malignant cells, preserving normal cells. Pomegranate, consumed as whole fruit, juice, or any form of derivates, possess anti-proliferative, pro-apoptotic, and/or anti-angiogenic effects superior to those observed with their isolated active compounds, suggesting therapeutic strategies that may depart from preference for pure single agents. There are several publications on the anticarcinogenic effects of pomegranate (Ahmed et al., 2005; Jeune et al., 2005; Malik et al., 2005; Syed et al., 2007; Lansky & Newman, 2007; Hajimahmoodi et al., 2008; Jurenka, 2008, Sartippour et al. 2008; Adams et al., 2010; Adhami et al., 2010; Faria & Calhau, 2010,2011; Miguel et al., 2010). Therefore, due to the vast explosion of interest in pomegranate as a functional food and therapeutic source the present work is launched to make a review that highlights anticarcinogenic activity of pomegranate and its products of recently published works.

4.2.1 Prevention of skin cancer

There is an urgent need to develop mechanism-based approaches for the prevention/therapy of lethal skin cancer (non-melanoma). Skin is the organ most accessible to sunlight, and directly suffers from the deleterious effects of ultraviolet (UV)1 radiation, that is known to accelerate aging changes, causing fine and coarse wrinkling, rough skin texture, dryness, telangiectasia and dyspigmentation, resulting in skin cell DNA damage (Afaq, 2011). The increase in incidinces of skin cancer due to constant exposure of skin to environmental carcinogens, such as chemical agents and ultraviolet radiation, provides a strong basis for chemoprevention (Gupta & Mukhtar, 2002). There is a considerable attention on the use of naturally occurring botanicals for their potential preventive effect against UV-mediated damages referred to as *photochemopreventive* effects (Afaq et al., 2005). In general, skin carcinogenesis, being a stepwise process of all three distinct stages, is an effective model for cancer chemoprevention (Richmond & Viner, 2003).

Hora et al. (2003) investigated pomegranate seed oil (PSO) stated that PSO appears to be a natural product with potential as a topical chemopreventive agent against skin cancer, through inhibition of PG biosynthesis and ornithine decarboxylase. PSO treatment did not delay the appearance of tumors, but significantly decreased the rate of tumor development, skin tumor multiplicity, and ornithine decarboxylase activity during 20 weeks of promotion. They stated that PSO, being rich in punicic acid, has inhibitory effect on PG biosynthesis, as well as inhibiting upstream eicosanoid enzyme, phospholipase A2.

Murthy et al. (2004) studied the wound healing activity of phenol-rich methanolic extract of dried pomegranate peel on the skin of Wistar rats. Following the application of the extract, formulated as a water-soluble gel, the animals treated with 5% gel showed complete healing after 10 days, whereas in rats treated with 2.5% gel, healing was observed on day 12, in contrast to the positive control animals receiving the blank gel, which took 16–18 days for complete healing. The animals treated with 2.5% gel showed moderate healing (55.8% and 40.8% healing compared with negative and positive controls, respectively), whereas the group treated with 5.0% gel showed good healing (59.5% and 44.5% healing compared with negative and positive controls, respectively). Histopathological studies supported the wound healing increased on application of the gels.

Afaq et al. (2005) showed that pretreatment of mouse skin with pomegranate fruit extract modulated the activation of mitogen-activated protein kinase (MAPKs) and nuclear factor kappa B (NF-κB), in the 12-*O*-tetradecanoylphorbol 13-acetate (TPA)-induced or ultra violet-B induced skin carcinogenesis model. Aslam et al. (2006) assessed the cosmeceutical value of pomegranate where aqueous fraction of the peel was shown to stimulate type I procollagen synthesis and inhibit MMP-1 production by human dermal fibroblasts. Syed et al. (2006) reported the remarkable photochemopreventive effects of pomegranate fruit extract (PFE) against UVA using normal human epidermal keratinocytes (NHEK) as a test system. PFE, extracted edible part of fruit with acetone, treatment was shown to inhibit UVA-induced phosphorylation of STAT3, ERK1/2 and AKT1 in human epidermal cells. In addition, the inhibitory effect of PFE on UVA-mediated phosphorylation of mTOR and p70S6K may have a regulatory effect on the rate of protein synthesis and activation of tumor cell proliferation.

In a study pretreatment of EpiDerm with pomegranate juice, oil or by-product resulted in marked inhibition in the number of cyclobutane primidine dimers (CPDs) and 8-hydroxy-2-deoxyguanosine (8-OHdG) positive cells, ultimately, showing a protective effect of against UVB-mediated DNA damage. UVB irradiation results in the induction in metalloproteinases (MMPs) which degrade extracellular matrix proteins, and eventually, cause skin wrinkling. It was shown that all three components of pomegranate were able to inhibit UVB-induced expressions of MMPs as well as MMP-2 and MMP-9 activity in the EpiDerm (Zaid et al., 2007). Cell culture and animal studies have also supported that intake of pomegranate is associated with decreased skin cancer risk (Pacheco-Palencia et al., 2008). Afaq et al. (2009) found that pretreatment of human reconstituted skin (EpiDermTM FT-200) with pomegranate-derived products inhibited UVB-induced CPDs and 8-OHdG as well as protein oxidation and proliferating cell nuclear antigen (PCNA) protein expression. In addition they reported an inhibition of UVB-induced metalloproteinases (collagenase, gelatinase, stromelysin, marilysin, elastase and tropoelastin).

George et al. (2011) examined the chemopreventive efficacy of pomegranate fruit extract (PFE) and diallyl sulfide (DAS), alone and in combination, using 2-stage mouse skin tumorigenesis model. PFE alone delayed onset and tumor incidence by 55%, while in PFE+DAS combination at low doses synergistically decreased tumor incidence more potentially (84%). In addition, regression in tumor volume was seen with continuous combinatorial treatment ($p < 0.01$). Mechanistic studies revealed that this inhibition was associated with decreased expression of phosphorylated ERK1/2, JNK1 and activated NF-κB/p65, IKKα, IκBα phosphorylation and degradation in skin tissue/tumor. Histological and cell death analysis also confirmed that combined PFE and DAS inhibit cellular proliferation and markedly induce apoptosis than the single agents.

4.2.2 Prevention of prostate cancer

Prostate cancer is the second-leading cause of cancer-related deaths in men in the World. *In vitro* studies stated several pomegranate products inhibit prostate cancer cell growth, induce apoptosis of several prostate cancer cell lines, suppress invasive potential of PC-3 cells, and decrease proliferation of DU-145 prostate cancer cells (Lansky et al., 2005a,b; Pantuck et al., 2006). Albrecht et al. (2004) showed that pomegranate seed oil (PSO) as well as polyphenols present in the pericarp and fermented juice suppress proliferation and invasion of several human prostate cancer cells, LNCaP, PC-3 and DU-145 across the matrigel matrix. Supra-additive, complementary and synergistic effects were proven in all models. Lansky et al (2005b) found equally combined amounts of pomegranate fermented juice, pomegranate pulp juice, cold-pressed pomegranate seed oil extracts resulted in a 99% suppression of DU-145 prostate cancer cell invasion across a matrigel matrix. Ellagic acid, caffeic acid, luteolin and punicic acid, important components of pomegranate significantly inhibited *in vitro* invasion of human PC-3 prostate cancer cells when employed individually.

Malik et al. (2005) showed that pomegranate fruit extract exhibited significant anti-proliferative and pro-apoptotic activity against highly aggressive human PC-3 cells. The cell growth inhibition was dose-dependent, and alterations were in the regulatory molecules responsible in the G1 phase of the cell cycle. Another molecular mechanism through which pomegranate fruit extract is capable of inducing apoptosis in prostate cancer cells may be up-regulation of Bax and down-modulation of Bcl-2. PFE intake was observed to significantly slow the progression of tumor growth in athymic nude mice implanted with androgen-responsive CWR22R-1 cells. Importantly, this tumor growth inhibition followed a significant decrease in the serum levels of PSA.

Pantuck et al. (2006) studied the effects of pomegranate juice consumption on prostate-specific antigen (PSA) progression in men with a rising PSA following primary therapy. A phase II, Simon two-stage clinical trial for eligible men patients with rising PSA after surgery or radiotherapy was conducted. The eligible patients had previous surgery or radiation therapy for prostate cancer, Gleason score ≤7, rising PSA value of 0.2-5.0 ng/mL, no prior hormonal therapy, and no evidence of metastases. Patients were treated with 8 ounces of pomegranate juice daily until disease progression. Mean PSA doubling time significantly increased with treatment from a mean of 15 months at baseline to 54 months posttreatment. *In vitro* assays comparing pretreatment and posttreatment patient serum on the growth of LNCaP showed a 12% decrease in cell proliferation and a 17% increase in apoptosis, a 23% increase in serum nitric oxide, and significant reductions in oxidative state and sensitivity to oxidation of serum lipids, after versus before pomegranate juice consumption.

Prostate cancer is dependent on circulating testosterone in its early stages and is treatable with surgery, radiation therapy, stereotactic radiosurgery, and proton therapy. Both androgen and androgen receptor (AR) are recognized risk factors in the development of prostate cancer (Heinlein & Chang, 2004). Reduction of circulating levels of androgens and suppression of AR are crucial for the treatment of prostate cancer as an elevated level of androgen causes enhancement of prostate cancer (Attard et al., 2006). Pomegranate extracts has been shown to inhibit both androgen-dependent and androgen-independent prostate cancer cell growth. Since androgen and AR play central roles throughout prostate cancer development Hong et al. (2008) examined the effects of pomegranate polyphenols, ellagitannin-rich extract and whole juice extract on the expression of genes for key androgen-synthesizing enzymes [HSD3B2 (3β-hydroxysteroid dehydrogenase type 2), AKR1C3 (aldo-keto reductase family 1 member C3) and SRD5A1 (steroid 5α reductase type 1)] and AR in LNCaP, LNCaP–AR and DU-145 human prostate cancer cells. Pomegranate polyphenols inhibited gene expression and AR most consistently in the LNCaP–AR cell line. Therefore, inhibition by pomegranate polyphenols of gene expression involved in androgen-synthesizing enzymes and the AR may be of particular importance in androgen-independent prostate cancer cells and the subset of human prostate cancers where AR is up-regulated.

Since the anticarcinogenic activity of ellagic acid, the main polyphenol in the pomegranate, has been shown on several cancer types Malik et al. (2011) evaluated the effect of ellagic acid treatment on the cell viability of human prostate cancer cells. They observed that ellagic acid (10-100 mol/L) treatment (48 h) of human prostate carcinoma PC3 cells resulted in a dose dependent inhibition of cell growth/cell viability. Ellagic acid caused cell growth inhibition which was accompanied by induction of apoptosis, as assessed by the cleavage of poly (ADP-ribose) polymerase (PARP) and morphological changes. Further, ellagic acid treatment was also found to result in significant activation of caspases, as shown by the dose dependent decrease in the protein expression of procaspase-3, -6, -8 and -9. This ellagic acid-mediated induction of apoptosis was significantly (80-90%) inhibited by the caspase inhibitor N-benzyloxycarbonyl-Val-Ala-Asp (OMe) fluoromethylketone (Z-VAD-FMK).

In a study, Koyama et al. (2010) investigated the relationship between pomegranate-induced apoptosis in human prostate cancer cells and the insuline-like growth factor (IGF)/IGF binding protein (IGFBP) system, as the IGF axis is critical for the regulation of apoptosis in many human cancer cell lines and IGFBPs in serum are responsible for regulation of IGF action, inhibition of cell proliferation and enhancement of apoptosis in many cell types, including prostate (Rajah et al., 1997) and breast (Gucev et al., 1996; Kim et al., 2004) cancers. They concluded that there are novel interactions between the IGF system and pomegranate-induced apoptosis, and pomegranate products modulate the tumor production and responsiveness to IGFs and the IGFBPs. Treatment of LAPC-4 prostate cancer cells with 10 μg/mL pomegranate extract, standardized to ellagitannin content (37% punicalagins by HPLC), resulted in inhibition of cell proliferation and induction of apoptosis. Co-treatment with pomegranate extract and IGFBP-3 revealed synergistic stimulation of apoptosis and additional inhibition of cell growth. The researchers also investigated the relationship between IGF-1 and pomegranate-induced apoptosis in 22RV-1 prostate cancer cells. Co-treatment with 100 ng/mL IGF-1 completely blocked apoptosis induction by pomegranate extract. In contrast, IGF-I failed to inhibit pomegranate-induced apoptosis in R^- cells, suggesting the importance of IGF-IR. POMx-treatment decreased Igf1 mRNA expression in a dose-dependent manner indicating that its actions also involve tumor-specific suppression of IGF-1.

4.2.3 Prevention of breast cancer

Along with enthusiastic efforts in early diagnosis, aggressive surgical treatment and application of additional non-operative modalities, the prognosis of breast cancer is stil chaotic. Pomegranate has been the target of several work in laboratories and cancer centres and known to have inhibition properties against diverse types of cancers. Recent review articles reported the laboratory and clinical evidence of cancer chemoprevention or treatment of pomegranate fruit, pomegranate juice, pomegranate seed and seed oil on prostate, breast, skin, colon, lung, oral and leukaemia cancers, through antioxidant, antiproliferation, antiangiogenesis and antiinflammatory mechanisms of action (Adhami et al., 2009,2010; Amin et al., 2009; Faria & Calhau, 2011; Johanningsmeier & Harris, 2011). They all reported that extracts of pomegranate or the juice are generally more active than individual or purified compounds.

The antiangiogenic potential of pomegranate was evaluated by Toi et al. (2003) where VEGF, interleukin-4 and migration inhibitory factor (MIF) were measured in the conditioned media of estrogen sensitive MCF-7, estrogen resistant MDA-MB-231 human breast cancer cells and MCF-10A immortalized human breast epithelial cells, grown in the presence or absence of pomegranate seed oil or fermented juice polyphenols. Polyphenols from fermented pomegranate juice, pericarp and oil were shown to inhibit endogenous active estrogen biosynthesis with subsequent inhibition of aromatase activity. VEGF was strongly downregulated in MCF-10A and MCF-7 cells, and MIF upregulated in MDAMB-231 cells, representing a marked potential for downregulation of angiogenesis by pomegranate fractions. Mehta & Lansky (2004) examined the effects of pomegranate fermented juice, cold pressed pomegranate seed oil extract and an HPLC-isolated peak (from the fruit extract-peak B), using the mouse mammary organ culture, an animal model of breast cancer having >75% accuracy to predict *in vivo* carcinogenesis. They showed that the purified chromatographic peak of pomegranate fermented juice polyphenols and pomegranate seed oil possesses greater chemopreventive potential than that previously reported by Kim et al. (2002). While fermented juice polyphenols effected a 42% reduction in the number of DMBA-induced cancerous lesions compared with control, purified compound, peak B, and pomegranate seed oil each effected an 87% reduction. Peak B is believed to be a phenolic compound with potent chemopreventative properties. Combination treatment of MCF-7 breast cancer cells with both pomegranate extracts and genistein was found to be more effective on inhibition and cytotoxicity than with single treatments (Jeune et al., 2005).

In an ethnobotanical study of medicinal plants in Chandauli District, Singh & Singh (2009) were able to document 40 medicinal plants belonging to 27 families by semi-structured interviews, field observations, preference and direct matrix ranking with traditional medicine practitioners. Pomegranate was found to be an ingredient of a powder for external treatment of breast cancer along with whole plant of *Vernonia cinerea* Less. (AS38) and leaves of *Crataeva nurvala.*

Epidemiological studies have demonstrated that elevated serum levels of the estrogens, mainly estrone and estradiol, and lower levels of sex hormone binding globulin, after menopause substantially increased the risk of breast cancer. After menopause, most circulating estrogen is derived from the conversion of adrenal androgens to estrone, and some of the estrone is further converted to estradiol, the most active estrogen in breast tissue. Sturgeon & Ronnenberg (2010) described the *in vitro* cell culture studies, animal studies and available data about the property of pomegranate to prevent breast cancer as well as the possible mechanisms involved. They reported that cyclooxigenase inhibition by the constituents of the pomegranate fruit, seed oils or pure compounds induce the decrease of PGE2 that known to downregulate aromatase expression, that converts adrenal androgens to estrone. Ellagic acid seems to exhibit apoptosis, inhibits activation of inflammatory pathways, and inhibits angiogenesis. However, these assays being performed in animal models need to be confirmed in humans.

Grossmann et al. (2010) found that punicic acid inhibited the proliferation of estrogen insensitive breast cancer cell line (MDA-MB-231) and an estrogen sensitive cell line developed from the MDA-MB-231 cells (MDA-ER 7), as well as induced apoptosis in both type of cells 86% and 91% respectively. They stated that punicic acid also disrupted mitochondrial membrane potential of both cell lines. Such antiproliferative effect of punicic acid on human breast cancer cells was due to lipid peroxidation of cells and activation of protein kinase C (PKC).

Tran et al. (2010) evaluated pomegranate seed linolenic acid isomers as selective estrogen receptor modulators (SERMs) *in vitro*. Punicic acid and α-eleostearic acid present in seed oil of pomegranate inhibited the IC_{50} estrogen receptors ERα and ERβ depending on the dose. At lower doses of punicic acid acted as agonist for both receptors and antagonist at higher concentrations. Both acids were effective in producing effective inhibition of cancer cell proliferation: MCF-7 (ER-positive human breast cancer cells) and MDA-MB-231 (ER-negative human breast cancer cells and are SERMs.

4.2.4 Prevention of colon cancer

Current treatment options in colorectal cancer such as surgical intervention and adjuvant chemotherapy have several limitations in counteracting the disease. Furthermore, at advanced stages the patients might be unresponsive to any form of treatment. In this regard, an optimal model for primary and secondary prevention in colon cancer, given the availability of effective screening procedures and a well-defined multi-step carcinogenic pathway, can be thought as the development of new cancer chemopreventive agents that could be employed to inhibit tumor development without causing systemic toxicity such as increasing the consumption of food containing anticarcinogenic compounds. Phytochemicals from pomegranate have been shown to inhibit colon cancer cell proliferation and apoptosis through the modulation of cellular transcription factors and signaling proteins (Mertens-Talcott & Percival, 2005; Seeram et al., 2006; Khan, 2009; Kasimsetty et al., 2010).

Kohno et al. (2004a,b) reported that dietary administration of pomegranate seed oil rich in conjugated linolenic acid markedly inhibited the development of azoxymethane-induced colonic adenocarcinomas in male F344 rats without causing any adverse effects. This was associated with an increased content of conjugated linoleic acid in the colon and liver and/or increased expression of peroxisome proliferator-activated receptor (PPAR)-protein in the non-tumor colon mucosa.

There is considerable evidence that the anticarcinogenic effect of pomegranate ellagitannins is mainly due to ellagic acid, which induces apoptosis in human colon cancer cell line via the intrinsic pathway with release of cytochrome *c* into the cytosol, activation of initiator caspase 9 and effector caspase 3 and down-regulation of B-cell lymphoma-extra large (Bcl-XL). In addition, pomegranate treated Caco-2 cells showed arrest in the S phase of the cell cycle, down-regulation of cyclins A and B1 and upregulation of cyclin E (Larossa et al., 2006).

Adams et al. (2006) examined the effects of pomegranate juice on inflammatory cell signaling proteins in the HT-29 human colon cancer cell line. In HT-29 colon cancer cells, at a concentration of 50 mg/L pomegranate juice significantly suppressed TNFalpha-induced COX-2 protein expression by 79%, total pomegranate tannin extract (TPT, 55%), and punicalagin 48% Cyclooxygenase-2 (COX-2) expression is increased via activation of nuclear factor kappa-B (NFKB) by tumor necrosis factor-alpha (TNF-Ot), an inflammatory cell signaling process that may be a cause of cancer initiation and progression. Additionally, pomegranate juice reduced phosphorylation of the p65 subunit and binding to the NFkappaB response element 6.4-fold. TPT suppressed NFK binding 10-fold, whereas punicalagin 3.6-fold. It was shown that inflammatory enzymes in colon cancer cells were inhibited by the pomegranate juice components. Ellagic acid, punicalagin and TPT failed to induce apoptosis in HT-29 and HCT-116 cells when treated at doses equivalent to found in pomegranate juice. They were only effective when treated at equivalent doses of 100μg/mL (Seeram et al., 2005).

In a seperate study, Boateng et al. (2007) examined the effect of pomegranate juice given access to 20%, before and after treatment with colon-specific chemical carcinogen, azoxymethanein to F-344 rats for 17 weeks. Pomegranate fruit juice reduced the number of aberrant cryptic foci (ACF) of the colon by 91% in male rats. Histopathology of rat colon after 17th week of treatment revealed a remarkable decrease in the number of large crypts in pomegranate juice-fed rats, and the number of crypts/ACF was also low. When compared to water melon and cranberry juices, pomegranate juice was found to be superior as an inhibitor of ACF in rat colon. Increase in weight gain and feed intake was observed in pomegranate fruit juice-fed rats, suggesting a possible protective effect against cancer cachexia.

Kasimsetty et al. (2010) investigated the colon cancer chemopreventive properties of pomegranate ellagitannins and their intestinal bacterial metabolites, urolithins, in HT-29 human colon cancer cells, and stated that the ellagitannins and urolithins released in the colon upon consumption of pomegranate juice in considerable amounts could potentially reduce the risk of colon cancer development, by inhibiting cell proliferation and inducing apoptosis. Ellagitannins and urolithins inhibited endocrine disrupter 2,3,7,8-tetrachlorodibenzo-*p*-dioxin (TCDD)-induced CYP1-mediated ethoxyresorufin-O-deethlyase (EROD) activity *in vitro* with IC_{50} values ranging from 56.7 μM for urolithin A to 74.8 μM for urolithin C. These compounds exhibited dose- and time-dependent decreases in cell proliferation and clonogenic efficiency of HT-29 cells.

In colon cancer, a large percentage of the tumour arises from activating mutations in the Wnt protein pathway. Sharma et al. (2010) studied the effects of urolitinins, ellagic acid and ellagitannin-rich fruit extracts on Wnt signalling in a human 293T cell line using a luciferase reporter of canonical Wnt pathway-mediated transcriptional activation. In the canonical Wnt pathway, the signal produced by the binding of Wnt ligands to cell surface receptors is transmitted through a cytoplasmic protein called disheveled (Dvl) to inhibit the activity of a complex of cellular proteins that phosphorylate β-catenin, and target it for destruction. Therefore, Dvl-mediated inhibition of the β-catenin destruction complex results in increased levels of cellular β-catenin and translocation of β-catenin into the nucleus, where β-catenin activates transcription factors of the LEF/TCF families and initiates transcription of target genes effective on tissue proliferation, differentiation and tumorigenesis. The researchers concluded that urolithins produced in the colon from ellagitannins present in pomegranate are inhibitors of the canonical Wnt signalling pathway at physiologically relevant concentrations.

4.2.5 Prevention of other cancer types

Eventhough there are advances in detection and therapy of cancer, the severe morbidity rate from cancer have not improved. Various parts of the pomegranate plant have been stated to exert selective antiproliferative effects on a lung, leukemia, stomach, bladder, oesaphagus and oral cancers (Lansky & Newman, 2007; Syed et al., 2007; Heber, 2008; Jurenka, 2008; Rahman et al., 2010; Khan & Mukhtar, 2010; Faria & Calhau 2011), through antioxidant, antiproliferation (growth inhibition, cell cycle disruption and apoptosis), antiangiogenesis and antiinflammatory mechanisms of action.

In vitro and *in vivo* studies revealed that pomegranate fruit extract (PFE) have chemopreventive/therapeutic potential of against lung cancer models (Khan et al., 2007a,b,2008). Normal human bronchial epithelial cells (NHBE) and human lung carcinoma A549 cells, in mice, were treated with pomegranate fruit extract (50–150 μg/ml) for 72 h. There was a significant decrease in the viability of A549 cells, however, only minimal effects were observed on NHBE cells. Pomegranate fruit extract treatment of A549 cells resulted in dose-dependent arrest of cells in G0/G1 phase of the cell cycle, which was associated with induction of WAF1/p21 and KIP1/p27 and accompanied by decrease in the expression of downstream cell cycle regulatory proteins (Khan et al., 2007a).

The effect of oral consumption of a human achievable dose of pomegranate fruit extract on tumor growth, progression and signaling pathways involved, was studied further in two other mouse lung tumor protocols. Benzo(a)pyrene [B(a)P] and N-nitroso-tris-chloroethylurea (NTCU) were used to induce lung tumors, and PFE was given in drinking water to A/J mice. Lung tumor yield was examined on the 84th day and 140 days after B(a)P dosing and 240 days after NTCU treatment. Mice treated with PFE and exposed to B(a)P and NTCU had statistically significant lower lung tumor multiplicities than mice treated with carcinogens only. Tumor reduction was 53.9% and 61.6% in the B(a)P+PFE group at 84 and 140 days, respectively, compared with the B(a)P group. The NTCU+PFE group had 65.9% tumor reduction compared with the NTCU group at 240 days. PFE treatment also resulted in inhibition of NF-κB, MAPK, and PI3K/Akt signaling. Treatment with B(a)P and NTCU caused increased phosphorylation of mTOR at Ser^{2448}, whereas PFE administration resulted in inhibition of phosphorylation of mTOR. This observation was significant since the mTOR integrates mitogenic signals and intracellular nutrient levels to activate 4EBP1 and p70S6K that control protein translation and cell cycle progression (Khan et al., 2007b).

Suzuki et al. (2001) investigated cytotoxicity of pomegranate seed oil and other plant seed oils containing conjugated linoleic acids in mouse tumors and human monocytic leukemia cells. They stated the cytotoxic effect of pomegranate seed oil (containing 9c,11t,13c-18:3), as well as tung seed oil (containing 9c,11t,13t-18:3) and catalpa seed oil (containing 9t,11t,13c-18:3), was much stronger than that of pot marigold seed oil (containing 8t,10t,12c-18:3), suggesting that the position of the double bond could be an important determinant for the cytotoxicity of conjugated inoleic acids.

Kawaii & Lansky (2004) examined the effect of flavonoid-rich pomegranate juice, pomegranate fermented juice and pomegranate pericarp extracts on HL-60 human leukemia cell differentiation and proliferation. *In vitro* assays confirmed that both the pomegranate fermented juice and pericarp extracts strongly promoted cellular differentiation and inhibited proliferation in HL-60 cell cultures; the effect of pomegranate juice on cellular differentiation was less significant. In view of the observations the authors stated the hypothesis of another mechanism by which pomegranate constituents impart an anticarcinogenic effect.

Mertens-Talcott & Percival (2005) investigated the interactions of ellagic acid and quercetin with resveratrol, with the hypothesis that the selected polyphenols would interact synergistically in the induction of apoptosis and reduction of cell growth in human leukemia cells (MOLT-4). They found significant interaction for the combination of ellagic acid with resveratrol, and alterations in cell cycle kinetics induced by single compounds and combinations were also observed. The authors concluded that the anticarcinogenic potential of foods containing polyphenols may not be based on the effects of individual compounds, but may involve a synergistic enhancement of the anticancer effects.

4.3 Other health effects

4.3.1 Antiinflammatory activity

Epidemiological evidence points that many cancers arise from sites of infection, chronic irritation and inflammation (Rakoff-Nahoum, 2006; Heber, 2008). The inflammatory response result in persistent oxidative stress orchestrates tumour microenvironment to microbial infection and mediates tissue repair and regeneration, which may occur due to infectious or non-infectious tissue damage.

Pomegranate and the selected chemical constituents isolated from juice, peel, and seed have been found to have a large range of effects: (i) inhibition of Cyclooxygenase-2 (COX-2) expression and ultimately eicosanoid biosynthesis (Schubert et al., 1999; Shukla et al., 2008); (ii) synergistic suppression of inflammatory cytokine expression (Adams et al., 2006); (iii) inhibition of matrix MMPs (Okamoto et al., 2004; Ahmad et al., 2005; Aslam et al., 2006).

In view of the antioxidant, anticarcinogenic and antiinflammatory properties of pomegranate phenolics and/or its derived metabolites, one could hypothesize that pomegranate and/or its derived metabolites have a beneficial effect on inflammation. Larrosa et al. (2010) evaluated the effects of pomegranate intake and its main microbiota-derived metabolite urolithin-A (UROA) on colon inflammation in a dextran sodium sulfate (DSS)-induced colon inflammation rat model and to assess whether UROA is the main anti-inflammatory compound. In addition, they examined the effect of the inflammation on the phenolic metabolism. DSS (5%) was administered for the five last days to Male Fisher rats, fed with 250 mg/kg day pomegranate extract or 15 mg/kg day UROA for 25 days. In both groups inflammation markers (iNOS, COX-2, PTGES and PGE2 in colonic mucosa) were decreased, the gut microbiota was modulated and the G1 to S cell cycle pathway was up-regulated. UROA group showed various down-regulated pathways, including that of the inflammatory response. Pomegranate extract, but not UROA, decreased oxidative stress in plasma and colon mucosa. Only UROA preserved colonic architecture. The normal formation of urolithins in pomegranate extract-fed rats was prevented during inflammation suggesting UROA could be the most active anti-inflammatory compound derived from pomegranate ingestion in healthy subjects, whereas in colon inflammation, the effects could be due to the nonmetabolized ellagitannin-related fraction.

Structure–activity relationships of natural products have been found to influence the various pharmacological functions. *In vitro* and *in vivo* antiinflammatory effects of *Punica granatum* Linne, a high phenolic content fruit, widely used as an antipyretic analgesic in Chinese culture, were investigated by Lee et al. (2010). Pomegranate has shown potential nitric oxide (NO) inhibition in liposaccaharide (LPS)-induced RAW 264.7 macrophage cells, with significant decrease in carrageenan-induced mice paw edema. Hydrolysable tannins, punicalagin, punicalin, strictinin A, and granatin B, inhibited NO production and inductible nitric oxide synthase (iNOS) expression in RAW 264.7 cells. Granatin B showed the strongest iNOS and COX-2 inhibitory effects, and exhibited these effects in the inhibition of paw swelling and the prostaglandin (PG) E2 level in carrageenan-induced mice.

Inflammatory disorders are due to excessive production of pro-inflammatory mediators such as TNFa, GM-CSF, IL-1, IL-6, IL-8, leukotriene B4 and PAF, the activity of inflammatory cells such as neutrophils, monocytes and macrophages, and excessive production of reactive oxygen species (ROS) (Nathan, 2006). Bachoual et al. (2011) investigated the effect of pomegranate peel aqueous extract (PPAE) on human neutrophil reactive oxygen species (ROS) production *in vitro* and on LPS-induced lung inflammation *in vivo* in mice. PPAE, in a concentration-dependent manner, inhibited luminol-amplified chemoluminescence of resting neutrophils and N-formyl-methionylleucyl- phenylalanine (fMLF)- or phorbol myristate acetate (PMA)-stimulated neutrophils. On the contrary, had no significant effect on superoxide anion generation, suggesting that it does not directly inhibit NADPH oxidase activity or activation pathways, or scavenge superoxide anions. *In vivo* studies showed that PPAE also attenuated LPS-induced lung inflammation in mice. Consequently PPAE found to inhibit neutrophil myeloperoxidase activity and attenuates LPS-induced lung inflammation in mice.

4.3.2 Cardiovascular health

Cardiovascular diseases (CVDs) are a leading cause of death and disability worldwide. Hypertension and atherosclerosis, a chronic inflammatory disease characterized by plaque formation in the large arteries, are major risk factors for CVDs, such as stroke, myocardial infarction and heart failure. In addition to genetic factors, age, body weight, blood pressure, dyslipidemia, physical inactivity and behavioural risk factors such as tobacco or alcohol use, diets that include high fat, salty food are thought to play an important role in the development of cardiovascular disease. Epidemiological data have clearly shown that independent risk factors for CVD are serum total cholesterol and low-density lipoprotein cholesterol (LDL-C) (Kannel et. al., 1986; Mirmiran et al., 2009). A large number of clinical trials have demonstrated in order to prevent these cardiovascular diseases from occurring, control of a patient's blood pressure is necessary, either by lifestyle modifications, medication(s) such as use of cholesterol-lowering statins, antihypertensive drugs and antiplatelet agents or both.

While modification of dietary patterns and increased physical activity constitute the primary preventive intervention in lowering coronary heart disease (CHD) and stroke, the role of plant-based bioactive compounds or phytochemicals has attracted much attention since there is a negative relationship between their consumption and CVDs (Hu, 2003; Dauchet et al., 2005; Nothlings et al., 2008). Pomegranate, being rich in flavonoids and ellagitannins, are potent antioxidants and antiinflammatory agents, thereby counteracting oxidative damage and inflammation which underlie the pathogenesis of CVD (Kaplan et al., 2001). Oxidative stress, the major contributor to CVD, is the build-up of highly reactive free radical species or the decrease of defence mechanisms to protect against biological damage by free radicals due to the imbalance between free radical formation and antioxidant status. Oxidative stress induces inflammation by acting on the pathways that generate inflammatory mediators like adhesion molecules and pro-inflammatory cytokines. The effect of reactive oxygen species (ROS) and reactive nitrogen species (RNS) on human health has been studied for decades, with results indicating increasing the risk of cancer, arthritis, degenerative eye and neurological disorders, as well as general aging (Aruoma, 1998). However, the attention has turned to the effect of these free radicals on CVD and related disorders; such as atherosclerosis, hypertension, hypercholesterolemia, type 2 diabetes, and heart failure (Hamilton et al., 2004).

Sumner et al. (2005) investigated the effect of daily consumption of pomegranate juice for 3 months on myocardial perfusion in patients who had coronary heart disease and myocardial ischemia in a randomized, placebo-controlled, double-blind study. The patients were given either 240 mL pomegranate juice (polyphenol content not specified) or a sports beverage of similar color, flavor, and caloric content daily for three months. Although both control and treatment patients demonstrated similar levels of stress-induced ischemia at baseline, at three months stress-induced ischemia decreased in the treatment group (from 4.5±3.1 to 3.7±3.7). In addition, angina episodes decreased 50% percent in the treatment group but increased 38% in the placebo group. The researchers concluded that pomegranate juice consumption resulted in a reduction in myocardial ischemia and improvement in myocardial perfusion.

Rosenblat et al. (2006) studied the antiatherosclerotic effects of a pomegranate by-product (PBP, which includes the whole pomegranate fruit left after juice preparation). Four-month-old E° mice with significant atherosclerosis were given PBP (17 or 51.5 μg of gallic acid equiv/kg/day) with an eight-fold higher polyphenol concentration than pomegranate juice for three months. Consumption of PBP by the mice resulted in a significant reduction in atherosclerotic lesion size by up to 57% and in MPM oxidative status as evidenced by a 27% decrease in total macrophage peroxide levels, a 42% decrease in cellular lipid peroxide levels, and a 19% decrease in peritoneal macrophage uptake of oxidized LDL (Ox-LDL).

Through *in vitro* and *in vivo* studies de Nigris et al. (2006) stated that the proatherogenic effects induced by perturbed shear stress can be also reversed by chronic administration of pomegranate fruit extract (PFE). The researcher investigated the effects of intervention with the PFE rich in polyphones (punicalagin, which is a potent antioxidant) on ELK-1, p-CREB, and endothelial nitric oxide synthase (eNOS) expression induced by high shear stress. Both the PFE and the regular pomegranate juice concentrate reduced the activation of ELK-1 and p-CREB and increased eNOS expression in cultured human endothelial cells and in atherosclerosis-prone areas of hypercholesterolemic mice. PFE and pomegranate juice increased cyclic GMP levels while there was no significant effect of both compounds on the conversion of L-arginine to L-citrulline. Administration of these compounds to hypercholesterolemic mice significantly reduced the progression of atherosclerosis and isoprostane levels and increased nitrates.

In a randomized, double-blind, parallel trial Davidson et al. (2009) assessed the influence of pomegranate juice consumption on anterior and posterior carotid intima-media thickness (CIMT) progression rates in subjects at moderate risk for coronary heart disease. Participants consumed 240 ml/day of pomegranate juice or a control beverage for up to 18 months. No significant difference in overall CIMT progression rate was observed between pomegranate juice and control treatments. In exploratory analyses, in subjects in the most adverse tertiles for baseline serum lipid peroxides, triglycerides (TGs), highdensity lipoprotein (HDL) cholesterol, TGs/HDL cholesterol, total cholesterol/HDL cholesterol, and apolipoprotein-B100, those in the pomegranate juice group had significantly less anterior wall and/or composite CIMT progression versus control subjects. They concluded that in subjects at moderate coronary heart disease risk, pomegranate juice consumption had no significant effect on overall CIMT progression rate but may have slowed CIMT progression in subjects with increased oxidative stress and disturbances in the TG-rich lipoprotein/HDL axis.

Endothelial apoptosis is a driving force in atherosclerosis development. Oxidized low-density lipoprotein (oxLDL) promotes inflammatory and thrombotic processes and is highly atherogenic, as it stimulates macrophage cholesterol accumulation and foam cell formation. In recent years ellagic acid has been the subject of intense research within the fields of cancer and inflammation, however, its protective effect against oxidized LDL-induced injury in vascular endothelial cells have not been clarified. Ou et al. (2010) investigated the anti-apoptotic effect of ellagic acid in human umbilical vein endothelial cells (HUVECs) exposed to OxLDL and explored the possible mechanisms. Pretreatment with ellagic acid (5–20 μM) significantly attenuated OxLDL-induced cytotoxicity, apoptotic features, and generation of ROS. In addition, the antiapoptotic effect of ellagic acid was partially inhibited by wortmannin (a PI3K inhibitor) and cavtratin (a specific endothelial NO synthase inhibitor). The alterations induced by OxLDL, however, were attenuated by pretreatment with ellagic acid. The inhibition of OxLDL-induced endothelial apoptosis by ellagic acid is due to its anti-oxidant activity and its ability to modulate the PI3K/Akt/eNOS signaling pathway upto a point.

4.3.3 Antidiabetic properties (glucose and lipid metabolism activity)

According to several review articles (Jurenka, 2008; Li et al., 2008; Yun, 2010) pomegranate flowers, containing abundant ellagitannins, was already prescribed in Unani and Ayurvedic systems of medicine as a remedy for diabetes. The protective effect of pomegranate flowers' extracts (PFLE) was investigated by some authors on blood glucose level, serum lipid profile, total cholesterol, LDL, pancreatic lipid peroxidation and activities of both enzymatic and non-enzymatic antioxidant status in diabetic rats (Huang et al., 2005a,b; Lei et al., 2007; Lan et al., 2009; Bagri et al., 2009). The authors reported that the increase in blood glucose level, total cholesterol, triglycerides, LDL-cholesterol, very low density lipoproteins, lipid peroxidation level with decrease in high density lipoprotein (HDL)-cholesterol, glutathione content and antioxidant enzymes namely, glutathione peroxidase, glutathione reductase, glutathione-S-transferase, superoxide dismutase and catalase can be reversed by administration of aqueous PFLE. PFLE was shown to activate PPAR-a, a cardiac transcription factor involved in myocardial energy production via fatty acid uptake and oxidation. PPAR-a activation decreased cardiac uptake and circulation of lipids. Decreases were observed in cardiac tissue triglycéride content at the end of the study and in plasma total cholesterol and NEFA after four weeks of treatment.These findinds suggest that pomegranate could be used as dietary supplement in the treatment and prevention of chronic diseases characterised by atherogenic lipoprotein profile, aggravated antioxidant status and impaired glucose metabolism.

Rosenblat et al. (2006) investigated the effect of 50 mL/day pomegranate juice for three months on oxidative stress, blood sugar, and lipid profiles in 10 type 2 diabetic patients, with a history of diabetes for 4–10 years, and 10 healthy controls. In diabetic patients, triglyceride levels were 2.8 times greater, (HDL) cholesterol was 28% lower, and hemoglobin AlC (HbAlC) values were 59% higher than in control patients. They stated that consuming pomegranate juice for three months did not significantly affect triglyceride, HDL cholesterol, HbAlC, glucose, or insulin values, but did lower serum C-peptide values by 23%, suggesting improved insulin sensitivity. Researchers concluded that despite the sugars naturally present in pomegranate juice, consumption did not adversely affect diabetic parameters but had a significant effect on atherogenesis via reduced oxidative stress.

Esmailzadeh et al. (2006) investigated the cholesterol-lowering effects of 40 g concentrated pomegranate juice on 22 type 2 diabetic patients (8 men and 14 women) for eight weeks. Statistically significant decreases were observed in total cholesterol, LDL cholesterol, total/HDL cholesterol ratio, and LDL/HDL ratio, which due in part to decreased absorption and increased fecal excretion of cholesterol, as well as possible affects on HMG-CoA reductase and sterol O-acyltransferase, two enzymes key to cholesterol metabolism.

Oleanolic acid, ursolic acid and gallic acid, active components contained in pomegranate flower (Li et al., 2008), have long been recognized to have antihyperlipidemic properties (Liu, 1995; Jang et al., 2008). Xu et al. (2009) speculated that PFLE might improve diabetes and obesity-induced fatty liver, and investigated the effects and underlying mechanisms of action of PFLE on hepatic lipid accumulation in ZDF rats with severe fatty liver and in human liver-derived HepG2 cell line. PFLE-treated ZDF rats showed reduced ratio of liver weight to tibia length, hepatic triglyceride contents and lipid droplets. These effects were accompanied by enhanced hepatic gene expression of peroxisome proliferator-activated receptor (PPAR)-alpha, carnitine palmitoyltransferase-1 and acyl-CoA oxidase (ACO), and reduced stearoyl-CoA desaturase-1. Incontrast, PFLE showed minimal effects on expression of genes responsible for synthesis, hydrolysis or uptake of fatty acid and triglycerides. PGF treatment also increased PPAR-alpha and ACO mRNA levels in HepG2 cells. The authors concluded that PFLE, an Unani medicine, ameliorates diabetes and obesity-associated fatty liver, at least in part, by activating hepatic expression of genes responsible for fatty acid oxidation.

There is growing evidence that paraoxnase (PON1) plays an important role in lipid metabolism, particularly in protecting LDL and HDL from oxidation in vitro, and thus lowering the risk of developing atherosclerosis, and the onset of cardiovascular disease (Mackness et al., 2000,2002). PON1 knockout mice exhibit about a two-fold increase in atherosclerosis (Rozenberg et al., 2003), whereas PON1 expression and activity can be modulated by dietary polyphenols i.e. LDL receptor deficient mice supplemented with quercitine (a polyphenol contained in pomegranate) and moderate ethanol inhibited the progression of atherosclerosis by upregulating the hepatic expression with concomitant increased serum PON1 activity (Gouédard et al., 2004; Leckey et al., 2010). Similarly, pomegranate polyphenols seem to have a specific transcriptional role in hepatocyte PON1 expression upregulation (Khateeb et al., 2010). Although it is known that diabetes is associated with increased oxidative stress and the development of atherosclerosis (Mooradian, 2009), no expression studies have been examined in a diabetic model that is fed with high fat. Therefore, Betanzos-Cabrera et al. (2011) investigated whether pomengranate juice induces PON1 gene expression and activity, especially in conditions known for affecting PON1 enzymatic function. The feeding of streptozotocin-induced diabetic mice with a high-fat diet supplemented daily with pomegranate juice significantly induced PON1 gene expression and activity. Interestingly, animals supplemented with pomegranate juice showed the lowest bodyweight. In addition, the pomegranate juice significantly reduced blood glucose but not triacylglycerols and cholesterol levels, demonstrating that pomegranate juice has a hypoglycemic effect.

4.3.4 Antimicrobial properties

Due to the increasing interest in natural antimicrobials and antioxidants derived from plant sources the investigation of pomegranate has also been an interesting scientific field for researchers, since the capacity of preventing infections of pomegranate extracts was well documented. Food-borne illnesses are still an important concern for both consumers, the food industry and food safety authorities, thus, the ongoing search for natural antimicrobials for prevention of food-borne illnesses is a vast exploring area for scientists. Antimicrobial activities of pomegranate have been studied by some researchers and the extent of inhibitory effect is always attributed to the pomegranate antioxidant activity that depends mainly on the phenolic and anthocyanin content of the fruit (Holetz et al., 2002; Braga et al., 2005; Mathabe et al., 2006; McCarrell et al., 2008; Al-Zoreky, 2009; Duman et al., 2009; Gould et al., 2009; Parashar et al., 2009; Panichayupakaranant et al., 2010, Orak et al., 2011). In a previous study, Opara et al. (2009) reported that the best activity against *Staphyloccocus aureus* and *Pseudomonas aeruginosa* were found in fruit peel compound punicalagin, particularly from Oman, which was coincident with the highest levels of vitamin C detected in these samples. Similar findings were reported by Salgado et al. (2009) and Dahham et al. (2010) in which antibacterial and antifungal activities of pomegranate peel extract (rind), seed extract, juice and whole fruit on the selected bacteria and fungi were investigated. The antimicrobial effectiveness of the extracts depends on the species of bacteria evaluated, the more sensitive being the Gram-positive species *S. aureus* and *Bacillus* sp. *along* with *Aspergillus niger*. Voravuthikunchai et al. (2006) tested pomegranate and seven other Thai medicinal plant extracts for *in vitro* activity against enterohemorrhagic *Escherichia coli (E. coli* O157:H7). An ethanolic pomegranate peel extract was shown to be both bacteriostatic and bacteriocidal, indicating it may be an effective adjunct treatment for *E. coli* O157:H7 infection.

The only human trials examining the antibacterial properties of pomegranate extracts have focused on oral bacteria (Sastravaha et al., 2003; Menezes et al., 2006). However, several *in vitro* assays demonstrate its bacteriocidal activity against several highly pathogenic and sometimes antibiotic-resistant organisms. Machado et al. (2002) evaluated the synergistic effect of a pomegranate methanolic extract with five antibiotics on 30 clinical isolates of methicilin-resistant *S. aureus* (MRSA) and methicillin-sensitive *S. aureus*. Antibiotics tested were. Although synergistic activity between the pomegranate extract and tested antibiotics (chloramphenicol, gentamicin, ampicillin, tetracycline, and oxacillin) was noted in the *S. aureus* isolates, synergy with ampicillin was the most pronounced. A combination of the two increased the lag time to bacterial growth by three hours and was also bacteriocidal as evidenced by a 72.5% reduction in methicillin-sensitive organisms and a 99.9% reduction in MRSA. Bialonska et al. (2009b) stated that commercial extract of pomegranate by-product provided by POM Wonderful (Los Angeles, CA) and punicalagins inhibited the growth of pathogenic clostridia and *S. aureus*. Nevertheless the probiotic lactobacilli and bifidobacteria were not affected by ellagitannins. These findings lead to the conclusion that the growth inhibition toward pathogenic bacteria could be attributed to the accumulation of ellagitannins in the large intestines, where they interact with complex gut microflora, and lower media pH due to the presence of punicalagins.

Su et al. (2010) stated that the combination of pomegranate juice and pomegranate polyphenols was also effective against food-borne viral infectivity and appear to be promising natural remedies for preventing or reducing human norovirus infections. In addition, pomegranate purified polyphenol extract inhibited influenza virus having also a synergistic effect with oseltamivir, since influenza continues to be a major cause of mortality and morbidity eventhough the applications of the vaccines and antiviral therapies (Haidari et al., 2009).

Johann et al. (2010) studying the activity of extracts of some plants used in Brazilian traditional medicine against the pathogenic fungus that causes this Paracoccidioidomycosis, *Paracoccidioides brasiliensis*, reported that the hexane extract of pomegranate stem exhibited better antifungal activity against the three clinical isolated than other parts of the plant or other fractions of the same plant.

Candida species, a normal component of the human biota in the gastrointestinal tract and oral and vaginal mucosa, can cause superficial infections such as thrush and vaginitis. Endo et al. (2010) reported that punicalagin isolated from pomegranate peels possessed strong activity against *Candida albicans* and *C. parapsilosis* as well as the combination of punicalagin and fluconazole showed a synergistic interaction. Tayel & El-Tras (2009) demonstrated that methanol, ethanol and water extracts of pomegranate peels were effective against *C. albicans* growth. In addition, they also proved that pomegranate peel extract aerosol was an efficient method for complete sanitizing of semi-closed places against *C. albicans* growth, and thereby could contribute for preventing *C. albicans* contamination and growth in suspected places. Ethnobotanical studies performed in Brazil had demonstrated the utilization of pomegranate in oral health since denture stomatitis is commonly associated with *C. albicans* and some other *Candida* species (Santos et al., 2009).

Dell'Agli et al. (2009) studied the *in vitro* antiplasmodial and antimalarial activity of methanolic extracts of a tannin-enriched fraction and of metabolites to estimate their curative efficacy and mechanisms of action. They conclude that methanolic extracts of pomegranate inhibited *Plasmodium falciparum* and *P. vivax* growth *in vitro*, and suggested that these might be attributed to the low bioavailability as well as the kinetic of conversion of ellagic acid to inactive metabolites urolithins.

5. Adverse effects and reactions/safety

Pomegranate and its products have a long history of use as food or ethnic medicine without adverse effects, and also it has GRAS (generally recognized as safe) status in the

USA. The published safety data is limited and no clinical or laboratory adverse events were reported. However, there are some publications on occurrence of allergic reactions when handling or ingestion of pomegranate fruit/seeds due to eliciting a type I hypersensitivity reaction, and thus it is crucial to advise consumers the side effects (McCutcheon et al., 2008).

6. Conclusion

Nowadays, it is widely accepted that the beneficial health effects of fruits and vegetables in the prevention of diseases are due to the bioactive compounds they contain.

Based on the explosion of interest in the numerous therapeutic properties over the last decade and *in vitro*, animal, and clinical trials pomegranate seems to be a promising food with well-defined therapeutic benefits. The epidomiological data suggests that the pomegranate fruit and its associated bioactive compounds such as phenolic acids, flavonoids, and tannins may possess a strong potential as a chemopreventive and possibly as new tools for preventive and possibly therapeutic interventions against various human cancers. This could have a direct practical implication to cancer patients if consumption of fruits like pomegranate can inhibit the process of carcinogenesis. Further studies should focus on the potential clinical usefulness of the agent through issues such as determining the optimal period and route of administration, systemic bioavailability, potent anticancer activity, optimal dosing and toxicity (if any) of the agent and single or combinatorial approach. In addition, the possible use of pomegranate extracts as a therapy or adjunct for prevention and treatment of several disease processes, such as diabetes, cardiovascular disease, atherosclerosis, inflammation, microbial infection, obesity, male infertility, Alzheimer underscores the need for more clinical research. Therefore, ongoing studies should focus on developing novel pomegranate derived products such as ready-to-eat pomegranate seeds, single-strength juices, juice concentrates, seeds in syrup, frozen seeds, and traditional products such as pomegranate pekmez, leather and molasses, to benefit from these constituents throughout a healthy life cycle.

7. References

Adams, L.S., Seeram, N.P., Aggarwal, B.B., Takada, Y., Sand, D. & Heber, D. (2006). Pomegranate Juice, Total Pomegranate Ellagitannins, and Punicalagin Suppress Inflammatory Cellsignaling in Colon Cancer Cells. *Journal of Agricultural and Food Chemistry*, Vol.54, No.3, pp.980-985, ISSN 0021-8561

Adams, L.S., Zhang, Y., Seeram, N.P., Heber, D. & Chen, S. (2010). Pomegranate Ellagitannin-derived Compounds Exhibit Antiproiferation and Antiaromatase Activity in Breast Cancer Cells In vitro. *Cancer Prevention Research*, Vol.3, No.1, pp.108-113, ISSN 1940-6207

Adhami, V.M., Khan, N. & Mukhtar, H. (2009). Cancer Chemoprevention by Pomegranate: Laboratory and Clinical Evidence. *Nutrition and Cancer*, Vol.61, No.6, pp.811-815, ISSN 0163-5581

Adhami, V.M., Khan, N. & Mukhtar, H. (2010). Prevention of Cancer with Pomegranate and Pomegranate Anthocyanins. In: *Berries and Cancer Prevention*, Stoner, G. & Seerelam, N.P. (Eds), pp.209-226, ISBN 1441975535, Springer

Adsule, R.N. & Patil, N.B. (1995). Pomegranate: In *Handbook of Fruit Science and Technology,* Salunke, D.K. & Kadam, S.S. (Eds), pp. 455-464, ISBN 0824796438, Marcel Dekkar, New York

Adsule, R.N., Kotecha, P.M. & Kadam, S.S. (1992). Preparation of Wine from Pomegranate. *Beverage Food World,* Vol.19, No.4, pp.13

Afaq, F. (2011). Natural Agents: Cellular and Molecular Mechanisms of Photoprotection. *Archives of Biochemistry and Biophysics,* Vol.508, No.2, pp.144-151, ISSN 0003-9861

Afaq, F., Saleem, M., Krueger, C.G., Reed, J.D. & Mukhtar, H. (2005). Anthocyanin- and Hydrolyzable Tannin-rich Pomegranate Fruit Extract Modulates MAPK and NF-kappaB Pathways and Inhibits Skin Tumorigenesis in CD-1 mice. *International Journal of Cancer,* Vol.113, No.3, pp.423-333, ISSN 1097-0215.

Afaq, F., Zaid, M.A., Khan, N., Dreher, M. & Mukhtar, H. (2009). Protective Effect of Pomegranate-Derived Products on UVB-Mediated Damage in Human Reconstituted Skin. *Experimental Dermatology,* Vol.18, No.6, pp.553-561, ISSN 1600-0625

Ahmed, S., Wang, N., Hafeez, B.B., Cheruvu, V.K. & Haqqi, T.M. (2005). *Púnica granatum L.* Extracts Inhibits IL-lBeta-induced Expression of Matrix Metalloptoteinases by Inhibiting the Activation of MAP Kinases and NF-kappaB in Human Chondrocytes in vitro. *Journal of Nutrition,* Vol.135, No.9, pp.2096-2102, ISSN 0022-3166

Akbarpour , V., Hemmati, K., Sharifani, M. & Sadr, Z.B. (2010). Multivariate Analysis of Physical and Chemical Characteristics in Some Pomegranate (*Punica granatum*) Cultivars of Iran. *Journal of Food, Agriculture and Environment,* Vol.8, No.1, pp.244-248, ISSN 1459-0255

Akiyama, H., Fujii, K., Yamasaki, O., Oono, T. & Iwatsuki, K. (2001). Antibacterial Action of Several Tannins Against *Staphylococcus aureus. Journal of Antimicrobial Chemotherapy,* Vol.48, No.4, pp. 487-491, ISSN 0305-7453

Akpinar-Bayizit, A. (2010). Analysis of Mineral Content in Pomegranate Juice by ICP-OES. *Asian Journal of Chemistry,* Vol.22, No.8, pp.6542-6546, ISSN 0970-7077

Alam, M.S., Alam, M.A., Ahmad, S., Najmi, A.K., Asif, M. & Jahangir, T. (2010). Protective Effects of *Punica granatum* in Experimentally-indoced Gastric Ulcers. *Toxicologicy Mechanism and Methods,* Vol.20, No.9, pp.572-578, ISSN 1537-6516

Albrecht, M., Jiang, W., Kumi-Diaka, J., Lansky, E.P., Gommersall, L.M., Patel, A., Mansel, R.E., Neeman, I., Geldof, A.A. & Campbell, M.J. (2004). Pomegranate Extracts Potently Suppress Proliferation, Xenograft Growth, and Invasion of Human Prostate Cancer Cells. *Journal of Medicine Food,* Vol.7, No.3, pp.274-283, ISSN 1096-620X

Al-Maiman, S.A. & Ahmad, D. (2002). Changes in Physical and Chemical Properties during Pomegranate (*Punica granatum* L.) Fruit Maturation. *Food Chemistry,* Vol.76, No.4, pp.437-441, ISSN 0308-8146

Alparslan, M. &Hayta, M. (2002). Rheological and Sensory Properties of Pekmez (grape molasses) / Tahin (sesame paste) blends. *Journal of Food Engineering.* Vol.54, No.1, pp.89-93, ISSN 0260-8774

Al-Said, F.A., Opara, L.U. & Al-Yahyai, R.A. (2009). Physico-chemical and Textural Quality Attributes of Pomegranate Cultivars (*Punica granatum* L.) Grown in the Sultanate of Oman. *Journal of Food Engineering,* Vol.90, No.1, pp. 129-134, ISSN 0260-8774

Altan, A. & Maskan, M. (2005). Rheological Behavior of Pomegranate (*Punica granatum* L.) Juice and Concentrate. *Journal of Texture Studies*, Vol.36, No.1, pp.68-77, ISSN 0022-4901

Al-Zoreky, N.S. (2009). Antimicrobial Activity of Pomegranate (*Punica granatum* L.) Fruit Peels. *International Journal of Food Microbiology*, Vol.134, No.3, pp.244–248, ISSN 0168-1605

Amakura, Y., Okada, M., Tsuji, S. & Tonogai, Y. (2000). Determination of Phenolic Acids in Fruit Juices by Isocratic Column Liquid Chromatography. *Journal of Chromatography A*, Vol. 891, No.1, pp.183-188, ISSN 0021-9673.

Amin, A.R.M.R., Kucuk, O., Khuri, F.R. & Shin, D.M. (2009). Perspectives for Cancer Prevention with Natural Compounds. *Journal of Clinical Oncology*, Vol.27, No. pp. 2712-2725, ISSN 0732-183X

Aruoma, O. I. (1998). Free Radicals, Oxidative Stress, and Antioxidants in Human Health and Disease. *Journal of the American Oil Chemists' Society*, Vol.75, No.2, pp.199-212, 0003-021X

Aslam, M.N., Lansky, E.P. & Varani, J. (2006). Pomegranate as a Cosmeceutical Source: Pomegranate Fractions Promote Proliferation and Procollagen Synthesis and Inhibit Matrix Metalloproteinase-1 Production in Human Skin Cells. *Journal of Ethnopharmacology*, Vol.103, No.3, pp.311–318, ISSN 0378-8741

Attard, G., Sarker, D., Reid, A., Molife, R., Parker, C. & de Bono, J.S. (2006). Improving the Outcome of Patients with Castration-resistant Prostate Cancer through Rational Drug Development. *British Journal of Cancer*, Vol.95, No.7, pp.767-774, ISSN 0007-0920

Aviram, M., Dornfeld, L., Rosenblat, M., Volkova, N., Kaplan, M., Coleman, R., Hayek, T., Presser, D. & Fuhrman, B. (2000). Pomegranate Juice Consumption Reduces Oxidative Stress, Atherogenic Modifications to LDL and Platelet Aggregation: Studies in Humans and in Atherosclerotic Apolipoprotein E-deficient mice. *The American Journal of Clinical Nutrition*, Vol.71, No.5, pp.1062-1076, ISSN 0002-9165.

Bachoual, R., Talmoudi, W., Boussetta, T., Braut, F. & El-Benna, J. (2011). An Aqueous Pomegranate Peel Extract Inhibits Neutrophil Myeloperoxidase *in vitro* and Attenuates Lung Inflammation in Mice. *Food and Chemical Toxicology*, Vol.49, No.6, pp.1224-1228, ISSN 0278-6915

Badenes, M.L., Martínez-Calvo, J. & Llácer, G. (1998). Analysis of Apricot Germplasm from the European Ecogeographical Group. *Euphytica*, Vol.102, No.1, pp.93-99, ISSN 0014-2336

Bagri, P., Ali, M., Aeri, V., Bhowmik, M., Sultana, S. (2009). Antidiabetic Effect of *Punica granatum* Flowers: Effect on Hyperlipidemia, Pancreatic Cells, Lipid Peroxidation and Antioxidant Enzymes in Experimental Diabetes. *Food and Chemical Toxicology*, Vol.47, No.1-2, pp.50-54, ISSN 0278-6915

Basu, A. & Penugonda, K. (2009). Pomegranate Juice: A Heart-Healthy Fruit Juice. *Nutrition Reviews*, Vol.67, No.1, pp.49-56, ISSN 0029-6643

Batta, A.K. & Rangaswami, S. (1973). Crystalline Chemical Components of Some Vegetable Drugs. *Phytochemistry*, Vol.12, No.1, pp.214-216, ISSN 0031-9422

Betanzos-Cabrera, G., Guerrero-Solano, J.A., Martínez-Pérez, M.M., Calderón-Ramos, Z.G., Belefant-Miller, H. & Cancino-Diaz, J.C. (2011). Pomegranate Juice Increases Levels of Paraoxonase1 (PON1) Expression and Enzymatic Activity in Streptozotocin-induced Diabetic Mice Fed with a High-fat Diet. *Food Research International*, Vol.44, No.5, pp.1381-1385, ISSN 0963-9969

Bialonska, D., Kasimsetty, S.G., Khan, S.I. & Ferreira, D. (2009a). Urolithins, Intestinal Microbial Metabolites of Pomegranate Ellagitannins, Exhibit Potent Antioxidant Activity in a Cell-Based Assay. *Journal of Agricultural and Food Chemistry,* Vol.57, No.21, pp.10181-10186, ISSN 0021-8561

Bialonska, D., Kasimsetty, S.G., Schrader, K.K. & Ferreira, D. (2009b). The Effect of Pomegranate (*Punica granatum* L.) by-products and Ellagitannins on the Growth of Human Gut Bacteria. *Journal of Agricultural and Food Chemistry,* Vol.57, No.18, pp.8344-8349, ISSN 0021-8561

Boateng, J., Verghese, M., Shackleford, L., Walker, L.T., Khatiwada, J., Ogutu, S., Jones, J., Guyton, M., Asiamah, D., Henderson, F., Grant, L., DeBruce, M., Johnson, A., Washington, S. & Chawan, C.B. (2007). Selected Fruits Reduce Azoxymethane (AOM)-induced Aberrant Crypt foci (ACF) in Fisher 344 Male Rats. *Food and Chemical Toxicology,* Vol.45, No.5, pp.725-732, ISSN 0278-6915

Borochov-Neori, H., Judeinstein, S., Tripler, E., Harari, M., Greenberg, A., Shomer, I. & Holland, D. (2009). Seasonal and Cultivar Variations in Antioxidant and Sensory Quality of Pomegranate (*Punica granatum L.*) Fruit. *Journal of Food Composition and Analysis,* Vol.22, No.3, pp.189-195, ISSN 0889-1575

Boukharta, M., Jalbert, G. & Castonguay, A. (1992). Efficacy of Ellagitannins and Ellagic Acid as Cancer Chemo Preventive Agents. *Bulletin of Liaison-Group Polyphenols,* Vol.16, pp.245-249, ISSN 0242-8466

Braga, L.C., Leite, A A.M., Xavier, K.G.S., Takahashi, J.A., Bemquerer, M.P., Chartone-Souza, E., Nascimento, A.M.A. (2005). Synergic Interaction between Pomegranate Extract and Antibiotics against *Staphylococcus aureus. Canadian Journal of Microbiology,* Vol.51, No.7, pp.541-547, ISSN 0008-4166

Chaturvedula, V., Prakash, S. & Prakash, I. (2011). Bioactive Chemical Constituents from Pomegranate (*Punica granatum*) Juice, Seed and Peel-A Review. *International Journal of Research on Chemistry and Environment,* Vol.1, No.1, pp.1-18, ISSN 0306-7319

Chidambara Murthy, K.N., Jayaprakasha, G.K. & Singh, R.P. (2002). Studies on Antioxidant Activity of Pomegranate *(Punica granatum)* Peel Extract Using *in vivo* Models. *Journal of Agricultural and Food Chemistry,* Vol.50, No.17, pp.4791-4795, ISSN 0021-8561

Dahham, S.S., Ali, M.N., Tabassum, H. & Khan, M. (2010). Studies on Antibacterial and Antifungal Activity of Pomegranate (*Punica granatum L.*). *American-Eurasian J. Agric. & Environ. Sci.,* Vol.9, No.3, pp.273-281, ISSN 1818-6769

Dai, Z., Nair, V., Khan, M. & Ciolino, H.P. (2010). Pomegranate Extracts Inhibits the Proliferation and Viability of MMTV-Wnt-1 Mouse Mammary Cancer Stem Cells In vitro. *Oncology Reports,* Vol.24, No.4, pp.1087-1091, ISSN 1021-335X

Das, A.K., Mandal, S.C., Banerjee, S.K., Sinha, S., Das, J., Saha, B.P. & Pal, M. (1999). Studies on Antidiarrheal Activity of *Punica granatum* Seed Extract in Rats. *Journal of Ethnopharmacology,* Vol.68, No.1-3, pp.205-208, ISSN 0378-8741

Dauchet, L., Amouyet, P., & Dallongeville, J. (2005). Fruit and Vegetable Consumption and Risk of Stroke. A Meta-analysis of Cohort Studies. Neurology, Vol.65, No.8, pp.1193-1197, ISSN 0028-3878

Davidson, M.H., Maki, K.C., Dicklin, M.R., Feinstein, S. B., Witchger, M., Bell, M., McGuire, D.K., Provost, J.C., Liker, H., Aviram, M. (2009). Effects of Consumption of

Pomegranate Juice on Carotid Intima–Media Thickness in Men and Women at Moderate Risk for Coronary Heart Disease. *The American Journal of Cardiology,* Vol.104, No.7, pp.936-942, ISSN 0002-9149

de Nigris, F., Williams-Ignarro, S., Botti, C., Sica, V., Ignarro, L.J., Napoli, C. (2006). Pomegranate Juice Reduces Oxidized Low-density Lipoprotein Downregulation of Endothelial Nitric Oxide Synthase in Human Coronary Endothelial Cells. *Nitric Oxide,* Vol.15, No.3, pp.259-63

Dell'Agli, M., Galli, G.V., Corbett, Y., Taramelli, D., Lucantoni, L., Habluetzel, A., Maschi, O., Caruso, D., Giavarini, F., Romeo, S., Bhattacharya, D. & Bosisio, E. (2009). Antiplasmodial Activity of *Punica granatum* L. Fruit Rind. *Journal of Ethnopharmacology,* Vol.125, No.2, pp. 279-285, ISSN 0378-8741

Demirozu, B., Sokmen, M., Ucak, A., Yilmaz, A. & Gulderen, S. (2002). Variation of Copper, Iron and Zinc Levels in Pekmez Products. *Bulletin of Enviromental Contamination and Toxicology,* Vol.69, No.3, pp.330-334, ISSN 1432-0800

Duman, A.D., Ozgen, M., Dayisoylu, K.S., Erbil, N. & Durgac, C. (2009). Antimicrobial activity of six pomegranate (*Punica granatum* L.) varieties and their relation to some of their pomological and phytonutrient characteristics. *Molecules,* Vol.14, No.3, pp.1808-1817, ISSN 1420-3049

Dumas, Y., Dadomo, M., Di Lucca, G. & Grolier, P. (2003). Effects of Environmental Factors and Agricultural Techniques on Antioxidant Content of Tomatoes. *Journal of the Science of Food and Agriculture,* Vol.83, No.5, pp.369-382, ISSN 0022-5142

Dutta, B.K., Rahman, I. & Das, T.K. (1998). Antifungal Activity of Indian Plant Extracts. *Mycoses,* Vol.41, No.11-12, pp. 535-536, ISSN 0933-7407

Elfalleh, W., Nasri, N., Marzougui, N., Thabti, I., M'Rabet, A., Yahya, Y., Lachiheb, B., Guasmi, F. & Ferchichi, A. (2009). Physico-chemical Properties and DPPH-ABTS Scavenging Activity of Some Local Pomegranate (*Punica granatum*) Ecotypes. *International Journal of Food Sciences and Nutrition,* Vol.60, No.s2, pp.197-210, ISSN 0963-7486

El-Nemr, S.E., Ismail, I.A. & Ragab, M. (2006). Chemical Composition of Juice and Seeds of Pomegranate Fruit. *Die Nahrung,* Vol.34, No.7, pp.601-606, ISSN 1613-4133

Endo, E.H., Cortéz, D.A.G., Ueda-Nakamura, T., Nakamura, C.V. & Filho, B.P.D. (2010). Potent Antifungal Activity of Extracts and Pure Compound Isolated from Pomegranate Peels and Synergism with Fluconazole against *Candida albicans. Research in Microbiology,* Vol.161, No.7, pp. 534-540, ISSN 0923-2508

Esmaillzadeh, A., Tahbaz, F., Gaieni, I., Alavi-Majd, H. & Azadbakht, L. (2006). Cholesterol-lowering Effect ot Concentrated Pomegranate Juice Consumption in Type II Diabetic Patients with Hyperlipidemia. *International Journal for Vitamin and Nutrition Reserach,* Vol.76, No.3, pp.147-151, ISSN 0300-9831

Evans, M.D., Dizdaroglu, M. & Cooke, M.S. (2004). Oxidative DNA Damage and Disease: induction, repair and significance. *Mutation Research,* Vol.567, No.1, pp.1-61, ISSN 0027-5107

Fadavi, A., Barzegar, M., Azizi, M.H. & Bayat, M. (2005). Physicochemical Composition of Ten Pomegranate Cultivars (*Punica granatum* L.) Grown in Iran. *Food Science and Technology International,* Vol.11, No.2, pp. 113-119, ISSN 1082-0132

Fadavi, A., Barzegar, M. & Azizi, H.M. (2006). Determination of Fatty Acids and Total Lipid Content in Oilseed of 25 Pomegranates Varieties Grown in Iran. *Journal of Food Composition and Analysis,* Vol.19, No.6-7, pp. 676-680, ISSN 0889-1575

Faria, A. & Calhau, C. (2010). Pomegranate in Human Health: An Overview. In: *Bioactive Foods in Promoting Health: Fruits and Vegetables,* Watson, R.R. & Preedy V.R.(Eds), pp.551-563, ISBN 9780123746283, Elsevier Science

Faria, A. & Calhau, C. (2011). The Bioactivity of Pomegranate: Impact on Health and Disease. *Critical Reviews in Food Science and Nutrition,* Vol.51, No.7, pp.626-634, ISSN 1040-8398

Festa, F., Aglitti, T., Duranti, G., Ricordy, R., Perticone, P. & Cozzi, R. (2001). Strong Antioxidant Activity of Ellagic Acid in Mammalian Cells *in vitro* Revealed by the Comet Assay. *Anticancer Research,* Vol.21, pp. 3903-3908, ISSN 0250-7005

Franco, R., Schoneveld, O., Georgakilas, A. G. & Panayiotidis, M. I. (2008). Oxidative Stress, DNA Methylation and Carcinogenesis. *Cancer Letters,* Vol.266, No.1 , pp.6-12, ISSN 0304-3835.

George, J., Singh, M., Srivastava, A.K., Bhui, K. & Shukla, Y. (2011). Synergistic Growth Inhibition of Mouse Skin Tumors by Pomegranate Fruit Extract and Diallyl sulfide: Evidence for Inhibition of Activated MAPKs/NF-κB and Reduced Cell Proliferation. *Food and Chemical Toxicology,* Vol.49, No.7, pp.1511-1520, ISSN 0278-6915

Gharzouli, K., Khennouf, S., Amira, S. & Gharzouli, A. (1999). Effects of Aqueous Extracts from *Quercus ilex* L. Root Bark, *Punica granatum* L. Fruit Peel and Artemisia Herba-alba Asso Leaves on Ethanol-induced Gastric Damage in Rats. *Phytotheraphy Research,* Vol.13, No.1, pp.42-45, ISSN 0951-418X

Gil, M., Tomas-Barberan, I., Hess-Pierce, F., Holcroft, B., D. M., & Kader, A. (2000). Antioxidant Activity of Pomegranate Juice and its Relationship with Phenolic Composition and Processing. *Journal of Agricultural and Food Chemistry,* Vol.48, No.10, pp. 4581-4589, ISSN 0021-8561

Gouédard, C., Barouki, R. & Morel,Y. (2004). Dietary Polyphenols Increase Paraoxonase 1 Gene Expression by an Aryl Hydrocarbon Receptor-dependent Mechanism. *Molecular and Cellular Biology,* Vol.24, No.12, pp. 5209-5222, ISSN 0270-7306

Gould, S.W., Fielder, M.D., Kelly, A.F., El Sankary, W., & Naughton, D.P. (2009). Antimicrobial Pomegranate Rind Extracts: Enhancement by Cu(II) and Vitamin C Combinations against Clinical Isolates of *Pseudomonas aeruginosa. British Journal of Biomedical Science,* Vol.66, No.3, pp.129-32, ISSN 0967-4845

Grossmann, M.E., Mizuno, N.K., Schuster, T. & Cleary, M.P. (2010). Punicic acid, a Fatty Acid from Pomegranate Seed Oil, Inhibits Breast Cancer Cell Proliferation. *Cancer Prevention Research,* Vol.3, No.1, pp.108-113, ISSN 1940-6207

Gucev, Z.S., Oh, Y., Kelley, K.M. & Rosenfeld, R.G. (1996). Insulin-like Growth Factor Binding Protein 3 MediatesRetinoic acid- and Transforming Growth Factor beta2-induced Growth Inhibition in Human Breast Cancer Cells. *Cancer Research,* Vol.56, No.7, pp.1545-1550, ISSN 0008-5472

Guo, C., Wei, J., Yang, J., Xu, J., Pang, W. & Jiang, Y. (2008). Pomegranate Juice is Potentially Better than Apple Juice in Improving Antioxidant Function in Elderly Subjects. *Nutrition Research,* Vol. 28, No.1, pp. 72-77, ISSN 0271-5317

Gupta, S. & Mukhtar, H. (2002). Chemoprevention of Skin Cancer: Current Status and Future Prospects. *Cancer and Metastasis Reviews,* Vol. 21, No.3-4, pp. 363-380,ISSN 0167-7659

Haidari, M., Ali, M., CasscellsIII, S.W. & Madjid, M. (2009). Pomegranate (*Punica granatum*) Purified Polyphenol Extract Inhibits Influenza Virus and has a Synergistic Effect with Oseltamivir. *Phytomedicine*, Vol.16, No.12, pp.1127-1136, ISSN 0944-7113

Hajimahmoodi, M., Oveisi, M.R., Sadeghi, N., Jannat, B., Hajibabi, M., Farahani, E., Akrami, M.R. & Namdar, R. (2008). Antioxidant Properties of Peel and Pulp Hydro Extract in Ten Persian Pomegranate Cultivars. *Pakistan Journal of Biological Science*, Vol.11, No.12, pp.1600-1604, ISSN 1028-8880

Hamilton, C. A., Miller, W.H., Al-Benna, S., Brosnan, M. J., Drummond, R.D., Mcbride, M.W. & Dominiczak, A.F. (2004). Strategies to Reduce Oxidative Stress in Cardiovascular Disease. *Clinical Science*, Vol.106, No.3, pp.219-234, ISSN 0143-5221

Hartman, R.E., Shah, A. & Fagan, A.M. (2006). Pomegranate Juice Decreases Amyloid Load and Improves Behavior in a Mouse Model of Alzheimer's disease. *Neurobiology of Disease*, Vol.24, No.3, pp.506-515, ISSN 0969-9961

Heber, D. (2008). Multitargeted Therapy of Cancer by Ellagitannins. *Cancer Letters*, Vol.269, No.2, pp.262–268, ISSN 0304-3835

Heinlein, C.A. & Chang, C. (2004). Androgen Receptor in Prostate Cancer. *Endocrine Reviews*, Vol.25, No.2, pp.276-308, ISSN 0163-769X

Holetz, F.B., Pessini, G.L., Sanches, N.R., Cortez, D.A.G., Nakamura, C.V. & Filho, B.P.D. (2002), Screening of Some Plants used in the Brazilian Folk Medicine for the Treatment of Infectious Diseases. *Memorias do Instituto Oswaldo Cruz*, Vol.97, No.7, pp.1027-1031, ISSN 0074-0276

Hong, M.Y., Seeram, N.P. & Heber, D. (2008). Pomegranate Polyphenols Down-regulate Expression of Androgen-synthesizing Genes in Human Prostate Cancer Cells over Expressing the Androgen Receptor. *Journal of Nutritional Biochemistry*, Vol.19, No.12, pp. 848-855, ISSN 0955-2863

Hora, J.J., Maydew, E.R., Lansky, E.P. & Dwivedi, C. (2003). Chemopreventive Effects of Pomegranate Seed Oil on Skin Tumor Development in CD_1 Mice. *Journal of Medicinal Food*, Vol.6, No.3, pp. 157-161, ISSN 1096-620X http://sciyo.com/articles/show/title/wind-power-integrating-wind-turbine-generators-wtg-s-with-energy-storage

Hu, F.B. (2003). Plant-based Foods and Prevention of Cardiovascular Disease: An overview. *The American Journal of Clinical Nutrition*, Vol.78, No.3, pp.544–551, ISSN 0002-9165

Huang, T. H. W., Peng, G., Kota, B. P., Li, G. Q., Yamahara, J., Roufogalis, B. D. & Li, Y. (2005a). Pomegranate Flower Improves Cardiac Lipid Metabolism in a Diabetic Rat Model: Role of Lowering Circulating Lipids. *British Journal of Pharmacology*, Vol.145, No.6, pp. 767-774, ISSN 1746-5381

Huang, T. H. W., Peng, G., Kota, B. P., Li, G. Q., Yamahara, J., Roufogalis, B. D. & Li, Y. (2005b). Antidiabetic Action of *Punica granatum* Flower Extract: Activation of PPAR-gamma and Identification of an Active Component. *Toxicology and Applied Pharmacology*, Vol.207, No.2, pp.160-169, ISSN 0041-008X

Incedayi, B., Tamer, E.C. & Copur, U. (2010). A Research on the Composition of Pomegranate Molasses. *Journal of Agricultural Faculty of Uludag University*, Vol.24, No.2, pp.37-47, ISSN 1301-3165

Jadeja, R.N., Thounaojam, M.C., Patel, D.K., Devkar, R.V., Ramachandran, A.V. (2010). Pomegranate (*Punica granatum* L.) Juice Supplementation Attenuates Isoproterenol-induced Cardiac Nerosis in Rats. *Cardiovascular Toxicology*, Vol. 10, No:3, pp. 174-180, ISSN: 1559-0259

Jafri, M. A., Aslam, M., Javed, K. & Singh, S. (2000). Effect of *Punica granatum Linn.* (flowers) on Blood Glucose Level in Normal and Alloxan-induced Diabetic Rats. *Journal of Ethnopharmacology,* Vol.70, No.3, pp.309-314, ISSN 0378-8741

Jahfar, M., Vijayan, K.K. & Azadi, P. (2003). Studies on a Polysaccharide from the Fruit Rind of *Punica granatum. Research Journal of Chemistry and Environment,* Vol.7, No.1, pp.43-50, ISSN 0972-0626

Jaiswal, V., DerMarderosian, A. & Porter, J.R. (2010). Anthocyanins and Polyphenol Oxidase from Dried Arils of Pomegranate (*Punica granatum L.*). *Food Chemistry,* Vol.118, No.1, pp. 11-16, ISSN 0308-8146

Jang, A., Srinivasan, P., Lee, N.Y., Song, H.P., Lee, J.W., Lee, M. & Jo, C.(2008). Comparison of Hypolipidemic Activity of Synthetic Gallic Acid-Linoleic Acid Ester with Mixture of Gallic Acid and Linoleic Acid, Gallic Acid, and Linoleic Acid on High-fat Diet Induced Obesity in C57BL/6 Cr Slc Mice. *Chemico-biological Interactions* Vol.174, No.2, pp.109-117, ISSN 0009-2797

Jeune, M.A., Kumi-Diaka, J. & Brown, J. (2005). Anticancer Activities of Pomegranate Extracts and Genistein in Human Breast Cancer Cells. *Journal of Medicinal Food,* Vol.8, No.4, pp. 469-475, ISSN 1096-620X

Johann, S., Cisalpino, P.S., Watanabe, G.A., Cota, B.B., de Siqueira, E.P., Pizzolatti, M.G., Zani, C.L. & de Resende, M.A. (2010). Antifungal Activity of Extracts of Some Plants used in Brazilian Traditional Medicine Against the Pathogenic Fungus *Paracoccidioides brasiliensis. Pharmaceutical Biology, Vol.* 48, No.3, pp. 388-396, ISSN 1388-0209

Johanningsmeier, S.D. & Harris, G.K. (2011). Pomegranate as a Functional Food and Nutraceutical Source. *Annual Review of Food Science and Technology,* Vol.2, pp.181-20, ISSN 1941-1413

Jurenka, J.S. (2008). Therapeutic Applications of Pomegranate (*Punica granatum L.*): A Review. *Alternative Medicine Review,* Vol.13, No.2, pp. 128–144, ISSN 1089-5159

Kannel, W.B., Neaton, J.D., Wentworth, D. (1986). Overall and Coronary Heart Disease Mortality Rates in Relation to Major Risk Factors in 325,348 Men Screened for the MRFIT. Multiple Risk Factors Intervention Trial. *American Heart Journal,* Vol.112, No.4, pp:825-836, ISSN 0002-8703

Kaplan, M., Hayek, T., Raz, A., Coleman, R., Dornfeld, L., Vaya, J. & Aviram, M. (2001). Pomegranate Juice Supplementation to Atherosclerotic Mice Reduces Macrophage Lipid Peroxidation, Cellular Cholesterol Accumulation and Development of Atherosclerosis. *Journal of Nutrition,* Vol.131, No.8, pp.2082-2089, ISSN 0022-3166

Kasimsetty, S.G., Bialonska, D., Reddy, M.K., Ma, G., Khan, S.I. & Ferreira, D. (2010). Colon Cancer Chemopreventive Activities of Pomegranate Ellagitannins and Urolithins. *Journal of Agricultural and Food Chemistry,* Vol.58, No.4, pp.2180-2187, ISSN 0021-8561

Kawaii, S. & Lansky, E.P. (2004). Differentiation-promoting Activity of Pomegranate *(Punica granatum)* Fruit Extracts in HL-60 Human Promyelocytic Leukemia Cells. *Journal of Medicinal Food,* Vol.7, No1, pp.13-18, ISSN 1096-620X

Kaya, A. & Sozer, N. (2005). Rheological Behaviour of Sour Pomegranate Juice Concentrates (*Punica granatum L.). International Journal of Food Science and Technology,* Vol.40, No.2, pp.223-227, ISSN 1365-2621

Khan, N., & Mukhtar, H. (2010). Cancer Chemoprevention. In: *Comprehensive Toxicology,* McQueen, C.A. (Ed.) pp.417-431, ISBN 978-0-08-046884-6 Elsevier, UK

Khan, N., Afaq, F. & Mukhtar, H. (2008). Cancer Chemoprevention through Dietary Antioxidants: Progress and Promise. Antioxidants Redox Signaling, Vol.10, No. 3, pp.475–510, ISSN 1523-0864

Khan, N., Afaq, F., Kweon, M.H., Kim, K. & Mukhtar, H. (2007b). Oral Consumption of Pomegranate Fruit Extract Inhibits Growth and Progression of Primary Lung Tumors in Mice. Cancer Research, Vol.67, No.7, pp. 3475-3482, ISSN 0008-5472

Khan, N., Hadi, N., Afaq, F., Syed, D.N., Kweon, M.H. & Mukhtar, H. (2007a). Pomegranate Fruit Extract inhibits Prosurvival Pathways in Human A549 Lung Carcinoma Cells and Tumor Growth in Athymic Nude Mice. Carcinogenesis, Vol.28, No.1, pp.163-173, ISSN 0143-3334

Khan, S.A. (2009). The Role of Pomengranate *(Punica granatum* L.) in Colon Cancer. *Pakistan Journal of Pharmaceutical Science,* Vol.22, No.3, pp. 346-348, ISSN 1011-601X

Khateeb, J., Gantman, A., Kreitenberg, A.J., Aviram, M. & Fuhrman, B. (2010). Paraoxonase 1 (PON1) Expression in Hepatocytes is Upregulated by Pomegranate Polyphenols: A Role for PPAR-gamma Pathway. *Atherosclerosis,* Vol.208, No.1, pp.119-125, ISSN 0021-9150

Kim, H.S., Ingermann, A.R., Tsubaki, J., Twigg, S.M., Walker, G.E. & Oh, Y. (2004). Insulin-like Growth Factor-binding Protein 3 induces Caspase-dependent Apoptosis through a Death Receptor-mediated Pathway in MCF-7 Human Breast Cancer Cells. *Cancer Research*, Vol.64, No.6, pp.2229-2237, ISSN 0008-5472

Kim, N.D., Mehta, R., Yu, W., Neeman, I., Livney, T., Amichay, A., Poirier, D., Nicholls, P., Kirby, A., Jiang, W., Mansel, R., Ramachandran, C., Rabi, T., Kaplan, B. & Lansky, E.. (2002). Chemopreventive and Adjuvant Therapeutic Potential of Pomegranate (*Punica granatum*) for Human Breast Cancer. *Breast Cancer Research Treatment,* Vol.71, No.3, pp.203-217, ISSN 1573-7217

Kohno, H., Suzuki, R., Yasui, Y., Hosokawa, M., Miyashita, K. & Tanaka, T. (2004b). Pomegranate Seed Oil Rch in Conjugated Linolenic Acid Suppresses Chemically Induced Colon Carcinogenesis in Rats. *Cancer Science,* Vol.95, No.6, pp.481-486, ISSN 1347-9032

Kohno, H., Yasui, Y., Suzuki, R., Hosokawa, M., Miyashita, K. & Tanaka, T. (2004a). Dietary Seed Oil Rich in Conjugated Linolenic Acid from Bitter Melon Inhibits Azoxymethane-induced Rat Colon Carcinogenesis through Elevation of Colonic PPAR Gamma Expression and Alteration of Lipid Composition. *International Journal of Cancer,* Vol.110, No.6, pp.896-901, ISSN 0020-7136

Koyama, S., Cobb, L.J., Mehta, H.H., Seeram, N.P., Heber, D., Pantuck, A.J. & Cohen, P. (2010). Pomegranate Extract Induces Apoptosis in Human Prostate Cancer Cells by Modulation of the IGF-IGFBP axis. *Growth Hormone & IGF Research,* Vol.20, No.1, pp.55-62, ISSN 1096-6374

Kryston, T. B., Georgiev, A. & Georgakilas, A.G. (2011). Role of Oxidative Stress and DNA Damage in Human Carcinogenesis. *Mutation Research,* Vol.711, No.1-2, pp.193-201, ISSN 0027-5107

Kulkarni, A. & Aradhya, S.(2005). Chemical Changes and Antioxidant Activity in Pomegranate Arils during Fruit Development. *Food Chemistry,* Vol.90, No.1-2, 319–324, ISSN 0308-8146

Lan, J., Lei, F., Hua, L., Wang, Y., Xing, D. & Du, L. (2009). Transport Behavior of Ellagic Acid of Pomegranate Leaf Tannins and Its Correlation with Total Cholesterol

Alteration in HepG2 cells. *Biomedical Chromatography,* Vol.23, No.5, pp.531-536, ISSN 0913-5685

Lansky, E.P. & Newman, R.A. (2007). *Punica granatum* (pomegranate) and Its Potential for Prevention and Treatment of Inflammation and Cancer. Journal of Ethnopharmacology, Vol.109, No.2, pp.177-206, ISSN 0378-8741

Lansky, E.P., Harrison, G., Froom, P. & Jiang, W.G. (2005a). Pomegranate (*Punica granatum*) Pure Chemicals Show Possible Synergistic Inhibition of Human PC-3 Prostate Cancer Cell Invasion Across Matrigel™. *Investigational New Drugs,* Vol.23, No.2, pp.121-122, ISSN 1573-0646

Lansky, E.P., Jiang, W., Mo, H., Bravo, L., Froom, P., Yu, W., Harris, N.M., Neeman, I., Campbell, M.J. (2005b). Possible Synergistic Prostate Cancer Suppression by Anatomically Discrete Pomegranate Fractions. *Investigational New Drugs,* Vol.23, No.1, pp.11-20, ISSN 1573-0646

Larrosa, M., González-Sarrías, A., Yáñez-Gascón, M.J., Selma, M.V., Azorín-Ortuño, M., Toti, S., Tomás-Barberán, F., Dolara, P. & Espín, J.C. (2010). Anti-inflammatory Properties of a Pomegranate Extract and its Metabolite Urolithin-A in a Colitis Rat Model and the Effect of Colon Inflammation on Phenolic Metabolism. *The Journal of Nutritional Biochemistry,* Vol.21, No.8, pp.717-725, ISSN 0955-2863

Larrosa, M., Tomas-Barberan, F.A., Espin, J.C. (2006).The Dietary Hydrolysable Tanin Punicalagin Releases Ellagic Acid that Induces Apoptosis in Human Colon Adenocarcinoma Caco-2 cells by Using the Mitochondrial Pathway. *The Journal of Nutritional Biochemistry,* Vol.17, No.9, pp. 611-625, ISSN 0955-2863

Lecerf, J.M. (2006) Pasteur Institute - Lille. Functional claims of article 13: Polyphenols in juices. References and Scientific Evidences.

Leckey, L.C., Garige, M., Varatharajalu, R., Gong, M., Nagata, T., Spurney, C.F. & Lakshman, R.M. (2010). Quercetin and Ethanol Attenuate the Progression of Atherosclerotic Plaques with Concomitant up Regulation of Paraoxonase1 (PON1) Gene Expression and PON1 Activity in LDLR-/- Mice. *Alcoholism: Clinical and Experimental Research,* Vol.34, No.9, pp.1535-1542, ISSN 1530-0277

Lee, C.J., Chen, L.G., Liang, W.L. & Wang, C.C. (2010). Anti-inflammatory Effects of *Punica granatum* Linne *in vitro* and *in vivo*. *Food Chemistry,* Vol.118, No.1-2, pp.315-322, ISSN 0308-8146

Lee, S.I., Kim, B.S., Kim, K.S,. Lee, S., Shin, K.S. & Lim, J.S. (2008). Immune-suppressive Activity of Punicalagin via Inhibition of NFAT Activation. *Biochemical and Biophysical Research Communications,* Vol.11, No.371, pp.799-803, ISSN 0006-291X

Lei, F., Zhang, X.N., Wang, W., Xing, D.M., Xie, W.D., Su, H. & Du, L.J. (2007). Evidence of Anti- obesity Effects of the Pomegranate Leaf Extract in High-fat Diet Induced Obese Mice. *International Journal of Obesity,* Vol.31, No.6, pp.1023-1029, ISSN 0307-0565

Li, Y., Guo, C., Yang, J., Wei, J., Xu, J. & Cheng, S. (2006). Evaluation of Antioxidant Properties of Pomegranate Peel Extract in Comparison with Pomegranate Pulp Extract. *Food Chemistry,* Vol.96, No.1-2, pp.254-260, ISSN 0308-8146

Li, Y., Qi, Y., Huang, T.H.W., Yamahara, J. & Roufogalis, B.D. (2008). Pomegranate Flower: A Unique Traditional Antidiabetic Medicine with Dual PPAR-α/-γ Activator Properties. *Diabetes Obesity and Metabolism,* Vol.10, No.1, pp.10-17, ISSN 1463-1326

Liu, J. (1995). Pharmacology of Oleanolic Acid and Ursolic Acid. *Journal of Ethnopharmacology,* Vol.49, No1, pp.57-68, ISSN 0378-8741

Longtin, R. (2003). The Pomegranate: Nature's Power Fruit? *Journal of the National Cancer Institute*, Vol.95, No.5, pp.346-348, ISSN 1460-2105

Machado, T.B., Leal, C.R., Amaral, A.C., Santos, K.R., Silva, M.G. & Kuster, R.M. (2002). Antimicrobial Ellagitannin of *Punica granatum* Fruits. *Journal of the Brazilian Chemical Society*, Vol.13, No.5, pp. 606-610, ISSN 0103-5053

Mackness, B., Mackness, M.I., Durrington, P.N., Arrol, S., Evans, A.E., McMaster, D., Ferrieres, J., Ruidavets, J.B., Williams, N.R. & Howard, A.N. (2000). Paraoxonase activity in two healthy populations with differing rates of coronary heart disease. *European Journal of Clinical Investigation*, Vol.30, No.1, pp.4–10, ISSN 0014-2972

Mackness, M. I., Mackness, B. M., & Durrington, P. N. (2002). Paraoxonase and Coronary Heart Disease. *Atherosclerosis Supplements*, 3, pp.49-55, ISSN 0021-9150

Madihassan, S. (1984). Outline of the Beginning of Alchemy and Its Antecedents. *American Journal of Chinese Medicine*, Vol.12, No.1, pp.32-42, ISSN 0192-415X

Maestre, J., Melgarejo, P., Tomas-Barberan, F.A. & Garcia-Viguera, C. (2000). New food products derived from pomegranate. In: *Production, Processing and Marketing of Pomegranate in the Mediterranean Region: Advances in Research and Technology*, P. Melgarejo-Moreno, J.J. Martínez-Nicolás and J. Martínez-Tomé, (Eds.), pp. 243–245, ISBN 2-85352-214-8 CIHEAM-IAMZ, Zaragoza.

Malik, A., Afaq, F., Sarfaraz, S., Adhami, V.M., Sved, D.N. & Mukhtar, H. (2005). Pomegranate Fruit Juice for Chemoprevention and Chemotherapy of Prostate Cancer. *Proceedings of the National Academy of Sciences USA*, Vol.102, No.40, pp.14813-14818, ISSN 1091-6490

Malik, A., Afaq, S., Shahid, M., Akhtar, K. & Assiri, A. (2011). Influence of Ellagic acid on Prostate Cancer Cell Proliferetion: A Caspase-Dependent Pathway. *Asian Pacific Journal of Tropical Medicine*, Vol.4, No.7, pp. 550-555, ISSN 1995-7645

Martin, O.A., Redon, C., Nakamura, A J., Dickey, J.S., Georgakilas, A.G. & Bonner, W.M. (2011). Systemic DNA Damage Related to Cancer. *Cancer Research*, Vol.71, No.10, pp.1-5, ISSN 0304-3835

Maskan, A., Kaya, S. & Maskan, M. (2002). Effect of Concentration and Drying Hot-Air and Microwave Drying. *Journal of Food Engineering*, Vol. 48, No.2, pp.169-175, ISSN 0260-8774

Mathabe, M.C., Nikolova, R., Lall, V.N. & Nyazema, N.Z. (2006). Antibacterial Activities of Medicinal Plants used for the Treatment of Diarrhoea in Limpopo Province, South Africa. *Journal of Ethnopharmacology*, Vol.105, No.2, pp.286-293, ISSN 0378-8741

McCarrell, E.M., Gould, S.W.J., Fielder, M.D., Kelly, A.F., Sankary, W.E. & Naughton, D.P. (2008). Antimicrobial Activities of Pomegranate Rind Extracts: Enhancement by Addition of Metal Salts and Vitamin C. *BMC Complementary and Alternative Medicine*, Vol.8, No.1, pp.64-70, ISSN 1472-6882

McCutcheon, A., Udani, J. & Brown, D.J. (2008). Proprietary Botanical Food Product, Scientific and Clinical Monograph for POM Wonderful® Pomegranate Juice. American Botanical Council. 20p. www.herbalgram.org

Mehta, R. & Lansky, E.P. (2004). Breast Cancer Chemopreventive Properties of Pomegranate (*Punica granatum*) Fruit Extracts in a Mouse Mammary Organ Culture. *European Journal of Cancer Prevention*, Vol.13, No.4, pp.345-355, ISSN 0959-8278

Melgarejo, P. & Artes, F. (2000). Organic Acids and Sugar Composition of Pomegranate Juice. *European Food Research Technology*, Vol.4, No.1, pp.30-31, ISSN 1438-2377

Menezes, S.M., Cordeiro, L.N. & Viana, G.S. (2006). *Púnica granatum* (pomegranate) Extract is Active Against Dental Plaque. *Journal of herbal pharmacotherapy,* Vol.6, No.1, pp.79-92, ISSN 1522-8940

Mertens-Talcott, S.U. & Percival, S.S. (2005). Ellagic Acid and Quercetin Interact Synergistically with Resveratrol in the Induction of Apoptosis and Cause Transient Cell Cycle Arrest in Human Leukemia Cells. *Cancer Letters,* Vol. 218, No.2, pp.141-51, ISSN 0304-3835

Miguel M.M., Neves, M.A. & Antunes, M.D. (2010). Pomegranate (*Punica granatum* L.): A medicinal Plant with Myriad Biological Properties - A Short Review. *The Journal of Medicinal Plants Research,* Vol. 4, No.25, pp. 2836-2847, ISSN 1996-0875

Miguel, M.G., Dandlen, S. & Neves, M.A. (2009). Antioxidant Activities of Flower Extract and Pomegranate Juice. *Acta Horticulturae (ISHS),* Vol.818, pp.389-394, ISSN 0567-7572

Mirdehghan, S.H. & Rahemi, M. (2007). Seasonal Changes of Mineral Nutrients and Phenolics in Pomegranate (*Punica granatum* L.) Fruit. *Scientia Horticulturae,* Vol.111, No.2, pp.120-127., ISSN 0304-4238

Mirmiran, P., Noori, N., Zavareh, M.B. & Azizi, F. (2009). Fruit and Vegetable Consumption and Risk Factors for Cardiovascular Disease. *Metabolism Clinical and Experimental,* Vol.58, No.4, pp.460-468, ISSN 0026-0495

Mooradian, A.D. (2009). Dyslipidemia in Type 2 Diabetes Mellitus. *Nature Clinical Practice Endocrinology & Metabolism,* Vol.5, No.3, pp. 150-159, ISSN 1745-8366

Mousavinejad, G., Emam-Djomeh, Z., Rezaei, K., Khodaparast, M.H.H. (2009). Identification and Quantification of Phenolic Compounds and Their Effects on Antioxidant Activity in Pomegranate Juices of Eight Iranian Cultivars. *Food Chemistry,* Vol.115, No.4, pp.1274-1278, ISSN 0308-8146

Mukhtar, H. & Ahmad, N. (1999). Cancer chemoprevention: Future Holds in Multiple Agents. *Toxicology and Applied Pharmacology,* Vol.158, No.3, pp.207-210, ISSN 0041-008X

Murthy, K.N.C., Jayaprakasha, G.K. & Singh, R.P. (2002). Studies on Antioxidant Activity of Pomegranate (*Punica granatum*) Peel Extract Using *in vivo* Models. *Journal of Agricultural and Food Chemistry,* Vol.50, No.17, pp. 4791-4795, ISSN 0021-8561

Murthy, K.N.C., Reddy, K.V. & Veigas, J.M. (2004). Study on Wound Healing Activity of *Punica granatum* peel. *Journal of Medicinal Food,* Vol.7, No.2, pp.256-259, ISSN 1096-620X

Narr Ben, C., Ayed, N. & Metche, M. (1996). Quantitative Determination of the Polyphenolic Content of Pomegranate Peel. *Zeitschrift für Lebensmittel-Untersuchung und –Forschung,* Vol.203, pp. 374-378, ISSN 1438-2377

Nathan, C. (2006). Neutrophils and Immunity: Challenges and Opportunities. *Nature Reviews of Immunology,* Vol.6, No.3, pp.173-82, ISSN 1474-1733

Nishikawa, M. (2008). Reactive Oxygen Species in Tumor Metastasis. *Cancer Letters,* Vol.266, No.1, pp.53-59, ISSN 0304-3835

Noda, Y., Kaneyuka, T., Mori, A. & Packer, L. (2002). Antioxidant Activities of Pomegranate Fruit Extract and Its Anthocyanidins: Delphinidin, Cyanidin, and Pelargonidin. *Journal of Agricultural and Food Chemistry,* Vol.50, No.1, pp.166-171, ISSN 0021-8561

Nothlings, U., Schulze, M. B., Weikert, C., Boeing, H., van der Schouw, Y. T., Bamia, C., Benetou, V., Lagiou, P., Krogh, V., Beulens, J. W., Peeters, P. H., Halkjaer, J., Tjonneland, A., Tumino, R., Panico, S., Masala, G., Clavel-Chapelon, F., de, Lauzon

B., Boutron-Ruault, M. C., Vercambre, M. N., Kaaks, R., Linseisen, J., Overvad, K., Arriola, L., Ardanaz, E., Gonzalez, C. A., Tormo, M. J., Bingham, S., Khaw, K. T., Key, T. J., Vineis, P., Riboli, E., Ferrari, P., Boffetta, P., Bueno-de-Mesquita, H. B., van der, A. DL, Berglund, G., Wirfalt, E., Hallmans, G., Johansson, I., Lund, E., & Trichopoulo, A. (2008). Intake of vegetables, legumes, and fruit, and risk for all-cause, cardiovascular, and cancer mortality in a European diabetic population. *The Journal of Nutrition*, Vol.138, No.4, pp.775-781, ISSN 0022-3166

Okamoto, T., Akuta, T., Tamura, F., Van Der Vliet, A., & Akaike, T. (2004).Molecular Mechanism for Activation and Regulation of Matrix Metalloproteinases during Bacterial Infections and Respiratory Inflammation. *Biological Chemistry,* Vol.385, No.11, pp.997-1006, ISSN 1431-6730

Opara, L.U., Al-ani, M.R. & Al-Shuaibi, Y.S. (2009). Physico-chemical Properties, Vitamin C Content, and Antimicrobial Properties of Pomegranate Fruit (*Punica granatum* L.). *Food Bioprocess Technology,* Vol. 2, No.3. pp.315-321, ISSN 1935-5130

Orak, H.H., Demirci, S., Gumus, T. (2011). Antibacterial and Antifungal Activity of Pomegranate (*Punica granatum* l.cv.) Peel. *Electronic Journal of Environmental, Agricultural and Food Chemistry,* Vol.10, No.3, pp. 1958-1969, ISSN 1579-4377

Oswa, T., Ide, A., Su, J.D., & Namiki, M. (1987). Inhibiting of Lipid Peroxidation by Ellagic Acid. *Journal of Agricultural and Food Chemistry,* Vol.35, No.5, pp.808-812, ISSN 0021-8561

Ou, H.C., Lee, W.J., Lee, S.D., Huang, C.Y., Chiu, T.H., Tsai, K.L., Hsu, W.C., Sheu, W. H.H. (2010). Ellagic Acid Protects Endothelial Cells from Oxidized Low-density Lipoprotein-induced Apoptosis by Modulating the PI3K/Akt/eNOS Pathway. *Toxicology and Applied Pharmacology,* Vol.248, No.2, pp.134-143, ISSN 0041-008X

Ovesná, Z., Vachálková, A., Horváthová, K., & Tóthová, D. (2004). Pentacyclic Triterpenoic Acids: New Chemoprotective Compounds Minireview. *Neoplasma,* Vol.51, pp.327-333, ISSN 1337-9569

Ozcan, T., Akpinar-Bayizit, A., Yilmaz-Ersan, L., Delikanli. B. & Yildiz, E. (2011). Bioavailability of Food Polyphenols. *International Food Congress-Novel Approaches in Food Industry,* İzmir, Turkiye, 26-29 May, 2011

Ozgen, M., Durgac, C., Serce, S. & Kaya, C. (2008). Chemical and Antioxidant Properties of Pomegranate Cultivars Grown in the Mediterranean Region of Turkey. *Food Chemistry,* Vol.11. No.3, pp.703-706, ISSN 0308-8146

Ozgul-Yucel, S. (2005). Determination of Conjugated Linolenic Acid Content of Selected Oil Seeds Grown in Turkey. *Journal of the American Oil Chemists' Society,* Vol.82, No.12, pp.893-897, ISSN 1558-9331

Pacheco-Palencia, L.A., Noratto, G., Hingorani, L., Talcott, S.T. & Mertens-Talcott, S.U. (2008). Protective Effects of Standardized Pomegranate (*Punica granatum* L.) Polyphenolic Extract in Ultraviolet-irradiated Human Skin Fibroblasts. *Journal of Agricultural and Food Chemistry,* Vol.56, No.18, pp.8434-8441, ISSN 0021-8561

Paladini, A.C., Marder, M., Viola, H., Wolfman, C., Wasowski, C. & Medina, J.H. (1999). Flavonoids and the Central Nervous System: from Forgotten Factors to Potent Anxiolytic Compounds. *The Journal of Pharmacy and Pharmacology,* Vol.51, No.5, pp.519-526, ISSN 2042-7158

Pande, G. & Akoh, C.C. (2009). Antioxidant Capacity and Lipid Characterization of Six Georgia- Grown Pomegranate Cultivars. *Journal of Agricultural and Food Chemistry,* Vol.57, No.20, pp.9427-9436, ISSN 0021-8561

Panichayupakaranant, P., Tewtrakul, S., Yuenyongsawad, S. (2010). Antibacterial, Anti-inflammatory and Anti-allergic Activities of Standardized Pomegranate Rind Extract. *Food Chemistry*, Vol.123, No.1, pp. 400-403, ISSN 0308-8146

Pantuck, A.J., Leppert, J.T., Zomorodian, N., Aronson, W., Hong, J., Barnard, R.J., Seeram, N., Liker, H., Wang, H., Elashoff, R., Heber, D., Aviram, M., Ignarro, L. & Belldegrun, A. (2006). Phase II Study of Pomegranate Juice for Men with Rising Prostate-specific Antigen following Surgery or Radiation for Prostate Cancer. *Clinical Cancer Research*, Vol.12. No.13, pp.4018-4026, ISSN 1557-3265

Parashar, A., Gupta, C., Gupta, S.K. & Kumar, A. (2009). Antimicrobial Ellagitannin from Pomegranate (*Punica granatum*) Fruits. *International Journal of Fruit Science*, Vol. 9, No.3, pp.226-231, ISSN 1553-8621

Park, H.M.., Moon, E., Kim, A.J., Kim, M.H., Lee, S., Lee, J.B., Park, Y.K., Jung, H.S., Kim, Y.B. & Kim, S.Y. (2010). Extract of Punica granatum Inhibits Skin Photoaging Induced by UVB Irradiation. *International Journal of Dermatology*, Vol.49, No.3, pp.276-282, ISSN 1365-4632

Perez-Vicente, A., Gil-Izquierdo, A. & Garcia-Viguera, C. (2002). *In vitro* Gastrointestinal Digestion Study of Pomegranate Juice Phenolic compounds, Anthocyanins, and Vitamin C. *Journal of Agricultural and Food Chemistry*, Vol.50, No.8, pp.2308-2312, ISSN 0021-8561

Petti, S. & Scully, C. (2009). Polyphenols, Oral Health and Disease: A Review. *Journal of Dentistry*, Vol.37, No.6, pp.413-423, ISSN 0300-5712

Poyrazoglu ,E., Gokmen, V. & Artik, N. (2002). Organic Acids and Phenolic Compounds in Pomegranates (*Punica granatum* L.) Grown in Turkey. *Journal of Food Composition and Analysis*, Vol.15, No.5, pp.567-575, ISSN 0889-1575

Prashanth, D.J., Asha, M.K. & Amit, A. (2001). Antibacterial Activity of *Punica granatum*. Fitoterapia, Vol.72, No.2, pp.171-173, ISSN 0367-326X

Pruthi, J.S. & Saxena, A.K. (1984). Studies on Anardana (dried pomegranate seeds). *Journal of Food Science and Technology*, Vol.21, No.5, pp.296, ISSN 0022-1155

Raffo, A., La Malfa, G., Fogliano, V., Madani, G. & Quaglia, G. (2006). Seasonal Variations in Antioxidant Components of Cherry Tomatoes (*Lyco-persicon esculentum* cv. Naomi F1). *Journal of Food Composition and Analysis*, Vol.19, No.1, pp.11-19, ISSN 0889-1575

Rahman, M.A., Amin, A.R.M.R., Shin. D.M. (2010). Chemopreventive Potential of Natural Compounds in Head and Neck Cancer. *Nutrition and Cancer*, Vol.62, No.7, pp.973-987, ISSN 0163-5581

Rajah, R., Valentinis, B. & Cohen, P. (1997). Insulin-like Growth Factor (IGF)-binding protein-3 induces Apoptosis and Mediates the Effects of Transforming Growth Factor-beta1 on Programmed Cell Death through a p53- and IGF-independent Mechanism. *Journal of Biological Chemistry*, Vol.272, No.18, pp.12181-12188, ISSN 0021-9258

Rakoff-Nahoum, S. (2006). Why Cancer and Inflammation? *Yale Journal of Biology and Medicine*, Vol.79, No.3-4, pp. 123-130, ISSN 0044-0086

Rettig, M.B., Heber, D., An, J., Seeram, N.D., Rao, J.Y., Liu, H., Klatte, T., Belldegrun, A., Moro, A., Henning, S.M., Mo, D., Aronson, W.J. & Pantuck, A. (2008). Pomegranate Extract Inhibits Androgen-independent Prostate Cancer Growth through a NuclearFactor-κB-dependent Mechanism. *Molecular Cancer Therapeutics*, Vol.7, No.9, pp.2662-2671, ISSN 1538-8514

Richmond, E. & Viner, J.L. (2003). Chemoprevention of Skin Cancer. *Seminars in Oncology Nursing*, Vol.19, No.1, pp.62-69. ISSN: 0749-2081

Rosenblat, M., Draganov, D., Watson, C.E., Bisgaier, C.L., La Du, B.N. & Aviram, M. (2003). Mouse Macrophage Paraoxonase 2 Activity is Increased whereas Cellular Paraoxonase 3Activity is Decreased under Oxidative Stress. *Arteriosclerosis, Thrombosis and Vascular Biology*, Vol.1, No.23, pp.468-474, ISSN 1079-5642

Rosenblat, M., Volkova, N., Coleman, R. & Aviram, M. (2006). Pomegranate by Product Administration to Apoiipoprotein e-deficient Mice Attenuates Atherosclerosis Development as a Result on Decreased Macrophage Oxidative Stress and Reduced Cellular Uptake of Oxidized low-density Lipoprotein. *Journal of Agricultural and Food Chemistry*, Vol.54, No.4, pp.1928-1935, ISSN 0021-8561

Rozenberg, O., Rosenblat, M., Coleman, R., Shih, D.M., & Aviram, M. (2003). Paraoxonase (PON1) Deficiency is Associated with Increased Macrophage Oxidative Stress Studies in PON1-knockout Mice. *Free Radical Biology & Medicine*, Vol.34, No.6, pp.774−784, ISSN 0891-5849

Sadeghi, N., Jannat, B., Oveisi, M.R., Hajimahmoodi, M. & Photovat, M. (2009). Antioxidant Activity of Iranian Pomegranate (*Punica granatum* L.) Seed Extracts. *Journal of Agriculture, Science and Technology*, Vol.11, Supplementary Issue, pp.633-638, ISSN 1680-7073

Salgado, L., Melgarejo, P., Meseguer, I. & Sánchez, M. (2009). Antimicrobial Activity of Crude Extracts from Pomegranate (*Punica granatum* L.). *Acta Horticulturae*, Vol.818, pp.257-264, ISSN 0567-7572

Santos, E.B., Dantas, G.S., Santos, H.B., Diniz, M.F.F.M. & Sampaio, F.C. (2009). Ethnobotanical Study of Medicinal Plants for Oral Health Problems in the City of Joao Pessoa, Brazil. *Brazilian Journal of Pharmacognosy*, Vol.19, No.1b, pp.321-324, ISSN 0102-695X

Sartippour, M.R., Seeram, N.P., Rao, J.Y., Moro, A., Harris, D.M., Henning, S.M., Firouzi, A., Rettig, M.B., Aronson, W.J., Pantuck, A.J. & Heber, D. (2008). Ellagitannin-rich Pomegranate Extract Inhibits Angiogenesis in Prostate Cancer *in vitro* and *in vivo*. *International Journal of Oncology*, Vol. 32, No.2, pp.475-480, ISSN 1791-2423

Sastravaha, G., Yotmicngnit, P., Booncong, P. & Sangrherapicikul, P. (2003). Adjunctive Periodontal Treatment with *Centella asiática* and *Punica granatum* Extracts. A Preliminary Study. *Journal of the International Academy of Periodontology*, Vol.5, No.2, pp.106-115, ISSN 1466-2094

Schubert, S.Y., Lansky, E.P. & Necman, I. (1999). Antioxidant and Eicosanoid Enzyme Inhibition Properties of Pomegranate Seed Oil and Fermented Juice Flavonoids. *Journal of Ethnopharmacology*, Vol.66, No.1, pp.11-17, ISSN 0378-8741

Sedelnikova, O.A., Redon, C.E., Dickey, J.S., Nakamura, A. J., Georgakilas, A.G. & Bonner, W.M. (2010). Role of Oxidatively Induced DNA Lesions in Human Pathogenesis. *Mutation Research*, Vol.704, No.1-3, pp.152-159, ISSN 0027-5107

Seeram, N.P., Adams, L.S., Henning, S.M., Niu, Y., Zhang, Y., Nair, M.G. & Heber, D. (2005). In vitro Antiproliferative, Apoptotic and Antioxidant Activities of Punicalagin, Ellagic acid and a Total Pomegranate Tannin Extract are Enhanced in Combination with Other Polyphenols as Found in Pomegranate Juice. *Journal of Nutritional Biochemistry*, Vol.16, No.6, pp.360-367, ISSN 0955-2863

Seeram, N.P., Henning, S.M., Zhang, Y., Suchard, M., Li, Z. & Heber, D. (2006). Pomegranate Juice Ellagitannin Metabolites are Present in Human Plasma and Some Persist in

Urine for up to 48 hours. *Journal of Nutrition*, Vol.136, No.10, pp.2481-2485, ISSN 0022-3166

Seppi, A. & Franciosi, A. (1980). Chemical Composition of Pomegranate Juice (*Punica granatum*): Amino Acid Contents. *Rivista della Società Italiana di Scienze dell'Alimentazione*, Vol.9, pp.211-212, ISSN 0391-4887

Sharma, M., Li, L., Celver, J., Killian, C., Kovoor, A. & Seeram, N.P. (2010). Effects of Fruit Ellagitannin Extracts, Ellagic Acid, and Their Colonic Metabolite, Urolithin A, on Wnt Signaling. *Journal of Agricultural and Food Chemistry*, Vol.58, No.7, pp. 3965-3969, ISSN 0021-8561

Shukla, M., Gupta, K., Rasheed, Z., Khan, K.A., & Haqqi, T.M. (2008). Bioavailable Constituents/metabolites of Pomegranate (*Punica granatum L*) preferentially Inhibit COX2 Activity ex vivo and IL-1beta-induced PGE2 Production in Human Chondrocytes in vitro. *Journal of Inflammation* (Lond), Vol.5, No.1, pp.9-19, ISSN 1078-7852

Singh, A. & Singh, P.K. (2009). An ethnobotanical study of medicinal plants in Chandauli district of Uttar Pradesh, India. *Journal of Ethnopharmacology*, Vol.121, No.2, pp 324-329, ISSN 0378-8741

Singh, D. & Sethi, V. (2003). Screening of Pomegranate Genotypes for the Preparation of Quality Grade Anardana. *Journal of Food Science and Technology*, Vol.40, No.2, pp.236-238, ISSN 0022-1155

Singh, D. & Singh, R.K. (2004). Processed Products of Pomegranate. *Natural Product Radiance.* Vol.3, No.2, pp.66-68, ISSN 0972-592X

Singh, R.P., Gupta, A.K. & Bhatia, A.K. (1990). Utilization of Wild Pomegranate in North-west Himalayas-Status and Problems. In:*Proc Nat Semi Production and Marketing of Indigenius Fruits*, pp.100-107, New Delhi, India.

Sivarajan, V.V. & Balachandran, I. (1994). *Ayurvedic Drugs and Their Plant Sources*. Oxford and IBH Publishing Co. Pvt. Ltd., ISBN 9788120408289, New Delhi, India

Sturgeon, S.R. & Ronnenberg, A.G. (2010). Pomegranate and Breast Cancer: Possible Mechanisms of Prevention. *Nutrition Reviews*, Vol.68, No.2, pp.122–128, ISSN 0029-6643

Su, X., Sangster, M.Y. & D'Souza, D.H. (2010). *In vitro* Effects of Pomegranate Juice and Pomegranate Polyphenols on Foodborne Viral Surrogates. *Foodborne Pathogens and Dis*ease, Vol.7, No.12, pp.1473-1479, ISSN 1535-3141

Sumner, M.D., Elliott-Eller, M., Weidner, G., Daubenmier, J.J., Chew, M.H., Marlin, R., Raisin, C.J. & Ornish, D. (2005). Effects of Pomegranate Juice Consumption on Myocardial Perfusion in Patients with Coronary Heart Disease. *The American Journal of Cardiology*, Vol.96, No.6, pp. 810-814, ISSN 0002-9149

Surh, Y.J. (2003). Cancer Chemoprevention with Dietary Phytochemicals. *Nature Reviews Cancer*, Vol.3, No.10, pp.768-780, ISSN 1474-175X

Suzuki, R., Noguchi, R., Ota, T., Abe, M., Miyashita, K.. & Kawada, T. (2001). Cytotoxic Effect of Conjugated Trienoic Fatty Acids on Mouse Tumor and Human Monocytic Leukemia Cells. *Lipids*, Vol.36, No.5, pp. 477-482, ISSN 0024-4201

Syed, D.N., Afaq, F. & Mukhtar, H. (2007). Pomegranate Derived Products for Cancer Chemoprevention. *Seminars in Cancer Biology*, Vol.17, No.5, pp.377-385, ISSN 1044-579X

Syed, D.N., Malik, A., Hadi, N., Sarfaraz, S., Afaq, F. & Mukhtar, H. (2006). Photo-chemopreventive Effect of Pomegranate Fruit Extract on UVA-mediated Activation of Cellular Pathways in Normal Human Epidermal Keratinocytes. *Photochemistry Photobiology,* Vol.82, No.2, pp.398-405, ISSN 0031-8655

Tayel, A.A. & El-Tras, W.F. (2009). Anticandidal Activity of Pomegranate Peel Extract Aerosol as an Applicable Sanitizing Method. *Mycoses,* Vol.52, No.2, pp.117-122, ISSN 0933-7407

Teodoro, T., Zhang, L., Alexander, T., Yue, J., Vranic, M. & Volchuk, A. (2008). Oleanolic Acid Enhances Insulin Secretion in Pancreatic b-cells. *FEBS Letters,* Vol.582, No.9, pp.1375-1380, ISSN 0014-5793

Tezcan, F., Gultekin-Ozguven, M., Diken, T., Ozcelik, B. & Erim, F.B. (2009). Antioxidant Activity and Total Phenolic, Organic Acid and Sugar Content in Commercial Pomegranate Juices. *Food Chemistry,* Vol.115, No.3, pp.873-877, ISSN 0308-8146

Thresiamma, K.C. & Kuttan, R. (1996). Inhibition of Liver Fibrosis by Ellagic Acid. *Indian Journal of Physiology and Pharmacology,* Vol.40, pp.363-366, ISSN 0019-5499

Toi, M., Bando, H., Ramachandran, C., Melnick, S.J., Imai, A., Fife, R.S., Carr, R.E., Oikawa, T. & Lansky, E.P. (2003) Preliminary Studies on the Anti-angiogenic Potential of Pomegranate Fractions in vitro and in vivo. *Angiogenesis* Vol.6, No.2, pp. 121-128, ISSN 0969-6970

Toor, R.K., Savage, G.P. & Lister, C.E. (2006). Seasonal Variations in the Antioxidant Composition of Greenhouse-grown Tomatoes. *Journal of Food Composition and Analysis,* Vol.19, No.1, pp.1-10, ISSN 0889-1575

Tran, H.N.A., Bae, S-Y., Song, B-H., Lee, B-H., Bae, Y-S., Kim, Y-H., Lansky, E.P. & Newman, R.A. (2010). Pomegranate (*Punica granatum*) Seed Linolenic Acid Isomers: Concentration-dependent Modulation of Estrogen Receptor Activity. *Endocrine Research,* Vol.35, No.1, pp.1-16, ISSN 0743-5800

Tsuyuki, H., Ito, S. & Nakatsukasa, Y. (1981). Lipids in Pomegranate Seeds. *Nihon Daigaku No-Juigakubu Gakujutsu Kenkyu Hokoku,* Vol.38, pp.141-148, ISSN 0016-5964

Turk, G., Sonmez, M., Aydin, M., Yuce, A., Gur, S., Yuksel, M., Aksu, E.H. & Aksoy, H. (2008). Effects of Pomegranate Juice Consumption on Sperm Quality, Spermatogenic Cell Density, Antioxidant Activity and Testosterone Level in Male Rats. *Clinical Nutrition,* Vol.27, No.2, pp.289-296, ISSN 0261-5614

Van Elswijk, D.A., Schobel, U.P., Lansky, E.P., Irth, H. & van der Greef, J. (2004). Rapid Dereplication of Estrogenic Compounds in Pomegranate (*Punica granatum*) using on-line Biochemical Detection Coupled to Mass Spectrometry. *Phytochemistry,* Vol.65, No.2, pp.233-241, ISSN 0031-9422

Vardin, H. & Abbasoglu, M. (2004). Nar Eksisi ve Narin Diger Degerlendirme Olanaklari. *Geleneksel Gidalar Sempozyumu,* Van, Turkiye, 23-24 September

Viuda-Martos, M., Fernández-López, J. & Pérez-Álvarez, J.A. (2010). Pomegranate and Many Functional Components as Related to Human Health: A Review. *Comprehensive Reviews in Food Science and Food Safety,* Vol.9, No.6, pp.635-654, ISSN 1541-4337

Voravuthikunchai, S.P. & Limsuwan, S. (2006). Medicinal Plant Extracts as anti-Escherichia coli O157:H7 Agents and their Effects on Bacterial Cell Aggregation. *Journal of Food Protection,* Vol.69, No.10, pp.2336-2341, ISSN 0362-028X

Wang, R., Ding, Y., Liu, R., Xiang, L. & Du, L. (2010). Pomegranate: Constituents, Bioactivities and Pharmacokinetics. In: *Fruit, Vegetable and Cereal Science and Biotechnology,* da Silva, J.A.T. (Ed), pp. 77-87, ISSN 1752-3419, Global Science Books

Wang, R., Wang, W., Wang, L., Liu, R., Ding, Y. & Du, L. (2006). Constituents of the Flowers of *Punica granatum*. *Fitoterapia*, Vol. 77, No. 7-8, pp. 534-537, ISSN: 0367-326X

Whitley, A.C., Stoner, G.D., Darby, M.V. & Walle, T. (2003). Intestinal Epithelial Cell Accumulation of the Cancer Preventive Polyphenol Ellagic acid—Extensive binding to Protein and DNA. *Biochemical Pharmacology*, Vol.15, No.66, pp.907-915, ISSN 0006-2952

Xu, K.Z., Zhu, C., Kim, M.S., Yamahara, J., Li, Y. (2009). Pomegranate Flower Ameliorates Fatty Liver in an Animal Model of Type 2 Diabetes and Obesity. *Journal of Ethnopharmacology*, Vol.123, No.2, pp.280-287, ISSN 0378-8741

Yilmaz, C. (2007). *Nar*. ISBN 978-975-8377-52-2, Hasad Yayıncilik, Istanbul, Turkiye

Yun, J.W. (2010). Possible Anti-obesity Therapeutics from Nature–A review. *Phytochemistry*, Vol. 71, No.14-15, pp. 1625-1641, ISSN 0031-9422

Zaid, M.A., Afaq, F., Khan, N. & Mukhtar, H. (2007). Protective Effects of Pomegranate derived Products on UVB-induced DNA Damage, PCNA Expression and MMPs in Human Reconstituted Skin. *Journal of Investigative Dermatology*, Vol.127, No.1, pp.143-153, ISSN 0022-202X

Zand, R.S., Jenkins, D.J. & Diamandis, E.P. (2000). Steroid Hormone Activity of Flavonoids and Related Compounds, *Breast Cancer Research and Treatment*, Vol.62, No1, pp.35-49, ISSN 0167-6806

Zarei, M., Azizi, M. & Bashir-Sadr, Z. (2011). Evaluation of Physicochemical Characteristics of Pomegranate (*Punica granatum L.*) Fruit during Ripening. *Fruits*, Vol.66, No.2, pp.121-129, ISSN 0248-129

Zhang, L., Fu, Q. & Zhang, Y. (2011). Composition of Antociyanins in Pomegranate Flowers and their Antioxidant Activity. *Food Chemistry*, Vol.127, No.3, pp.1444-1449, ISSN 0308-8146

Ziech, D., Franco, R., Georgakilas, A.G., Georgakila, S., Malamou-Mitsi, V., Schoneveld, O., Pappa, A. & Panayiotidis, M.I. (2010). The Role of Reactive Oxygen Species and Oxidative Stress in Environmental Carcinogenesis and Biomarker Development. *Chemico-Biological Interactions*, Vol.188, No.2, pp.334-339, ISSN 0009-2797

Section 3

Strategies for Treatment and Advances from the Clinic

14

Strategic Communication for Cancer Prevention and Control: Reaching and Influencing Vulnerable Audiences

Gary L. Kreps
George Mason University
USA

1. Introduction

Strategic health communication efforts can help reduce cancer risks, incidence, morbidity and mortality, and improve quality of life for at-risk populations. However, providing relevant information about cancer prevention and control to vulnerable populations is fraught with difficulties. Just the ability to get members of at-risk populations to pay attention to information provided about cancer can often be a challenge. Most people do not want to hear or think about cancer unless they are forced into it because they or someone they care about has been diagnosed with some form of the dreaded disease. Since the term "cancer" is surrounded by a significant stigma in modern society that equates cancer with death and suffering, communication about cancer makes many people uncomfortable, forcing them to think about their potential to suffer and die.[1] Strategic cancer prevention and control communication campaigns should be designed to overcome the pervasive social stigma that influences public attitudes towards cancer education.

The good news for health communicators is that the extremely negative social stigma surrounding cancer as an unavoidably deadly disease does not reflect the reality of cancer care in the modern world. Increasingly, those who are diagnosed with cancers are able to get helpful treatments and live productive lives as cancer survivors. Some public health scholars have suggested that with the advent of viable cancer treatments, cancer is becoming a chronic, rather than a terminal, disease due to increases in long-term cancer survivorship.[1] There are also many good evidence-based health promotion strategies available to help people reduce their risks for developing cancers, to help them detect cancers early when the cancers can be most effectively treated, and to get the best care for living with cancer.[2] However, consumers who have elevated cancer risks need access to the relevant information about cancer prevention and control to make their best health promoting decisions. While the pervasive negative social stigma surrounding cancers makes communicating about cancer prevention very difficult to do well, cancer communication efforts can be strategically planned and executed to encourage key audiences to attend to and respond to relevant cancer prevention information. Access to relevant and persuasive health information is essential for helping vulnerable population members reduce their risks for cancer-related morbidity and mortality by guiding evidence-based decision-making about cancer prevention and control.

In addition to the negative stigma surrounding cancer and the reluctance to communicate about cancer, the complex nature of cancer etiology and treatment needs to be attended to when disseminating relevant cancer prevention and control information to health care consumers. Helping consumers make sense of the complexity of cancer-related information can often be a major challenge for consumers. Many consumers perceive cancer as one general disease and do not clearly differentiate between the unique forms, stages, and responses to different forms of cancer. Yet, cancer is not just one health care problem, but a complex set of diseases. The word cancer is an umbrella term that refers to a broad range of different forms and stages of cancer. These different forms of cancer typically are caused by a range of different factors, affect different parts of the body in unique ways, are displayed in distinct ways, produce a variety of symptoms and effects, are detected and treated in very different ways, and are likely to result in quite distinct prognoses depending on the kind of cancer diagnosed, its stage of detection, the treatments that are available, and the unique health histories and other co-morbidities experienced by the specific individuals who are confronting the cancer diagnosis.

The terminology and concepts related to cancer research and care can also be quite complicated, making it difficult to communicate relevant cancer information fully and clearly. It is not easy for most laypersons to understand the science behind cancer prevention and control recommendations. This can be especially problematic when communicating with representatives of vulnerable populations, such as many immigrants, people with limited education, those with lower socioeconomic status, some minority group members, and elderly individuals who may have limited levels of health literacy. [1] The need for effective communication about cancer risks, early detection, prevention, care, and survivorship is particularly acute for these at-risk populations, yet it is also tremendously challenging.[2] Effective cancer communicators must develop culturally sensitive communication strategies for addressing health literacy challenges, explaining cancer information clearly to targeted audiences, and promoting full understanding about how to use the relevant information to promote cancer prevention and control. Strategic cancer communication efforts can help reduce the many uncertainties concerning cancer for at-risk consumers. It can provide vulnerable consumers with a rationale for making informed health decisions. It can facilitate participation in cancer prevention and control efforts, empowering consumers to engage in relevant health behaviors, such as adopting healthy living activities (such as recommendations for exercise, nutrition, and risk avoidance), and to seek early detection and screening tests. It can also encourage consumers to seek the best treatments for cancer and to cooperate with prescribed therapeutic regimens.[2]

However effective cancer communication efforts are further complicated by the sense of fatalism about cancer control that is widely held by many members of at-risk populations. Data reported from recent administrations of the Health Information National Trends Survey (HINTS) conducted by the National Cancer Institute suggest that many members of the American public believe there is little that can be done to prevent cancers and even less that can be done to treat cancers once they are diagnosed.[2] A large numbers of HINTS respondents reported that they are confused by all the different recommendations they encounter concerning cancer prevention and control and are not sure what to do to reduce their risks for contracting cancers. [2] The range of competing recommendations about cancer that consumers often encounter gives them the impression that "everything causes cancer." What is worse, consumers report that the recommendations they hear concerning cancer prevention and control seem to change all the time, further confusing them. [2] To counter these communication challenges, cancer communicators should develop clear, easy to understand, and consistent communication strategies for breaking through the confusion. They need to reduce the inertia caused by public fatalism concerning cancer with the use of engaging and persuasive messages that motivate adoption of evidence-based cancer prevention recommendations. This chapter examines the challenges to communicating relevant cancer prevention and control information to vulnerable populations and suggests best practices for designing meaningful messages and effectively using relevant media to reduce cancer-related health disparities and to promote public health.

2. Vulnerable populations and health communication

Communication is the central social process in health promotion and care for informing cancer prevention and control for vulnerable populations.[1,2] The process of communication is the primary social mechanism used to both seek and deliver cancer care. Communication is the primary process for delivering cancer education and influencing cancer-related health behaviors. Communication is the coordinating process used to manage health care delivery systems. It is also the social process used to establish and reinforce health policies and practices. Health care consumers and providers depend upon communication to gather relevant health information for guiding evidence-based health decision making, encouraging participation in health care and health promotion activities, reducing uncertainty about cancers and increasing understanding about relevant health issues, as well as promoting needed cooperation and collaboration to achieve health goals.

Vulnerable populations are those groups of health care consumers who are most likely to suffer significantly higher levels of morbidity and mortality from cancers than other segments of the general population. [3] These vulnerable population members are typically the poorest, least well educated, and most disenfranchised members of modern society, including members of many immigrant and minority groups, the elderly, the socio-economically deprived, the disabled, and people suffering from serious chronic diseases. [3] Many members of these vulnerable populations are likely to experience key health communication barriers such as health literacy challenges, limited access to and ability to use key channels of communication (such as new information technologies), as well as suffer from serious social and economic problems that can limit their ability to get needed care and to follow cancer prevention and control recommendations. [4,5] There are a broad range of significant health risks confronting members of vulnerable populations today, including risks from cancers, heart disease, diabetes, stroke, HIV/AIDS, and other serious health threats.[6,7] Effective health communication is needed to help those members of the public who are at greatest risk (most vulnerable) for suffering from these health threats to recognize, minimize, and respond effectively to potential health problems.[8,9]

It is particularly important to effectively communicate clear, accurate, and persuasive information about cancer prevention and control to audiences who are at greatest risk for negative cancer outcomes, those who suffer from cancer health disparities.[10,11,12,13] Unfortunately, current efforts to educate the most vulnerable segments of society about cancer prevention and control strategies have been insufficient to significantly reduce cancer incidence, morbidity, and mortality for members of these groups by helping them make informed decisions about their best health care and health promotion choices. [15,16,17,18] The need for effective communication about cancer risks and responses is particularly acute, yet also tremendously challenging, for reaching vulnerable health care consumers.[19,20] These vulnerable population members are heir to serious disparities in cancer-related health outcomes, resulting in alarming levels of cancer-related morbidity and mortality, especially in comparison to the rest of the public.[19,21,22] The cultural barriers and health literacy challenges faced by many members of vulnerable populations, who are often immigrants, as well as non-native and substandard English speakers, readers, and writers, creates significant barriers to accessing and making sense of relevant cancer-related information.[23,24,25] These consumers are often confused and misinformed about the causes, preventive strategies, early detection procedures, and the treatments for different forms of cancer, which serves to exacerbate their poor cancer-related health outcomes.[25]

Members of vulnerable populations who are likely to suffer from significant cancer-related health disparities are desperately in need of relevant, accurate, and timely health information about cancer prevention and control.[26,27,28] Some vulnerable group members, such as elderly health care consumers, have elevated risks for contracting different forms of cancer, while other vulnerable group members, such as African American women, are more likely to die from breast cancer than other women.[3,16,25,26] Many members of immigrant populations in the US are non-native English speakers and encounter serious language and health belief barriers that necessitate adaptive, culturally-sensitive communication strategies to provide them with needed cancer-related health information.[27,28,29,30] Furthermore, consumers with serious and chronic medical conditions, as well as individuals who confront physical and mental disabilities, are often particularly vulnerable to health risks and have unique communication needs that must to be adequately addressed to provide them with the relevant health information they need to preserve their health.[31] Strategic, adaptive, and culturally-sensitive health communication information dissemination programs are needed for reducing cancer-related health disparities by providing vulnerable consumers with relevant and persuasive health information to help them evaluate health risks, make informed health care decisions, and direct their health behaviors.

3. Focus on cultural issues

Vulnerable consumers' unique cultural backgrounds and orientations have powerful influences on their communication practices that must be carefully accounted for when designing and implementing strategic cancer communication efforts.[32] It is critically important to identify and examine the relevant cultural issues that are likely to influence the ways consumers, particularly members of vulnerable populations, respond to communication about cancer prevention and control. [27,29,31] Several of the key cultural variables that influence cancer communication outcomes include the unique health beliefs, values, norms, and expectations that different consumers bring to health situations that influence their cancer-related health decisions and behaviors.[26] It is also important to assess consumers' culturally-based language skills and orientations, their health literacy levels (both their levels of literacy for language and numbers), their motivations to seek health information, their unique media use patterns, and their social network memberships.[33,34] Examination of these key cultural factors can provide relevant information for determining how to best design and deliver key messages for effectively communicating complex health information to diverse and vulnerable populations.[27,20,31] Culturally-sensitive health communication is essential to providing vulnerable consumers with relevant information about cancer prevention, screening, and treatment strategies.[30,31]

The best cancer communication education efforts begin with careful analysis of the critical cultural factors that influence the health beliefs and behaviors of targeted members of at-risk groups, since these cultural factors will also influence these consumers' reception and response to cancer prevention messages. It is important to identify the current levels of relevant cancer-related knowledge, strongly-held health beliefs, and primary health goals of key audience members before composing communication strategies. By determining what consumers know and don't know about cancer, health campaign strategist can guide the design of cancer-related health messages to help fill consumers' cancer information gaps and to correct any misconceptions these consumers may have concerning cancer prevention and control. Too often health communication efforts are based on very good intentions, but extremely limited audience data, so health promotion campaign do not hit the mark, failing to provide consumers with the information they most need. Without collecting good background information about audience members' cultural beliefs, attitudes, expectations, and behaviors, it is very difficult to develop health promotion messages that will be appropriate and influential for targeted audiences. The best health promotion messages are carefully designed to speak to audience members' unique cultural experiences. The messages employ familiar language and provide compelling culturally-rich examples to illustrate key points.

It is also important to carefully assess the level of communication skills and the unique communication orientations of targeted audience members. By learning about the communication skills and orientations of key audiences, campaign planners can design messages that will be easily understood by member of these audiences. They can employ communication channels for delivering the messages that will be easy to use and comfortable for audience members to access. They can also identify and use appropriate information sources to deliver cancer prevention and control messages who are likely tol be perceived as interesting and credible by members of key target audiences.

4. Strategic health communication design

Health education messages must be carefully designed to be effective. The critical factor in strategic message design is adapting health education messages to meet the unique needs and communication orientations of specific audiences. This means that effective health communication efforts should adopt a consumer orientation to health education.[35,36] Careful audience analysis is essential to identify the salient consumer characteristics that can be used for guiding message design.[37,38]

Good audience analysis research will help answer a variety of important questions for guiding cancer prevention and control efforts. These questions are likely to examine a number of relevant communication factors about members of targeted audiences. For example, what are the typical message exchange and information sharing processes employed by targeted groups of consumers? Who do these consumers typically talk to and acquire health related information from? Who do they trust? How do they receive and provide social support? What are their predispositions for interpreting cancer prevention and control messages? What are most influential factors for persuading members of targeted groups to attend to and respond positively to health messages? Which communication channels do members of these targeted groups prefer to use? What are the best ways to provide these consumers with feedback about their health behaviors that can promote and reinforce health behavior changes? What are the most influential communication strategies for developing cooperative and trusted relationships with members of targeted groups? The best health communication intervention programs will be designed to be responsive to audience communication patterns. They will be relevant to audience needs and interests. They will be easily accessible to targeted audience members. The messages will be culturally appropriate for key audience members. Messages and communication strategies will be adaptive to changing social situation. The messages provided will also be motivational and reinforcing, as well as engaging, interesting, and interactive.

Messages should be designed to appeal to key beliefs, attitudes, and values of targeted audience members, using familiar and accepted language, interesting images, and vivid examples to illustrate key points.[29] It is wise to pre-test sample health education messages with representatives of targeted audiences to make sure the messages hit the intended mark with these audiences before implementing health communication intervention programs. Formative evaluation data gathered through message pre-testing is essential to refining health education messages.[39] This is a form of user-centered design, where health education messages are shaped and refined by actively gathering feedback about campaign design from representatives of the actual audiences who are being targeted in health communication interventions.[39] Pre-testing is also a strategy for helping to increase audience participation in health education efforts. This active participation can not only help to increase the cultural sensitivity of health communication efforts, but can also enhance audience members receptivity to and cooperation with health promotion efforts.[39] Involving consumers, their family members, key members of their social networks, and community representatives can increase support and social encouragement for paying attention to, accepting, and utilizing health education messages.[40,41,42]

To be effective at presenting cancer prevention and control information it is wise to design multiple, reinforcing strategic messages that will be delivered at several points in time over different complementary channels of communication for reaching, influencing, and reinforcing vulnerable audiences with health education information. This multiple complementary message strategy builds from the communication principles of redundancy and reinforcement to enhance message exposure and impact.[43] Multiple, reinforcing cancer prevention and control messages can help to capture audience attention by providing these consumers with relevant information at several points of time. This strategy helps to reinforce message content by repeating key ideas. This also helps to illustrate key health education concepts. The use of vivid imagery in health communication interventions through the use of powerful narrative and visual illustrations can also reinforce message content, especially for audiences with limited health literacy, as well as audience members who have problems with numeracy (understanding numerically presented information) that may make it difficult for them to comprehend statistics and numerical risk estimates.[39,40,44,45,46,47]

Tailored communication is a powerful approach for designing customized health messages to meet the unique needs and backgrounds of specific individuals.[48] Tailored approaches provide specific customized messages to an individual that match the person's unique background, beliefs, and orientations. Key bits of an individual's background information, such as the person's name, age, cultural memberships, or health status are gathered and included in the specific health messages sent to that person. For example, a tailored message might state, "Research has shown that mammograms should be scheduled every other year for a woman of your age, race, and family history with breast cancer Helen." By including specific key information about Helen's background in the message, the information becomes much more interesting and relevant for her. Typically, tailored communication systems employ interactive computer systems that can be used to gather relevant background information from consumers concerning key communication variables (age, race, gender, occupation, health history, etc.) through questions posed to these individuals, including questions eliciting information about individual demographics, psychographics, and health beliefs/behaviors. Once key background information is gathered from the individual, the information is used to select specific messages stored in a library of messages that match the unique background features of the individuals selected to receive health education messages. In this way, information about the individual health risks and orientations of a specific consumer, for example an elderly, African-American, male, with a history of prostate cancer and diabetes, will automatically be selected and used to provide content-appropriate health information to the individuals through a tailored health information communication system. As the consumer continues to interact with the tailored health information system, providing the system with additional background information, a tailored communication computer program can store and catalog this information to continually refine the content of message sent to this consumer to match his or her unique personal characteristics and interests.

In addition to developing strategic messages that match the cultural orientations of at-risk consumers, it is critically important to determine the most effective communication channels for reaching targeted populations of consumers. The best communication channels to utilize are those that are close, familiar, and easily accessible for targeted audience members.[49] For example, it is important to employ communication channels that are easy for members of the intended audience to use. It would be a serious error to develop an online health education website for consumers who do not have access to computers or who are not sophisticated computer users. Communication channels that are dramatic and memorable can have strong influences on audience attention and interpretation of health messages.[49] Health educators should consider using communication channels that can be accessed over time, channels that can retain important information for later review, and even interactive channels that can enable consumers to ask questions and receive clarifications about complex health information. The best strategic communication designs use interactive channels where consumers can provide feedback and ask questions to clarify the information provided. Multiple overlapping communication channels can present complementary messages that are reinforcing over time and delivered by multiple credible sources.

It is important to decide what the best sources are for delivering key messages about cancer prevention and control strategies to different audiences.[39] It is crucial to identify the most credible sources of health information for members of the intended audiences.[49] Decisions need to be made about whether it is best to utilize familiar sources of information, expert sources, or perhaps peer communication as the most influential ways to provide cancer-elated health information to different audiences. Just as with the use of strategic messages, it is a good idea to pre-test the use of different information sources and different communication channels with targeted audiences.[39] Message testing research that examines the impact of different communication sources on targeted audience members can help strategic communicators make good decisions about the best representatives to employ to deliver health information to different audiences.

5. Evaluating health communication interventions

Evaluation research should be a basic process that is built in to all cancer prevention and control communication efforts.[50] Cancer communication efforts should always begin with careful needs analysis and audience analysis to identify the best goals, targets, and strategies for communication interventions. The messages designed and channels identified for delivering cancer prevention and control messages should be carefully tested with representatives from targeted groups to make sure they communicate effectively to these groups and provide them with the intended information. Message testing can also be used to refine and improve message strategies as a form of formative research. Usability testing is also a useful formative research strategy for testing consumer access to, comfort with, and ability to effectively use communication channels and tools.

A critical juncture in communicating risk and benefit information to vulnerable audiences is evaluating how well different communication strategies work to educate targeted audiences about important health issues.[50] It is important to assess how well consumers really understand the risks and benefits that are being communicated and what differences communication programs are making in promoting informed consumer decision-making. A first step in evaluating the outcomes of communication efforts is to establish clear baseline measures of consumer understanding before introducing new health education programs. These baseline measures can be used as a starting point for tracking the influences of communication efforts on consumer attitudes, beliefs, and behaviors concerning cancer prevention and control.[45] Feedback mechanisms, such as consumer surveys, focus groups, hotlines, help-desks, and comment cards, can be introduced as integral parts of communication interventions for tracking and evaluating consumer understanding of health messages, as well as their reaction to campaign strategies. The data gathered through these feedback mechanisms can be used to refine health communication programs and track progress in health education. Evaluation research can track the influences of communication efforts on consumer beliefs, behaviors, and even their physiological outcomes. Furthermore, it is important to conduct cost-benefit analyses to determine whether cancer prevention and control communication interventions are cost-effective. (See Figure 1 for a summary of the different forms of evaluation research that should be used to inform strategic cancer communication interventions).

6. Policy and practice implications for strategic communication

What policies and best practices are needed to guide effective communication efforts about cancer prevention and control to vulnerable populations? First and foremost, communication interventions to educate vulnerable populations need to be strategic and evidence-based. Cancer communication is too complex a process to be handled without careful planning

Needs Analysis Research	What is the nature of the health issue, problem or disparity that needs to be addressed? What are the likely causes of the problem? What are the negative outcomes of the problem? What needs to be changed to address this problem? What are the ideal goals to be achieved for improving this situation?
Audience Analysis Research	Who are the key target audiences who are affected by this health problem? What are the target group members' unique beliefs, attitudes, values, and experiences related to this issue? What are their communication skill levels and orientations to this issue? Can these groups be segmented into homogenous sub-groups?
Message Testing Research	What language level is most effectively understood by members of the target audience? What numerical examples will make sense to members of this audience? Which messages resonate with audience members, are interesting, memorable, and persuasive? What narrative examples resonate with this audience?
Channel Testing Research	Which channels of communication are most familiar to audience members? How easy are different communication channels for audience members to use? How likely is it for audience members to access and pay attention to different communication channels. Which channels are likely to work well together?
Source Credibility Testing	Which information sources will be deemed as trustworthy and credible to target audience members? How attractive are different potential message sources for audience members? Which sources will audience members pay attention to? Which sources will be most persuasive?
Usability Testing	How easily can target audience members use the different media selected for delivering health messages? Can they navigate through the different levels of information presented via these different media? Can they find the most relevant health information and the information they are most interested in?
Formative Evaluation Research	How well are strategic communication strategies working with targeted audience members? How are the audience members reacting to key messages and communication strategies? Are there unintended reactions to the health education efforts? Is there a need to change communication strategies to better meet audience needs or respond to changing conditions?
Summative Evaluation Research	How effective was the communication strategy for achieving established health goals? Did the communication effort influence health beliefs, values, attitudes, and behaviors? Did the effort influence cancer incidence, early detection, treatment, morbidity, quality of life, and survivorship? Was the communication program cost-effective?

Fig. 1. The Functions of Evaluation Research for Informing Strategic Cancer Communication Interventions.

and data. It is also critical for health educators to adopt culturally sensitive communication practices to reach and influence vulnerable populations. Community participative communication interventions are a valuable strategy for integrating consumers' perspectives into cancer education efforts and building community commitment to health communication interventions.[41,42] It is a good idea to consider introduction of relevant communication technologies, such as tailored information systems, to support health education efforts.[19] It is also a good idea to incorporate health communication training for both health care providers (educators) and consumers to enhance the quality of cross-cultural communication efforts.[20,51]

Strategic communication efforts can promote cancer prevention and control for at-risk populations. To achieve these goals efforts must be taken to develop evidence-based communication campaigns to increase awareness about prevention. These campaigns must be designed to persuade members of at-risk groups to adopt prevention recommendations, change negative health habits, and adopt healthy lifestyles. Communication campaigns should be designed not only to initiate these healthy behavior changes, but to also reinforce and sustain behavior changes over time. Campaigns should be designed to increase awareness about the importance of developing healthy lifestyles and engaging in regular recommended cancer screening and early detection activities. Efforts should be taken to implement and promote easily accessible and affordable screening programs. Screening practices should be monitored to refine and improve screening programs and promotion activities.

7. Conclusion

Several lessons have been learned from past efforts to increase the effectiveness of cancer communication interventions with vulnerable populations.[20,29,26] These lessons include the importance of:

- Gathering full audience and needs information to guide health communication efforts.
- Testing message and channel strategies to refine communication activities.
- Using close, familiar, and frequently used communication channels.
- Developing vivid, engaging, and moving messages for interventions.
- Involving and empowering vulnerable and at-risk consumers in health communication efforts;
- Developing inter-organizational partnerships to support intervention efforts;
- Providing appropriate training and support for both consumers and providers;
- Designing culturally appropriate messages and materials for communication efforts;
- Focusing on the family and the community for delivering and reinforcing messages, and;
- Providing consumers with choices and options for promoting their health.
- Evaluating the influences of communication interventions to refine and improve efforts.

The development and implementation of strategic health communication interventions holds great promise for promoting cancer prevention and control for vulnerable populations. By investing in the development of strategic cancer communication efforts we can develop an infrastructure for disseminating relevant cancer information. We can test new strategies, models, and tools for designing effective strategic communication interventions to reduce cancer-related health disparities. We can also encourage the adoption of best practices for cancer prevention and control.

8. Acknowledgment

I acknowledge the support of my current colleagues at George Mason University's Center for Health and Risk Communication and my former colleagues in the Health Communication and Informatics Research Branch at the National Cancer Institute for their input and encouragement in helping me refine the ideas presented in this chapter.

9. References

[1] Kreps, G.L., & Sivaram, R. (2008). The central role of strategic health communication in enhancing breast cancer outcomes across the continuum of care in limited-resource countries. *Cancer,* Vol. *113(S8),* pp. *2331-2337*

[2] Kreps, G.L. (2008). Strategic use of communication to market cancer prevention and control to vulnerable populations. *Health Marketing Quarterly.* Vol. *25(1/2), pp.* 204-216

[3] Kreps, G.L. (2006). Communication and racial inequities in health care. *American Behavioral Scientist,* Vol. *49(6). pp. 760-774*

[4] Kreps, G.L., & Sparks, L. (2008). Meeting the health literacy needs of vulnerable populations. *Patient Education and Counseling. Vol. 71(3),*pp. 328-332

[5] Neuhauser, L., & Kreps, G.L. (2008). Online cancer communication interventions: Meeting the literacy, linguistic, and cultural needs of diverse audiences. *Patient Education and Counseling,* Vol. *71(3),* pp. 365-377

[6] Singh, G.K. & Hiatt, R.A. (2006). Trends and disparities in socioeconomic and behavioural characteristics, life expectancy, and cause-specific mortality of native-born and foreign-born populations in the United States, 1979–2003. *International Journal of Epidemiology. Vol.*35, pp. 903-919

[7] Kunitz, S.J. & Pesis-Katz, I. (2005). Mortality of white Americans, African Americans, and Canadians: The causes and consequences for health of welfare state institutions and policies. *Milbank Quarterly. Vol.*83, pp. 5-39

[8] Haider, M. (2005). *Global public health communications: Challenges, perspectives, and strategies.* Jones & Bartlett Publishers, ISBN-13: 9780763747763, Sudbury, MA.

[9] Kreps, G.L. (2003). The impact of communication on cancer risk, incidence, morbidity, mortality, and quality of life. Health Communication. Vol.15, pp. 163-171

[10] Morris L.A., & Aikin, K.J. (2001). The "Pharmokinetics" of patient communications. Drug Informatics Journal. Vol.35, pp. 509–527

[11] Patel, V.L., Branch, T., & Arocha, J.F. (2002). Errors in interpreting quantities as procedures: The case of pharmaceutical labels. Int J Med Informatics. Vol.65, pp. 193-211

[12] Chandra, A., Malcolm, N., & Fetters, M. (2003). Practicing health promotion through pharmacy counseling. Health Promotion Practice. Vol.4, pp. 64-71

[13] Moisan, J., Gaudet, M., Grégoire, J.P., & Bouchard, R. (2002). Non-compliance with drug treatment and reading difficulties with regard to prescription labelling among seniors. Gerontology. Vol.48, pp. 44-51

[14] Kreps, G.L. (2005). Communication and racial inequities in health care. American Behavioral Scientist. Vol49, pp. 1-15

[15] Thomas, S.B., Fine, M.J, & Ibrahim, S.A. (2004). Health disparities: The importance of culture and health communication. American Journal of Public Health. Vol.94, p. 2050

[16] Ashton, C.M., Haidet, P., Paterniti, D.A., Collins, T.C., Gordon, H.S., O'Malley, K., Petersen, L.A., Sharf, B.F., Suarez-Almazor ,M.E., Wray, N.P., & Street, R.L. (2003). Racial and ethnic disparities in the use of health services. Journal of General Internal Medicine. Vol. 18, pp. 146-152

[17] Freeman, H.P. (2004). Poverty, culture, and social injustice: Determinants of cancer disparities. CA: Cancer Journal for Clinicians. Vol 54, pp. 72-77

[18] Kreps, GL. (1996). Communicating to promote justice in the modern health care system. *Journal of Health Communication*. Vol.1, pp. 99-109.

[19] Chang, B.L., Bakken, S., Brown, S.S., Houston, T.K., Kreps, G.L., Kukafka, R., Safran, C., & Stavri, P.Z. (2004). Bridging the digital divide: Reaching vulnerable populations. *Journal of the American Medical Informatics Association*. Vol.11(6), pp. 448-457

[20] Kreps, G.L. (2005). Disseminating relevant information to underserved audiences: Implications from the Digital Divide Pilot Projects. *Journal of the Medical Library Association*. Vol.*93(4)*, pp. *65-70*

[21] Koo, M.M., Krass, I., & Aslani, P. (2003). Factors influencing consumer use of written drug information. *Annals of Pharmacotherapy*. Vol.37, pp. 259-267

[22] Gazmararian, J.A., Williams, M.V., Peel, J., & Baker, D.W. (2003). Health literacy and knowledge of chronic disease. *Patient Education and Counseling*. Vol.51, pp.267-275.

[23] Praska, J.L, Kripalani, S., Seright, A.L., Jacobson, T.A.. (2005). Identifying and assisting low-literacy patients with medication use: A survey of community pharmacies. *Annals of Pharmacotherapy*. Vol.39, pp. 441-445

[24] Wolf, M.S., Davis, T.C., Tilson, H.H., Bass, P.F., & Parker, R.M. (2006). Misunderstanding of prescription drug warning labels among patients with low literacy. *American Journal of Health-System Pharmacies*. Vol.*63, pp.* 1048-1055

[25] Kreps, G.L. (1990). A systematic analysis of health communication with the aged. In: Giles H, Coupland N, Wiemann JM, eds. *Communication, health, and the elderly*. Fulbright Series No. 8., University of Manchester Press, ISBN 0-7190-3174-5, p 135-154, Manchester, England

[26] Kreps, G.L. (1986). Health communication and the elderly. *World Communication*. Vol.*15. pp. 55-7.*

[27] Chew, L.D., Bradley, K.A., & Boyko, E.T. (2004). Brief questions to identify patients with inadequate health literacy. *Family Medicine*. Vol.36, pp. 588-594

[28] Hardin, L.R. (2005). Counseling patients with low health literacy. *American Journal of Health-System Pharmacies*. Vol.62, pp. 364-365

[29] Kreps, G.L. (2006). One size does not fit all: Adapting communication to the needs and literacy levels of individuals. *Annals of Family Medicine (online)*. 2006; http://www.annfammed.org/cgi/eletters/4/3/205

[30] Parker, R., & Kreps, G.L. (2005). Library outreach: Overcoming health literacy challenges. *Journal of the Medical Library Association*. Vol*93(4), pp. 78-82*

[31] Kreps, G.L., & Kunimoto, E. (1994). *Effective communication in multicultural health care settings*. Sage Publications, ISBN-10: 0803947143, Newbury Park, CA

[32] Kreuter, M.W., & McClure, S.M. (2004). The role of culture in health communication. *Annual Reviews of Public Health*. Vol.*25, pp.* 439-455

[33] Youmans, S.L., & Schillinger, D. (2003). Functional health literacy and medication use: The pharmacist's role. *Annals of Pharmocotherapy*. Vol.*37, pp.* 1726-1729

[34] Andrus, M.R., & Roth, M.T. (2002). Health literacy: A review. *Pharmacotherapy*. Vol.22, pp. 282-302

[35] Trewin, V.F., & Veitch, G.B. (2003). Patient sources of drug information and attitudes to their provision: A corticosteroid model. *Pharmacy World Science*. Vol.25, pp. 191-196

[36] Pilnick, A. (2003). Patient counseling" by pharmacists: Four approaches to the delivery of counseling sequences and their interactional reception. *Social Science and Medicine*. Vol.56, *pp.* 835-849

[37] Kreps, G.L. (1996). Promoting a consumer orientation to health care and health promotion. *Journal of Health Psychology*. Vol.*1, pp. 41-48.*

[38] Kreps, G.L. (2002). Enhancing access to relevant health information. In: Carveth R, Kretchmer, SB, Schuler, D eds. *Shaping the network society: Patterns for participation, action, and change*. CPSR, OL 19478014M, pp. 149-152, Palo Alto, CA

[39] Maibach, E.W., & Parrott, R., (Eds). (1995). *Designing health messages: Approaches from communication theory and public health practice*. Sage Publications, ISBN 0803953984, Thousand Oaks, CA

[40] Kinzie, M.B., Cohn, W.F., Julian, M.F., & Knaus, W.A. (2002). A user-centered model for web site design: Needs assessment, user interface design, and rapid prototyping. *Journal of the American Medical Informatics Association*, Vol.9, pp. 320-330

[41] Minkler, M. (2000). Using participatory action research to build healthy communities. *Public Health Reports*. Vol.115(2-3), pp. 191-197

[42] Minkler, M., & Wallerstein, N., (Eds.). (2002). *Community based participatory research for health*. Jossey-Bass, ISBN 0787964573, Indianapolis, IN

[43] Donohew, L., Lorch, E.P., & Palmgreen, P. (1998). Applications of a theoretic model of information exposure to health interventions. *Human Communication Research*. Vol.24, pp. 454–468

[44] Dowse, R., & Ehlers, M. (2005). Medicine labels incorporating pictograms: Do they influence understanding and adherence. *Patient Education and Counseling*. Vol.58, pp. 63-70

[45] Gustafsson, J., Kälvemark S, Nilsson, G., & Nilsson, J.L.G. (2005). Patient information leaflets – patients comprehension of information about interactions and contraindications. *Pharmacy World Science*. Vol.27, pp. 35-40

[46] Hwang, S.W., Tram, C.Q.N., & Knarr, N. (2005). The effect of illustrations on patient comprehension of medication instruction labels. *BMC Family Practitioner*. Vol.6, pp.26-32

[47] Knapp, P., Raynor, D.K., Jebar, A.H., & Price, S.J. (2005). Interpretation of medication pictograms by adults in the UK. *Annals of Pharmocotherapy*. Vol.39, pp. 1227-1233

[48] Rimer, B.K., & Kreuter, M.W. (2006). Advancing tailored health communication: A persuasion and message effects perspective. *Journal of Communication*. Vol.56(s1), pp. S184–S201

[49] Maibach, E.W., Kreps, G.L., Bonaguro, E.W. (1993). Developing strategic communication campaigns for HIV/AIDS prevention. In Ratzan S ed. *AIDS: Effective health communication for the 90s*. Taylor and Francis, ISBN: 156032273X, p 15-35, Washington, D.C.

[50] Kreps, G.L. (2002). Evaluating new health information technologies: Expanding the frontiers of health care delivery and health promotion. *Studies in Health Technology and Informatics*. Vol.80, pp. 205-212

[51] Coleman, C.L. (2003). Examining influences of pharmacists' communication with consumers about antibiotics. *Health Communication*. Vol.15, pp. 79-99

15

Early Detection: An Opportunity for Cancer Prevention Through Early Intervention

D. James Morré and Dorothy M. Morré
MorNutech, Inc. West Lafayette, IN, USA

1. Introduction

Cancer is the second leading disease cause of death in the United States. A group of more than 100 different and distinctive diseases, cancer may involve any tissue of the body. Estimates are that there were over 1.5 million cases in 2010 in the United States alone. Only a small fraction (less than 20%) of cancers are diagnosed at a localized stage where curative therapy is effective. Most cancers are diagnosed only after the primary tumor has already metastasized so that chemotherapy is required for treatment. Hence, early detection is a favored opportunity to reduce cancer mortality. By detecting cancer in its very earliest stages when perhaps only a small number of cells are present, it is possible that early intervention will be effective in preventing further development of the incipient cancer thereby resulting in what might be viewed as curative prevention.

Despite advances in early detection of major forms of human cancer (prostate, breast, lung, colon, leukemia, lymphoma), more often than not, cancers have developed to a sufficiently late stage at the time of detection to preclude most opportunities for curative therapy (Altekruse et al., 2010). The problem is exacerbated for pancreatic cancer where clinical symptoms invariably are delayed until the disease state is well advanced beyond metastatic spread. A need for early detection remains as one of the most important challenges at the forefront of cancer research, treatment and prevention.

2. Approach

2.1 Early detection

Ecto-Nicotinamide Adenine Dinucleotide Oxidase Disulfide-Thiol Exchanger 2 (ENOX2) (GenBank accession no. AF207881; Chueh et al., 2002) also known as Tumor-Associated Nicotinamide Adenine Dinucleotide Oxidase (tNOX) is ideally suited as a target for early diagnosis of cancer as well as for early preventive intervention (Fig. 1). The proteins are expressed on the cell surface of malignancies and detectable in the serum of patients with cancer (Cho et al., 2002). ENOX2 proteins are terminal hydroquinone oxidases of plasma membrane electron transport. From the standpoint of early intervention, they are important in the growth and enlargement of tumor cells (Morré and Morré, 2003a; Tang et al., 2007, 2008). Our approach using ENOX2, as a target for both early detection and for early interventions, is based on these properties (Cho et al., 2002; Morré and Morré, 2003a;

reviewed by Davies and Bozzo, 2006). While ENOX2 presence provides a non-invasive approach to cancer detection, without methodology to identify cancer site-specific ENOX2 forms, it offered no indication as to cancer type or location.

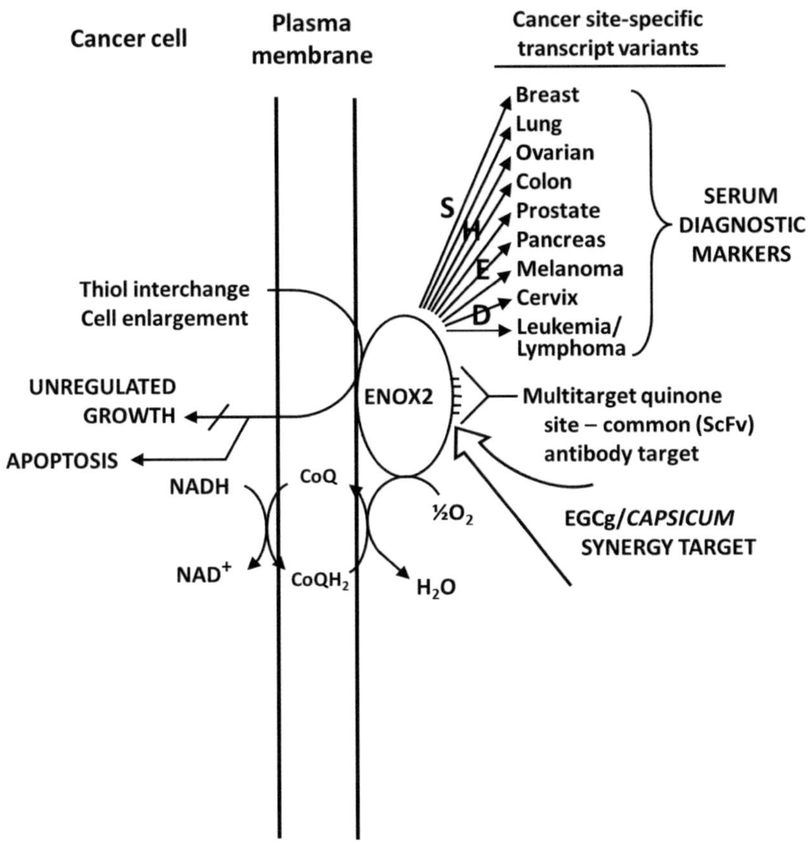

Fig. 1. Schematic representation of the utility of the ENOX2 family of cancer-specific, cell surface proteins for early diagnosis and early intervention of cancer. Cancer site-specific transcript variants of ENOX2 are shed into the serum to permit early detection and diagnosis. The ENOX2 proteins of origin at the cell surface act as terminal oxidases of plasma membrane electron transport functions essential to the unregulated growth of cancer. When the ENOX2 proteins are inhibited, as for example through EGCg/*Capsicum* synergies, the unregulated growth ceases and the cancer cells undergo programmed cell death (apoptosis).

The opportunity to simultaneously determine both cancer presence and cancer site emerged as a result of 2-dimensional gel electrophoretic separations where western blots with a pan ENOX2 recombinant single chain variable region (ScFv) antibody carrying an S tag (Fig. 2) was employed for detection (Hostetler et al., 2009; Hostetler and Kim, 2011). The antibody cross reacted with all known ENOX2 forms from hematological and solid tumors of human origin but, of itself, did not differentiate among different kinds of cancers. Analyses using this antibody, when combined with two-dimensional gel electrophoretic separation, revealed specific ENOX2 species possibly as transcript variants, each with a characteristic molecular weight and isoelectric point indicative of a particular form of cancer (Hostetler et al., 2009; Table l).

ENOX transcript variants of specific molecular weights and isoelectric points are produced uniquely by patients with cancer. The proteins are shed into the circulation and have the potential to serve as definitive, non-invasive and sensitive serum markers for early detection of both primary and recurrent cancer in at risk populations with a low incidence of false positives, as they are molecular signature molecules produced specifically by cancer cells and absent from non-cancer cells.

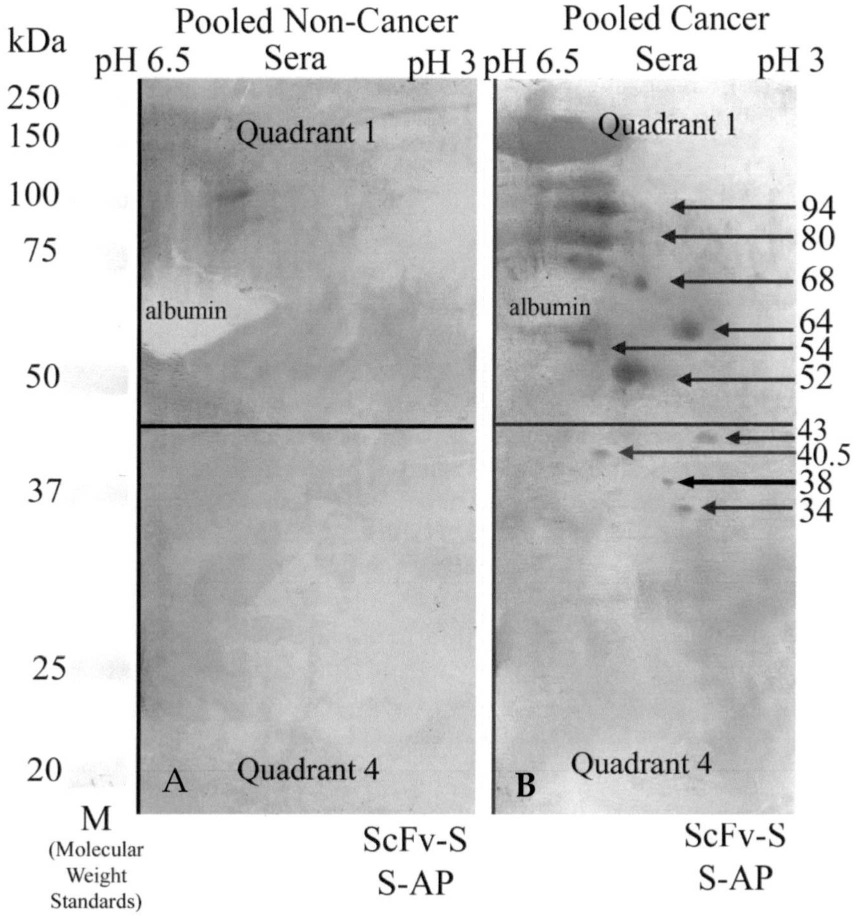

Fig. 2. 2-Dimensional gel/western blot of ENOX2 transcript variants comparing pooled non-cancer (A) and pooled cancer representing major carcinomas plus leukemias and lymphomas (B) patient sera. The approximate location of unreactive (at background) albumin is labeled for comparison. ENOX2 reactive proteins are restricted to quadrants I and IV. Detection uses recombinant scFv-S (S-tag peptide: His-Glu-Ala-Ala-Lys-Phe--Gln-Arg-Glu-His) antibody with alkaline phosphatase linked antiS protein. The approximately 10 ENOX2 transcript variants of the pooled cancer sera are absent from non-cancer (A) and are cancer site-specific as indicated in Fig. 3. From Hostetler et al. (2009).

Cancer	Sera analyzed	Molecular weight	Isoelectric point, pH
Cervical	18	94 kDa	5.4
Ovarian	41	80 and 40.5 kDa	4.2 and 4.1
Prostate	70	75 kDa	6.3
Breast/Uterine	55	64 to 68 kDa	4.5
Non-small cell lung	83	54 kDa	5.1
Small cell lung	22	52 kDa	4.3
Pancreatic	24	50 and 52 kDa	4.3 and 3.9
Colon	55	52 and 34 kDa	4.3 and 3.9
Lymphoma, Leukemia	16	45 kDa	3.9
Melanoma	12	38 kDa	5.1

Table 1. Sera from patients with different cancers exhibit distinct patterns of ENOX2 isoforms with characteristic molecular weights and isoelectric points (pH). Updated from Hostetler et al. (2009).

2.2 Early intervention

As the 2-D-western blot protocol detects cancer early, well in advance of clinical symptoms, the opportunity to combine early detection with early intervention as a potentially curative prevention strategy for cancer by eliminating the disease in its very earliest stages is unique. The approach to early intervention is based on previous work in cell culture models showing that ENOX2 proteins are required to support the unregulated growth that typifies cancer cells. If the growth function of ENOX2 is blocked for 48 to 72 h, the cancer cells cannot enlarge following division, cannot pass the checkpoint in G_1 that monitors cell size and eventually undergo programmed cell death (apoptosis) (Morré and Morré, 2003b; De Luca et al., 2010) as diagrammed in Figure 1. Among the early intervention strategies under investigation are several targeted to ENOX2, production of ENOX2-directed vaccines being one promising example. Recombinant ENOX2 peptides that exhibit cancer specificity are employed as antigens. Other forms of ENOX2-directed therapeutic interventions under study include use of dietary modulators (Morré et al., 2009b). Most advanced are studies with herbal mixtures of green tea and powders of ground chili peppers (*Capsicum* species) from efficacious pepper sources (e.g. guajillo or ancho) with levels of capsaicin, the pungent principle of chili peppers, sufficiently low so as to not cause discomfort.

3. Results

3.1 Early detection

Analytical 2-D gel electrophoresis and immunoblotting of ENOX proteins from a mixed population of cancer patients (cervical, breast, ovarian, lung and colon carcinomas, leukemias and lymphomas) revealed multiple species of acidic proteins of molecular weights between 34 and 100 kDa in quadrants I and IV (Fig 2B), none of which were present in sera of non-cancer patients (Fig. 2A) (Hostetler et al., 2009). Separation in the first dimension was by isoelectric focusing over the pH range of 3 to 10 and separation in the second dimension was by 10 percent SDS-PAGE. Isoelectric points of the ENOX2 transcript variants were in the range of 3.9 to 6.3. The principal reactive proteins other than the ENOX2 forms were a 53 kDa isoelectric point pH 4.1, mostly phosphorylated α1-antitrypsin inhibitor (α2-HS-glycoprotein; fetuin A) (Labeled "R" in Fig. 5) which served as a convenient loading control and isoelectric point reference and a 79-85 kDa, isoelectric point pH 6.8 serotransferrin which served as a second point of reference for loading and as an isoelectric point reference (Table 2). The two cross reactive reference proteins are present in a majority of sera and plasma of both cancer and non-cancer subjects. Albumin and other serum proteins do not react. On some blots, the recombinant scFv was weakly cross-reactive with heavy (ca. 52 kDa) and light (ca. 25 kDa) immunoglobulin chains.

ENOX2	EEMTETK400ETEESA406LVS
Alpha-1-antitrypsin inhibitor	GTDCVAK211EATEAA216KCN
Serrotransferrin	CLDGTRK589PVEEYA595NCH

Table 2. Protein sequence similarity between ENOX2 and the two reference proteins α1- anti-trypsin inhibitor and serrotransferrin reactive with the pan ENOX2 scFv recombinant antibody. Regions of similarity are restricted to a 7 amino acid sequence (underlined) adjacent in ENOX2 to the E394EMTE398 quinone inhibitor-binding site.

Sera from individual patients with various forms of cancer were analyzed by 2-D gel electrophoresis and immunoblotting to assign each of the ENOX2 isoforms of Fig. 2 to a cancer of a particular tissue of origin (Table 1). Sera of breast cancer patients contained only the 64 to 68 kDa ENOX2 (Fig. 3D; Fig. 5 arrow) and the α1-antitrypsin inhibitor reference protein (Fig. 5). Sera from cervical cancer patients contained the 94 kDa ENOX2 transcript variant (Fig. 3A). Sera from ovarian cancer patients contained ENOX1 transcript variants of 80 kDa and 40.5b kDa (Fig. 3B). Sera from patients with prostate cancer contained one or more 75 kDa ENOX2 transcript variants resulting in small variations in isoelectric points (Fig. 3C). Sera from patients with non-small cell lung carcinoma contained a 52 kDa ENOX2 transcript variant while sera from non-small cell lung carcinoma patients contained a 52 kDa ENOX2 transcript variant (Fig 3E;F; Fig 4). Simultaneous presence of ENOX2 transcript variants of both 50 and 52 kDa characterized sera of pancreatic cancer patients (Fig. 3G) whereas sera of colon cancer patients contained ENOX2 transcript variants of 52 kDa and 43 kDa (Fig. 3H). Fig. 3I from sera of a patient with non-Hodgkin's lymphoma illustrates the 45 kDa ENOX2 transcript variant of low isoelectric point characteristic of leukemias and lymphomas. Sera of patients with malignant melanoma contained an ENOX2 transcript variant of 38 kDa (Fig. 3J).

Particularly relevant are observations where the 64 to 68 kDa ENOX2 transcript variant (pH 4.5) of sera correlated with disease presence in both late (Stage IV) (Fig. 5A) and early (Stage I) (Fig. 5E) disease and in Stage IV recurrence (Fig. 5C) but was absent from sera of non-cancer (normal) volunteers (Fig. 5B) or in survivors free of disease for one to five years (Fig. 5D). Additionally, the 64 to 68 kDa breast cancer-specific transcript variant does not apply to a subset of breast cancer patients but appears to be widely present. Analyses of sera of more than 55 patients with active disease including 20 Stage I and Stage II breast cancer patients all tested positive.

Unlike most published cancer markers, cancer-specific ENOX2 variants are not simply present as elevated levels of a serum constituent present in lesser amounts in the absence of cancer. The cancer-specific ENOX2 transcript variants result from cancer-specific expression of alternatively spliced mRNAs (Tang et al., 2007; 2008). Neither the splice variant mRNAs nor the ENOX2 isoform proteins are present in detectable levels in non-cancer cells or in sera of subjects without cancer (Table 1).

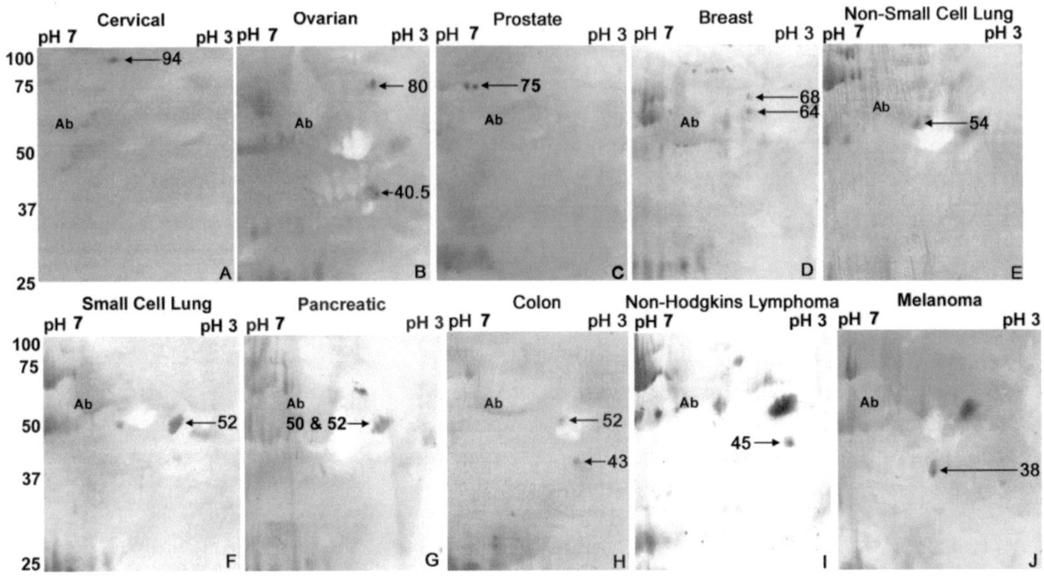

Fig. 3. Western blots of 2-D gel electrophoresis/western blots of sera from cancer patients analyzed individually. Cancer sites are presented in the order of decreasing molecular weight of the major transcript variant present. A. Cervical cancer. B. Ovarian cancer C. Prostate cancer. D. Breast cancer. E. Non-small cell lung cancer. F. Small cell lung cancer. G. Pancreatic cancer. H. Colon cancer. I. Non-Hodgkins lymphoma. J. Melanoma. The approximate location of unreactive (at background) albumin (Ab) is labeled for comparison. Approximately 180 non-cancer patient sera were analyzed in parallel without evidence of proteins indicative of specific transcript variants. From Hostetler et al. (2009).

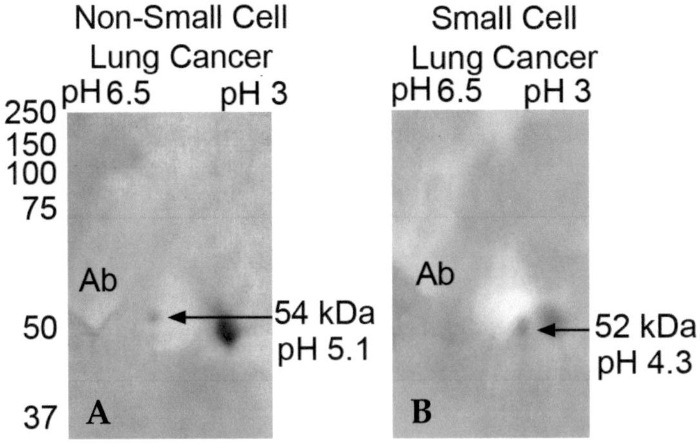

Fig. 4. Analytical gel electrophoresis and immunoblot of patient sera. A Sera from a patient with non-small cell lung cancer contains a 54 kDa ENOX2 transcript variant, pH 5.1 (arrow). B. Sera from a patient with small cell lung cancer contains the 52 kDa, isoelectric point pH 4.3 is transcript variant (arrow). The reference spots to the right, M_r 52 kDa and isoelectric point pH 4.1 is α1-antitrypsin. Albumin and other serum proteins are unreactive.

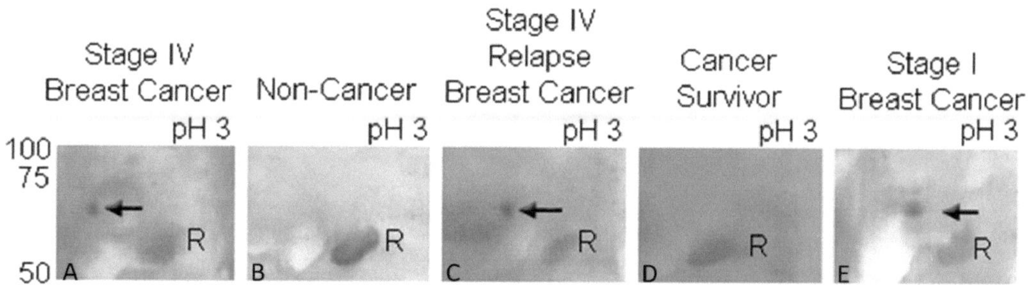

Fig. 5. 2-D gel electrophoretic separations and detection of ENOX2 transcript variants specific for breast cancer by western blotting of patient sera. Arrow = 66 to 68 kDa breast cancer specific transcript variant. R = 52 kDa, isoelectric point pH 4.1 α1-antitrypsin inhibitor reference spot.

Findings from a separate study with small cell and non-small cell lung cancer suggest that the 2-D-western blot test detects cancer presence as early as 5 to 7 years in advance of the appearance of clinical symptoms. This supposition is based mainly on our analysis of two special cancer panels of sera obtained through the Early Detection Research Network (EDRN) of the National Cancer Institute. One panel consisted of about 20 known lung cancer patient sera and 35 control patient sera. Using the 2-D-western blot protocol to identify specific ENOX2 isoforms, we successfully identified all 20 of the known lung cancer patient sera. However, unexpectedly, a high incidence of ENOX2 presence was encountered in sera from the "control" group which were obtained from a community screening study. From additional information obtained through the EDRN, 16 of the 17 positive control subject samples where our findings specifically indicated lung cancer (the lung cancer ENOX2 markers were found) were smokers with smoking histories in the range of 15 to 88 pack-years. However, the anticipated incidence of undetected lung cancers in such a population would be in the order of 10% or less rather than nearly 50%. Since the aberrant ENOX2 transcript variants associated with lung cancer are single molecular species produced only by lung cancer, the possibility was raised that lung cancer was being detected much earlier than was currently possible by other methods. The indications might be as early as 5 to 7 years before clinical symptoms, based on the estimated 20 year development time for lung cancer expression between carcinogen exposure and a clinically evident cancer (Petro et al., 2000) as diagrammed in Figure 6.

Similar results were obtained with a panel of female subjects at risk for breast and ovarian cancer. An analysis of a panel of 127 sera in a Biomarker Reference Set for Cancers in Women also provided through the Early Detection Research Network of the National Cancer Institute support our indications that the 2-D gel-western blot system is able to detect cancer presence 5 to 7 years in advance of clinical symptoms. The panel consisted of samples pooled from 441 women in 12 different gynecologic and breast disease categories plus 115 sera from age-matched control women. Of the 127 sera samples in the panel, 29 tested positive for breast cancer and another 16 tested positive for ovarian cancer. Since the aberrant transcript variants are single molecular species produced by specific cancers such as lung, breast or ovarian, the findings suggest that cancer was being detected in the control popuation much earlier than is currently possible by other methods. As estimated for lung cancer, the indications might be as much as 5 to 7 years before clinical symptoms based on the development time estimated for breast as well as lung cancer expression between a cancer causing event and clinically evident disease (Weinberg, 2007).

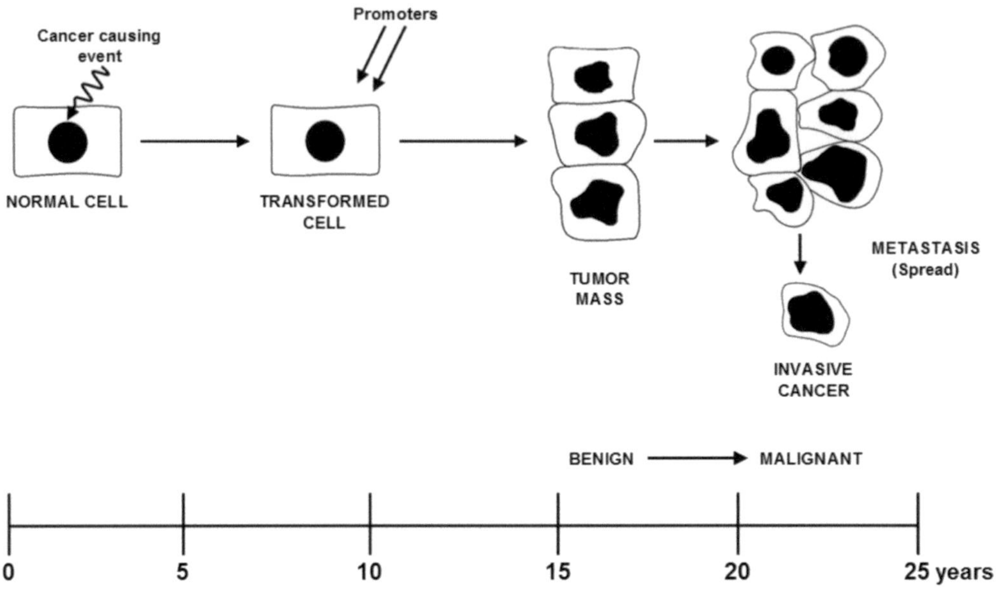

Fig. 6. Interpretive diagram to illustrate the various stages of cancer progression (estimated to require as long as 20 y) beginning with a cancer-causing event (initiation) through development of a clinically defined malignancy.

4. Discussion

4.1 Significance

Cells in tissues and organs are continuously subjected to oxidative stress and free radicals as well as other potential cancer initiating events on a daily basis (Kryston et al., 2011). Cells normally withstand these attacks but some result in cancer causing events to initiate the rather long (est. 20 y) development phase prior to clinical symptoms (Fig. 6). Our hypothesis is that ENOX proteins being critical to the unregulated growth of cancer will be shed into sera well in advance of clinical symptoms as the rationale for the proposed early detection strategy. The essential role of ENOX2 in unregulated cancer growth provides the basis for early intervention.

Early detection coupled with early intervention as diagrammed in Figure 1 raises the possibility of an important paradigm shift in cancer management toward early diagnosis and treatment options vastly different from those currently employed to deal primarily with advanced cancer. Consequently, the treatment of cancer might evolve from a primarily acute to a more chronic setting with monitoring and less invasive treatments. Reducing surgery, radiation and chemotherapy, as well as shortened hospital stays based on less invasive and less costly interventions afforded by very early detection would be expected to have a significant impact on reducing health care costs world wide.

Applications of the diagnostic methodology to post surgery patients is expected to help determine which patients still harbor residual disease following surgery and will require chemotherapy and which patients are free of disease where chemotherapy could be delayed or averted. The expectation is that the 2-D gel-western blot protocol will indicate that chemotherapy might be avoided or delayed in many patients (cancer survivors) where no evidence of disease is indicated. Additionally, the assay might be employed in patients with no clinical evidence of disease to monitor for recurrence.

4.2 ENOX2 cloning and tissue distribution

ENOX2 was expression cloned (Chueh et al., 2002) (Genbank Accession No. AF207881) using a monoclonal antibody that recognizes only a common ENOX2 epitope near the cancer drug-binding site (Cho et al., 2002) and from which the pan ENOX2 scFv recombinant antibody was derived (Kim, 2011). This binding site contains a conserved 5 amino acid (EMTEE) motif (Table 2). Based on biochemical (drug inhibition of activity) and immunological evidence, this EEMTE drug binding motif in Exon 5 appears to be common to all ENOX2 forms and absent from the amino acid sequence of the constitutive ENOX1 proteins characteristic of both cancer and non-cancer cells.

The presence of ENOX2 proteins in sera of cancer patients represents an origin due to shedding from the patient's cancer (Wilkinson et al., 1996). The presence of the ENOX2 proteins has been demonstrated in a number of human tumor tissues and xenografts (mammary carcinoma, prostate cancer, neuroblastoma, colon carcinoma, and melanoma). However, serum analysis indicates a much broader association with cancer. ENOX2 proteins are ectoproteins reversibly bound at the outer leaflet of the plasma membrane (Morré, 1995). As is characteristic of other examples of ectoproteins (sialyl and galactosyl transferases, dipeptidylamino peptidase IV, etc.), the ENOX2 proteins are shed, appearing in soluble form in conditioned media of cultured cells and in patient sera (Wilkinson et al., 1996; Morré et al., 1997). The ENOX2 transcript variants from sera exhibit the same degree of drug responsiveness as do the membrane-associated forms (Morré and Reust, 1997; Morré et al., 1997). With sera from more than 200 breast cancer patients, the majority (ca. 196), were found to exhibit the drug-responsive activity. In contrast, no drug-responsive activities were found with sera from healthy volunteers or sera from patients with diseases other than cancer (cardiac, arthritis and other inflammatory diseases, gastric ulceration, emphysema, various non-malignant blood disorders). As such the antitumor drug-responsive ENOX2 activities represent novel cell surface properties potentially associated with most, if not all, forms of human cancer to confirm their appropriateness as appropriate biomarkers for serum or plasma detection and diagnosis of cancer. ENOX2 proteins are robust and highly resistant to heat and protein degradation which enhances their utility as non-invasive markers for cancer detection and diagnosis (Morré and Morré, 2003a).

ENOX2 proteins are absent or present at levels below the limits of detection (less than 10 picomoles/ml of serum) from sera of healthy volunteers or patients with diseases other than cancer. Circulating ENOX2 has been detected based on drug response of ENOX activity of sera of more than 500 cancer patients representing all major forms of human cancer including leukemias and lymphomas (Morré and Reust, 1997; Morré et al., 1997).

4.3 Very early detection and diagnosis is unique to ENOX2 transcript variants

Many cancers are detected only after clinical symptoms present and often after the cancer has spread leaving chemotherapy as perhaps the only resource for treatment. Tomographic or x-ray methods may detect before clinical symptoms present but only after a tumor mass has already formed. There appear to be few, if any, on-going indications of opportunities either for early cancer detection or for early intervention. Various genomic, transcriptomic and/or proteomic analyses, while of potential utility for tissue analyses of biopsy material, have thus far failed to provide new and reliable non-invasive serum indicators of cancer occurrence (Goncalves and Bertucci, 2011) despite continued promise offered by circulating microRNAs (Wu et al., 2011). A relatively small percentage of all cancers can be attributed to predisposing genes such as *BRACA1, BRACA2* and less frequently *p53* and *PTEN* (Lee et al., 2010) for 5 to 10% of all breast cancers. While indicative of cancer risk, predisposing genes do not necessarily signal cancer presence.

4.4 Early intervention strategy based on green tea- *Capsicum* synergies

The potential benefits of early detection will not be fully realized without some opportunity for early curative or preventive intervention. As an early intervention strategy, findings suggest that a decaffeinated green tea extract containing 98% tea catechins of which 40% are EGCg and a *Capsicum* powder in the ratio of 25 parts tea extract plus 1 part *Capsicum* powder, available on line as Capsol-T (www.Capsol-T.com) and under commercial development by Stratum Nutrition, a division of Novus International, St. Charles, Mo under the brand name TeaFense may induce apoptosis as a means to eliminate early stage cancer when only a small number of cells are present prior to development of clinical symptoms. The ENOX proteins are responsible for the increase in cell size following cell division. After cell division, a minimum cell size must be reached or cell division stops and after several days, the cells undergo programmed cell death (apoptosis). Cancer cells with blocked ENOX2 activity are not able to enlarge and are thus directed towards apoptosis. The growth inhibition is due mainly to cell cycle arrest in G_1 (stage of cell division before DNA is replicated). EGCg inhibits growth of cancer cells in culture and in implanted tumors in mice (Li et al., 2010). The growth of implanted tumors was inhibited in a dose-dependent manner at doses of 0.1%, 0.3% and 0.5% in the diet.

Morré and Morré (2003b) have described synergy of decaffeinated green tea and a commercially available *Capsicum* preparations containing anti-cancer vanilloids (Capsibiol-T) at a ratio of 25:1 which resulted in a 100-fold increase in killing of cultured cancer cell lines compared to green tea alone. The current food grade *Capsicum*-green tea product (Capsol-T®) gives equivalent results. EGCg, when combined with other catechins also found in green tea, is superior to EGCg alone (Morré et al., 2003).

Evidence from laboratory studies with cancer cells in culture indicate that one 250 mg capsule of Capsol-T® every 4 h is equivalent to drinking 16 cups of green tea every 4 h. The need for 1 capsule of Capsol-T® every 4 h is predicated on pharmacokinetic information (Janle et al., 2008) and the knowledge that the inhibition of ENOX2 by Capsol-T® is reversible (Morré et al., 2000). In order to have therapeutic efficacy in selective killing of cancer cells, findings with cultured cancer cells show that the catechins must be present in the culture medium at a level of about 100 nM and to inhibit ENOX2 continuously at that level for a period of 48 to 72 h (Morré et al., 2000). If EGCg, for example, is removed and replaced by EGCg-free media, even after 8 h, cancer cells in vivo resume normal rates of growth. Similarly, normal rates of growth are resumed as EGCg is cleared from the culture medium and/or metabolized. Even in cell culture, the EGCg may not survive in the media for more that a few h at nanomolar concentrations. The cancer cells in vitro must be inhibited from growing for at least 48 and perhaps up to 72 h in order for apoptosis to be induced by EGCg in a majority of the cancer cells present.

Feasibility of an efficacious dosing schedule is indicated from studies with rats (Janle et al., 2008). The results from the animal study are consistent with epidemiological studies in humans and animal experiments where cancer benefit has been ascribed to drinking at least 10 cups of green tea per day without adverse effects (Fujiki, 1999; Nakachi et al., 2000). Green tea polyphenols are absorbed after oral administration and reach their highest plasma levels after about 1 to 2 h after dosing both in rats (Unno and Takeo, 1995; Zhu et al., 2000; Janle et al., 2008) and in humans (Warden et al., 2001). In the rat, the levels of EGCg reached of 12.3 nmoles/ml in plasma (12.3 µmolar) 60 min after a single oral administration of 500 mg/kg body weight of EGCg (Nakagawa, 1997), which is more than 100 times the effective dose to stop the growth of tumor cells. The studies by Yang (1997) show that the concentration of EGCg in the blood after 2-3 cups of green tea reached a maximum of about 0.6 µM.

In human studies of ingested catechins, 0.2% of the ingested EGCg and 0.2% to 1.3% of ingested (-)-epigallocatechin (EGC) were found in plasma 90 min after ingestion (Nakagawa et al. 1997). Van het Hof et al. (1999) determined the half life for plasma levels of individuals drinking 8 cups of tea per day for 3 days to be 4.8 h for green tea and 6.9 h for black tea. After ingestion of green tea by human volunteers, C_{max} values were observed 1.4 to 2.4 h after injection with a half life of 5 to 5.5 h (Yang et al., 1998). These observations provided the rational basis for dosing at regular intervals of 4 h with the Capsol-T product. Formulated for sustained release, the expectation is that two 500 mg capsules of 50% material per day, one in the morning and one in the evening will prove to be sufficient.

Tea catechins especially EGCg in combination with *Capsicum* have been characterized as specific ENOX2 inhibitors inducing apoptotic cell death in cancer but not in non-cancer cells (Morré et al., 2000; Chueh et al., 2004; Morré et al., 2009a). Safety and efficacy are well documented (Cooper et al., 2005). Safety has been the subject of a series of reports dealing with genotoxic, acute, dermal, sub-chronic short-term, teratogenic and reproductive assays (e.g. Isbrucker et al., 2006a,b,c). Capsol-T® is both caffeine- and vitamin K-free and free of herbicide, pesticide and/or heavy metal residues. Tea as a food form is generally recognized as safe by the U.S. Food and Drug Administration (National Cancer Institute Fact Sheet).

Oral green tea extracts have been studied in human cancer patients. Pisters et al. (2001) did a phase 1 study with a commercially available but not decaffeinated green tea source given 1 or 3 times daily for 4 weeks to 6 months Doses of 0.5 to 5.05 g/m^2 per day and 1.0-2.2 g/m^2 three times per day were tested in 49 cancer patients. The maximum tolerated dose of 4.22 g/m^2 was limited primarily by caffeine levels easily avoided with decaffeinated green tea.

In a series of open label sequential trials with Capsol-T® summarized by Morré and Morré (2006), 36% of participants with advanced cancer reported significant prolongation of life and/or remained alive at the time of the analysis. Another 32 reported improvement while the remaining 32% experienced a normal course of their disease. Most in the last category were diagnosed very late in the development of their disease such that an inability even to comply with six capsule per day taken one every four hours became problematic. Preliminary human studies on patients (compassionate intervention) with severe head and neck carcinomas who were treated with a commercial preparation of the dietary supplement Capsibiol-T containing the mixture of decaffeinated green tea and modified chili peppers (*Capsicum* sp.), generated results that indicated a positive role for herbal mixtures of green tea and *Capsicum* for clinical use to eliminate cancer cells from the body (Fernandez et al., 2003).

5. References

Altekruse SF, Kosary CL, Krapcho M, Neyman N, Aminou R, Waldron W, Ruhl J, Howlader N, Tatalovich Z, Cho H, Mariotto A, Eisner MP, Lewis DR, Cronin K, Chen HS, Feuer EJ, Stinchcomb DG, Edwards BK (eds).: SEER Cancer Statistics Review, 1975-2007, National Cancer Institute. Bethesda, MD, 2010.

Cho N, Chueh PJ, Kim C, Caldwell S, Morré DM, Morré DJ: Monoclonal antibody to a cancer-specific and drug-responsive hydroquinone (NADH) oxidase from the sera of cancer patients. Cancer Immunol Immunother 51:121-129, 2002.

Chueh PJ, Kim C, Cho N, Morré DM, Morré DJ: Molecular cloning and characterization of a tumor-associated, growth-related, and time-keeping hydroquinone (NADH) oxidase (tNOX) of the HeLa cell surface. Biochemistry 41:3732-3741, 2002.

Chueh, PJ, Wu, LY, Morré DM, Morré DJ: tNOX is both necessary and sufficient as a cellular target for the anticancer actions of capsaicin and the green tea catechin (-)-epigallocatechin-3-gallate. BioFactors 20:249-263, 2004.

Cooper RD, Morré DJ, Morré DM: Medicinal benefits of green tea: Part II. Review of anticancer properties. J Altern Comp Med 11:639-652, 2005.

Davies SL, Bozzo J: Spotlight on tNOX: A tumor-selective target for cancer therapies. Drug News Prospect 19:223-225, 2006.

De Luca T, Morré DM, Morré DJ: Reciprocal relationship between cytosolic NADH and ENOX2 inhibition triggers sphingolipid-induced apoptosis in HeLa cells. J Cell Biochem 110:1504-1511, 2010.

Fernandez, RF, Ganzon D: Use of green tea *Capsicum* supplement (Capsibiol-T) as adjuvant cancer treatment. Phillipine Soc Ontolaryngol Head Neck Surg 18:171-177, 2003

Fujiki H: Two stages of cancer prevention with green tea. J Cancer Res Clin Oncol 125:589-597, 1999.

Goncalves A, Bertucci F: Clinical application of proteomics in breast cancer: State of the art and perspectives. Med Princ Pract 204:4-18, 2011.

Hostetler B, Kim C: Patent GB2441860. Detecting neoplasia specific tNOX isoforms, 2011.

Hostetler B, Weston N, Kim C, Morré DM, Morré DJ: Cancer site-specific isoforms of ENOX2 (tNOX), a cancer-specific cell surface oxidse. Clin Proteomics 5:46-51, 2009

Isbrucker RA, Bausch J, Edwards JA, Wolz E: Safety studies on epigallocatechin gallate (EGCg) preparations. Part 1: Genotoxicity, Food Chem Toxicol 44:626-635, 2006a.

Isbrucker RA, Edwards JA, Wolz E, Davidovich A, Bausch J: Safety studies on epigallocatechin gallate (EGCg) preparations. Part 2: Dermal, acute and short-term toxicity studies. Food Chem Toxicol 44: 636-650, 2006b.

Isbrucker RA, Edwards JA, Wolz E, Davidovich A, Bausch J: Safety studies on epigallocatechin gallate (EGCg) preparations. Part 3. Teratogenicity and reproductive toxicity studies in rats. Food Chem Toxicol 44:651-661, 2006c.

Janle E, Morré DM, Morré DJ, Zhou Q, Chang H, Zhu Y: Pharmacokinetics of green tea catechins in extract and sustained-release preparations. J Dietary Suppl 5:248-263, 2008.

Kim C: Patent GB2442553B, Single chain pan ECTO-NOX variable region (ScFv) antibody, coding sequence and methods, 2011.

Kryston TB, Georgiev A, Georgakilas AG: Role of oxidative stress and DNA damage in human carcinogenesis. Mutat Res 711:193-201, 2011.

Li GX, Chen YK, Hou Z, Xiao H, Jin H, Lu G, Lee MJ, Liu B, Guan F, Yang Z, Yu A, Yang CS: Pro-oxidative activities and dose-response relationship of (-)-epigallocatechin-3-gallate in the inhibition of lung cancer cell growth: a comparative study *in vivo* and *in vitro*. Carcinogenesis 31:902-910, 2010.

Lee E, Park SK, Park B., Kim S-W, Lee MH, Ahn S-H, Son BH, Yoo K-Y, Kang D: Effect of *BRCA1/2* mutation on short-term and long-term breast cancer survival: a systematic review and meta-analysis. Breast Cancer Res Treat 122:11-25, 2010.

Morré DJ: NADH oxidase activity of HeLa plasma membranes inhibited by the antitumor sulfonylurea N-(4-methylphenylsulfonyl)-N-(4-chlorophenyl)urea (LY181984) at an external site. Biochim Biophys Acta 1240:201-208, 1995.

Morré DJ, Morré DM: Cell surface NADH oxidases (ECTO-NOX proteins) with roles in cancer, cellular time-keeping, growth, aging and neurodegenerative diseases. Free Radic Res 37:795-808, 2003a.

Morré DJ, Morré DM: Synergistic *Capsicum*-tea mixtures with anticancer activity. J Pharm Pharm 55:987-994, 2003b.

Morré DJ, Morré DM: Catechin-vanilloid synergies with potential clinical applications in cancer. Rejuv Res 9:45-55, 2006

Morré DJ, Reust T: A circulating form of NADH oxidase responsive to the antitumor sulfonylurea N-4-methylphenylsulfonyl-N'-4-chlorophenylurea LY181984 specific to sera from cancer patients. J Bioenerg Biomemb 29:281-289, 1997.

Morré DJ, Wilkinson FE, Kim C, Cho N, Lawrence J, Morré DM, McClure D: Antitumor sulfonylurea-inhibited NADH oxidase of cultured HeLa cells shed into media. Biochim Biophys Acta 1280:197-206, 1996.

Morré DJ, Caldwell C, Mayorga A, Wu LY and Morré DM: NADH oxidase activity from sera altered by capsaicin is widely distributed among cancer patients. Arch Biochem Biophys 342: 224-230, 1997.

Morré DJ, Bridge A, Wu LY, Morré DM: Preferential inhibition by (-)-epigallocatechin-3-gallate of the cell surface NADH oxidase and growth of transformed cells in culture. Biochem Pharmacol 60:937-946, 2000.

Morré DJ, Morré DM, Sun H, Cooper R, Chang J, Janle EM: Tea catechin synergies in inhibition of cancer cell proliferation and of a cancer-specific cell surface oxidase (ECTO-NOX). Pharmacol Toxicol 92:234-241, 2003.

Morré DJ, Geilen CC, Welch AM, Morré DM: Response of carcinoma in situ (actinic keratosis) to green tea concentrate plus *Capsicum*. J Dietary Suppl 6:385-389, 2009a.

Morré DJ, Morré DM, Brightmore R: Omega-3 but not omega-6 unsaturated fatty acids inhibit the cancer-specific ENOX2 of the HeLa cell surface with no effect on the constitutive ENOX1. J Dietary Suppl 7:154-158, 2009b.

Nakachi K, Matsuyama S, Miyake S, Sugaruma M, Imai K: Preventive effects of drinking green tea on cancer and cardiovascular disease: Epidemiological evidence for multiple targeting prevention. BioFactors 13:49-54, 2000.

Nakagawa KMT: Absorption and distribution of tea catechin, (-)-epigallocatechin-3-gallate, in the rat. J Nutr Sci Vitaminol 43:679-584, 1997,

Nakagawa K, Okuda S, Miyazawa T: Dose-dependent incorporation of tea catechins, (-)-epigallocatechin-3-gallage and (-)-epigallocatechin, into human plasma. Biosci Biotechnol Biochem 61:1981-1985, 1997,

National Cancer Institute Fact Sheet, Tea and Cancer Prevention: Strengths and Limits of Evidence, 2010.

Petro R, Darby S, Deo H, Silcocks P, Whitley E, Doll R: Smoking, smoking cessation, and lung cancer in the UK since 1950: combination of national statistics with two case-control studies. Br Med J 321:323-329, 2000.

Pisters KM, Newman RA, Coldman B, Shin DM, Khuri FR,Hong WK, Glisson BS, Lee JS: Phase 1 trial of oral green tea extract in adult patients with solid tumors. J Clin Oncol 19:1830-1838, 2001.

Tang X, Tian Z, Chueh PJ, Chen S, Morré DM, Morré DJ: Alternative splicing as the basis for specific localization of tNOX, a unique hydroquionone (NADH) oxidase, to the cancer cell surface. Biochemistry 46:12,337-12,346, 2007.

Tang X, Morré DJ, Morré DM: Antisense experiments demonstrate an exon 4 minus splice variant mRNA as the basis for expression of tNOX, a cancer-specific cell surface protein. Oncol Res 16:557-567, 2008.

Unno T, Takeo T: Absorption, distribution, elimination of tea polyphenols in rats. Absorption of (-) -epigallocatcechin gallate into the circulation system of rats. Biosci Biotechnol Biochem 59:1558-1559, 1995.

van het Hof KH, Wiseman SA, Chang CS, Tijburg BM: Plasma and lipoprotein levels of tea catechins following repeated tea consumption. Proc Soc Exp Biol Med 320:203-209, 1999.

Warden BA, Smith LA, Beecher GR, Balentine DA, Clevidence BA: Catechins are bioavailable in men and women drinking black tea throughout the day. J Nutr 131:1731-1737, 2001

Weinberg RA: The Biology of Cancer, Fig. 11.1, p. 400 (Courtesy of Hong WK compiled from SEER Cancer Statistics Review), Garland Science, 2007.

Wilkinson FE, Kim C, Cho NM, Chueh PJ, Leslie S, Moya-Camarfena S, Wu LY, Morre DJ, Morre DJ: Isolation and identification of a protein with capsaicin-inhibited NADH oxidase activity from culture media conditioned by growth of HeLa cells. Arch Biochem Biophys 336:275-282, 1996.

Wu Q, Lu Z, Li H, Lu H, Guo L, Ge Q: Next-generation sequencing of microRNAs for breast cancer detection. J Biomed Biotechnol, Article ID 597145, 2011.

Yang CS: Inhibition of carcinogenesis by tea. Nat Clin Proc Cardiovasc Med 389:134-135, 1997.

Yang CS, Chen L, Lee MJ, Balentine D, Kyo MC, Schantz SP: Blood and urine levels of tea catechins after ingestion of different amounts of green tea by human volunteers, Cancer Epidemiol Biomarkers Prev 7:679-684, 1998.

Zhu M, Chen Y, Li RC: Oral absorption and bioavailability of tea catechins. Planta Med 66:444-447, 2000.

16

Creating a Sustainable Cancer Workforce: Focus on Disparities and Cultural Competence

Maureen Y. Lichtveld, Lovell Jones,
Alison Smith, Armin Weinberg,
Roy Weiner and Farah A. Arosemena
*Tulane University, MD Anderson Cancer Center, C-Change,
Life Beyond Cancer Foundation
USA*

1. Introduction

While the role of culture in addressing health care disparities in general and, cancer health disparities specifically is increasingly recognized, a systemic approach aimed at bolstering the cultural competence of our nation's health care workforce is absent. Among the health outcomes, the impact of this gap is most pronounced in cancer. Ample scientific evidence exists affirming that eliminating cancer health disparities requires a multi-sectorial approach. The lack of cultural competence among frontline providers - physicians, nurses, pharmacists, health educators – is only compounded by the cancer workforce crisis, a national threat to assuring quality cancer care to a growing vulnerable and increasingly culturally diverse global population. Traditional solutions to the health care workforce crisis in general and that of the cancer workforce specifically have largely failed because of a silo- rather than a systems approach, focusing on one specific segment of the workforce or one specific aspect of cancer care. Furthermore, much of those efforts were limited to addressing the quantitative aspect of the problem – increase the number of cancer care professionals, ignoring the equally important qualitative component- assuring a health care workforce, *competent* in providing cancer care across the cancer spectrum to culturally diverse populations. (C-Change 2008; Lichtveld 2009)

The cancer workforce is faced with various obstacles as cancer prevalence and mortality rates swell worldwide and cancer patients and survivors are directly affected by the shortage in a workforce to provide care. Compounding the shortfall in health prevention and clinical care, the disproportionate impact of cancer on minorities and disadvantaged populations has been apparent for decades with few innovative cancer care delivery models implemented. A growing body of evidence indicates that in addition to race, and geo-socio-economic parameters, culture is a strong influencing factor on cancer outcomes.(Grouse 2005; Chin, Walters et al. 2007; Fisher, Burnet et al. 2007) Converting the role culture plays in eliminating cancer health disparities from a barrier to an asset, requires cultural competence from those providing care across the entire cancer care continuum – from prevention to survivorship. (Lichtveld 2009)

2. Racial, cultural and ethnic disparities in cancer care

Global health disparities is a critical area of concern and intensifies the issue of cancer in developed and developing countries.(Jones, Chilton et al. 2006; Kawahara, Masui et al. 2010) Cancer is the leading cause of death worldwide with mortality rates spiking in low- and middle- income countries.(Linkov, Padilla et al. 2010) Medical care alone cannot adequately improve health related quality of life or reduce cancer disparities without also addressing where and how people live.(Subban, Terwoord et al. 2008) As countries become more culturally diverse, taking action to train the future cancer workforce to better serve their changing communities is a top priority. (Dogra, Reitmanova et al. 2010) Public & private health systems need to move beyond identifying problems to development of novel interventions and their implementation. Additionally, genuine efforts need to be made to offer culturally & linguistically appropriate services to the world's most vulnerable populations.

Addressing global cancer health disparities requires a holistic solution to a complex and interdependent set of patient, provider, and health system factors. Through educational interventions, projects can aim to position the health care system to effectively serve patients and communities of color. The state of the cancer workforce displays a grim picture, with several shortages including oncologists, pharmacists and nurses. These shortages can be characterized as supply and demand determinants; the demand for oncologists – the lifetime probability of developing cancer is 1 in every 2 men and 1 in every 3 women - is expected to exceed supply by 25%-30% by 2020. Against this backdrop, bolstering the basic cancer care competency knowledge and skills of medical, nursing and pharmacy students is essential as an evidence-based prevention priority and sustainable capacity for cancer care.(C-Change 2008; Smith, Tyus et al. 2009)

Cancer health disparities in low- and middle- income countries provides a uniquely rich platform for educational interventions as reflected by the large number of physicians, nurses and pharmacists serving resource-challenged and underserved populations. By "mainstreaming" cultural competence-embedded cancer care education into health professions curricula, a competent cadre of health care providers produced as a result of revised competencies and cancer education curricula has a "ready practice setting" to implement those skills in a fashion that is measurable.

3. A balanced perspective: understanding the social determinants of health

To elucidate the global perspective of lower-resourced communities, the Social-Ecological Model of Health provides an applicable theoretical framework. The model proposes that individual health is influenced by biological and genetic functioning, social and familial relationships, the built environment, and broader psychosocial and economic factors (Figure 1). Health is influenced by multiple facets in the physical and social environment; the environment itself is multidimensional, incorporating social, physical, actual or perceived elements as discrete attributes or constructs. An individual's environment is influenced by the interaction with people who share that environment. Person-environment interactions occur in cycles in which people influence their settings; these changes in turn influence health behaviors.(Stokols 1996)

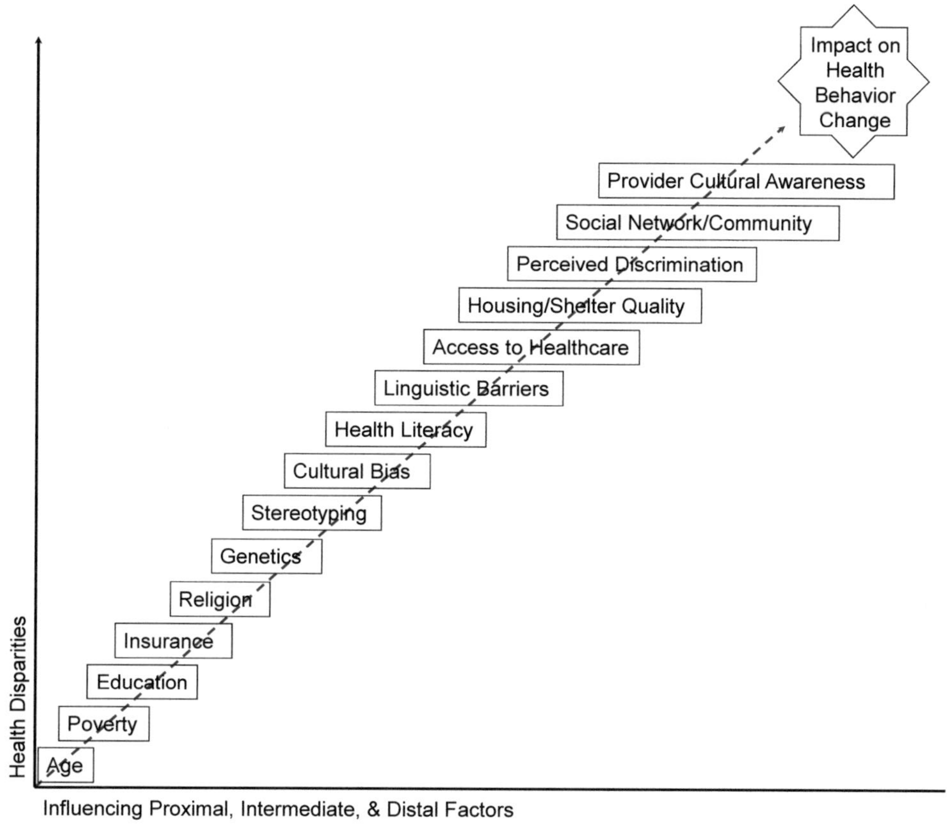

Fig. 1. Social-ecological model: reversing the social determinants that widen the healthy divide.

Social determinants are inextricably linked with socioeconomic disparities that impact every phase of the cancer care spectrum from screening to palliative care. (Smedley, Stith et al. 2003) Despite the United States nationally acclaimed decreases in breast and cervical cancer mortality due in large part to early screening and better therapeutics, African American Hispanic and American Indian/Alaska Native (AI/AN) populations have not enjoyed these same benefits. African American and Hispanic women have higher breast and cervical cancer mortality respectively despite similar screening rates to White women. Colorectal cancer screening rates are also lower while advanced stage at diagnosis higher within African American and Hispanic people. Treatment disparities are particularly concerning. The absolute proportion of African American and Hispanic women receiving radiation therapy less than 1 year after breast conserving therapy is 12% lower in African American and 19% lower in Hispanic women. There is no stable data for AI/AN women. (Natale Pereira, Enard et al. 2011) African American women with breast cancer were less likely to receive full course chemotherapy (Griggs, Sorbero et al. 2003)and more likely to receive non-standard chemotherapy regimens (OR 1.93 [1.11 - 3.36]). (Griggs, Culakova et al. 2007; Griggs, Culakova et al. 2007)This correlated with stage of disease i.e. Stage II and III OR 2.82 (2.01 - 3.95) and 7.95 (4.06-15.98) respectively, and lower education levels i.e. less than high school OR 3.24 (1.17 - 9.0), high school graduate OR 1.8 (1.08-3.0). These data in part, may explain the lower survival rates in African American and Hispanic women although data in Hispanic women is lacking. System factors pose significant problems with lower proportions of Hispanic women reporting timely receipt of appointments (35 vs. 49%) and higher proportion reporting difficulty in getting care when needed compared to White women (66 vs. 55.8%). Higher poverty rates, lower insurance rates and higher discontinuously insured rates, decreased English proficiency when compared to White populations characterize African American and/or Hispanic populations. (Smith Bindman, Miglioretti et al. 2006; Elkin, Ishill et al. 2010; Miranda, Wilkinson et al. 2011) Effective cancer care cannot be delivered without a multi-tiered approach that effectively links and integrates the patient with all components of the cancer care delivery system. Patient navigation is a promising strategy that can affect this.

4. Addressing adversity: linking cultural competence to health disparities

Over the past three decades, efforts to meaningfully address health disparities have largely focused on exhaustive characterization and definition of health disparities through multiple lenses - community, social, demographic, environmental, economic, race/ethnicity, gender, age, disabilities - with significantly less attention, until recently, to outcomes and effective interventions to reduce and/or alleviate them. In part this results from the complexity of developing and implementing interventions that can effectively and seamlessly leverage opportunities and traverse barriers within and between the health care system, provider, patient, academic and at large community components. The economic climate is forcing a 'lean thinking' approach to intervention development that focuses on innovative process and resource reallocation that will lead to measured and sustainable improvement in health outcomes. (Womack and Jones 2003) The Patient Protection and Affordable Care Act (PPACA Public Law 111-148), though imperfect and controversial, is an important first step in systemic funding to address health disparities. Furthermore, relevant outcome evaluation that goes beyond traditional metrics is central to development and assessment of effective interventions. Past naïve and archaic approaches focusing on one sector of the health care system, trusting that passive diffusion will decrease disparities throughout the entire system have failed. The health care crisis will continue to mandate an integrated, non-silo approach that meaningfully incorporates traditional (physicians, nurses, pharmacists, health educators) and emerging non-traditional (navigators, community health workers) into traditional and most importantly, non-traditional highly innovative and meaningfully integrate roles within the health care team and care delivery model.

4.1 Cultural competence: the devil is in the details

Culture, "the integration of patterns of human behavior that includes language, thoughts, communications, actions, customs, beliefs, values and institutions of different racial, ethnic, religious or social groups" is a powerful lens through which patients make virtually every health care decision. (Matthews-Juarez and Weinberg 2004) Cultural competence, "acquiring and integrating knowledge, awareness and skills about culture and cultural differences that enables Health Care Professionals to provide optimal care to patients from different racial ethnic and cultural backgrounds", a bidirectional requisite for oncology providers and their patients has been largely overlooked within the clinical continuum.

Treatment outcome starts with the patient's first encounter with the health care system. The quality of that encounter, distinct from customer service, significantly impacts the subsequent patient-provider relationship, ultimate partnership, adherence to treatment recommendations, quality of life during treatment and the survivorship continuum. Qualitative factors have an equal if not greater role than quantitative information in patient decision making. Therefore, the qualitative approach that the provider chooses to communicate the quantitative information is paramount. The provider must understand the culture through which the patient relates and understands information about medical and social aspects of the disease process and treatment.

Cultural nuances differ ethnically as well as geographically a factor which becomes especially important when dealing with populations in various phases of acculturation in a country or community. For example, in the United States, all phases of the patient-provider interaction center on the implicit understanding that the patient will make the ultimate treatment decision. In certain Hispanic cultures, the husband might make the ultimate decision while in Asian culture, the eldest son will be the decision maker. In African American culture, the children and spouse collectively drive the treatment decisions of the patient. Failure to address these decision makers through all phases of the patient encounter and decision making process will negatively impact on the overall quality of the provider-patient relationship and ultimately treatment compliance by creating an environment of mistrust and devaluing the patient and their support system.

Understanding how people from different cultures actually make treatment decisions is critical. In western culture, the process is linear- treatment discussion, research treatment options via internet/publications, analyze the data and reach a decision within a defined, usually short, timeframe. If the provider does not realize that the doctor's opinion rather than the research process may be the deciding factor for Hispanic patients, that the American Indian patient may want to discuss their condition with the tribal elders or healer, that African American patients may want to discuss their options with the family matriarch/patriarch and obtain *their* treatment decisions before informing the provider of the patient's treatment decision then the delay in treatment decision will not 'make sense'. Furthermore, the questions posed to the provider through the patient may in fact emanate from these other individuals. This can result in mismatched patient-provider expectations leading to miscommunication and narrow, biased interpretations of how 'capable' a given patient may be to 'understand' their treatment.

Subtle aspects of the patient encounter engagement process are important. African American patients expect direct eye contact as lack thereof conveys the message that the provider cannot be trusted. Conversely, Asian patients will avoid eye contact as direct eye contact is a sign of disrespect to the provider who is perceived, in that setting to have higher status. Conversely, listening to the provider's treatment discussion with closed eyes does not signify disinterest or information/emotional overload for the Japanese patient but indicates that the provider has the patient's full attention. Failing to directly address the husband of a Hispanic woman when making treatment recommendations is an insult to her husband. The importance of cultural competence in the provider patient partnership cannot be overstressed and is critical to effectively address health disparities.

4.2 Eliminating disparities and enhancing diversity in clinical trials

The improvement in health status in a community, region or country can be measured in many ways. Sir Michael Marmot, WHO Chair of the Commission on Social Determinants of Health, posits that the health care system accounts for about 20% of this.(Wilkinson and Marmot 2003) Improved health status is greatly impacted through social policy such as controlling access to tobacco or designing communities that provide conditions that support walking rather than dependence on mass transit. Such environmental interventions do not eliminate the need or benefit of required individual application or adoption of preventive behaviors such as smoking cessation, increased exercise, better dietary choices, or breast feeding.

However, when someone is diagnosed with a life threatening disease like cancer, it is no longer a question of how to prevent an occurrence; it is time to provide access to the best quality of care. For this, the process of informed decision making begins with their clinician, and what do they offer? What are they required to offer? Unfortunately, there is less participation in clinical trials and often the clinician's failure to provide information as a part of their care options is at the root of the problem. Yet there are many others in the cancer workforce that have an equally important role in guiding patients, supporting their decision making process, and helping them as participants if they choose to enter a clinical trial.

Clinical trials are a critical resource for developing new lifesaving drugs as well as better prevention, diagnostic, and treatment methods. However, numerous demographic groups are underrepresented in cancer clinical trials. These include racial and ethnic minorities, the elderly, women, children and adolescents, low income and uninsured individuals, rural residents, and individuals with disabilities.

There is no single reason why the evidence consistently demonstrates widespread disparities in clinical trial participation. Rather, multiple factors coalesce to produce a system that features such disparities. Accordingly, the Eliminating Disparities in Clinical Trials (EDICT) Project sought to model an approach that would not merely address individual contributing variables, but would instead analyze the problem and proposed solutions via a systematic, multi-level approach.(ICC 2009)

Each of the more than 300 EDICT participants represented one or more of the many stakeholders who encountered the multiple factors that produce underrepresentation in clinical trials. For example, concerns of scientific validity suggest that protocol design include, from the outset, recognition of patterns of disease burden and, where appropriate, reflect those patterns in recruitment and retention strategies. In addition, members of underrepresented populations consistently report mistrust of medical and research professionals, in contrast to local community healthcare workers, who are rarely involved with clinical research. Finally, the mistaken belief that appropriate representation in clinical trials requires larger expenditures in conducting the trial(s) justifies the unwarranted assumption that ameliorating disparities in clinical trials is cost-ineffective.

These examples demonstrate how the factors contributing to the problem of disparities in clinical trials operate at different levels, across different sectors, and involve different stakeholders. The primary initial result of the EDICT Project is the 33 Policy Recommendations. There are both data and theory strongly suggesting that if relevant stakeholders implemented even a minority of the recommendations, disparities in clinical trials could be substantially reduced. Because of this complexity, eliminating disparities in clinical trials requires a multi-level systems approach and certainly one that requires the creation of a fully engaged and competent workforce. (Wilkinson and Marmot 2003; ICC 2009)

The EDICT Credo can serve as a framework for training and sustaining a workforce that ensures the appropriate inclusion of under-represented populations are ameliorated in the future. The following beliefs guide the work of the EDICT Project:

- All individuals will have the opportunity and necessary support to participate voluntarily in clinical trials for which they are eligible.
- Participants and researchers will understand and promote the benefits of diversity in clinical trials.
- Results from clinical research will benefit the participants' communities and society at large.(ICC 2009)

Creating such a workforce will require attention to barriers related to researchers, referring physicians, and the recruitment process itself. For example, racial/ethnic minorities are underrepresented among researchers. Community physicians are often unaware of clinical trial opportunities and experience excessive administrative or financial burden related to clinical trials. Additional barriers include lack of institutional interest, infrastructure, staff time, sufficiently skilled research coordinators, and training in culturally competent communication skills related to clinical trial recruitment.

A competent workforce should be capable of understanding frequent patient barriers to recruitment that are exacerbated for underrepresented groups. These barriers include poor understanding of the research and its related risk; transportation difficulties and caregiver availability; participant fatigue and inconvenience; general lack of awareness that clinical trials are an option; mistrust due to previous unethical research experiences; cultural, linguistic, and literacy issues; inadequate paid work leave, childcare, or insurance coverage; misidentification of race/ethnicity; and relocations, extended visits, or return to countries of origin.

While helping potential participants to "navigate" their way into, through, and after the clinical trial process is critical to improving inclusion of these groups in cancer research. The task is complicated by the fact that there are multiple professionals and paraprofessionals involved in recruitment and retention of participants in clinical trials at different points of contact along the continuum of cancer care. These include, but are not limited to, clinical researchers, research administrators, community health workers and promotoras,, nurses, patient navigators, physicians who refer patients, physician assistants, and social workers to name a few.

The Department of Health and Human Services (DHHS) Office of Minority Health (OMH) developed National Standards for Culturally and Linguistically Appropriate Services (CLAS) in 2000. The CLAS-And Clinical Trials (CLAS-ACT) Project helps to assess how well CLAS Standards are implemented in a single clinical trial or study as well as across multiple trials in an organization. CLAS-ACT materials may also be used to train research staff and administrators about CLAS standards. These standards are a straightforward method to support taking one significant step in providing a cancer workforce in general but in particular for those involved in clinical research they can be instrumental in bringing the research experience into a comparable position with overall access to health care services in general.

"Imagine that you possess an indicator for a disease or illness that has nothing to do with your body. It is not a genetic predisposition to acquire cancer or a vice that raises the probability of contracting some dread disease, though estimates of its health risks have placed it on par with having diabetes. It has nothing to do with the environmental pollutants you are exposed to or whether you can afford health care. It is not a physical susceptibility that renders you more easily reachable by the clutches of pathology. No, this indicator of health hinges on certain learned abilities and skills, and it is a barrier to health that is totally within the health field's power and resources to lift. The condition hinted at above is the inability to speak English proficiently in the United States."(Bustillos 2009)

Correcting for this will not be easy. Little data exists on issues such as this in the clinical research enterprise. What will be important is the ability to recognize that it will be both a combination of policy and programs that culminate in a competent corps of health care workers. Indeed as an evidence base is developed we must recall that those currently in the cancer workforce can make a significant step by striving for cultural competence. The nature of funding and conducting randomized clinical trial research is changing to reflect the evolution of the science base, the need to increase diversity among study participants, to establish trust among certain communities by acknowledging the need for social justice and health equity, and of course the globalization of drug development and emerging markets. In response, there are significant efforts underway to address the barriers to participation in clinical trials, which remain low.(Wilkinson and Marmot 2003)

The National Cancer Institute recently conducted research with oncology professionals that identified unmet accrual needs. As a result they have developed a comprehensive platform for accrual resources, AccrualNet.(NCI 2011) Their methodology used a variety of techniques including literature and resource searches to identify the content for the site. Certainly, as noted throughout EDICT's recommendations, designing interventions to support a broader the workforce must meet different barriers AccrualNet represents a unique, centralized comprehensive-solution platform to systematically capture accrual knowledge for all stages of a clinical trial. It is designed to foster a community of practice by encouraging users to share additional strategies, resources, and ideas.(NCI 2011)

For those who recognize the importance of clinical trials there is an opportunity to educate, encourage, and inform others. It is important to learn how to intervene with members of the cancer workforce who today have the ability to increase awareness about clinical trials and provide patients the opportunity to consider participation in a clinical trial. We need to make this part of our education and training of future workforce, if not, we are likely to have medicine's role in improving the quality of life diminish rather than flourish.

The lesson of EDICT is that there are many things that need our attention if we are truly to overcome the barriers to increasing participation in clinical trials. However, it is clear that if those (our cancer workforce) who can do something will, ultimately we will succeed.

5. Revitalization of cancer care: cancer competencies framework

Nearly all of the professional disciplines that play a role in the delivery of comprehensive cancer services are experiencing a shortage including physicians, nurses, social workers, pharmacists, public health workers, researchers, technologists, and cancer registrars. The rising incidence of cancer, an aging population, and an increased rate of cancer survivorship all predict an increased demand for health services. These trends threaten our ability to provide timely and comprehensive cancer care. Many cancer-focused organizations are investing in efforts to expand the number of cancer specialists in anticipation of a worsening cancer workforce crisis.

5.1 Building a cultural bridge through a competency-based approach

Complementing other national efforts focused on the recruitment and retention of oncology health professionals, C-Change pursued the Cancer Core Competency Initiative to develop standards and tools for strengthening the cancer knowledge and skills of non-oncology health professionals, including generalist and other non-oncology specialists. Defining the core competencies needed by all members of the health workforce represents one important approach toward expanding the cancer workforce (Figure 2). A multi-disciplinary panel of national leaders and experts developed competency standards spanning the continuum of cancer care, basic cancer science, and communication and collaboration. Implementation tools included a logic model and curriculum validation template.(C-Change 2008; Smith, Tyus et al. 2009)

Continuum of Care
Prevention | Early Detection | Treatment | Survivorship | Palliative Care
Basic Cancer Science
Etiology | Epidemiology | Clinical Trials | Cancer Surveillance
Communications & Collaboration
Inter-disciplinary Care | Psychosocial Communication
Cross-Cultural Communication

Fig. 2. Scope of competency standards.

In an effort to test this approach, a grant program invited applicants from any academic, healthcare, cancer coalition, or voluntary/advocacy organization to apply the standards and tools to address a specific need in the professionals and, ultimately, the patients that they serve. Four grant-funded sites implemented the C-Change Cancer Core Competency Program in their organization by utilizing this rigorous set of competency standards, curriculum design tools, and evaluation methods to create their own programs. Each of the grant sites focused on a unique combination of a cancer topic, discipline, education/experience level, and practice setting.(C-Change 2008)

	Audrain Medical Center (MO)	Marshall University School of Medicine (WV)	University of Pittsburg Medical Center (PA)	California University of Pennsylvania (PA)
Cancer Topic	Skin cancer prevention and early detection	Breast cancer screening and patient communication	Survivorship	Cancer-related depression and anxiety
Healthcare Discipline	Nurses	Physicians	Physicians, Advanced Practice Nurses	Social Workers
Level of Education & Experience	Practicing professionals, Nurses, AD, BSN, MSN	Students, Year 2 Medical School	Practicing professionals, Masters	Graduate students, Practicing professionals/ field faculty, BSW, MSW
Practice Setting	Rural, Public health field workers	Academic training program	Urban/Rural, Primary care clinics	Rural, Social service agencies

Table 1. Scope of pilot site competency initiatives.

	Iowa Cancer Coalition (ICC)	University of Florida (UF)	Virginia Commonwealth University (VCU)	South Puget Intertribal Planning Agency (SPIPA)
Cancer Topic	Palliative and end-of-life care Hospice care	Pain and cancer-related symptoms and management resources	Pain management in pediatric patients	Culture-specific cancer pain
Healthcare discipline	Nurses, Medical Assistants	Physicians, Nurses, Social Workers, Office Staff	Medical Students, Pediatric Residents	Native Health Workers
Type / Level of education and experience	Practicing professionals AD, BSN Certificate	Practicing professionals MD, RN, MSW, Diploma	Students, Pre-Professional	Variable education and training as "lay" community health worker
Practice Setting	Rural long term care facilities	Rural health, primary care clinics (mostly Federally Qualified Health Centers)	Pediatric Clinic and Medical Center	Native American communities

Table 2. Scope of pain and palliative care grant site competency.

The pilot sites reported that the methods were flexible and useful when addressing various cancer topics, with a wide variety of disciplines, and within different organizational settings. Measureable gains in knowledge, skills, and attitudes were realized by all sites. In addition, all four pilot sites experienced benefits beyond those derived by the participant including positive effects such as professional development, institutional visibility, and community relations. A full description of the standards, tools, and pilot site results can be found at www.cancercorecompetency.org. (C-Change 2008)

As a continuation of this innovative program, C-Change invited grant applicants for a more focused purpose of strengthening the cancer pain and palliative care knowledge, skills, and attitudes of non-oncology health professionals. Program activities could focus on any relevant organization, discipline, or geographic area. This initiative was guided by a multidisciplinary, multi-sector advisory committee and managed by C-Change staff. Funding for the grant awards was provided through a generous donation from the Purdue Pharma L.P.

Through a collaborative process, four new grant sites worked with C-Change to plan and implement their programs. Again, the sites reported that the methods were flexible and useful when addressing various cancer topics, with a wide variety of disciplines, and within different organizational settings. Measurable gains in knowledge, skills, and attitudes were realized by all sites.

5.2 Cultural competency focus

One of the eight grant recipients, the South Puget Intertribal Planning Agency (SPIPA), indicated a specific cultural focus in meeting the needs of the population they serve. They recognized the need to understand cultural experiences and beliefs in order to equip health professionals with the most productive language, tools, and approach to reaching individuals at risk for and living with cancer.(C-Change 2010) The South Puget Intertribal Planning Agency (SPIPA), a Tribally-chartered nonprofit organization serves five Tribes, Chehalis, Nisqually, Shoalwater Bay, Skokomish, and Squaxin Island near Seattle, Washington. SPIPA's grant application described their aim to improve pain and palliative care management for community members.(C-Change 2010) They illustrated the existing cancer burden to their community in terms familiar to most health professionals:

"According to the Washington State Cancer Registry, American Indians/Alaska Natives (AI/ANs) have the highest incidence and mortality rate of cancer incidence of any racial group in our state[1]. Geographically the SPIPA service population is located in the area of Washington that has had higher than expected total cancer deaths for each year individually and for all years combined. For 2000-2004 combined, the relative risk (rr) was 1.14, or 14% more cancer deaths than expected; this equals about *290 excess deaths* per year. Survival is poorer in small rural towns compared to urban and large rural cities/towns. [2] The reservations served by the Tribal clinics are considered to serve rural populations; the majority is considered Health Professional Shortage Areas (HPSA)."(C-Change 2010)

5.3 Pre-assessment and program planning

The statistics alone were daunting, but as the planning process unfolded, cultural nuances emerged that made achieving their initial program goal more challenging. As part of the initial needs assessment process, the project leaders conducted a series of talking circles (focus groups) with each tribe. Initially, they gathered feedback that revealed some of the prevailing beliefs of the community, "[f]or Native Elders, pain is not discussed until it is severe, pain is believed to always accompany cancer, and it is not believed that it can be relieved, although traditional healers can help. Many have addiction concerns or concerns about being perceived as 'drug seekers'." This feedback was consistent with previous observations and reinforced the need to address myths in the competency training.(C-Change 2010)

Feedback that was not expected revealed a culturally-driven difference in basic vocabulary. The word "pain" had a different meaning to tribal members than what is typically understood to mean an unpleasant physical or emotional sensation occurring in varying degrees of severity as a consequence of injury or disease. The word "pain" meant historical trauma from past injustices experienced by Native Americans. Upon further inquiry, the term "discomfort" was a more accurate word for physical symptoms and the term "distress" was a more meaningful word for emotional symptoms. (C-Change 2010)

Initially, the program aimed to strengthen the competency of traditional western medical providers who serve the native community, but the need to empower native health workers with knowledge, skills, and tools to build a bridge between the patient and the medical provider emerged as a more strategic starting point.(C-Change 2010)

Project leaders refined the program goals and audience accordingly to: 1) Address community and patient understanding of cancer pain (distress and discomfort) assessment, communication and management of that distress and discomfort for survivors and caregivers in Native communities; 2) Improve communication and understanding about cancer pain, cancer related distress and discomfort, and palliative care, among Tribal members, their caregivers and the Tribal Health system by providing a common language; 3) Prepare a cadre of community members, targeting caregivers, at the local community level who will be community resources for cancer pain and can effectively provide peer level education within their communities and clinics; and 4) Empower Native people experiencing cancer pain to raise this quality-of-life issue with their health care providers.(C-Change 2010)

The competency goals set for participant included:

- Manage symptoms of the cancer pain, distress and discomfort / provide culturally appropriate tools for describing distress
- Describe the methods used to identify pain throughout the progression of the disease
- Differentiate between acute and chronic pain symptoms
- Perform pain assessment / train "Wellness Workers" (caregivers) on performing culturally tailored pain assessment
- Explain and explore the different treatment options for pain - including culturally appropriate as well as medical best practices
- Perform a pain related history taken during physical examination; teach patients how to document/ journal pain

Using a logic model, the program leaders designed an interactive workshop that would be delivered by trusted community members to an audience of community "Wellness Workers," caregivers, peer educators, and advocates as well as cancer patients and survivors. The objectives, inputs, outputs, outcomes (short-, medium-, and long-term), and impact are illustrated in Table 3.(C-Change 2010)

5.4 Workshop content and tools

The workshop content addressed the distinction between cancer discomfort, distress, and historical pain; the importance of treating pain as part of the healing process; myths about addiction; ways to communicate pain; and obstacles to seeking pain management in the

SPIPA
CCCP

Addressing Culture-Specific Pain Management: Creating a Common Ground between Community Members and Caregivers to Address Native American Cancer Pain and Palliative Care

Objectives/Aims:	Inputs	Outputs	Outcomes	
Aim #1: Improve community and patient knowledge of cancer pain/distress assessment, communication and management for survivors and caregivers in Native communities, **Aim #2:** Improve ability to communicate about cancer pain, cancer related distress and palliative care between Tribal members, their caregivers and the Tribal Health system	**Course Materials:** Community input on curriculum (CCCP Advisory and Support groups) Unbroken Circle AI/AN Pain Mgt. Training **Presenters:** Oncology Nursing Association U. of Washington Traditional Healers **Other Assistance/resources:** Native People for Cancer Control **Communication Tools:** Community input on assessment tools Unbroken Circle assessment tools Cancer Pain Foundation resources SPIPA customized assessment tools	**Major Activities:** Formative Assessment of community needs Pre/post survey Training Curriculum Training Post assessment with support groups Final Report **Participation:** 25 AI/AN Wellness Workers AI/AN cancer pain training team, trainers and partners **Materials:** Cancer pain assessment tools collected and/or developed Digital stories as examples of communication	AIM #1	**Short term:** Improved knowledge of cancer related pain, discomfort and stress by AI/AN patients and caregivers Improved knowledge of treatment options for cancer pain and discomfort
			AIM #2	**Medium term:** Increased acceptance of cancer patients to work with health care team to address cancer related pain Culturally appropriate cancer pain assessment tools used by patient and caregivers to document pain Culturally appropriate mechanism for communicating cancer pain to health care providers implemented Improved communication about cancer pain between those with cancer and their caregivers
			AIM #1 and 2	**Long term:** Caregivers, patients & providers have improved core competency in culturally appropriate cancer pain assessment Curriculum, tools and resources available and used by othe AI/AN communities to improve communication about cancer pain between patients, caregivers and providers
Impact: AI/AN cancer patients are able to assess and communicate cancer related pain/distress to their caregiver and health care team *Every provider will ask the patient for their pain assessment checklist/journal*				

Table 3. SPIPA logic model.

health system. In preparation for the workshop, two important tools were developed, video segments of cancer survivors discussing their discomfort and distress and a pain journal. The videos were an important way to convey the patient experience with familiar community members and reinforced the importance of expressing, rather than suppressing, pain symptoms.

The pain journal was specially designed to provide a place for patients to record their symptoms and a tool to share their symptoms with their medical providers. The journal contains a variety of resources that prompt a patient to record onset, quality, intensity, duration, and the effect of relief interventions. The prompts included anatomical diagrams, vocabulary lists to describe the pain sensations, functional assessment of activities of daily living, and checklists to inventory other symptoms. In addition to addressing aspects of "discomfort," the journal also explored aspects of "distress" with functional and mood assessment tools.(C-Change 2010)

The CCCP (Comprehensive Cancer Control Program) Advisory Council made a specific recommendation to create a customized pain barometer, mirroring the classic Wong-Baker faces (Figure 3). They commissioned a local artist, Peter Boome, to create a culturally meaningful rendition of this scale using traditional Salish faces. The scale provided a more culturally familiar image and more direct connection to their pain experience. In a broader sense, the knowledge and tools for expressing pain provided in the workshop gave participants "permission" to talk about a subject that was not a cultural norm. (C-Change 2010)

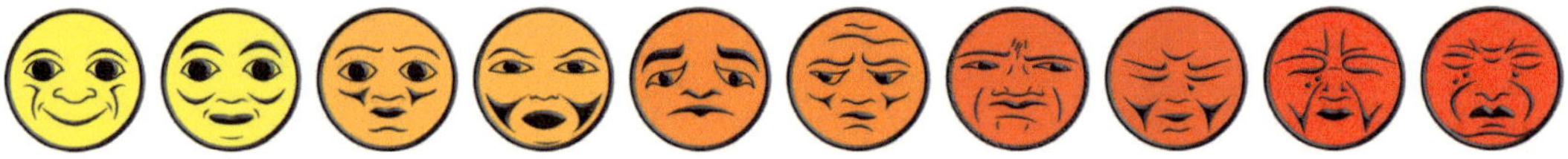

Fig. 3. Pain Barometer.

5.5 Evaluation methods and outcomes

Evaluation methods for the workshop training including a pre- and post-tests for participants, which included questions assessing perceptions, knowledge, and skills. The perception questions assessed changes in confidence in knowledge, ability to recognize distress and discomfort, and ability to communicate symptoms. Knowledge questions assessed definitions of types of discomfort and distress and common interventions to address these symptoms. Skills questions assessed the ability to report symptoms clearly and completely.

In total, 102 people participated in one of the five workshops held for each of the tribes. This represents approximately 3.5% of the combine populations of these communities. Confidence scores increased dramatically from pre- to post test, ranging from 129-233% change on individual questions. Knowledge and skills questions showed modest improvements averaging a 7.4% change. Upon further reflection, the program leaders recognized the role that the timing, format, and reading skills of the participants may have played in these results. During the workshop, the faculty used interactive verbal true/false questions to assess comprehension which anecdotally reflected a much stronger gain in knowledge and skills. When asked about the impact of the training experience, 68% of respondents were "very" or "extremely likely" to change their caregiving as a result of the training. Eighty-seven percent were "very" or "extremely likely" to recommend the training to a friend.(C-Change 2010)

5.6 Conclusions

The impact of the workshop series has had a longer lasting and broader impact than expected. SPIPA has produced and distributed journals since the training within and beyond the SPIPA communities. In addition, they have received inquiries from other AI/AN communities interested in hosting a similar workshop. With these initial successes, they are turning back to their original goal of providing competency-based training for culturally appropriate pain management to western medical providers who serve the SPIPA community. The initial investment in the knowledge and skills of native healthcare workers and caregivers should provide an important cultural competency bridge for bringing patients and care providers together to improve patient outcomes

6. A roadmap towards culturally competent community based participatory cancer care

To date, health systems research has focused disproportionately more on health services research than community-based public health systems research. Likewise, funding for Community Based Participatory Research (CBPR) is orders of magnitude less than traditional biomedical research. In both instances failure to make progress is complex and advocating for one type of research over the other is counterproductive and may hurt rather than help strengthen the science base required to address cancer health disparities. Perhaps the most fundamental root cause of health disparities is infrastructure in general and the health infrastructure specifically: where you live indeed determines your health.

The three core components of the health infrastructure- workforce, organizational setting, and health system capacity- directly influence a community's health status. Overlaying this already complex relationship is the need to deliver culturally competent care to in our case communities with a historic burden of cancer health disparities. Figure 4 presents a multidimensional framework depicting the relationship among the three core components in the context of delivering culturally competent cancer care.

The most important perquisite for successful culturally competent care is the collaboration and active participation of the community. Rather than focusing on a community's needs only, asset-driven participation fulfills a pivotal role to inform the development of a culturally competent cancer care workforce on one hand and to embed community assets as an important component of the health system capacity portfolio on the other. Reciprocally, neighborhood community health centers can embed culturally competent care and serve as an anchor of community sustainability. This enriched portfolio can also form the nurturing professional workplace setting of a culturally competent health workforce. In turn, this workforce can also stimulate transformation leading to a better functioning culturally competent health system. This framework also allows for cultural *targeting*—focusing on a culturally-specific population—as well as culturally *tailoring* a health intervention or program to maximize community benefits. This conceptual framework goes beyond the role of cultural leverage in interventions to allow for assessing not only the impact of a health action or intervention as a silo effort; rather it operationalizes the three core components as one interconnected health system: the community as health seeking beneficiaries, the health workforce as providers of culturally competent care, and the health system as the locus of health services within communities.(Fisher, Burnet et al. 2007) This interconnected system will facilitate what has eluded many cancer health disparities scientists to date: transforming impact ascertainment of health intervention from behavioral outcomes to functional health status. This paradigm shift will result in targeting the community rather than the individual to benchmark impact.

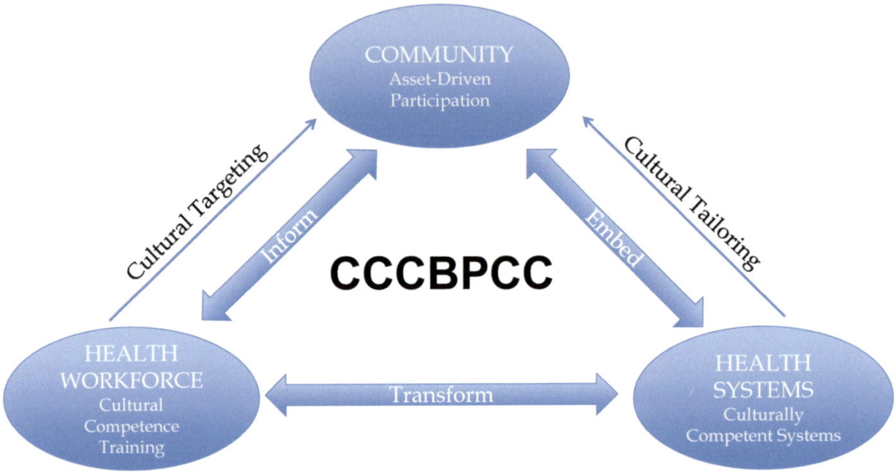

Fig. 4. Culturally competent community based participatory cancer care.

6.1 Creating a culturally competent cancer care workforce: forces of change and opportunities

Among the plethora of challenges are three forces of change directly affecting developing a cadre of culturally competent cancer care providers: the new primary care practice, the rapidly changing demographics, and cancer as a global chronic disease burden. The "new" primary care practice represents a "back to the future" phenomenon in some instances- the primary care physician's role becomes one of a communicator who empowers, informs, and engages patients in their care.(Fiscella and Epstein 2008) Team-based care requires skills in leadership, management, and coordination and a medical home as a one stop health care shop. Among the projected cancer care beneficiaries are two synergistic socio-demographic trends: an increase of minority populations, and a widening of the disparities gap, despite current, yet insufficient investments in research.(Hobbs and Stoops 2002) For over a decade, the relationship between cultural competence and health disparities has been well documented.(Brach and Fraser 2000; Betancourt, Green et al. 2003; Goode, Dunne et al. October 2006) Increasingly, developing nations are faced with diseases of the "developed world" and resource limitations rendering many such governments incapable of caring for their people. For example, cancer is the third leading cause of mortality in the Caribbean Region surpassed only by cerebro- and cardiovascular disease.(Phillips, Jacobson et al. 2007) Approximately 50% of cancer mortality occurs in developing countries and 60 to 70% of new cases are projected in those countries by 2020 (Jones et al 2006). In the case of cancer, developing nations lack the resources to provide even the basic components of the cancer care continuum including screening mammography and radiation therapy. While there is a growing visibility regarding each of these three forces of change no comprehensive effort to derive community-based solutions has been undertaken to date.

From a health workforce perspective, efforts to counteract these forces have largely amounted to a number of training courses targeting practicing health care providers, "special" courses or lectures on cultural competence for those still in the pipeline, and research efforts which often last only until the end of the funding period. Exemplary exceptions targeting the practicing health workforce such as the cancer care competency case studies from C-Change are included in this chapter. The Interprofessional Education Collaborative spearheaded by the Association of American Medical Colleges (AAMC), and consisting of the Association of Schools of Public Health, American Association of Colleges of Nursing, American Association of Colleges of Osteopathic Medicine, American Association of Colleges of Pharmacy, American Dental Education Association has recently published a transdisciplinary competency model to guide the education of the represented disciplines with the desired outcome of more holistic frontline practice.(IPEC 2011) This signals an increasing realization that discipline-specific graduates may not adequately perform on today's practice frontline. A more persistent demand is coming from the increasingly culturally diverse consumers of graduate health education: the " is there and app for this" generation is not only calling for a change in instructional delivery, but is also more in tune with its future customers and the global health threats facing them.

6.2 A core set of cultural competencies for medicine and public health

AAMC and ASPH are engaged in a collaborative partnership to develop a set of core cultural competencies appropriate for medical-, public health students and those in other health-related educational institutions to bolster the delivery of health care services especially to underserved, diverse populations.(Lichtveld 2010) The overarching aims of the initiative were: to illustrate cultural competence as an effective cross over topic area for students in both academic medicine and public health; to demonstrate how cultural competence can advance health disparities research in medical and public health education; and to provided most needed examples of how to incorporate cultural competencies into curricula and practica to graduate more culturally competent practitioners. There are several unique features to this joint effort: there is full agreement from both organizations that the emphasis should be on embedding cultural knowledge, skills, and attitudes medicine and public health education and practice rather than creating separate, standalone courses; The explicit anticipated outcome is a patient-centered approach in a community setting embracing both the customers of medicine and public health in a holistic fashion; the competencies were designed deliberately broad to not only allow for integration and tailoring within the scope of practice but also support pedagogical approaches accommodating the progressive stages of learning. Therefore, the competency set is not intended to be implemented in its entirety giving schools of medicine and public health flexibility in application while providing benchmarks of learning performance.

The competencies are categorized in three domains: knowledge- focusing on educational learning outcomes-, skills- representing practice competencies-, and attitudes. Included in the competency set are bridging competencies, logically linking one domain to the other,

	KNOWLEDGE	SKILLS	ATTITUDES
At the completion of the program of study, (medical and public health) students will be able to	Define the dimensions of culture to include language, sexual orientation, gender, age, race, ethnicity, disability, beliefs, socio-economic status, and educational attainment.	Identify one's own assets and learning needs related to cultural competence.	Demonstrate willingness to apply the principles of cultural competence.
	Differentiate health, health care, health care systems, and health disparities,	Incorporate culture as a key component of patient, family, and community history.	Appreciate how cultural competence contributes to the practice of medicine and public health.
	Identify cultural factors that contribute to overall health and wellness.	Integrate patients/ families/ communities cultural perspective(s) in developing treatment/ interventions.	Appreciate that becoming culturally competent involves life-long learning.
	Describe the contributions of culture and resiliency to positive health outcomes.	Apply (community) constituent/ patient -centered principles to earn trust and credibility.	Demonstrate willingness to assess the impact of one's own culture, assumptions, stereotypes, and biases on the ability to provide culturally competent care and service.
	Examine factors that contribute to health disparities, particularly social, economic, environmental, health systems, and access.	Conduct culturally appropriate risk and asset assessment, management, and communication with patients and populations.	Demonstrate willingness to explore cultural elements and aspects that influence decision making by patients, self, and colleagues.
	Identify health disparities that exist at the local, state, regional, national and global level.	Contribute to the planning, implementation, and evaluation of culturally competent interventions.	Demonstrate willingness to collaborate to overcome linguistic and literacy challenges in the clinical and community encounter (note—this could be an example of a bridging comp).
	Recognize that cultural competence alone does not address health care disparities.	Communicate in a culturally competent manner with patients, families, and communities.	Appreciate the influence of institutional culture on learning content, style, and opportunities of professional training programs.
	Describe the elements of effective communication with patients, families, communities, peers and colleagues.	Employ self-reflection to evaluate the impact of one's practice.	
	Describe strategies to communicate with limited English proficient patients and communities, such as working with trained medical interpreters or translated materials.	Work effectively in a trans-disciplinary setting/team.	
	Describe the role of community engagement in healthcare and wellness.	Demonstrate shared decision-making.	
	Assess the impact of acculturation and immigration on healthcare and wellness.	Analyze illness conditions and health outcomes of concern at the patient and community level.	
	Articulate cultural humility, cultural diversity, and cultural competence and their roles in ongoing professional development.	Engage community partners in actions which promote a healthy environment and healthy behaviors.	
	Describe the values and limitations of evidence-based literature on understanding the health of individuals and communities	Communicate with colleagues, patients, families, and communities about health disparities and health care disparities.	
	Articulate the roles and functions of local health departments, community partners and organizations.	Establish equitable partnerships with local health departments, faith and community-based organizations, and leaders to develop culturally appropriate outreach and interventions.	

Table 4. Cultural competencies for students in medicine and public health.

often incorporating more than one domain. For example, a student's ability to "describe the elements of effective communication with patients, families, communities, peers and colleagues" requires both attaining the requisite knowledge as well as demonstrating the skill to successfully implement the role of communicator. In the context of cancer diagnosis and treatment, patient-physician communication can profoundly influence decision-making and consequently health outcome (Smith, Lichtveld, 2007). For example, recognizing cultural beliefs and practices guides health care providers to negotiate rather than demand a given course of treatment. Successful patient -physician encounters require both interpersonal- as well as instrumental communication (Manfredi et al 2010). Therefore, while *knowledge* about aspects of interpersonal communication such as respect will help make a patient feel more comfortable with the physician, instrumental communication is the dimension which most influences a patient's decision-making regarding cancer treatment for example—emphasizing a demonstration of effective communication *skills*.

A series of transdisciplinary case studies currently in development will accompany the competencies listed below in Table 4 to demonstrate the translation into learner level-specific educational modalities.

7. Applications in the field

Patient navigation is an emerging component of the cancer care delivery team and system that offers an innovative solution to decrease cancer health disparities by bridging the chasm between access to and optimal utilization of services through sustainable and culturally relevant mechanisms. Embedding cultural competence in medical education has been a long-standing objective, reinforced by the painful disparity in outcomes that perpetuate excess morbidity and mortality among underserved minority populations (Betancourt 2003; Smedley, Stith et al. 2003; Betancourt 2006; Betancourt 2006). This section will discuss the role of culturally competent patient navigation and cultural competence training in the era of health reform.

7.1 Navigation

There is perhaps no other area in health care in which active patient participation through screening, diagnosis and treatment phases is as important as in cancer care. Cancer treatment is multidisciplinary (radiation, chemotherapy, surgery) and requires the patient, in equal partnership with the oncology provider, to make complex treatment decisions and participation in clinical trials - decisions that can impact survival. Cancer centers are highly specialized and therefore quite distinct from the broadly focused community based medicine environment. Primary care practitioners may be reluctant to actively engage oncology team physicians due to unfamiliarity with cancer treatment approaches, protocols and successful cancer center navigation and therefore unable to provide needed support. Navigators can bridge the gap in cultural competence, health care access and coordination, insurance coverage and continuity, prevention and early detection and treatment.

For patients, the navigator operates in two environments- health care system and caring companion and provides "insider" information about system access and navigation and advocacy while simultaneously building trust that will extend to the larger health care system. Navigators who are representative community members who understand the culture in the patient and provider communities and function within a biospychosocial theoretical framework (Engel 1977; King, Miranda et al. 2010) are critical in facilitating effective bidirectional patient provider communication and, most importantly, treatment *partnership*.(Carroll, Lardiere et al. 2010)

Patient perception of health care system and services access directly correlate with utilization. Navigators who know the local environment can navigate financial/insurance issues, cultural beliefs and language barriers, childcare and transportation issues, identification of a medical home and provide the necessary patient education and support to assure healthcare access and continuity of care. (Dohan and Schrag 2005) Utilization of screening and early detection has improved but remains problematic in rural and minority populations. This is the point within the health care delivery system at which the navigator can have the highest, sustainable community impact. Patient navigation is critical within the Federally Qualified Health Centers which provide services to high needs populations. Navigators connect patients with education, outreach, screening, diagnosis and treatment resources and provide advice tailored to individual patient needs. Studies to evaluate navigation effectiveness are underway.

7.1.1 Evaluating navigation effectiveness

Navigation has improved survival via detection of early stage disease, better follow-up of abnormal screening and diagnostic tests through reduction in the time interval between tests, improved utilization and treatment adherence to multidisciplinary cancer treatment regimens and clinical trial participation. Navigation has also resulted in improved patient satisfaction with respect to health care delivery, decreased anxiety as well as doctor and waiting time concerns. (Guadagnolo, Dohan et al. 2011) Patient outcome evaluation is critical for assessing the effectiveness of navigation. Most efforts have targeted screening and diagnosis aspects of cancer care i.e. number of people served, screening tests and biopsies performed, cancers diagnosed etc. However, identification of successful navigation strategies that result in *sustained* improvements in access, utilization and health behaviors, requires the identification and utilization of tailored metrics that better qualitatively and quantitatively evaluate quality of care from the system, provider and patient perspectives. Candidate treatment tracking metrics include receipt of appropriate radiation and/or adjuvant chemotherapy after cancer surgery, guideline concordant treatment rates and adherence to treatment regimens, care coordination (provider notification, discussion at multidisciplinary tumor conference, receipt and type of ancillary services, medication and devices. Patient reported care metrics could include satisfaction with cancer related care and navigation, functional health status and symptom burden, coping skills and co-morbidity, quality of life during treatment and palliative care.

7.1.2 Financing navigation

The Patient Protection and Affordable Care Act (PPACA) addressed 4 key issues: prevention and early detection, access and coordination, insurance coverage and continuity and diversity and cultural competency. The PPACA provided infrastructure development support through grant funding to establish medical homes for Medicaid patients with chronic diseases, community based, interdisciplinary teams to provide support services to primary care practices and health care provider consortiums to coordinate and integrate health care services for low income under- and uninsured populations which collectively will enable comprehensive, multidisciplinary case management. Navigator integration into the PPACA infrastructure will create sustainable changes in the health care system and promote health behavior modification. Most importantly, it establishes a matrix structured platform that will reward innovation in streamlining health care delivery, promote the development of fiscally accountable and efficient health care delivery and in the mid and long term the resurrecting a "healthy America".

7.2 Embedding cultural competence in cancer care education

Substantive training relevant to culturally competent communication in schools of medicine, nursing, dentistry, public health and social work has been an elusive goal, awaiting, perhaps, consensus agreement on competencies as a framework upon which to build an evidence based curriculum (Beach, Price et al. 2005; Lichtveld, Boulton et al. 2008) Yet, health care preparation in all disciplines acknowledges and emphasizes shared decision making as the effective method by which patients receive the best care and, long term, the best outcomes (O'Connor, Wennberg et al. 2007; King, Eckman et al. 2011) Why then is there a reluctance to launch curricula in cultural competence - a fundamental component of communication aimed at shared decision making?

It is generally acknowledged that the effectiveness of health care provider communication is dependent on the health literacy of the patient and the ability of the provider to a.) recognize the level of health literacy and b.) tailor the communication appropriately (Dewalt, Berkman et al. 2004; Weiss, May et al. 2005) There are well-established health literacy tools to guide providers in tailoring communication. Understanding health literacy and the tools available for assessment is a key element to successful training in cultural competency (Shaw, Huebner et al. 2009) Moreover, knowledge of health literacy and its importance in achieving the level of communication that results in shared decision making is a "prerequisite" for embracing cultural competence. A recent study by Price-Haywood, et al. (2010) combined the evaluation of special physician training by a measure of effectiveness - cancer screening behavior - in patients stratified by their health literacy score. (Price-Haywood, Roth et al. 2010). The model was colon cancer screening, a preventive behavior that is an excellent paradigm for shared decision making since there are several acceptable options for screening. The physician training based on attention to health literacy alone was successful measured by surrogate-reported progressive change in physician behavior and communication during the study period. An important finding, however, was that the low health literacy patients did not feel satisfied with the communication of risk reduction with screening, though the "trained" physicians rated their communication as effective (Price-Haywood, Harden-Barrios et al. 2011) Moreover, the early results demonstrate that patient screening behavior among the low health literacy patients had not changed at 1 year of follow-up. The investigators acknowledge the need to enrich the physician training based on the racial, ethnic, and cultural characteristics of the patient population.

The lack of linkage between training in communication and positive changes in patient outcomes seems to plague educators, psychologists, and health service researchers

(Betancourt 2010; Lie, Lee-Rey et al. 2011) Ineffective curricula, as measured by positive changes in health outcome, thus far appear to be common to both health literacy and cultural competence training. Despite academic "longing", there has not been evidence based tools that can guide health care workers to influence health behavior in a manner that improves outcomes. The literature is rife with "assessments", but outcome thus far belies success.

Nevertheless, some ongoing efforts are encouraging. Lichtveld and colleagues are planning to build a curriculum based on healthcare provider competencies. The 'competencies' will provide the metrics to measure the didactic effectiveness of the curriculum. A second order of assessment will determine linkage between health outcomes and provider/learner achievement. Price-Haywood proposes a physician practice guide and didactic curriculum built on self-expressed needs and expectations of the target population obtained through analysis of information obtained from focus groups of various health literacy.

What is most encouraging is the movement from assessment to plans for action and measurement of health outcomes. (Chun 2010; Echeverri, Brookover et al. 2010; Kamaka 2010; Wilkerson, Fung et al. 2010; Crenshaw, Shewchuk et al. 2011) These evolving tools will enrich the health care provider and enhance the relationship between diverse patients and the health care system. The next five years should be exciting as these tools, guides, and curricula emerge. Today, however, health care providers remain confronted by their ineffectiveness in normalizing the disparate outcomes and their impotence in fostering better health behaviors among their patients. What can the 2012 graduate from medical school, dental school, nursing school, pharmacy school and school of public health do to optimize communication and shared decision making? (Kumagai and Lypson 2009) As we enter the era of "team care" the challenge intensifies because responsibility may become diffuse. The team leader should be the primary care giver with the appropriate knowledge base. The team leader should assess and define the patient's knowledge base and then - and only then - involve the appropriate team members to work with the patient. The team leader should begin by asking the patient to ask any questions and to speak his understanding of his condition and the advice he has received. Often, the patient is or should be accompanied by family or friends who will play an important role in the shared decision making. These principles are fundamental to all courses teaching history, physical examination, and medical decision making. Our professional schools should reinforce the fundamental didactics while preparing for the enhancements which will come from ongoing research into more effective, more focused communication and more elegant science that will combine to contribute to the elimination of outcome disparity.

8. Acknowledgement

C-Change would like to acknowledge John Simmons, Program Coordinator for SPIPA and Jennifer Olson, MPH, MA, Epidemiologist, SPIPA CCC Project, for their leadership and technical guidance on SPIPA's competency grant project; C-Change's Pain & Palliative Care Competency Advisory Committee for their leadership and expertise; and Purdue Pharma L.P. for their generous funding. For a full report from all of the competency projects see www.cancercorecompetency.org.

About C-Change: The vision/mission of C-Change is to eliminate cancer as a major public health problem at the earliest possible time by leveraging the expertise and resources of its members. C-Change is a 501(c)3 organization comprised of leaders from public, private, and not-for-profit organizations. The organization convenes multi-sector leaders in the cancer community to address issues that we cannot affect alone. For more information about C-Change visit www.c-changetogether.org.

9. References

Beach, M. C., E. G. Price, et al. (2005). "Cultural Competence: A Systematic Review of Health Care Provider Educational Interventions." Medical Care 43(4): 356-373.

Betancourt, J., A. Green, et al. (2003). "Defining cultural competence: a practical framework for addressing racial/ethnic disparities in health and health care." Public health reports 118(4): 293-302.

Betancourt, J. R. (2003). "Cross-cultural medical education: conceptual approaches and frameworks for evaluation." Academic Medicine 78(6): 560-569.

Betancourt, J. R. (2006). "Cultural Competence and medical education: many names, many perspectives, one goal." Academic Medicine 81(6): 499-501.

Betancourt, J. R. (2006) "Improving quality and achieving equity: the role of cultural competence in reducing racial and ethnic disparities in health care." The Commonwealth Fund.

Betancourt, J. R. (2010). "Commentary: Linking cultural competence training to improved health outcomes: Perspectives from the field." Academic Medicine 85(4): 583-585.

Brach, C. and I. Fraser (2000). "Can Cultural Competency Reduce Racial And Ethnic Health Disparities? A Review And Conceptual Model." Medical Care Research and Review 57(suppl 1): 181-217.

Bustillos, D. (2009). "Limited English Proficiency and disparities in research " J Law Medical Ethics 37(1): 28 -37.

C-Change (2008). Addressing the Cancer Workforce Crisis Using a Competency-Based Approach with Non-Oncology Health Professionals.

C-Change (2010). C-Change Cancer Pain & Palliative Care Core Competency Initiative. Addressing Culture-Specific Pain Management: Creating a Common Ground between Community Members and Caregivers to Address Native American Cancer Pain and Palliative Care J. Simmons, South Puget Intertribal Planning Agency Comprehensive Cancer Control Program.

Carroll, M. J., JA, M. Lardiere, et al. (2010). "Innovation Networks for Improving Access and Quality Across the Healthcare Ecosystem." Telemedicine Journal and e-Health 16(1): 107–111.

Chin, M. H., A. E. Walters, et al. (2007). "Interventions to Reduce Racial and Ethnic Disparities in Health Care." Medical Care Research and Review 64(5 suppl): 7S-28S.

Chun, M. B. (2010). "Pitfalls to avoid when introducing a cultural competency training initiative." Medical Education 44(6): 613-620.

Crenshaw, K., R. M. Shewchuk, et al. (2011). "What should we include in a cultural competence curriculum? An emerging formatice evaluation process to foster curriculum development." Academic Medicine 86(3): 333-341.

Dewalt, D. A., N. D. Berkman, et al. (2004). "Literacy and health outcome: a systematic review of the literature." Journal of General Internal Medicine 19(12): 1228-1239.

Dogra, N., S. Reitmanova, et al. (2010). "Teaching Cultural Diversity: Current Status in U.K., U.S., and Canadian Medical Schools." Journal of General Internal Medicine 25(0): 164-168.

Dohan, D. and D. Schrag (2005). "Using navigators to improve care of underserved patients: Current practicies and approaches." Cancer 104: 848-855.

Echeverri, M., C. Brookover, et al. (2010). "Nine constructs of cultural competence for curriculum development." American Journal of Pharmaceutical Education 74(10): 181.

Elkin, E., N. Ishill, et al. (2010). "Geographic access and the use of screening mammography." Medical Care 48(4): 349-356.

Engel, G. L. (1977). "The Need for a New Medical Model: A Challenge for Biomedicine." Science 196(4286): 129-136.

Fiscella, K. and R. M. Epstein (2008). "So Much to Do, So Little Time: Care for the Socially Disadvantaged and the 15-Minute Visit." Arch Intern Med 168(17): 1843-1852.

Fisher, T. L., D. L. Burnet, et al. (2007). "Cultural Leverage." Medical Care Research and Review 64(5 suppl): 243S-282S.

Goode, T. D., M. C. Dunne, et al. (October 2006). The Evidence Base for Cultural and Linguistic Competency in Health Care, The Commonwealth Fund.

Griggs, J., E. Culakova, et al. (2007). "Social and racial differences in selection of breast cancer adjuvant chemotherapy regimens." Journal of clinical oncology 25(18): 2522-2527.

Griggs, J., E. Culakova, et al. (2007). "Effect of patient socioeconomic status and body mass index on the quality of breast cancer adjuvant chemotherapy." Journal of clinical oncology 25(3): 277-284.

Griggs, J., M. E. S. Sorbero, et al. (2003). "Racial disparity in the dose and dose intensity of breast cancer adjuvant chemotherapy." Breast cancer research and treatment 81(1): 21-31.

Grouse, L. (2005) "Reducing disparities in cancer healthcare." Benchmarks.

Guadagnolo, B. A., D. Dohan, et al. (2011). "Metrics for evaluating patient navigation during cancer diagnosis and treatment : Crafting a policy-relevant research agenda for patient navigation in cancer care." Cancer 117(15 Suppl): 3563-3572.

Hobbs, F. and N. Stoops (2002). U.S. Census Bureau, Census 2000 Special Reports, Series CENSR-4. Demographic Trends in the 20th Century. Washington, DC.

ICC (2009). Eliminating Disparities in Clincal Trials (EDICT) Project: Executive Summary Report from Eight Community Dialogue Meetings Houston, Baylor College of Medicine.

IPEC (2011). Core competencies for interprofessional collaborative practice: Report of an expert panel. Washington, DC, Interprofessional Education Collaborative.

Jones, L., J. Chilton, et al. (2006). "Between and within: international perspectives on cancer and health disparities." Journal of clinical oncology 24(14): 2204-2208.

Kamaka, M. L. (2010). "Designing a cultural competency curriculum, asking the stakeholders." Hawaii Medical Journal 69(6 Suppl 3): 31-34.

Kawahara, N., T. Masui, et al. (2010). "What Should We Do to Raise Awareness on the Issue of Cancer in the Global Health Agenda?" Japanese Journal of Clinical Oncology 40(suppl 1): i82-i85.

King, D., P. Miranda, et al. (2010). "Addressing cancer health disparities using a global biopsychosocial approach." Cancer 116(2): 264-269.

King, J. S., M. H. Eckman, et al. (2011). "The potential of shared decision making to reduce health disparities." Journal of Law, Medicine and Ethics: 30-33.

Kumagai, A. K. and M. D. Lypson (2009). "Beyond cultural competence: critical consciousness, social justice and multicultural education." Academic Medicine 84(6): 782-787.

Lichtveld, M. (2009). "Making cultural competence work for cancer prevention: fact of fiction." Journal of Cancer Education 24(Supplement 2): 20-21.

Lichtveld, M. (2010). Cultural Competence Education for Students in Medicine and Public Health. Patients and Populations: Public Health in Medical Education. ASPH and AAMC. Cleveland, OH.

Lichtveld, M., M. Boulton, et al. (2008). "From Competencies to Capacity: Assessing the National Epidemiology Workforce." Public Health Reports (1974-) 123(ArticleType: research-article / Issue Title: SUPPLEMENT 1: Competency-Based Epidemiologic Training in Public Health Practice / Full publication date: 2008 / Copyright © 2008 Association of Schools of Public Health): 128-135.

Lie, D. A., E. Lee-Rey, et al. (2011). "Does cultural competency training of health professionals improve patient outcomes? A systematic review and proposed algorithm for future research." Journal of General Internal Medicine 26(3): 317-325.

Linkov, F., N. Padilla, et al. (2010). "Global Networking of Cancer and NCD Professionals Using Internet Technologies: The Supercourse and mHealth Applications." J Prev Med Public Health 43(6): 472-478.

Matthews-Juarez, P. and A. D. Weinberg (2004). Cultural competence in cancer care: A health care professionals passport, Baylor College of Medicine.

Miranda, P., A. Wilkinson, et al. (2011). "Policy implications of early onset breast cancer among Mexican-origin women." Cancer 117(2): 390-397.

Natale Pereira, A., K. Enard, et al. (2011). "The role of patient navigators in eliminating health disparities." Cancer 117(15 Suppl): 3541-3550.

NCI. (2011). "Accrual Net - A Resource and Professional Community for Clinical Trial Accrual." Retrieved August 24, 2011, from http://accrualnet.acscreativeclients.com/.

O'Connor, A. M., J. E. Wennberg, et al. (2007). "Toward the "tipping point": Decision aids and informed patient choice." Health Affairs 26(3): 716-725.

Phillips, A. A., J. S. Jacobson, et al. (2007). "Cancer Incidence and Mortality in the Caribbean." Cancer Investigation 25(6): 476-483.

Price-Haywood, K. G. Roth, et al. (2010). "Cancer risk communication with low health literacy patients: a continuing medical education program." Journal of General Internal Medicine 25(Sippl 2): S126 - S129.

Price-Haywood, E. G., J. Harden-Barrios, et al. (2011). Health information needs and predictors of cancer screening status among patients with limited literacy. American Association for Cancer Research 4th Annual Cancer Health Disparities Conference, Washington, DC.

Shaw, S. J., C. Huebner, et al. (2009). "The role of culture in health literacy and chronic disease screening and management." Journal of Immigrant Minor Health 11(6): 460-467.

Smedley, B. D., A. Y. Stith, et al. (2003). Unequal Treatment: Confronting racial and ethnic disparities in health care, The National Academies Press.

Smith, A. P., S. L. Tyus, et al. (2009). "A Competency-Based Approach To Expanding the Cancer Care Workforce: Proof of Concept." MEDSURG Nursing 18(1): 39-49.

Smith Bindman, R., D. Miglioretti, et al. (2006). "Does utilization of screening mammography explain racial and ethnic differences in breast cancer?" Annals of Internal Medicine 144(8): 541-553.

Stokols, D. (1996). "Translating social ecological theory into guidelines for community health promotion." American Journal of Health Promotion 10(4): 282-298.

Subban, J., N. Terwoord, et al. (2008). "With or without intent: How racial disparities prevent effective implementation of care." The Journal of Nutrition, Health & Aging 12(10): 770S-775S.

Weiss, B. D., M. Z. May, et al. (2005). "Quick assessment of literacy in primary care: the newest vital sign." Annals of Family Medicine 3(6): 514-522.

Wilkerson, L., C. C. Fung, et al. (2010). "Assessing patient-centered care: One approach to health disparities education." Journal of General Internal Medicine 25(Suppl 2): S86-90.

Wilkinson, R. and M. Marmot, Eds. (2003). Social determinants of health: The solid facts, 2nd Edition. Copenhagen, The World Health Organization.

Womack, J. P. and D. T. Jones (2003). Lean Thinking: Banish waste and create wealth in your corporation, Free Press.

17

The Changing Landscape of Prostate Cancer Chemoprevention: Current Strategies and Future Directions

Jason M. Phillips and E. David Crawford
University of Colorado Division of Urology
USA

1. Introduction

Current controversy exists regarding the role of chemopreventative agents for prostate cancer. However, prostate cancer's role in our society remains prevalent. Prostate cancer continues to be the leading cause of newly diagnosed male cancers in the United States. In 2011, the American Cancer Society estimated 241,740 new cases and 28,170 deaths from prostate cancer.[1] Only lung cancer has more male cancer deaths. Current treatment strategies such as surgery, radiation, chemotherapy and hormone therapies have been successful in decreasing prostate cancer related morbidity and mortality. However, the physician's armamentarium is focused on treating existing prostate cancer and not preventing it. Despite the prolongation of life for patients with prostate cancer, each therapy carries a side effect profile.

Due to improved early detection, prostate cancer is now often identified at an earlier stage and grade. Newly diagnosed tumors are often organ confined and slow growing. However, once a patient's PSA laboratory value is abnormal, he will most likely receive a prostate biopsy for diagnosis. Given the fact that less than 10% of Americans select active surveillance, screening starts a snowball effect that usually "buys" a treatment. It is well known that treatment including radical prostatectomy or radiation has been shown to overtreat prostate cancer in as many as 30-50% of patients.[2] Morbidity, including incontinence and impotence can significantly affect a patient's quality of life. In addition, the knowledge of prostate cancer may cause emotional, financial and physical harm.[3,4] Given that the US male population faces a 16.7% lifetime risk of prostate cancer, prostate cancer is an ideal candidate for prevention strategies.

Cancer chemoprevention focuses on the use of natural or synthetic agents to suppress, delay, or prevent the development of tumors. Natural substances have long been utilized with varying results for prostate cancer prevention. More recently in the 2000s, 5-alpha reductase inhibitors (5-ARI) have also been used. These substances have focused on both primary prevention and secondary prevention. Primary prevention focuses on deferring or preventing the presence of cancer prior to cancer formation. Secondary prevention focuses on preventing premalignant lesions from progressing to cancer. For prostate cancer, secondary prevention focuses on preventing the progression of high grade prostate epithelial neoplasia (HGPIN).

In December of 2010, the Federal Drug Administration's (FDA) Oncology Drugs Advisory Committee (ODAC) reviewed 5-ARI's indication for the prevention of prostate cancer in men at increased risk for prostate cancer. This committee ruled against the use of 5-ARI's for the use of prostate chemoprevention. Advocacy groups have since issues statements disagreeing with the FDA's ruling, highlighting the fact that controversy continues to exist. The goal of this paper is to examine the available agents and the current environment.

2. Current chemopreventative agents - pharmaceuticals and micronutrients

The ideal chemopreventative agent should be minimally expensive, nontoxic and effective. Having multiple preventative benefits is considered a plus; however it should not potentiate other causes of morbidity or mortality. Pharmaceutical agents, most notably 5-ARIs, and micronutrients have been studied to better establish their potential role in cancer prevention.

2.1 Pharmaceuticals

Finasteride and dutasteride are both 5-ARI medications used to successfully inhibit prostate growth. These two agents are both currently accepted for treating benign prostatic hypertrophy (BPH). The difference between the two medications is minimal, however potentially significant. 5-α-Reductase has two isoenzymes. Finasteride inhibits the type 2 isoenzyme while dutasteride inhibits both the type 1 and type 2 isoenzymes. Dutasteride thus has more complete inhibition of DHT, roughly 90% as compared to finasteride's 70% reduction of serum DHT.[5,6] It has been proposed that expression of the type 1 isoenzyme is increased with prostate cancer while the type 2 isoenzyme is unaffected with prostate cancer.[7] 5-ARI medications focus on inhibiting androgen receptor (AR) activation. Research on BPH has shown that consistent use of finasteride or dutasteride decreases prostatic volume 30% and reduce PSA levels 50-60%.[8] Both 5-ARI medications have been tested for chemopreventative benefits with multicenter, randomized, double blind, placebo controlled trials. The thrust of this paper will discuss the 5-ARI medications and their current role in prostate cancer prevention.

Other pharmaceutical agents potentially used for prostate cancer prevention include statins, nonsteroidal anti-inflammatory drugs (NSAIDS), and toremifene. Statins inhibit HMG-CoA, the rate limiting step of cholesterol synthesis. Statin use over 2 years has been associated with a decrease in prostate specific antigen.[9] By inhibiting prostatic cellular growth and promoting apoptosis, statins also decrease cellular growth. No large double blind study has evaluated the effect of statin use on prostate cancer but a meta-analysis did find a protective effect.[10] Further studies are needed to substantiate current evidence.

NSAIDS inhibit cyclooxygenase-2 (COX-2), which is a key enzyme found in prostate cancer which converts arachidonic acid to prostaglandins. Experimental evidence demonstrated a regression of PIN after NSAID use, but the planned trial with rofecoxib was withdrawn after safety concerns.[11,12]

Selective estrogen modulators (SERMs) are best known for their effects on breast cancer. Toremifene has decreased prostate cancer in the TRAMP model. A phase 2b study found that 20mg doses of toremifene resulted in a 48% decrease in prostate cancer at one year.[13] However, the phase III trial demonstrated no significant risk reduction.[14]

2.2 Micronutrients

Micronutrients have long been sought after to provide a chemotherapeutic benefit for the development or prevention of prostate cancer. Antioxidants in vitro can inhibit cellular proliferation, induce apoptosis and modulate genes leading to the suppression of prostatic tumor. [15,16] The largest scale trial on micronutrients was for selenium and vitamin E in the Selenium and Vitamin E Cancer Prevention Trial (SELECT).

The interest in selenium began with the Nutritional Prevention of Cancer Trial, which used oral selenium for nonmelanoma skin cancer. Men were randomized to selenium versus placebo and were found to have a 65% reduction in prostate cancer incidence after a 4.5 year follow up. Vitamin E interest developed after a 32% reduction in prostate cancer in the Alpha-Tocopherol, Beta-Carotene Cancer Prevention Trial (ATBC) trial, which was a double blind randomized placebo controlled trial for lung cancer incidence and mortality.

These studies paved the way for the SELECT trial, published in 2009, which was a randomized, placebo controlled population based primary prevention trial focused on the effects of selenium and vitamin E on preventing prostate cancer. SELECT randomized 35,533 men to four treatment arms: selenium with placebo, selenium with vitamin E, Vitamin E with placebo, placebo with placebo. Study supplements included 200 micrograms l-selenomethionine, 400mg racemic alpha-tocopherol and an optional multivitamin containing no selenium or vitamin E. Eligible men were at least 50 years of age for African-Americans, at least 55 for Caucasians, negative DRE, PSA less than 4ng/mL, and normal blood pressure.

The primary endpoint was the presence of prostate cancer found on for cause biopsies. The indications for biopsy were not indicated in the protocol and were at the discretion of the physician.

During the second interim analysis seven years after initiation of the trial, the independent Data and Safety Monitoring Committee recommended discontinuation of the SELECT because the data demonstrated no significant differences between groups. No statistically significant effects were reported on primary or secondary analyses of the data, suggesting no prostate cancer prevention benefits from selenium or vitamin E.[17] Unfortunately, selenium and vitamin E, which initially demonstrated promise, was eventually found to not have a significant effect on preventing prostate cancer. [17-19]

Other chemopreventative micronutrients include lycopene, green tea, soy, DIM and curcumin. Molecular targets these agents affect include nuclear factor-KB, AKt, Wnt, Hedgehog and Notch.[20]

Lycopene is a biologically occurring carotenoid that is a potent antioxidant. It has been shown to be associated with lower prostate cancer risk in a number of epidemiologic studies.[21] Using the preclinical TRAMP mouse model, prostate cancer was significantly decreased 60% vs. 95% (P=.01). However, no correlation was found with prostate cancer in a PLCO trial examining 29,000 men.

Green tea contains several catechins believed to inhibit oncogenesis and provide antioxidants. Epidemiologic studies between Asian men with a high intake of green tea first suggested that green tea may provide a protective benefit against prostate cancer. Three clinical trials suggest a benefit.[22] A small clinical trial (n=60) using oral green tea catechins (GTC) found that patients with HGPIN randomized to GTC vs. placebo had no change in PSA levels, but did have less progression of prostate cancer: 1 patient vs. 9 patients progress.[23]

Soy, like green tea, was also found to demonstrate lower prostate cancer in epidemiologic studies between diets high in soy versus western diets. The benefit is potentially a 70% reduction of prostate cancer.[24] Soy affects signaling pathways, specifically Wnt and Hh signaling. Randomized studies are currently being performed.

DIM (the dimeric product of indole-3-carbinol) is found in a variety of plants and has been shown to inhibit alpha reductase suggesting that it may have an inhibitory role in prostate cancer. Curcumin is a bioavailable agent in turmeric and is also an alpha reductase inhibitor. Other regulators along the tumor pathway are inhibited by these two substances. Clinical trials are required to evaluate their effects.

Currently no biologically available micronutrients have been proven to provide chemoprevention benefits of prostate cancer. As such, current patient recommendations are to eat healthy foods and pursue healthy lifestyle changes.[25]

3. Review of 5-ARI chemoprevention trials

We reviewed the multicenter randomized double blind studies focused on 5-ARI usage versus placebo for prostate cancer chemoprevention including the Prostate Cancer Prevention Trial (PCPT) and the Reduction by Dutasteride of Prostate Cancer Events (REDUCE). Table 1 compares their study design.

Trial	Population	Risk Category	Agent	Target	Reported
Prostate Cancer Prevention Trial (PCPT)	n = 18,882	PSA <3.0 ng/mL DRE Normal	Finasteride (Merck)	Type 1 5-ARI	2008
Reduction by Dutasteride of Prostate Cancer Events Trial (REDUCE)	n = 8,229	PSA 2.5-10 ng/mL DRE Normal	Dutasteride (GlaxoSmithKline)	Type 1,2 5-ARI	2009

Table 1. Comparison of PCPT & REDUCE trials.

3.1 Prostate Cancer Prevention Trial (PCPT)

The Prostate Cancer Prevention Trial was the first large multicenter randomized double blind prostate prevention trial using a 5-ARI. In 2003, 18,882 men, 55 years or older with a PSA level less than 3.0ng/mL and a normal digital rectal exam (DRE) were randomized for seven years to finasteride 5mg daily or placebo.

Of the men who participated, 48%, or 9060 men were included in the final analysis. Enrollment criteria included men 55 years or older who were free of prostate cancer, no other significant co morbidities, and an American Urological Association symptom score (AUA-SS) of less than 20. Eligible participants were required to have a PSA less than 3.0ng/ml, normal DRE, adherent to the study protocol and no side effects during placebo. Men were contacted every three months for medical event evaluation and were seen by the study site every six months for side effect evaluation and medication refills. Annual PSA and DRE were performed. Biopsy was recommended if the DRE was abnormal or PSA was greater than 4.0ng/ml in the placebo arm or 2.0 times PSA (adjusted to 2.3x in year 4) in the finasteride arm. At the completion of the trial in year seven, all participants were recommended to undergo an end of study prostate biopsy with at least six cores. All biopsies were reviewed by a blinded pathologist.

The primary endpoint of the study was the prevalence of prostate cancer as diagnosed by biopsy for cause or end of study biopsies. Prostate cancer was found in 24.4% of the placebo group (1,147/4,692) and 18.4% of the finasteride group (803/4,368), representing a 24.8% risk reduction (CI 19-31, $p<0.001$). Finasteride's relative benefit was found across all groups including age, race/ethnicity, family history and entry PSA. In addition, Finasteride also reduced the risk of HGPIN compared to placebo.

Interestingly, tumors with a Gleason grade of 7-10, high grade tumors, were found to be more prevalent in the finasteride group (37%), 280 of 757 graded tumors, as compared to the placebo group (22%), 237 of 1,068 graded tumors. This was statistically significant ($P<.001$). The increased prevalence of high grade tumors in the treatment group has generated tremendous speculation and sub-analysis. Forty of the excess high grade tumors were found in the "for cause" biopsies, clinically indicated due to increasing PSA or changes in the DRE.

Secondary analyses have found a detection bias demonstrating a net reduction in high-grade cancers and a 53% reduction in low grade cancers.[26] However, due disagreement in the medical community regarding finasteride's effect on high-grade cancers, it was not given a new indication for prostate cancer prevention.

3.2 The Reduction by Dutasteride of Prostate Cancer Events (REDUCE)

Published in the *New England Journal of Medicine* in April of 2010, the REDUCE trial, was a 4-year multicenter, randomized, double-blind, placebo-controlled, parallel-group study. 8,231 men were randomized equally to dutasteride 0.5mg daily versus placebo. This trial was begun prior to the completion of the PCPT trial. Eligible patients were randomized to receive either Dutasteride or placebo. There has never been a large randomized trial comparing finasteride to dutasteride for the prevention of prostate cancer.

An important distinction between dutasteride and finasteride is the effect on 5-alpha reductase. Unlike finasteride, dutasteride affects the expression of both type 1 and type 2 isoenzymes of 5-alpha reductase inhibitors. Animal studies demonstrate that compared to finasteride, dutasteride has an increased reduction in both DHT and tumor growth.[27] Dutasteride, then, theoretically could enhance the anti-tumor effect.

Eligible participants were required to be 50-75 years old, have a serum PSA between 2.5ng/mL-10mg/mL for men aged 50-60 years or 3.0-10ng/mL for men aged >60 years, and had undergone a prostate biopsy within six months of enrollment. Men were excluded if they had more than one biopsy, had prostate cancer of any grade, HGPIN, atypical small acinar proliferation, or a prostate volume of more than 80 grams, had previous prostate surgery of any kind, or had an international prostate symptom score (IPSS) of 25 or higher.

During the trial 6726 men (82.6%) underwent at least 1 biopsy and 1516 men (22.5%) were diagnosed with prostate cancer. The primary endpoint was the presence of prostate cancer detected on biopsy 2 or 4 years after treatment. Biopsies performed out of the protocol were considered protocol independent biopsies. Other important endpoints included Gleason score, tumor volume, percent of positive biopsy cores, presence of HGPIN, and presence of small acinar proliferation. BPH endpoints were also evaluated.

The dutasteride arm represented an absolute risk reduction of 5% and a relative risk reduction of 23% (857 in the placebo arm versus 659 in the dutasteride arm, P<.001). This benefit was across all subgroups including age, family history, PSA level, prostate volume, or body mass index. The odds ratio for prostate cancer, detected on biopsy, with dutasteride as compared with placebo was 0.60 for all tumors (P<.001) and 0.62 for Gleason scores of 7 to 10 (P<.001).

Low grade tumors (Gleason 5, 6) were statistically higher in the placebo group (617 in placebo vs. 437 in dutasteride, P<0.001). The evidence of premalignant lesions was also decreased. HGPIN had a relative risk reduction of 39% (p<0.001) and small acinar proliferation (ASAP) had a relative risk reduction of 21% (p=0.04).

For high grade tumors, REDUCE demonstrated no significant overall increase in Gleason score 7 to 10, high grade, cancers. This was different from the PCPT, which alarmingly showed an increase in high grade cancer. Overall, there were 220 tumors with a Gleason score of 7 to 10 among 3299 men in the dutasteride group and 233 among 3407 men in the placebo group (P=0.81).

For the Gleason grade 8-10 tumors, there was no overall statistical difference looking at biopsies from all four years: 19 in placebo vs. 29 in dutasteride (P = .15). However, focusing on the second round of biopsies during years 3 and 4 of the study demonstrated a statistical increase in high grade tumors as compared to placebo. There were 12 tumors with a Gleason score of 8 to 10 in the dutasteride group, as compared with only 1 in the placebo group (P=0.003).[28] The authors speculate that this was caused by more frequent early detection of low grade tumors in the placebo group that might have progressed if left untreated. As expected, dutasteride also demonstrated improved outcomes with BPH. Prostate volume, acute urinary retention and BPH related surgery, and urinary tract infections were all significantly reduced in the dutasteride group.

The REDUCE trial, like the PCPT, demonstrated a significant effect on low grade cancers (Gleason 5, 6), but did not appear to alter the prevalence of high grade cancers. Overall it was well tolerated but did have significant effects on libido, erectile dysfunction, and semen volume.

3.3 Controversy: high grade tumor risk and generalizability

The effects of 5ARI's on low grade cancer is consistent across both the PCPT and the REDUCE trials. However, each trial demonstrates a trend towards high grade disease. Initially, the authors from the PCPT concluded that the risk of finasteride on high grade tumors was uncertain. They recommended finasteride not be used as a chemopreventative agent.[29]

Secondary analyses based on the PCPT data were then performed to better understand the conclusions drawn from the data. These authors concluded that biases due to prostate specific antigen (PSA), digital rectal exam (DRE), and prostate volume detection were responsible for a trend towards increased detection of higher grade tumors found in the "for cause" biopsies for the finasteride arm of the PCPT trial. Consequently, the "end of study" biopsies showed no increased risk of high grade tumor.[30] The increased sensitivity of digital rectal exam performed while a patient is on finasteride has also been shown to increase sensitivity for detecting nodules. Detection increased from 16% to 21% (P=.015).[31]

Finally, PSA sensitivity for detecting prostate cancer increased with the use of 5-ARIs. Both finasteride and dutasteride reduce the PSA laboratory value by approximately half. Consequently, PSA performs better (is more sensitive) in detecting high grade tumors.[32] For the PCPT, for cause biopsies due to a higher PSA level artificially selected for more biopsies to be taken from the treatment group. Prostate volume decreases with finasteride use thus allowed for a larger percentage of the gland to be sampled due to the ratio of the needle to the prostate. The PCPT did not stratify on prostate volume size and it is unclear if this theoretical bias altered the trend towards high grade tumors.

A reevaluation of the PCPT data adjusted for prostate sampling density and baseline PSA levels found that the finasteride group actually had a small net reduction in high grade cancers and a 53% decrease in low grade tumors.[26] A subsequent analysis of the PCPT data using end point prostatectomy instead of prostate biopsy demonstrated a 16% reduction in high grade tumor. At the time of prostatectomy, significant upstaging of cancer was detected in the placebo group but not in the treatment group. In fact, the misclassification of true high-grade disease (to low-grade disease on biopsy) was significantly lower for finasteride (34.6%) than for placebo (52.6%).[33] Finally, another study looking at 500 patients who underwent prostatectomy demonstrated a high-grade cancer rates of 8.2% (placebo) versus 6.0% (finasteride), a 27% risk reduction (RR, 0.73; 95% CI, 0.56-0.96; P = 0.02) with finasteride.[34] The authors concluded that it finasteride probably does not cause high grade cancers, and may in fact improve the detection of them.

The REDUCE trial proved that there was no overall difference for high grade tumors between dutasteride and placebo during the entire study. However subgroup analyses demonstrated a trend towards Gleason 8-10 tumors in the dutasteride group study (19 in placebo vs. 29 in dutasteride, P = .15). In addition the statistically significant increase of high grade tumors in years 3 and 4 was alarming (1 in placebo vs. 12 in dutasteride, P = .003). The authors of the study concluded that the increased number of high grade tumors was due to the increased detection bias in the dutasteride arm as well as removal of low grade cancer in years one and two in the placebo arm. Post hoc analyses similar to the ones performed on the PCPT are pending.

3.4 Current political environment of 5-ARI

In December of 2010, the Federal Drug Administration's Oncology Drugs Advisory Committee (ODAC) reviewed 5-ARI's indication for the prevention of prostate cancer in men at increased risk for prostate cancer. GlaxoSmithKline submitted an application to add prostate cancer prevention as an indication for dutasteride, and Merck submitted an application to alter the labeling for finasteride to reflect a more favorable safety profile with regard to preventing prostate cancer.

ODAC analyzed the results from the PCPT and REDUCE trials. They concluded that the majority of cancers prevented were low risk, thus providing no evidence of prostate cancer mortality reduction. Also, the controversy with the potential increase in high grade cancers could not be overlooked. Their conclusion was based on the fact that the risks of high-grade cancer were potentially real and could not be explained entirely by volume grade bias, increased sensitivity of PSA and DRE or removal of low-grade cancers. Finally, since the both REDUCE and the PCPT trials utilized end-of-study biopsies, the trial results were not yet generalizable to the US population. ODAC voted against the new indication for dutasteride (yes = 2, no = 14, abstain = 2) and against the new labeling for finasteride (yes = 0, no = 17, abstain = 1).

Due to ODAC's ruling, the FDA does not currently support the use of 5-ARIs for prostate cancer chemoprevention. After the decision made by ODAC, a publicly funded clinical trials cooperative group, SWOG (Southwest Oncology Group), released a statement disagreeing with ODAC's decision to not use 5-ARIs for the prostate cancer prevention.[35]

Clearly, disagreement remains after the publication of the two trials. GlaxoSmithKline has subsequently announced that it is withdrawing applications for similar approval in other countries.[36] More long term data is needed to help experts agree on a consensus although we doubt that any further trials will be done with these agents to prevent prostate cancer. And likely because the other trials mentioned above have been negative, future trials for chemoprevention of prostate cancer will be rare.

3.5 Economic impact of prostate chemoprevention

Current economic assessments for chemoprevention are based on varying assumptions that take into account data from the PCPT, treatment costs, and life expectancy. In addition, variations on the model include how the PCPT data is integrated into the model. For example, PCPT high grade disease can include projections based on the actual data set or based on a data set adjusted for biases.

To be effective, chemoprevention for cancer should cost roughly $100,000 or less per life year (LY) saved due to low adoption rates when cost is greater than $100,000/yr and high when cost is less than $20,000/yr .[37] Svatek *et al* used SEER data to estimate real world incidence and analyzed the cost-effectiveness of finasteride. Their group concluded that finasteride was too expensive at $578,000 to $1,107,000 USD per LY saved.[38]

Subsequent studies supported that chemoprevention was too expensive and estimated the expense per LY saved at up to $1.6 million.[39] However, an analysis on quality adjusted life-years (QALYs) based on PCPT prevalence rates showed a lower cost per LY due to higher PCPT prevalence rates. This analysis demonstrated $122,000 per QALY saved.[40] If finasteride is assumed to not increase the incidence of high grade cancers, then the analysis demonstrated $112,000 per QALY saved. Thus more patients benefit from chemoprevention. These analyses were based on the current price of finasteride at $66/month. If finasteride becomes less expensive, then the cost per QALY has the potential to drop significantly. Similarly, one study evaluated dutasteride based on the REDUCE study data and concluded that it too was not cost effective as a general chemopreventative agent.[41]

Currently chemoprevention with either finasteride or dutasteride is not cost effective. The identification of a high risk subgroup would potentially decrease the cost to benefit ratio thus making chemoprevention feasible from an economic standpoint. In addition, decreasing the cost of either 5-ARI has the potential to make chemoprevention feasible.

4. Discussion

Currently the only proven chemopreventative agents for prostate cancer are finasteride and dutasteride with up to a ~24% reduction in prostate cancer (24% PCPT, 23% REDUCE). However, as discussed earlier, the perceived risk of high grade cancers and the unclear long term benefit for low grade cancers has caused the ruling against the use of 5-ARI's for chemoprevention. Reanalysis of the Prostate Cancer Prevention Trial (PCPT) does not support this ruling and suggests that high-grade cancer is not associated with finasteride therapy and that prostatectomy is the only definitive diagnosis for the evaluation for prostate cancer.[42] In addition, the effects of PSA, DRE and prostate volume bias will continue to make interpretation of the data difficult.[43]

It is important to note that as many of 30% of clinically insignificant cancers on first biopsy are then upstaged on second biopsy to become significant cancers. Consequently, the long term benefits of preventing low grade disease are uncertain.[44] Also, by reducing the incidence of low grade disease, the potential for decreasing the "burden of treatment" is uncertain. But in the US environment where greater than 90% of men diagnosed with prostate cancer seek treatment, it is clear that individuals who have low grade cancer prevented will benefit.[45]

Despite evidence from the PCPT and REDUCE trials, there does not appear to be a trend towards prescribing 5-ARIs for the prevention of prostate cancer. Approximately 64% of Urologists and 80% of primary care providers never prescribe finasteride for prostate cancer chemoprevention. Over half of Urologists reported concerns for inducing high grade tumors. In addition, half of the primary care physicians were not aware 5-ARIs could be used for chemoprevention.[46] With the current ruling by ODAC, it is likely that physicians will trend away from prescribing 5-ARI medications for chemoprevention.

Further analyses are required to pinpoint the subgroup population that will benefit most and the timing that is required to be effective. The PCPT revealed a high prevalence of prostate cancer, but no reliable markers were available to determine who would benefit most from biopsy or treatment. REDUCE prospectively collected samples to retrospectively analyze potential biomarkers but has not yet identified a subgroup that would yet benefit from dutasteride prevention.[47]

In the current political environment, the adoption of 5-ARI medications is slim due to the uncertainty surrounding finasteride and dutasteride. Further analysis into subgroups of patients may reveal that 5-ARIs are clinically significant and economically available for at risk individuals. Maybe then, the benefits of 5-ARI medications will outweigh their uncertainty regarding high risk disease. In the meantime, investigations into new biomarkers, nutritional supplements and other pharmacologic agents may elicit a potential solution to the perplexing problem of primary prevention.

5. References

[1] Siegel R, Naishadham D, Jemal A. Cancer statistics, 2012. CA Cancer J Clin 2012;62:10-29.

[2] Etzioni R, Penson DF, Legler JM, et al. Overdiagnosis due to prostate-specific antigen screening: lessons from U.S. prostate cancer incidence trends. J Natl Cancer Inst 2002;94:981-90.

[3] Vignati G, Giovanelli L. Standardization of PSA measures: a reappraisal and an experience with WHO calibration of Beckman Coulter Access Hybritech total and free PSA. Int J Biol Markers 2007;22:295-301.

[4] Dale W, Bilir P, Han M, Meltzer D. The role of anxiety in prostate carcinoma: a structured review of the literature. Cancer 2005;104:467-78.

[5] Titus MA, Gregory CW, Ford OH, 3rd, Schell MJ, Maygarden SJ, Mohler JL. Steroid 5alpha-reductase isozymes I and II in recurrent prostate cancer. Clin Cancer Res 2005;11:4365-71.

[6] Frye SV. Discovery and clinical development of dutasteride, a potent dual 5alpha-reductase inhibitor. Curr Top Med Chem 2006;6:405-21.

[7] Thomas LN, Lazier CB, Gupta R, et al. Differential alterations in 5alpha-reductase type 1 and type 2 levels during development and progression of prostate cancer. Prostate 2005;63:231-9.

[8] Marberger M. Drug Insight: 5alpha-reductase inhibitors for the treatment of benign prostatic hyperplasia. Nat Clin Pract Urol 2006;3:495-503.

[9] Mener DJ. Prostate specific antigen reduction following statin therapy: Mechanism of action and review of the literature. IUBMB Life;62:584-90.

[10] Bonovas S, Filioussi K, Sitaras NM. Statin use and the risk of prostate cancer: A metaanalysis of 6 randomized clinical trials and 13 observational studies. Int J Cancer 2008;123:899-904.

[11] Smith MR, Manola J, Kaufman DS, Oh WK, Bubley GJ, Kantoff PW. Celecoxib versus placebo for men with prostate cancer and a rising serum prostate-specific antigen after radical prostatectomy and/or radiation therapy. Journal of clinical oncology : official journal of the American Society of Clinical Oncology 2006;24:2723-8.

[12] Narayanan BA, Narayanan NK, Pittman B, Reddy BS. Regression of mouse prostatic intraepithelial neoplasia by nonsteroidal anti-inflammatory drugs in the transgenic adenocarcinoma mouse prostate model. Clin Cancer Res 2004;10:7727-37.

[13] Price D, Stein B, Sieber P, et al. Toremifene for the prevention of prostate cancer in men with high grade prostatic intraepithelial neoplasia: results of a double-blind, placebo controlled, phase IIB clinical trial. J Urol 2006;176:965-70; discussion 70-1.

[14] Hamilton RJ, Freedland SJ. 5-alpha reductase inhibitors and prostate cancer prevention: where do we turn now? BMC medicine 2011;9:105.

[15] Dong Y, Zhang H, Hawthorn L, Ganther HE, Ip C. Delineation of the molecular basis for selenium-induced growth arrest in human prostate cancer cells by oligonucleotide array. Cancer Res 2003;63:52-9.

[16] Zhao H, Dupont J, Yakar S, Karas M, LeRoith D. PTEN inhibits cell proliferation and induces apoptosis by downregulating cell surface IGF-IR expression in prostate cancer cells. Oncogene 2004;23:786-94.

[17] Lippman SM, Klein EA, Goodman PJ, et al. Effect of selenium and vitamin E on risk of prostate cancer and other cancers: the Selenium and Vitamin E Cancer Prevention Trial (SELECT). JAMA 2009;301:39-51.

[18] Duffield-Lillico AJ, Dalkin BL, Reid ME, et al. Selenium supplementation, baseline plasma selenium status and incidence of prostate cancer: an analysis of the complete treatment period of the Nutritional Prevention of Cancer Trial. BJU international 2003;91:608-12.

[19] Heinonen OP, Albanes D, Virtamo J, et al. Prostate cancer and supplementation with alpha-tocopherol and beta-carotene: incidence and mortality in a controlled trial. J Natl Cancer Inst 1998;90:440-6.
[20] Sarkar FH, Li Y, Wang Z, Kong D. Novel targets for prostate cancer chemoprevention. Endocr Relat Cancer;17:R195-212.
[21] Thompson IM. Chemoprevention of prostate cancer: agents and study designs. J Urol 2007;178:S9-S13.
[22] Johnson JJ, Bailey HH, Mukhtar H. Green tea polyphenols for prostate cancer chemoprevention: a translational perspective. Phytomedicine;17:3-13.
[23] Bettuzzi S, Brausi M, Rizzi F, Castagnetti G, Peracchia G, Corti A. Chemoprevention of human prostate cancer by oral administration of green tea catechins in volunteers with high-grade prostate intraepithelial neoplasia: a preliminary report from a one-year proof-of-principle study. Cancer Res 2006;66:1234-40.
[24] Jacobsen BK, Knutsen SF, Fraser GE. Does high soy milk intake reduce prostate cancer incidence? The Adventist Health Study (United States). Cancer Causes Control 1998;9:553-7.
[25] Venkateswaran V, Klotz LH. Diet and prostate cancer: mechanisms of action and implications for chemoprevention. Nat Rev Urol;7:442-53.
[26] Cohen YC, Liu KS, Heyden NL, et al. Detection bias due to the effect of finasteride on prostate volume: a modeling approach for analysis of the Prostate Cancer Prevention Trial. J Natl Cancer Inst 2007;99:1366-74.
[27] Xu Y, Dalrymple SL, Becker RE, Denmeade SR, Isaacs JT. Pharmacologic basis for the enhanced efficacy of dutasteride against prostatic cancers. Clin Cancer Res 2006;12:4072-9.
[28] Andriole GL, Bostwick DG, Brawley OW, et al. Effect of dutasteride on the risk of prostate cancer. N Engl J Med;362:1192-202.
[29] Scardino PT. The prevention of prostate cancer--the dilemma continues. N Engl J Med 2003;349:297-9.
[30] Roehrborn CG. Prevention of prostate cancer with finasteride. N Engl J Med 2003;349:1569-72; author reply -72.
[31] Thompson IM, Tangen CM, Goodman PJ, et al. Finasteride improves the sensitivity of digital rectal examination for prostate cancer detection. J Urol 2007;177:1749-52.
[32] Thompson IM, Chi C, Ankerst DP, et al. Effect of finasteride on the sensitivity of PSA for detecting prostate cancer. J Natl Cancer Inst 2006;98:1128-33.
[33] Pinsky P, Parnes H, Ford L. Estimating rates of true high-grade disease in the prostate cancer prevention trial. Cancer Prev Res (Phila) 2008;1:182-6.
[34] Redman MW, Tangen CM, Goodman PJ, Lucia MS, Coltman CA, Jr., Thompson IM. Finasteride does not increase the risk of high-grade prostate cancer: a bias-adjusted modeling approach. Cancer Prev Res (Phila) 2008;1:174-81.
[35] http://swog.org/visitors/newsletters/2010/12/index.asp?a=spotlight.
[36] GSK statement on Avodart™ (dutasteride) for prostate cancer risk reduction. http://wwwgskcom/media/pressreleases/2011/2011_pressrelease_10043htm.
[37] Laupacis A, Feeny D, Detsky AS, Tugwell PX. Tentative guidelines for using clinical and economic evaluations revisited. CMAJ 1993;148:927-9.

[38] Svatek RS, Lee JJ, Roehrborn CG, Lippman SM, Lotan Y. The cost of prostate cancer chemoprevention: a decision analysis model. Cancer Epidemiol Biomarkers Prev 2006;15:1485-9.
[39] Zeliadt SB, Etzioni RD, Penson DF, Thompson IM, Ramsey SD. Lifetime implications and cost-effectiveness of using finasteride to prevent prostate cancer. Am J Med 2005;118:850-7.
[40] Svatek RS, Lee JJ, Roehrborn CG, Lippman SM, Lotan Y. Cost-effectiveness of prostate cancer chemoprevention: a quality of life-years analysis. Cancer 2008;112:1058-65.
[41] Svatek RS, Lotan Y. Cost utility of prostate cancer chemoprevention with dutasteride in men with an elevated prostate specific antigen. Cancer Prev Res (Phila) 2011;4:277-83.
[42] Strope SA, Andriole GL. Update on chemoprevention for prostate cancer. Curr Opin Urol;20:194-7.
[43] Crawford ED, Andriole GL, Marberger M, Rittmaster RS. Reduction in the risk of prostate cancer: future directions after the Prostate Cancer Prevention Trial. Urology;75:502-9.
[44] Berglund RK, Masterson TA, Vora KC, Eggener SE, Eastham JA, Guillonneau BD. Pathological upgrading and up staging with immediate repeat biopsy in patients eligible for active surveillance. J Urol 2008;180:1964-7; discussion 7-8.
[45] Cooperberg MR, Broering JM, Carroll PR. Time trends and local variation in primary treatment of localized prostate cancer. Journal of clinical oncology : official journal of the American Society of Clinical Oncology 2010;28:1117-23.
[46] Hamilton RJ, Kahwati LC, Kinsinger LS. Knowledge and use of finasteride for the prevention of prostate cancer. Cancer Epidemiol Biomarkers Prev;19:2164-71.
[47] Andriole G, Bostwick D, Brawley O, et al. Chemoprevention of prostate cancer in men at high risk: rationale and design of the reduction by dutasteride of prostate cancer events (REDUCE) trial. J Urol 2004;172:1314-7.

18

Prevention and Therapeutic Strategies in Endometrial Cancer

Dan Ancuşa[1], Gheorghe Furău[2], Adrian Carabineanu[1], Răzvan Ilina[1], Octavian Neagoe[1] and Marius Craina[1]
[1]*University of Medicine and Pharmacy „Victor Babeş" Timişoara,*
[2]*"Vasile Goldiş" Western University of Arad,*
Romania

1. Introduction

Endometrial cancer is the most common gynecological cancer in developed countries. Endometrial cancer primarily affects postmenopausal women, with a median age at diagnosis of 60 years approximately 25% of women are premenopausal at diagnosis and up to 5% of these are below the age of 40 years [Orr, 1997].

2. Clinico-anatomopathological characteristics

17 studies covering 10,572 women showed a prevalence of a malignancy within endometrial polyps in postmenopausal women about 5.42% compared to 1.70% in premenopausal women [Lee, 2010]. Endometrial neoplasia was identified in 214 of 3,946 women with endometrial polyps who were postmenopausal compared with 68 of 3,997 premenopausal women (relative risk 3.86). There were 4,967 women with symptomatic bleeding and 195 from them (4.15%) had neoplastic polyps compared with 85 of 3,941 (2.16%) without normal bleeding, according to the report (relative risk 1.97). Looking at the increased risks seen with postmenopausal status and abnormal bleeding, this did not seem to be additive. Polyp size did not appear to be associated with malignancy. Women with hereditary nonpolyposis colorectal cancer (HNPCC) syndrome have a markedly increased risk of endometrial cancer compared with women in the general population. Among women who are HNPCC mutation carriers, the estimated cumulative incidence of endometrial cancer ranges from 20% to 60% [Morrow, 1991; Goff, 1994]. In terms of histopathology, endometrial cancer can be considered as two types: type I, endometrioid, most commonly seen in 80-90% of cases and type II, and all other forms nonendometrioide serous. Endometrial carcinoma has three architectural degrees, depending on Solid to glandular component rate (for grade 1 is <5% and >50% for grade 3). That tipycally will be arised in younger obese women, hyper lipidemia, and signs of hyperestrogenism (exogenous or endogenous). Serous carcinomas are high-grade carcinomas. Comprising -1% of endometrial adenocarcinomas, the clear cell carcinomas are rare. There is an increasing of them in thinner, older women and show no hormonal risk factors. The endometrial carcinomas type I are commonly diagnosed at an early stage and have a favorable prognosis, often only surgically treated; recurrences are usually local (the most common site is pelvis) and curable very frequently with tumor-

directed radiotherapy. The carcinomas type II from endometrial are present with metastatic disease at diagnosis and carry a poorer prognosis (Soslow 2007). Complex or simple hyperplasia could be associated with cellular atypia. We can subdivide them into mild atypia (nuclear enlargement and rounding with evenly dispersed chromatin) or moderate atypia (clumped chromatin, larger nuclear size, prominent nucleoli). There is a low likelihood of hyperplasia without atypia, either simple or complex (1%, 3%) of progressing to carcinoma. In contrast, atypical endometrial hyperplasia is believed to be the direct precursor to endometrioid carcinoma [Bokhman, 1983; Soslow, 1997]. An investigation by The Gynecologic Oncology Group found that from19% to 62% of endometrial biopsy. There is an association between endometrial hyperplasia and invasive endometrial cancer postoperative. (Merisio, 2005) Complex and simple hyperplasia can be treated with only progestative therapy, whereas hysterectomy is mandatory for patients with atypical hyperplasia. Atypical hyperplasia regresses after treatment with progestational therapy in 60% to 95% of patients [Randall, 1997].

In patients with atypical hyperplasia and the high risk of progression to endometrium carcinoma, hysterectomy is the standard treatment. For women who desire a fertility preserving therapy should be reserved progestative therapy for six months (Trimble, 2006).

The risk factors of endometrioid cancer are late menopause, continuous anovulation (e.g., polycystic ovarian syndrome), obesity and nulliparity. Additional risk factors may be related to estrogenic effects, a high-fat diet, tamoxifen use, early menarche. Endometrioid adenocarcinomas frequently show genetic instability, typically found in patients with hereditary nonpolyposis colon cancer and mutations (the b-catenin gene is more frequently mutated in carcinomas with squamous differentiation). Serous carcinomas are characterized by chromosomal instability and p53 mutations. Clear cell carcinomas have absent reactivity for estrogen and progesterone receptors and low immunoreactivity for p53. After an initial assessment, necessary treatment of the disease, this depends on its stage of development and disease risk (the risk of recurrence and metastasis).

2.1 Assessment

Assessment of myometrial invasion is to specify the page, the possible extension to the pelvic organs and distance and tumor grade. This evaluation consisted of noninvasive preoperative investigations (imaging) and invasive (biopsy curettage). CT scans have poor sensitivity and specificity in detecting the depth of myometrial invasion, cervical and parametrial involvement, and lymph node metastases [Zerbe, 2000]. MRI appears to be the best imaging modality for preoperative assessment of myoinvasion [Kinkel, 2009]. MRI presents an overall staging accuracy of 85% [Hricak, 1991]. In addition, whilst more accurate than CT, the limitations of MRI in detecting myometrial invasion must be considered [Kinkel, 1999]. In one institutional review of endometrial cancer, 30% of tumors were found to be at an advanced stage and 24% of women had high-grade tumors [Bandyopadhyay, 2008]. Another study of 301 women with stage I endometrial cancer reported that the negative predictive value of MRI for myometrial invasion was 49.2% [Suh, 2009]. The use of PET/ CT is reported in small prospective series to have a high negative predictive value for nodal metastases [Frumovitz, 2004; Signorelli, 2009; Picchio, 2010]. Park demonstrated that PET/CT had a sensitivity of 69.2%, specificity of 90.3%, positive predictive value of 42.9%, and negative predictive value of 96.6 % [Park, 2008].

Endometrial cancer is generally staged according to the International Federation of Gynecology and Obstetrics (FIGO) system. Since 1988, the FIGO system has recommended surgical staging with systematic pelvic and para-aortic lymphadenectomy. In May 2009, a new FIGO staging system was published, but most of studies are based on the old classification (Tables 1). Some centers use intraoperative frozen section analysis of the uterus based upon histological grade, type and depth of myometrial invasion and appears significantly better than MRI scanning in the assessment of myometrial invasion. [Furukawa, 2010].

Stage	**Involvement**
Stage I	Tumor confined to the corpus uteri
IA	No or less than half myometrial invasion
IB	Invasion equal to or more than half of the myometrium
Stage II	Tumor invades cervical stroma, but does not extend beyond the uterus Endocervical glandular involvement alone should be considered as stage I
Stage III	Local and/or regional spread of the tumor
IIIA	Tumor invades the serosa of the corpus uteri and/or adnexae†
IIIB	Vaginal and/or parametrial involvement†
IIIC	Metastases to pelvic and/or para-aortic lymph nodes†
IIIC 1	Positive pelvic nodes
IIIC 2	Positive para-aortic lymph nodes ± positive pelvic lymph nodes
Stage IV	Tumor invades bladder and/or bowel mucosa, and/or distant metastases
IVA	Tumor invasion of bladder and/or bowel mucosa
IVB	Distant metastases, including intra-abdominal metastases ± inguinal nodes

*Positive cytology should be reported separately without changing the stage [Pecorelli, 2009].

Table 1. FIGO staging of endometrial cancer

2.2 Risk assessment

Multiple factors have been identified for relative high risk of recurrence in apparent early-stage disease: histological subtype, grade 3 histology, myometrial invasion ‡50%, lymphovascular space invasion (LVSI), lymph node metastases and tumor diameter >2 cm.

Stage I can be subdivided into three risk categories [Fiorelli, 2008]:

Low risk:	stage IA (G1 and G2) with endometrioid type
Intermediate risk:	stage IA (G3) with endometrioid type
	stage IB (G1 and G2) with endometrioid type
High risk:	stage IB (G3) with endometrioid type
	all stages with non-endometrioid type

2.3 Surgical staging

Full staging endometrial cancer can be performed surgically [Pecorelli, 2009]. In addition to data related to uterine tumor, surgical research can provide data about state and pelvic lymph lomboaortic by lymphadenectomy. Studies of women undergoing full pelvic lymphadenectomy report rates of occult pelvic lymph node disease ranging from 8 to 28% depending on grade and depth of myometrial invasion [Zivanovic, 2009; Lin, 2008]. Lymphadenectomy causes significant morbidity in approximately 11% of cases [Nunns, 2000]. Pelvic MRI and sentinel lymph node evaluation appear equally effective in detecting pelvic node metastases although the ability to detect the sentinel node varies significantly between studies [Selman, 2008]. Hirahatake reported that para-aortic lymph node metastases in 2.5% of stage IA, 8.5% of stage IB, and 15.7% of stage II endometrial cancers [Hirahatake, 1997]. Mariani and Tanaka reported a direct correlation between pelvic and para-aortic lymph node involvement [Mariani, 2004; Tanaka, 2006]. In a study of 291 endometrial cancer patients by Goudge 18% were upgraded postoperative [Goudge, 2004]. Ben-Shachar reported that tumor was upgraded in 19% of 181 patients with a preoperative grade 1 tumor [Ben-Shachar, 2005]. The results of surgical staging also led to adjuvant treatment in 12% of patients who were found to have extrauterine disease or other high-risk characteristics [Ben-Shachar, 2005].

3. Prevention

Pain was the most common complain in patients with recurrent disease, in the follow-up of endometrial cancer patients, followed by vaginal bleeding, general malaise, loss of weight and intestinal complaints (Zhang, 2010). The routine use of the Pap smear and systematic radiography are not clinically justified in the follow-up of patients with endometrial carcinoma (Agboola, 1997; Morice, 2001). In Lynch syndrome, the current gynecologic carcinoma screening guidelines include annual endometrial sampling and transvaginal ultrasonography beginning at age 30-35 years (178). Primary prevention by using a progesterone device in utero, such as the Mirena IUCD is an alternative approach. This merits full evaluation (Hitchener, 2006). Prophylactic hysterectomy and bilateral salpingoophorectomy should be offered as risk-reducing surgery to women aged 35 years or older who do not wish to preserve fertility. Schmeler et al. reported a retrospective analysis with known germ line mutations associated with Lynch syndrome. There were sixty-one participants who underwent prophylactic hysterectomy and were compared to over 200 matched controls with similar mutations that did not have preventive surgery. In 33% of the controls was eventually diagnosed the endometrial cancer, with no cases in the prophylactic group (Schmeler, 2006). There was detected asymptomatic muscle invasive endometrial carcinoma by Pistorius et al, in two of four women who underwent prophylactic hysterectomy after requiring surgery for Lynch syndrome related colorectal carcinoma (Schmeler, 2006). In 2006, a multiinstitutional, matched case-control study found that prophylactic bilateral salpingoophorectomy and hysterectomy preventive strategy in women with HNPCC syndrome [Schmeler, 2006]. Most cases of endometrial cancer cannot be prevented, but women can take some measures to reduce their risk of developing endometrial cancer. Risks might be reduced with using oral contraceptives controlling obesity and controlling diabetes.

In addition, women who are considering estrogen replacement therapy should talk to their doctors to assess their risk of endometrial cancer. Use of combination oral contraceptives (birth control pills) decreases the risk of developing endometrial cancer.

Women who use oral contraceptives at some time have half the risk of developing endometrial cancer as women who have never used oral contraceptives.

This protection occurs in women who have used oral contraceptives for at least 12 months, and continues for at least 10 years after oral contraceptive use. The protection is most notable for women who have never been pregnant.

Edward Giovannucci, M.D., Sc.D., Professor of Nutrition and Epidemiology at the Harvard School of Public Health, said coffee is emerging as a protective agent in cancers that are linked to obesity, estrogen and insulin. Giovannucci, along with Youjin Je, a doctoral candidate in his lab, and colleagues observed cumulative coffee intake in relation to endometrial cancer in 67,470 women who enrolled in the Nurses' Health Study. During the course of 26 years of follow-up, researchers documented 672 cases of endometrial cancer. Drinking more than four cups of coffee per day was linked with a 25 percent reduced risk for endometrial cancer. Drinking between two and three cups per day was linked with a 7 percent reduced risk [Giovannucci, 2005]. A similar link was seen in decaffeinated coffee, where drinking more than two cups per day was linked with a 22 percent reduced risk for endometrial cancer.

Hormone and lifestyle factors explain up to 80% of risk for endometrial cancer. The investigators found that women who were normal weight and active had a reduction in risk of 73%, compared with inactive women who were overweight (BMI above 25 kg/m^2). Women who were normal weight but inactive had a 55% lower risk for endometrial cancer than inactive women who were overweight. Women who were overweight but active had a 38% lower risk for endometrial cancer.

Aspirin has been shown in vitro to inhibit endometrial cancer cell growth through the induction of apoptosis in a dose-dependent manner [Arango, 2001].

Other NSAIDs have also been shown to reduce endometrial cancer cell proliferation and induce apoptosis in a dose- and time-dependent manner [Gao, 2004; Li, 2002].

African-american women with advanced stage endometrial cancer have lower survival rates than white women with the disease even when both groups receive similar treatments, according to a study published online September 25, 2006, in the journal Cancer .

4. Therapeutic strategies

4.1 Molecularly targeted treatments

One of the major challenges in endometrial cancer treatment remains the current inability to effectively prevent distant metastasis in women with deeply myoinvasive, high-grade or biologically aggressive tumors (e.g., serous and clear cell cancers). One potential target in serous tumors is HER_2 [Konecny, 2009; Villella, 2006; Flemimg, 2003]. The monoclonal antibody trastuzumab binds to HER-2 and can reduce growth in cell lines that overexpress HER-2. Epidermal growth factor receptor (also known as c-erbB-1). One strategy to tackle tumor growth is to target angiogenesis,. The main factor controlling angiogenesis is VEGF. The most well known of these is bevacizumab, a monoclonal antibody against VEGF-A. A study of single-agent bevacizumab in women with recurrent endometrial cancer demonstrated a 15% response rate and a median progression-free survival of 4 months, although approximately 36% of women had a progression-free survival of 6 months [Konecny, 2009].

A number of other antiangiogenic agents are currently being tested as single agents in Phase II trials. These include VEGF–Trap and small-molecule inhibitors of VEGF receptors [Hayes, 2009; Hayes, 2010].

One of the main challenges will be getting the more promising drugs into the clinic. Development of these newer drugs is expensive and costs will therefore be high. Whether there is a therapeutic role for lymphadenectomy in nonendometrioid tumors remains an unanswered. It has been possible to provide clear guidance with respect to the use of radiotherapy following the completion and publication of several key trials in this area, and treatment is now applied on an individualized patient basis. The investigators found that women who were normal weight and active had a reduction in risk of 73%, compared with inactive women who were overweight (BMI above 25 kg/m^2). Women who were normal weight but inactive had a 55% lower risk for endometrial cancer than inactive women who were overweight. Women who were overweight but active had a 38% lower risk for endometrial cancer.

4.2 Treatment of localized disease

In the case of a low-risk disease evolution, with tumor confined to the uterus, non-aggressive treatment is required, while high-risk disease require evolution untreatment multimodal radiochimiotherapy. Treatment of localized disease is mainly surgical and consists of a total hysterectomy with bilateral anexectomy as or no lymphadenectomy. The problem is the continuing debate and systematic lombo-aortic lymphadenectomy role. Lymphadenectomy can be selectively performed in women at highest risk of nodal metastases (deeply invasive or high-grade tumors) [Mariani, 2008]. Lymphadenectomy causes morbidity in approximately 11% of cases [Nunns, 2000]. In an effort to decrease the morbidity that results from lymphadenectomy, the sentinel node approach has been successfully employed. If the sentinel node is pathologically negative for metastasis, all downstream nodes should also be negative and would not require dissection. This technique yielded an overall detection rate of 82%-89% [Niikura, 2004; Delaloye, 2007]. Presently the sentinel lymph node biopsy in endometrial cancer is still an investigational technique. Studies of women undergoing full pelvic lymphadenectomy report rates of occult pelvic lymph node disease ranging from 8 to 28% depending on grade and depth of myometrial invasion [Creasman, 1987; Chi, 2008]. At present there is great uncertainty regarding what is the optimal adjuvant treatment for localized endometrial cancer. The use of adjuvant therapy for endometrial cancer depends on the patient's estimated risk of recurrence. Novel techniques for the delivery of radiation, including intensity-modulated radiation therapy and tomotherapy are promising technologies to improve the therapeutic index for patients receiving combined therapy [Lian, 2008; Salama, 2006; Beriwal, 2006]. A number of trials are ongoing to examine novel biologic and target therapies for women with endometrial cancer [Konecny, 2008; Kamat, 2007; Wright, 2007; Ozbudak, 2008; Morrison, 2006]. Systemic treatment for metastatic and relapsed disease may consist of endocrine therapy or cytotoxic chemotherapy.

4.3 Surgical treatment

The surgical approach for the treatment of endometrial cancer has traditionally been laparotomy. In the last years, the use of minimally invasive techniques is widely accepted by many authors. A recent publication of the GOG LAP2 study has shown similar operative outcomes in the minimally invasive surgery group [Walker, 2010]. Authors have reported that the economic benefits of laparoscopy [Scribner, 1999]. Laparoscopy seems to provide equivalent results in terms of disease-free survival and overall survival compared with laparatomy, with further benefit: shorter hospital stay, less use of pain killers, lower rate of complications and improved quality of life. An increasing number of studies have shown no difference in survival or recurrence between laparoscopy and laparatomy surgery, in early- and advanced-stage endometrial cancer [Eltabbakh, 2002; Holub, 2002; Nezhat, 2008]. Recent reports have examined robotically assisted hysterectomy in the treatment of gynecologic malignancies [Advincula, 2006]. The robotic approach could be a 'benefit' in obese women. (Boggess, 2008], but access to the high para-aortic area appears to be limited compared with the laparoscopic or open surgical approaches [Soliman, 2010]. When surgery is not feasible due to medical contraindications (5–10% of patients), external radiation therapy with or without intracavitary brachytherapy to the uterus and vagina is suitable for individual clinical use [Colombo, 2011]. In three trials women treated with laparoscopic hysterectomy were compared with 193 women treated with open surgery and there appears to be no significant difference in either disease-free or overall survival [Lin, 2008; Palomba, 2009].

4.4 Surgical treatment in stage I endometrial cancer

The standard surgical treatment for stage I endometrial cancer is radical hysterectomy and bilateral anexectomy with or without lymphadenectomy. In young women with stage IA endometrial carcinoma is proposed to preserve fertility, based on the hysteroscopic resection of the tumor followed by hormone therapy regimen of megestrol acetate (160 mg/day) [Mazzon, 2010]. The role of systematic pelvic lymphadenectomy is in current debate. Mariani states that patients with stage I endometrial cancer, excluding stage IA–IB G1, systematic lymphadenectomy did not improve disease-free or overall survival [Mariani 2000]. In the ASTEC randomized trial, women with endometrial cancer confined to the uterus and pelvic lymphadenectomy was no evidence of benefit on overall survival or recurrence-free survival [Blake, 2009]. The authors recommended that systematic pelvic lymphadenectomy cannot be recommended in women with stage I endometrial cancer. Lymphadenectomy is highly important for determining a prognosis and in tailoring adjuvant therapies. Prognostic factors for para-aortic spread are similar to those for pelvic nodal disease and include depth of myometrial invasion and the presence of lymphovascular space invasion [Fotopoulou, 2010; Park, 2010; Nomura, 2006]. Many authors suggest a lymphadenectomy for intermediate–high risk endometrial cancer (stage IA G3 and IB) [Colombo, 2011]. Lymph node sampling did not appear to confer a survival benefit in patients with stage IA, grade 1 or 2 tumors, but improved survival in patients with grade 3 [Trimble, 1998]. External beam radiation has been shown to reduce the rate of locoregional recurrence in intermediate-risk endometrial cancer. The Postoperative Radiation Therapy in Endometrial Cancer (PORTEC) trial randomly assigned 715 women with endometrial cancer stage IB grade 2-3 tumors or stage IC grade 1-2 tumors who underwent surgery treatment to whole pelvic radiotherapy versus no further treatment. After 10 years of follow-up there was a reduction in vaginal recurrences from 15 to 4% but no difference in survival [Creutzberg, 2000]. Aalders and collaborators published the results of 540 women with stage I endometrial cancer that underwent surgical treatment and vaginal brachytherapy and were randomized to whole pelvic radiation versus observation. Pelvic control was improved with the addition of radiotherapy, but there were no survival differences at 5 years [Aalders, 1980]. Nout publish the results of a randomized clinical trial (PORTEC-2) comparing vaginal brachytherapy and external beam radiation in intermediate-risk patients [Nout, 2010]. This study showed no any difference in overall survival or progression-free survival (PFS). The quality of life was better in the vaginal brachytherapy treatment. Radiation of patients who underwent hysterectomy with comprehensive lymphadenectomy improves local control and disease-free survival, but did not affect overall survival. (Keys, 2004) but is associated with appreciable toxicity [Creutzberg, 2000; Keys, 2004]. ESMO Guidelines Working Group 2011 recommended in stage IB G1-2 with negative prognostic factors pelvic radiotherapy and/or adjunctive chemotherapy could be considered [Colombo, 2011]. Endometrial cancer stage I with grade 3 tumors combination chemotherapy to pelvic radiotherapy require. Platinum-based chemotherapy can be considered in stage I G3 with adverse risk factors (patient age, lymphovascular space invasion and high tumor volume) platinum-based adjuvant chemotherapy for early (stage I) disease improves PFS and overall survival. Two trials, one Italian and one Japanese in high-risk patients comparing five courses of cisplatin, doxorubicin and cyclophosphamide with external pelvic radiation reported no difference between therapies in terms of PFS or overall survival [Maggi, 2006; Susumu, 2008]. Chemotherapy appeared superior to pelvic radiotherapy in patients with stage IC, aged >70 years with outer half myometrial invasion, with grade 3, or with stage I disease and positive peritoneal cytology [Maggi, 2006]. In a Cochrane Collaboration review of adjuvant radiotherapy for stage I, external-beam radiotherapy resulted in a 72% reduction in pelvic relapses, a reduction in death in patients with multiple high-risk factors (stage IC and grade 3 tumors) did not translate into a reduction in distant metastatic [Kong, 2007].

4.5 Surgical treatment in stage II endometrial cancer

Traditionally, the surgical approach consists of radical hysterectomy with bilateral salpingo-oophorectomy and systematic pelvic lymphadenectomy with or without paraaortic lymphadenectomy. In stage II, lymphadenectomy is essential to guide surgical staging and adjuvant therapy. Para-aortic dissection should aim to remove the nodes to level of the mesenteric artery up to the renal vessels, rather than restricting dissection to the level of the inferior mesenteric artery. Large retrospective nonrandomized studies demonstrated that women, who have a para-aortic dissection, have improved outcomes, with increased overall survival [Chan, 2006; Chan, 2007]. Authors show that women at intermediate or high risk of disease recurrence should have pelvic and para-aortic lymphadenectomy and no benefit was seen in low-risk patients [Todo, 2010]. ESMO suggests that adjuvant treatment in stage II consists of pelvic radiotherapy and vaginal brachytherapy. If prognostic factors (grade 1–2 tumor, myometrial invasion <50%, LVSI and complete surgical staging) are negative-brachytherapy alone. If prognostic factors are negative it is feasible chemotherapy with/without radiation [Colombo, 2011].

Chemotherapy appeared superior to pelvic radiotherapy in patients with stage II with a significantly higher overall survival and progression-free survival and the rate of pelvic recurrence was the same (7%). (Susumu, 2008) Platinum-based chemotherapy can be considered in this stage. In retrospective series that platinum-based adjuvant chemotherapy for stage II disease improves PFS and overall survival [Soliman, 2010].

4.6 Surgical treatment in stage III-IV endometrial cancer

Maximal surgical debunking is imperative in patients with a good performance status. The surgical approach consists of anterior and posterior pelvic exenteration. For distant metastatic disease, palliative surgery could be considered in patients with a good performance. If positive nodes: radiotherapy. If metastatic disease: chemotherapy-radiotherapy for palliative treatment [Colombo, 2011]. Traditionally, treatment for women with stage III endometrial cancer has relied on radiotherapy while women with stage IV disease have been treated with palliative chemotherapy [Ross, 2008; Denschlag, 2007; Mariani, 2006]. 396 women with stage III or IV disease were randomized to postoperative whole abdominal radiation versus chemotherapy with doxorubicin and cisplatin. Patients in the chemotherapy group had a statistically significant increased progression-free (42 vs 38%) and overall survival (53 vs 42%) [Gallion, 2003]. Agents for endometrial cancer appear to be doxorubicin and cisplatin. Response rates to single-agent doxorubicin alone are generally in the range of 17-25% [Carey, 2006; Gallion, 2003]. Two prospective randomized trials have demonstrated a superior response rate to doxorubicin and cisplatin as compared with doxorubicin alone, however, with similar survival rates [Thigpen, 1994; Thigpen, 2004, Aapro, 2003]. When carboplatin is associated with cisplatin, is reported a response rate of greater than 40% [Akram, 2005; Dimopoulos, 2000; Sovak, 2006; Secord, 2007]. Given this provocative data, doxorubicin plus paclitaxel was investigated by the GOG (GOG 163) as an alternative to doxorubicin and cisplatin for women with advanced or recurrent disease. Doxorubicin, cisplatin and paclitaxel demonstrated a significant improvement in response rate, progression free and overall survival, but toxicity was much higher with the three drug regimen [Fleming, 2004]. The combination with cisplatin and doxorubicin or cisplatin, doxorubicin and paclitaxel for women with stage III and IV completely resected endometrial cancer appeared equivalent [Alvarez, 2007; Bruzzone, 2004]. Patients with stage IIIC underwent adjuvant treatment with paclitaxel and concurrent pelvic radiation therapy. Overall survival was 81% at 3 years with a median time to relapse of 19 months [Mangili, 2006]. In a similar design, Greven and colleagues reported on 46 patients with endometrial adenocarcinoma with greater than 50% myometrial invasion, stromal invasion of the cervix, or extrauterine disease confined to the pelvis and/or positive peritoneal cytology that underwent postoperative adjuvant treatment with pelvic radiation therapy, vaginal brachytherapy and concurrent cisplatin and paclitaxel. Survival at 4 years was 85% [Greven, 2006].

4.7 Locoregional recurrence

Radiation therapy is standard treatment for vaginal recurrence (external beam plus vaginal brachytherapy). There is high rates in local control, complete response (CR) and 5-year survival is 50%. Surgery is the treatment of choice for pelvic recurrence, or radiation therapy, while for regional pelvic recurrences it is radiation therapy, associated if possible with chemotherapy.

The combination of Doxorubicin, Cisplatin, and Paclitaxel was found to produce an improvement in progression free survival for patients with recurrent endometrial cancer, compared with the two drug combination of Doxorubicin and Cisplatin [Fleming, 2000]. When using adjuvant chemotherapy without adjuvant radiation therapy in patients with advanced-stage endometrial cancer, 40% of women experienced a pelvic relapse at 3 years

[Mundt, 2001]. Five year local control rate of 54%, disease specific survival of 51%, and overall survival of 44% has been reported in a group of patients with locoregional recurrence who made radiotherapy alone [Sears, 1994]. The tumors tend to become resistant to progestational therapy, but may offer a prolonged complete response interval [Fiorica, 2000]. For first-line chemotherapy combinations regimens are preffered of recurrent endometrial cancer.

4.8 Advanced disease

There is no agreement on the standard treatment for women with advanced endometrial cancer. A combination of optimally debulked, radiotherapy and chemotherapy is employed. Metastatic endometrial cancer can be effectively treated with progestational agents. Response rates ranged from 40% with grade 1 disease and 0% with Broder's grade 4 lesions. [Podratz, 1985]. ESMO recommended hormonal therapy for endometrioid histologies only with overall response 25% [Colombo, 2011]. Chemotherapy alone determines a response rate of 40%. The most commonly used are compounds, antracyclines and taxanes, alone and in combination. Paclitaxel-based combination regimens are preffered for first-line chemotherapy of advanced endometrial cancer. The consistent response rate was only for paclitaxel>20% [Colombo, 2011]. The paclitaxel-containing regimens demonstrated a response rate > 60% and a possibly prolonged survival. GOG shows that patients with metastatic endometrial carcinoma require pelvic irradiation with or without paraaortic irradiation, followed by cisplatin, doxorubicin and paclitaxel (Randall, 2006).

4.9 Papillary serous carcinoma and clear cell carcinoma

Papillary serous and clear cell carcinoma require total hysterectomy, bilateral salpingoophorectomy, pelvic and paraaortic lymphadenectomy, omentectomy, appendectomy and peritoneal biopsies. There is more aggressiveness with higher rates of metastatic disease and lower 5-year survival rates. The same chemotherapy regimens usually used for ovarian cancer could be also used in women with advanced or recurrent papillary serous or clear cell uterine cancer. Papillary serous endometrial carcinomas have not been considered to be hormone responsive [Colombo, 2011].

5. References

Aalders, J.; Abeler, V.; Kolstad, P.; Onsrud, M. (1980). Postoperative external irradiation and prognostic parameters in stage I endometrial carcinoma: clinical and histopathologic study of 540 patients. *Obstetrics and Gynecology,* Vol. 56, No.4, (October, 1980), 419-427.

Aapro MS, van Wijk FH, Bolis G et al. (2003). Doxorubicin versus doxorubicin and cisplatin in endometrial carcinoma: definitive results of a randomised study (55872) by the EORTC Gynaecological Cancer Group. *Annals of Oncology,* Vol. 14, No.3, (March, 2003), pp. 441-448.

Advincula AP. (2006). Surgical techniques: robot-assisted laparoscopic hysterectomy with the da Vinci surgical system. *International Journal of Medical Robotics,* Vol. 2, No.4, (December, 2006), pp. 305-311.

Agboola O. O., E. Grunfeld, D. Coyle, and G. A. Perry, (1997).Costs and benefits of routine follow-up after curative treatment for endometrial cancer, *Canadian Medical Association Journal,* vol. 157, no. 7, pp. 879–886.

Akram T, Maseelall P, Fanning J. (2005). Carboplatin and paclitaxel for the treatment of advanced or recurrent endometrial cancer. *American Journal of Obstetrics and Gynecology,* Vol. 192, No.5, (May, 2005), pp. 1365-1367.

Alvarez Secord A, Havrilesky LJ, Bae-Jump V et al. (2007). The role of multi-modality adjuvant chemotherapy and radiation in women with advanced stage endometrial cancer. *Gynecologic Oncology,* Vol. 107, No.2, (November, 2007), pp. 285-297.

Arango HA, Icely S, Roberts WS, Cavanagh D, Becker JL. (2001). Aspirin effects on endometrial cancer cell growth *Obstetrics and Gynecology,* Vol. 97: 423 –427.

Bruzzone M, Miglietta L, Franzone P, Gadducci A, Boccardo F. (2004). Combined treatment with chemotherapy and radiotherapy in high-risk FIGO stage III-IV endometrial cancer patients. *Gynecologic Oncology,* Vol. 93, No. 2, (May, 2004), pp. 345-352.

Bandyopadhyay S, Arabi H, Thirabanjasak D, Quddus MR, Lawrence WD, Fehmi RA. (2008). Endometrial cancer diagnosed in young patients is not always a low-risk cancer. *Modern Pathology,* Vol. 21, pp. 900.

Ben-Shachar I, Pavelka J, Cohn DE, et al. (2005). Surgical staging for patients presenting with grade 1 endometrial carcinoma. *Obstetrics and Gynecology,* Vol. 105, No. 3, (March, 2005), pp. 487-493.

Beriwal S, Jain SK, Heron DE et al. (2006). Clinical outcome with adjuvant treatment of endometrial carcinoma using intensity-modulated radiation therapy. *Gynecologic Oncology,* Vol. 102, No. 2, (May, 2006), pp. 195-199.

Blake P, Swart AM, Orton J et al. (2009). Adjuvant external beam radiotherapy in the treatment of endometrial cancer (MRC ASTEC and NCIC CTG EN.5 randomised trials): pooled trial results, systematic review, and meta-analysis. *Lancet,* Vol. 373, (January, 2009), pp. 137–146.

Boggess JF, Gehrig PA, Cantrell L et al. (2008). A comparative study of 3 surgical methods for hysterectomy with staging for endometrial cancer: robotic assistance, laparoscopy, laparotomy. *American Journal of Obstetrics and Gynecology,* Vol. 199, No. 4, (October, 2008), pp. 360. e1–9.

Bokhman, J.V. (1983). Two pathogenetic types of endometrial carcinoma, *Gynecologic Oncology,* vol. 15, no. 1, (February, 1983), pp. 10–17.

Creutzberg CL, van Putten WL, Koper PC et al. (2000). Surgery and postoperative radiotherapy versus surgery alone for patients with stage-1 endometrial carcinoma: multicentre randomised trial. PORTEC Study Group. Post Operative Radiation Therapy in Endometrial Carcinoma. *Lancet,* Vol. 355, No. 9213, (April, 2000), 1404-1411.

Carey MS, Gawlik C, Fung-Kee-Fung M, Chambers A, Oliver T. (2006). Systematic review of systemic therapy for advanced or recurrent endometrial cancer. *Gynecologic Oncology,* Vol. 101, No.1, (April, 2006), pp.158-167.

Chan JK, Wu HS, Cheung MK, Shin JY, Osann K, Kapp DS. (2007). The outcomes of 27,063 women with unstaged endometrioid uterine cancer. *Gynecologic Oncology,* Vol. 106, No. 2, (August, 2007), pp. 282–288.

Chan JK, Cheung MK, Huh WK et al. (2006). Therapeutic role of lymph node resection in endometrioid corpus cancer - a study of 12,333 patients. *Cancer*, Vol. 107, No. 8, 1823–1830.

Colombo, N.; Preti, E.; Landoni, F.; Carinelli, S.; Colombo, A.; Marini, C. (2010). Endometrial cancer: ESMO Clinical Practice Guidelines for diagnosis, treatment and follow-up. *Annals of Oncology*, Vol. 21 (Supplement 5), (May, 2010), pp. vi41–vi45.

Creasman WT, Morrow CP, Bundy BN, Homesley HD, Graham JE, Heller PB. (1987). Surgical pathological spread patterns of endometrial cancer - a Gynecologic Oncology Group study. *Cancer*, Vol. 60, No. 8, (October, 1987), pp. 2035–2041.

Chi DS, Barakat RR, Palayekar MJ et al. (2008).The incidence of pelvic lymph node metastasis by FIGO staging for patients with adequately surgically staged endometrial adenocarcinoma of endometrioid histology. *International Journal of Gynecological Cancer*, Vol. 18, No. 2, (March-April, 2008), pp. 269–273.

Delaloye JF, Pampallona S, Chardonnens E, et al. (2007). Intraoperative lymphatic mapping and sentinel node biopsy using hysteroscopy in patients with endometrial cancer. *Gynecologic Oncology*, Vol. 106, No.1, (April, 2007), pp.89-93.

Denschlag D, Tan L, Patel S, Kerim-Dikeni A, Souhami L, Gilbert L. (2007). Stage III endometrial cancer: preoperative predictability, prognostic factors, and treatment outcome. *American Journal of Obstetrics and Gynecology*, Vol. 196, No. 6 (June, 2007), pp. 546 e1- e7.

Dimopoulos MA, Papadimitriou CA, Georgoulias V et al. (2000). Paclitaxel and cisplatin in advanced or recurrent carcinoma of the endometrium: long-term results of a Phase II multicenter study. *Gynecologic Oncology*, Vol. 78, No.1, (July, 2000), pp. 52-57.

Eltabbakh GH. (2002). Analysis of survival after laparoscopy in women with endometrial carcinoma. *Cancer*, Vol. 95, No. 9, (November, 2002), pp.1894-1901.

Fiorica JV, Thigpen JT, Gersell D, et al. (2000). A phase II study of recurrent and advanced endometrial carcinoma treated with alternating courses of megestrol acetate (Megace) and tamoxifen citrate (Nolvadex). *Procedings of American Society Clinical Oncology*.

Fleming GF, Brunetto VL, Cella D et al. (2004). Phase III trial of doxorubicin plus cisplatin with or without paclitaxel plus filgrastim in advanced endometrial carcinoma: a Gynecologic Oncology Group Study. *Journal of Clinical Oncology*, Vol. 22, No.11, (June, 2004), 2159-2166.

Fotopoulou C, Savvatis K, Kraetschell R, Schefold JC, Lichtenegger W, Sehouli J. (2010). Systematic pelvic and aortic lymphadenectomy in intermediate and high-risk endometrial cancer: lymph-node mapping and identification of predictive factors for lymph-node status. *European Journal of Obstetrics, Gynecology and Reproductive Biology*, Vol. 149, No. 2, (April, 2010), pp. 199–203.

Frumovitz M, Slomovitz BM, Singh DK et al. (2004). Frozen section analyses as predictors of lymphatic spread in patients with early-stage uterine cancer. *Journal of the American College of Surgeons*, Vol. 199, No. 3, (September, 2004), pp. 388–393.

Furukawa N, Takekuma M, Takahashi N, Hirashima Y. (2010). Intraoperative evaluation of myometrial invasion and histological type and grade in endometrial cancer: diagnostic value of frozen section. *Archives of Gynecology and Obstetrics*, Vol. 281, No. 5, (May, 2010), pp. 913–917.

Gallion HH, Brunetto VL, Cibull M et al. (2003). Randomized Phase III trial of standard timed doxorubicin plus cisplatin versus circadian timed doxorubicin plus cisplatin in stage III and IV or recurrent endometrial carcinoma: a Gynecologic Oncology Group Study. *Journal of Clinical Oncology*, Vol. 21, No.20, (October, 2003), pp. 3808-3813.

Gao J, Niwa K, Sun W, et al. (2004). Non-steroidal anti-inflammatory drugs inhibit cellular proliferation and upregulate cyclooxygenase-2 protein expression in endometrial cancer cells. *Cancer Science*, Vol.95, pp.901–907.

Giovannucci Edward, M.D., Harvard School of Public Health, *NCI Cancer Bulletin*, March 29, 2005.

Goudge C, Bernhard S, Cloven NG, et al. (2004). The impact of complete surgical staging on adjuvant treatment decisions in endometrial cancer. *Gynecologic Oncology*, Vol. 93, No.2, (May, 2004), pp.536-539.

Goff BA, Kato D, Schmidt RA, Ek M, Ferry JA, Muntz HG, et al. (1994). Uterine papillary serous carcinoma: patterns of metastatic spread. *Gynecologic Oncology*, Vol. 54, (September, 1994), pp.264-268.

Greven K, Winter K, Underhill K, Fontenesci J, Cooper J, Burke T. (2006). Final analysis of RTOG 9708: adjuvant postoperative irradiation combined with cisplatin/paclitaxel chemotherapy following surgery for patients with high-risk endometrial cancer. *Gynecologic Oncology*, Vol. 103, No.1, (October, 2006), pp. 155-159.

Hirahatake K, Hareyama H, Sakuragi N, et al. (1997). A clinical and pathologic study on para-aortic lymph node metastasis in endometrial carcinoma. *Journal of Surgical Oncology* , Vol. 65, No.2, (June, 1997), pp. 82-87.

Kitchener H. (2006). Management of endometrial carcinoma, *European Journal of Surgical Oncology*, vol. 32, no. 8, pp. 838–843.

Hayes MP, Douglas W, Ellenson LH. (2009). Molecular alterations of EGFR and PIK3CA in uterine serous carcinoma. *Gynecologic Oncology*, Vol. 113(3), pp. 370–373.

Hayes MP, Ellenson LH. (2010). Molecular alterations in uterine serous carcinoma. *Gynecologic Oncology*, Vol. 116(2), pp. 286–289.

Holub Z, Jabor A, Bartos P, et al. (2002). Laparoscopic surgery for endometrial cancer: long-term results of a multicentric study. *European Journal of Gynecologic Oncology* Vol. 23, No.4, pp. 305-310.

Hricak H, Rubinstein LV, Gherman GM, et al. (1991). MR imaging evaluation of endometrial carcinoma: results of an NCI cooperative study. *Radiology*, Vol. 179, No. 3, pp. 829-832.

Jessica L. Fiorelli; Thomas J. Herzog; Jason D. Wright. (2008). Current Treatment Strategies for Endometrial Cancer. *Expert Reviews in Anticancer Therapy*. Vol. 8, No.7, (July, 2008), pp.1149-1157.

Kamat AA, Merritt WM, Coffey D et al. (2007). Clinical and biological significance of vascular endothelial growth factor in endometrial cancer. *Clinical Cancer Research*, Vol. No. 24, (December, 2007), pp. 7487-7495.

Keys HM, Roberts JA, Brunetto VL et al. (2004). A Phase III trial of surgery with or without adjunctive external pelvic radiation therapy in intermediate risk endometrial adenocarcinoma: a Gynecologic Oncology Group study. *Gynecological Oncology* Vol. 92, No. 3, (March, 2004), 744-751.

Kinkel K, Kaji Y, Yu KK et al. (1999). Radiologic staging in patients with endometrial cancer: a meta-analysis. *Radiology,* Vol. 212, No. 3, (September, 1999), pp. 711–718.

Kitchener H, Redman CW, Swart AM, Amos CL. (2006). ASTEC - a study in the treatment of endometrial cancer: a randomised trial of lymphadenectomy in the treatment of endometrial cancer. *Society of Gynecologic Oncologists.*

Kinkel K, Forstner R, Danza FM et al. (2009). Staging of endometrial cancer with MRI: guidelines of the European Society of Urogenital Imaging. *European Radiology,* Vol. 19, No. 7, (July, 2009), pp. 1565–1574.

Konecny GE, Venkatesan N, Yang G et al. (2008). Activity of lapatinib a novel HER2 and EGFR dual kinase inhibitor in human endometrial cancer cells. *British Journal of Cancer*, Vol. 98, No. 6, (March, 2008), 1076-1084.

Konecny GE, Santos L, Winterhoff B et al. (2009). HER2 gene amplification and EGFR expression in a large cohort of surgically staged patients with nonendometrioid (type II) endometrial cancer. *British Journal of Cancer,* 100(1), pp. 89–95.

Kong A, Johnson N, Cornes P et al. (2007). Adjuvant radiotherapy for stage I endometrial cancer. *Cochrane Database Systematic Reviews*, Vol. 18, No.2, (April, 2007), CD003916.

Lee, R. Saunders. (2003). Endometrial Polyp More Likely Cancer If Women Are Bleeding, Women's Health Study. *International Journal of Obesity and Related Metabolic Disorders,* Vol. 27, No. 12, pp. 1447-52, 2003.

Li HL, Zhang HW, Chen DD, Zhong L, Ren XD, St-Tu R. JTE-522, a selective COX-2 inhibitor, inhibits cell proliferation and induces apoptosis in RL95 - 2 cells. (2002). *Acta Pharmacologica Sinica,* Vol. 23, pp.631 - 637.

Lian J, Mackenzie M, Joseph K et al. (2008). Assessment of extended-field radiotherapy for stage IIIC endometrial cancer using three-dimensional conformal radiotherapy, intensity-modulated radiotherapy, and helical tomotherapy. *International Journal of Radiation Oncology, Biology, Physics,* Vol. 70, No.3, (March, 2008), pp.935-943.

Lin F, Zhang QJ, Zheng FY et al. (2008). Laparoscopically assisted versus open surgery for endometrial cancer - a meta-analysis of randomized controlled trials. *International Journal of Gynecological Cancer,* Vol. 18, No.6, (November-December, 2008), pp.1315–1325.

Maggi R, Lissoni A, Spina F et al. (2006). Adjuvant chemotherapy vs radiotherapy in high-risk endometrial carcinoma: results of a randomised trial. *British Journal of Cancer,* Vol. 95, No.3, (August, 2006), pp. 266-271.

Mangili G, De Marzi P, Beatrice S et al. (2006). Paclitaxel and concomitant radiotherapy in high-risk endometrial cancer patients: preliminary findings. *BMC Cancer,* No. 6, 198.

Mariani A, Webb MJ, Keeney GL et al. (2000). Low-risk corpus cancer: islymphadenectomy or radiotherapy necessary? *American Journal of Obstetrics and Gynecology,* Vol. 18, (June, 2000), pp.1506–1519.

Mariani A, Keeney GL, Aletti G, et al. (2004). Endometrial carcinoma: paraaortic dissemination. *Gynecologic Oncology,* Vol.92, No.3, pp. 833-838.

Mariani A, Dowdy SC, Cliby WA et al. (2006). Efficacy of systematic lymphadenectomy and adjuvant radiotherapy in node-positive endometrial cancer patients. *Gynecologic Oncology,* Vol. 101, No. 2, (May, 2006), pp. 200-208.

Mariani A, Dowdy SC, Cliby WA et al. (2008). Prospective assessment of lymphatic dissemination in endometrial cancer: a paradigm shift in surgical staging. *Gynecologic Oncology*, Vol. 109, No.1, (April, 2008), pp. 11-18.

Mazzon, I.; Corrado, J.; Masciullo, D.; Morricone, D.; Fernandina, G. (2010). Conservative surgical management of stage IA endometrial carcinoma for fertility preservation, *Fertility and Sterility*, vol. 93, no. 4, (March, 2010), pp. 1286–1289.

Merisio, C., Berretta, R., de Ioris, A. et al. (2005). Endometrial cancer in patients with preoperative diagnosis of atypical endometrial hyperplasia, *European Journal of Obstetrics Gynecology and Reproductive Biology*, vol. 122, no. 1, (September, 2005), pp. 107–111.

Morice P., Levy-Piedbois C., S. Ajaj et al. (2001). Value and cost evaluation of routine follow-up for patients with clinical stage I/II endometrial cancer, *European Journal of Cancer*, vol. 37, no. 8, pp. 985–990.

Morrow CP, Bundy BN, Kurman RJ, Creasman WT, Heller P, Homesley HD, Graham JE. (1991). Relationship between surgical-pathological risk factors and outcome in clinical stage I and II carcinoma of the endometrium: a gynecologic oncology group study. *Gynecologic Oncology*, Vol. 40, (January, 1991), pp. 55-65.

Morrison C, Zanagnolo V, Ramirez N et al. (2006). HER-2 is an independent prognostic factor in endometrial cancer: association with outcome in a large cohort of surgically staged patients. *Journal of Clinical Oncology*, Vol. 24, No.15, (May, 2006), pp. 2376-2385.

Mundt AJ, McBride R, Rotmensch J, Waggoner SE, Yamada SD, Connell PP. (2001). Significant pelvic recurrence in high-risk pathologic stage I-IV endometrial carcinoma patients after adjuvant chemotherapy alone: implications for adjuvant radiation therapy. *International Journal of Radiation Oncology, Biology, Physics*, Vol. 50, No. 5, (August, 2001), pp.1145-1153.

Nezhat F, Yadav J, Rahaman J, et al. (2008). Analysis of survival after laparoscopic management of endometrial cancer. *Journal of Minim Invasive Gynecology*, Vol. 15, No.2, (March-April, 2008), pp. 181-187.

Nomura H, Aoki D, Suzuki N et al. (2006). Analysis of clinicopathologic factors predicting para-aortic lymph node metastasis in endometrial cancer. *International Journal of Gynecological Cancer*, Vol. 16, No.2, (March-April, 2006), pp. 799–804.

Nout RA, Smit VT, Putter H et al. (2010). Vaginal brachytherapy versus pelvic external beam radiotherapy for patients with endometrial cancer of high-intermediate risk (PORTEC-2): an open-label, non-inferiority, randomised trial. *Lancet*, Vol. 375, (March, 2010), pp. 816–823.

Nunns D, Williamson K, Swaney L, Davy M. (2000). The morbidity of surgery and adjuvant radiotherapy in the management of endometrial carcinoma. *International Journal of Gynecological Cancer*, Vol. 10, No. 3, (May, 2000), pp. 233–238.

Niikura H, Okamura C, Utsunomiya H, et al. (2004). Sentinel lymph node detection in patients with endometrial cancer. *Gynecologic Oncology*, Vol. 92, No. 2, (February, 2004), pp.669-674.

Orr JW, Holiman JL, Orr PF. (1997). Stage I corpus cancer: is teletherapy necessary? *American Journal of Obstetrics and Gynecology*, Vol.176, (April, 1997), pp. 777-89.

Ozbudak IH, Karaveli S, Simsek T, Erdogan G, Pestereli E. (2008). Neoangiogenesis and expression of hypoxia-inducible factor 1α, vascular endothelial growth factor, and glucose transporter-1 in endometrioid type endometrium adenocarcinomas. *Gynecologic Oncology,* Vol. 108, No.3, (March, 2008), pp. 603-608.

Palomba S, Falbo A, Mocciaro R, Russo T, Zullo F. (2009). Laparoscopic treatment for endometrial cancer: a meta-analysis of randomized controlled trials (RCTs). *Gynecologic Oncology,* Vol. 112, No. 2, (February, 2009), pp. 415–421.

Park JY, Kim EN, Kim DY, et al. (2008). Comparison of the validity of magnetic resonance imaging and positron emission tomography/computed tomography in the preoperative evaluation of patients with uterine corpus cancer. *Gynecologic Oncology,* Vol. 108, No. 3, (March, 2008), pp. 486-492.

Park JY, Kim DY, Kim JH, Kim YM, Kim YT, Nam JH. (2010). The role of pelvic and/or para-aortic lymphadenectomy in surgical management of apparently early carcinosarcoma of uterus. *Annals of Surgical Oncology,* Vol. 17, No.3, (March, 2010), pp. 861–868.

Pecorelli S. Revised FIGO staging for carcinoma of the vulva, cervix, and endometrium. (2009), *International Journal of Gynecological Obstetrics,* Vol. 105, No. 2, pp. 103–104.

Picchio M, Mangili G, Samanes Gajate AM et al. (2010). High-grade endometrial cancer: value of [(18)F]FDG PET/CT in preoperative staging. *Nuclear Medicine Communications,* Vol. 31, No.6, (June, 2010), pp. 506–512.

Podratz KC, O'Brien PC, Malkasian GD Jr, Decker DG, Jefferies JA, Edmonson JH. (1985). Effects of progestational agents in treatment of endometrial carcinoma. *Obstetrics and Gynecology,* Vol. 66, (July, 1985), pp.106-110.

Randall T.C. and Kurman, R.J. (1997). Progestin treatment of atypical hyperplasia and well-differentiated carcinoma of the endometrium in women under age 40, *Obstetrics and Gynecology,* Vol. 90, No. 3, (September, 1997), pp. 434–440.

Randall, M.E, Filiaci, V.L., Muss, H.et al. (2006). Randomized phaseIII trial of whole-abdominal irradiation versus doxorubicin and cisplatin chemotherapy in advanced endometrial carcinoma: a gynecologic oncology group study, *Journal of Clinical Oncology,* Vol. 24, No. 1, (January, 2006), pp. 36–44.

Rossi PJ, Jani AB, Horowitz IR, Johnstone PA. (2008). Adjuvant brachytherapy removes survival disadvantage of local disease extension in stage IIIC endometrial cancer: a SEER registry analysis. *International Journal of Radiation Oncology, Biology, Physics,* Vol. 70, No. 1, pp. 134-138.

Salama JK, Mundt AJ, Roeske J, Mehta N. (2006). Preliminary outcome and toxicity report of extended-field, intensity-modulated radiation therapy for gynecologic malignancies. *International Journal of Radiation Oncology, Biology, Physics,* Vol. 65, No. 4, pp. 1170-1176.

Scribner DR Jr, Mannel RS, Walker JL, et al. (1999). Cost analysis of laparoscopy versus laparotomy for early endometrial cancer. *Gynecologic Oncology,* Vol. 75, No.3, (December, 1999), pp. 460-463.

Selman TJ, Mann CH, Zamora J, Khan KS. (2008). A systematic review of tests for lymph node status in primary endometrial cancer. *BMC Womens Health,* Vol. 8, (May, 2008), No. 8.

Sovak MA, Hensley ML, Dupont J et al. (2006). Paclitaxel and carboplatin in the adjuvant treatment of patients with high-risk stage III and IV endometrial cancer: a retrospective study. *Gynecologic Oncology,* Vol. 103, No.2, (November, 2006), pp. 451-457.

Secord AA, Havrilesky LJ, Carney ME et al. (2007). Weekly low-dose paclitaxel and carboplatin in the treatment of advanced or recurrent cervical and endometrial cancer. *International Journal of Clinical Oncology,* Vol. 12, No.1, (February, 2007), pp. 31-36.

Sears JD, Greven KM, Hoen HM, Randall ME. (1994). Prognostic factors and treatment outcome for patients with locally recurrent endometrial cancer. *Cancer,* Vol. 74, (August, 1994), pp. 1303-1308.

Signorelli M, Guerra L, Buda A et al. (2009). Role of the integrated FDG PET/CT in the surgical management of patients with high risk clinical early stage endometrial cancer: detection of pelvic nodal metastases. *Gynecologic Oncology,* Vol. 115, No.2, (November, 2009), pp.231–235.

Soliman PT, Frumovitz M, Spannuth W et al. (2010). Lymphadenectomy during endometrial cancer staging: practice patterns among gynecologic oncologists. *Gynecologic Oncology,* Vol. 119, No. 2, (November, 2010), pp. 291–294.

Susumu N, Sagae S, Udagawa Y et al. (2008). Randomized Phase III trial of pelvic radiotherapy versus cisplatin-based combined chemotherapy in patients with intermediate- and high-risk endometrial cancer: a Japanese Gynecologic Oncology Group study. *Gynecologic Oncology,* Vol. 108, No. 1, (January, 2008), pp. 226-233.

Soslow, R.A., Bissonnette, J.P., Wilton,A. et al. (2007). Clinicopathologic analysis of 187 high-grade endometrial carcinomas of different histologic subtypes: similar outcomes belie distinctive biologic differences, *American Journal of Surgical Pathology,* vol. 31, no. 7, (July, 2007), pp. 979–987.

Suh DS, Kim JK, Kim KR et al. (2009). Reliability of magnetic resonance imaging in assessing myometrial invasion absence in endometrial carcinoma. *Acta Obstetrica Gynecologica Scandinavica,* Vol. 88, No.9, pp. 990–993.

Tanaka H, Sato H, Miura H, et al. (2006). Can we omit para-aorta lymph node dissection in endometrial cancer? *Japanese Journal of Clinical Oncology,* 2006, Vol. 36, No.9, (July, 2006), pp. 578-581.

Thigpen JT, Brady MF, Homesley HD et al. (2004). Phase III trial of doxorubicin with or without cisplatin in advanced endometrial carcinoma: a gynecologic oncology group study. *Journal of Clinical Oncology,* Vol. 22, No.19, pp. 3902-3908.

Thigpen JT, Blessing JA, DiSaia PJ, Yordan E, Carson LF, Evers C. (1994). A randomized comparison of doxorubicin alone versus doxorubicin plus cyclophosphamide in the management of advanced or recurrent endometrial carcinoma: a Gynecologic Oncology Group study. *Journal of Clinical Oncology,* Vol. 12, No. 7, (July, 1994), pp. 1408-1414.

Todo Y, Kato H, Kaneuchi M, Watari H, Takeda M, Sakuragi N. (2010). Survival effect of para-aortic lymphadenectomy in endometrial cancer (SEPAL study): a retrospective cohort analysis. *Lancet,* Vol. 375, No. 9721, (April, 2010), pp. 1165–1172.

Trimble, C.L.; Kauderer, J.; Zaino, R. et al. (2006). Concurrent endometrial carcinoma in women with a biopsy diagnosis of atypical endometrial hyperplasia: a gynecologic oncology group study, *Cancer,* vol. 106, no. 4, (February, 2006), pp. 812–819.

Trimble EL, Kosary C, Park RC. (1998). Lymph node sampling and survival in endometrial cancer. *Gynecologic Oncology,* Vol. 71, No.3, (December, 1998), pp. 340-343.

Walker J, Piedmonte M, Spirtos N et al. (2009). Recurrence and survival after randomization to laparoscopy versus laparotomy for comprehensive surgical staging of uterine cancer (Gynecologic Oncology Group LAP2). *Gynecologic Oncology,* Vol. 117, No.2, (November, 2009), 393-393.

Villella JA, Cohen S, Smith DH, Hibshoosh H, Hershman D. (2006). HER-2/neu overexpression in uterine papillary serous cancers and its possible therapeutic implications. *International Journal of Gynecological Cancer* 16(5), 1897-1902.

Wright JD, Powell MA, Rader JS, Mutch DG, Gibb RK. (2007). Bevacizumab therapy in patients with recurrent uterine neoplasms. Anticancer Research 27(5B), (September-October, 2007), pp. 3525-3528.

Zerbe MJ, Bristow R, Grumbine FC, et al. (2000). Inability of preoperative computed tomography scans to accurately predict the extent of myometrial invasion and extracorporal spread in endometrial cancer. *Gynecologic Oncology,* Vol. 78, No.1, (July, 2000), pp.67-70.

Zivanovic O, Carter J, Kauff ND, Barakat RR. (2009). A review of the challenges faced in the conservative treatment of young women with endometrial carcinoma and risk of ovarian cancer. *Gynecologic Oncology,* Vol. 115, No. 3, (December, 2009), pp. 504-509.

Zhang Y,Wang J, Controversies in theManagement of Endometrial Carcinoma Obstetrics and Gynecology International Volume 2010, Article ID 862908, 16 pages, doi:10.1155/2010/862908.

19

Reducing False Positives in a Computer-Aided Diagnosis Scheme for Detecting Breast Microcalcificacions: A Quantitative Study with Generalized Additive Models

Javier Roca-Pardiñas[1], María J. Lado[1], Pablo G. Tahoces[2] and Carmen Cadarso Suárez[2]
[1]*University of Vigo*
[2]*University of Santiago de Compostela*
Spain

1. Introduction

Breast cancer continues to be one of the most usual cancers in the world (Siegel et al., 2011). The primary signs that indicate the presence of breast cancer are masses and microcalcifications. Masses can be defined as three-dimensional structures demonstrating convex outward borders, usually evident on two orthogonal views. Microcalcifications are relevant radiologic signs of irregular shape, varying size, and located in an inhomogeneous background of parenchymal tissues. While individual microcalcifications are not, in most cases, clinically significant, clustered microcalcifications appear in 30%-50% of breast cancers (Murphy & DeSchryver, 1978). Moreover, the distribution of the calcification should be specified as grouped, linear, segmental, regional, or diffuse.

It has been demonstrated that an early diagnosis of breast cancer can dramatically reduce the mortality rates. Mammography continues to be the most effective technique for an early detection of the disease, and it is recommended every 1-2 year for women aged between 40-50 years old, and every year for women over 50 years of age. Furthermore, mammography screening should not only be based on age and family history of breast cancer, but also on breast density, among other factors (Schousboe et al., 2011). In fact, mammographic sensitivity for breast cancer can significantly decrease with increasing breast density (Mandelson et al., 2000).

It also deserves comment that radiologists do not detect all the breast cancers present in the mammograms. In fact, the cancers missed at mammographic screening can be categorized into different groups, such as screening errors; minimal sign present; radiographically occult; or radiographically occult at diagnosis (Van Dijck et al., 1993). To minimize the percentage of missed cancers, an independent double reading of mammograms can be an interesting option for increasing the number of breast cancers that are detected at screening mammography (Duijm et al., 2007).

In the last decades, digital mammography has emerged as a promising technique that offers the possibility of a second-opinion consultation, or computer-aided detection (CAD) schemes to assist radiologists in the detection of radiological features that could point to those different pathologies (Banik et al., 2011; Hupse & Karssemeijer, 2009 ; Lado et al., 2001).

Nowadays, utility of CAD systems has been already demonstrated, and there are several computerized systems dedicated to detection and diagnosis tasks approved by the Food and Drug Administration (FDA), such as Second Look (CADx Medical Systems, Inc) (approved in 2002), MammoReader (Intelligent Systems Software, Inc) (approved in 2002), or the Kodak Mammography CAD Engine (Eastman Kodak Company) (approved in 2004).

It is clear that, in order to automatically detect lesions, it could be very useful to learn from the radiologists' experience, as well as to quantify the different image features employed by the clinicians to perform their diagnosis. Even although a computer system will never reach the specialists knowledge level, its ability to detect and classify abnormalities can be improved analyzing the existing differences between the human observer and the computer (Kuprinski & Nishikawa, 1997). It becomes necessary to understand both the medical image contents and the process developed by radiologists for analyzing the information. Given the difficult task of interpreting mammograms by radiologists, the CAD mammographic systems are addressed to limited goals, such as the detection and classification of masses and microcalcifications.

It must be indicated that CAD systems, dedicated to detect abnormalities not only in the breast but also in other medical fields (Doi, 2007), produce suspicious areas that should be identified as lesions or false detections, in order to avoid confusing the clinicians when analyzing the areas detected by the computer. Because of this, a significant stage in nearly all the CAD schemes consists in reducing the number of false positives, by the application of different algorithms and diverse statistical methods(Lado et al., 2006; Tourassi et al., 2005).

There are several models, usually employed by the CAD systems in any field to reduce false detections, such as linear discriminant analysis (LDA) (Yoshida et al., 2002), neural networks (Park et al., 2011), or generalized additive models (GAMs) (Lado et al., 2006). However, reduction of false positives can be a difficult task if an inadequate method or algorithm is selected, this leading to incorrect results, by rejecting correct detections while keeping false positives. Because of this, researchers should pay much attention to the reduction of false positives step.

One of the most important aspects to be considered when the diagnostic imaging systems are analyzed is the evaluation of their diagnostic performance. To perform this task, receiver operating characteristic (ROC) curves are the method usually selected, since they indicate the trade-off between sensitivity and specificity, available from a diagnostic system describing the inherent discrimination capability of these systems (Metz, 1986).

The method of ROC curves can be generalized for the diagnostic performance of both the human observers and the CAD systems. In fact, a large amount of automated systems dedicated to the early detection and diagnosis cancer are frequently evaluated employing ROC methodology, not only in the field of breast lesions (Obuchowski, 2005), but also in nearly any type of cancer or disease (Keotan et al., 2002; Li et al., 2005).

In previous works (Lado et al., 2006; 2008) GAMs were applied to the reduction of false positives in CAD systems dedicated to the detection of microcalcifications. In the first work (Lado et al., 2006), the main goal was to overcome the limitations imposed by LDA in the type of variable participating in the reduction of false positives. To perform this task, nonlinear classifiers were used, and the methodology was evaluated employing empirical ROC. Results yielded an improvement in sensitivity close to 3%, while the average number of false positive detections was reduced in 0.5 per image.

One of the limitations present in this previous work was that no factors were used in the study. Factors can be defined as categorical variables, such as, for example, type of breast tissue (fatty or dense), than can clearly affect the diagnosis of clusters of microcalcifications, as stated before (Mandelson et al., 2000), and should be taken in consideration, because the response of a continuous covariate may vary across groups defined by levels of a given factor. This indicates that the continuous covariates can behave different in absence/presence of several factors, this producing the corresponding factor-by-curve effects.

To overcome the limitations imposed by the absence of factors in GAMs, the second work (Lado et al., 2008) introduced in the analysis factors and their interactions with continuous variables in the reduction step. The results obtained showed an increase in the sensitivity from more than 2%, while the false positive rate was drastically reduced to the half.

In this work, we propose a new approach to reduce false clustered microcalcifications, employing GAMs and GLMs, which is based on the extraction of several features from the detected clusters, corresponding to both fatty and dense mammograms, and the automated study to discover different behaviours and influences among the covariates (microcalfication features) present in the analysis.

The software programs employed to perform the analysis were developed using `R` (`http://www.r-project.org/`), an open source software idiom for statistical computing and graphics, which is being used by an increasing number of researchers. Moreover, the R language is distributed under the GNU project, and can run on a wide variety of UNIX, Windows and MacOSX platforms. It is mainly characterized by its core functionality and its high extensibility via the packages, which can be easily downloaded and installed from the CRAN family of Internet sites.

Results show an increase of the sensitivity of the automated system, this leading to a better diagnosis of the disease, not confusing the radiologists by indicating normal areas as suspicious regions, thus reducing the number of biopsies to be performed.

The paper is organized as follows: Section 1 gives a detailed introduction about the breast cancer problem, the automated detection employing CAD systems, and the limitations in detection derived from the use of several features, as well as several solutions and methods employed to perform this task; Section 2 gives an overview about the GLMs and GAMs and the interactions among variables; Section 3 presents the database employed, as well as the CAD system developed for detecting microcalcifications. The database of selected features and the study employing GAMS are presented in Section 4. Section 5 shows and discusses the results obtained. Finally, Section 6 provides the main conclusions of the work. An Appendix also presents the source code developed in `R` language for performing the GAM analysis.

2. Generalized additive models

In this work, we are interested in predicting the presence or absence of a lesion, using a regression model for binary response. Explicitly, let Y be a binary (0/1) response variable, and $\mathbf{X} = (X_1, \ldots, X_q)$ the q-vector of the associated continuous covariates. In this framework, denoting by $p(\mathbf{X}) = p(Y = 1|\mathbf{X})$, the logistic generalized linear models (GLM) (McCullagh & Nelder, 1989) takes the form:

$$p(\mathbf{X}) = p(Y = 1|\mathbf{X}) = \frac{\exp\left(a_0 + a_1 \cdot X_1 + \ldots + a_q \cdot X_q\right)}{1 + \exp\left(a + a_1 \cdot X_1 + \ldots + a_q \cdot X_q\right)} \quad (1)$$

where $(a_0, a_1, \ldots, a_q)$ is a vector of coefficients. In some instances, GLMs can be very restrictive, since they assume linearity in the covariates. This constraint can be avoided by replacing the linear index $\eta = a_0 + a_1 \cdot X_1 + \ldots + a_q \cdot X_q$ with a non-parametric structure. Accordingly, here we shall concentrate on the generalized additive model (GAM) (Hastie & Tibshirani, 1990), which is a generalization of the GLM, by introducing one-dimensional, non-parametric functions instead of linear components. Specifically, GAMs express the conditional mean

$$p(\mathbf{X}) = p(Y = 1|\mathbf{X}) = \frac{\exp\left(a + f_1(X_1) + \ldots + f_p(X_q)\right)}{1 + \exp\left(a + f_1(X_1) + \ldots + f_p(X_q)\right)} \quad (2)$$

where a is a constant and f_j is the unknown smooth partial function or effect curve associated to each continuous covariate X_j. Note that identification is guaranteed by introducing a constant a into the model and requiring a zero mean for the partial functions. The GAM is widely used as an extension of the traditional GLMs (McCullagh & Nelder, 1989) specially when continuous covariates are present. The GAM is more flexible than the GLM, since the researcher does not assume a parametric form for the effects of the continuous covariates, but only assumes that these effects may be represented by arbitrary unknown smooth functions. The GAMs are easy to interpret, because the additive components simply describe the influence of each covariate separately. Several contributions to GAMs can be found in the literature. Hastie and Tibshirani discussed various approaches using smoothing splines (Hastie & Tibshirani, 1990). Wood introduced a numerical procedure based on regression splines (Wood, 2006). Nowadays, there exists standard software, such as the `mgcv` package in `R`, to fit this model.

A generalization of the "pure" GAM in (2) is the GAM with "factor-by-curve" interactions. In this type of model, the relationship between Y and each of the continuous covariates X_j may vary among the subsets defined by the levels $1, \ldots, L$ of a categorical covariate Z (called factor). Explicitly, in the the factor-by-curve logistic GAM the effect of each covariate X_j can be expressed as

$$f_j(Z, x) = \begin{cases} f_j^1(x) \text{ if } Z = 1 \\ \vdots \\ f_j^M(x) \text{ if } Z = M \end{cases}$$

In this way, the effect of each continuous covariate X_j is descomposed in the effects f_j^l associated to each level l $(1, \ldots, L)$ of the factor Z .

3. Database and CAD system

3.1 Mammogram selection

The mammogram database was constituted by 174, mammograms containing 77 clusters of microcalcifications, proven by biopsy, each mammogram having no more than one cluster.

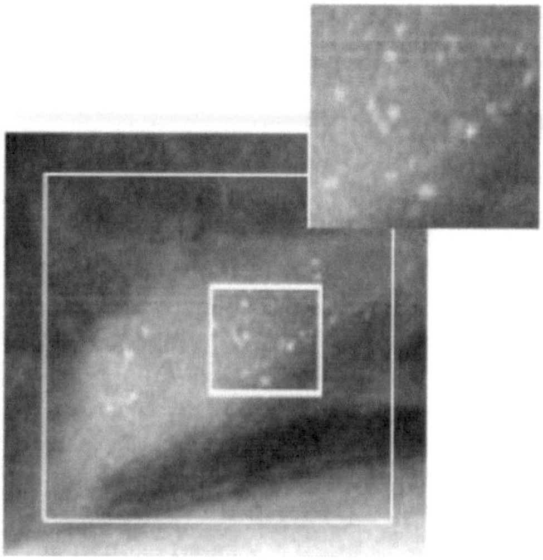

Fig. 1. Region of a mammogram containing a cluster of microcalcifications, delimited by the white square, and a zoomed window containing some microcalcifications

The cases were randomly selected from the mammographic screening program, currently underway, from 1992, at the Galicia Community (Spain). This program is integrated in the European Network of Reference Centers for Breast Cancer Screening.

The average radiation dose employed for the craniocaudal projections was 1.26 mGy, and 1.49 mGy for mediolateral oblique projection. The radiological classification criteria followed the guidelines stated by the Breast Imaging Reporting and Data System (BI-RADS), which establishes the following groups: a) category 0: need additional imaging evaluation; b) category 1: negative; c) category 2: benign finding, noncancerous; d) category 3: probably benign finding, short-interval follow-up suggested; e) category 4: suspicious abnormality, biopsy considered; f) category 5: highly suggestive of malignancy, appropriate action needed.

All the images were digitized at a resolution of 2000x2500 pixels and 4096 gray levels employing a Lumiscan 85 laser scanner (Lumysis Inc., Sunnyvale, CA).

Two experienced radiologists, by consensus, categorized the mammograms into two groups, according to the breast tissue, resulting in 118 dense mammograms, the rest (56) being classified as fatty mammograms. Theses two experts also marked the location of each cluster of microcalcification in the digital images, being this marks stored on truth data files, in terms of x and y directions. These data truth archives were used to compare the experimental results, obtained with the use of the computerized system to detect microcalcifications, with the true position of the clusters. Figure 1 shows a region of a mammogram containing clustered microcalcifications.

3.2 CAD system

To detect the clusters of microcalcifications, a CAD system was developed and extensively described elsewhere (Lado et al., 2001). Briefly, the method is a five-step process that includes (Figure 2): a) detection of the breast border, employing a tracking algorithm that computes the gradient of gray levels; b) application of wavelet transform to enhance

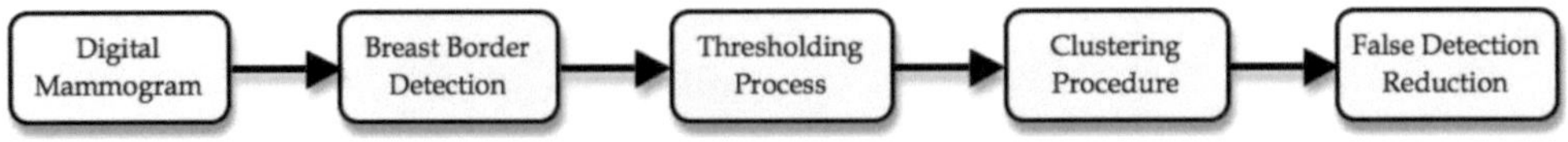

Fig. 2. Scheme of the CAD system for detecting microcalcifications

microcalcifications, by dividing each mammogram into vertical lines, and applying wavelet transform to each lines. As a result, and after applying a local thresold to the wavelet image, a binary image containing the possible seed (origin) points of microcalcifications was obtained; c) gray level thresholding to extract the possible microcalcifications, and application of contrast-size test and morphologic operators, including a region growing algorithm "to grow" the microcalcifications from the corresponding seed points; d) clustering procedure to group the microcalcifications, following the criteria given by Kopans (Kopans, 1989), that considers a cluster of microcalcifications as five or more signals within a region of 1 cm2 of area; and 5) reduction of false positives, employing different techniques.

4. Feature extraction and GAM study

When the CAD system previously described was applied over the complete dataset of fatty and dense mammograms, 72 true positives (TPs) were detected, but the system yielded 740 false detections or positives (FP). This means a sensitivity of 93.5% (72/77) at a false positive rate of 4.25 FPs/image.

At this moment, even although the sensitivity produced by the automated system is really promising, it is needed to understand the importante of maintaining a reduced number of false detections, in order to not confuse the radiologist by suggesting normal areas as suspicious, and to reduce the number of biopsies to be performed. Our system arosed a high number (4.25) of false detections per image. Beacuse of this, a FP reduction step becomes necessary and fundamental.

To reduce false detections, various features of the detected clusters (true and false positives) were extracted:

1. avglbreast (X1): average gray level value of the breast image containing the detected region, ranging from 0 to 4095 (mean value of 2765.08±275.97).
2. avglROI (X2): average gray level value of the region of interest (ROI) containing the detected region, ranging from 0 to 4095 (mean value of 2976.70±359.61).
3. avglcluster (X3): average gray level value of the pixels belonging to the detected microcalcifications, ranging from 0 to 4095 (mean value of 3080.32±340.91).
4. avgldist (X4): average distance among the detected microcalcifications in each cluster, measured in pixels (mean value of 74.69±34.63).
5. dimx and dimy (X5 and X6): x and y dimensions of the ROI containing the detected cluster (mean values of 85.25ś70.76 and 82.91±69.48, respectively).
6. size (X7): size of each detected cluster, in pixels (mean value of 10356.02±24558.54).
7. size/avgldist (X8): relationship between the size and the mean distance among microcalcifications for a cluster mean value of 99.26±133.51).
8. size/avglcluster (X9): relationship between the size and the distribution of gray level values of a cluster (mean size of 3.34±7.56).

9. dif1 (X10): difference in gray level values between the average gray level value of the cluster, avglcluster, and the average gray level value of the ROI, avglROI (mean size of 103.63±73.16).
10. dif2 (X11): difference in gray level values between the average gray level value of the cluster, avglcluster, and the average gray level value of the breast image, avglbreast (mean size of 315.25±300.00).

The response of the model was the binary variable `true` (0/1): a value of 0 indicates that the detected cluster is a false positive. If true equals 1, the detected cluster corresponds to a real cluster, and it is a correct detection.

The analysis of the previous feature values was performed employing GAMs, and considering as the factor added to the model the breast tissue (BT), corresponding either to dense tissue (d) or to fatty tissue (f), as previously classified by the radiologists. Explicity we have considered the following GAM:

$$p(BT,\mathbf{X}) = p(\text{true} = 1|\mathbf{X}) = \frac{\exp\left(a + f_1(BT,X_1) + \ldots + f_{11}(BT,X_{11})\right)}{1 + \exp\left(a + f_1(BT,X_1) + \ldots + f_{11}(BT,X_{11})\right)} \tag{3}$$

with $f_j(BT,x) = f_j^d(x)$ for dense tissue and $f_j(BT,x) = f_j^f(x)$ for fatty tissue.

As stated before, the present work was an attempt to improve the sensitivity of our computerized system by trying the discriminatory capability of different subsets of covariates. A question that tends to arise in regression models of type (3) is that of determining the best subset or subsets of q ($q < 11$) predictors, which will establish the model or models with the best discrimination capacity. As a general rule, as an increasing number of variables are added to the model, the "apparent" fit of the observed data will be improved. However, these estimates are not always satisfied, due to various reasons. On the one hand, inclusion of irrelevant variables would increase the variance of the estimates, thereby amounting to a loss of the predictive capacity of the model; and on the other, inclusion of many variables would mean that the model would be difficult to interpret.

To choose the model, we have used an automatic fordward stepwise selection procedure. This procedure selects the model containing the best subset of q variables that would provide the best discrimination capacity, and eliminates the remainder from the model, according to an optimal criterion based on the use of the ROC curve. The area under the ROC curve (AUC) is one of the most widely used criteria for comparing the performance of a series of binary response regression models. The ROC curve relies on false/true-positive/negative tests, where sensitivity is the proportion of event responses that were predicted to be events and specificity is the proportion of non- event responses that were predicted to be non-events. The plot of sensitivity (i.e., hit rate) versus 1-specificity (i.e., false alarm rate) is the ROC curve; the area under this curve measures the accuracy of the detection system and does not require any assumptions concerning either the shape or form of the underlying signal and noise distributions (Saveland & Neuenschwander, 1990). This statistic is a threshold-independent measure of model discrimination, where 0.5 suggests no discrimination, 0.7-0.8 suggests acceptable discrimination, and 0.8-0.9 suggests excellent discrimination (Hosmer & Lemeshow, 2000).

To obtain the corresponding AUCs for various and different covariate subsets, the models (3) were trained on half of the outputs of the detection scheme, which resulted in 36 true positives and 370 false detections, corresponding to 90 mammograms. The cases employed for training the technique were randomly extracted from the total number of outputs of the CAD scheme. The models were finally tested on the other half of the cases: 36 true positives and 370 false positives (84 mammograms) that had not been used at the initial training stage. The performances of the developed GAMs and GLMs, with the different feature values, were analyzed employing ROC analysis, and considering as the decision variable the estimated probabilities obtained with the models.

To obtain the corresponding AUCs for various and different covariate subsets, the models (3) were trained on half of the outputs of the detection scheme, randomly extracted from the total number of outputs of the CAD system. The models were finally tested on the other half of the cases that had not been used at the initial training stage. The performances of the developed GAMs and GLMs, with the different feature values, were analyzed employing ROC analysis, and considering as the decision variable the estimated probabilities obtained with the models.

5. Results and discussion

This research work aimed at studying how the different features extracted from true and false positive clusters of microcalcifications behave in presence of categorical covariates and factors that can influence and even condition their behaviour. The main goal is, in this way, to discriminate between true clusters and false detections.

The interactions among the different variables were considered in the study. Previously to the selection of variables, correlation among the different covariates was calculated in Table (1).

	X1	X2	X3	X4	X5	X6	X7	X8	X9	X10	X11
X1	100	56	54	-1	-3	-4	-21	-30	-1	-4	-4
X2	56	100	98	-2	0	-2	-35	60	2	1	-3
X3	54	98	100	1	4	4	-16	64	6	6	2
X4	-1	-2	1	100	74	75	19	3	65	64	66
X5	-3	0	4	74	100	67	20	7	82	88	83
X6	-4	-2	4	75	67	100	25	8	83	86	84
X7	-21	-35	-16	19	20	25	100	1	22	25	23
X8	-30	60	64	3	7	8	1	100	9	10	6
X9	-1	2	6	65	82	83	22	9	100.	93	100
X10	-4	1	6	64	88	86	25	10	93	100	94
X11	-4	-3	2	66	83	84	23	6	100	94	100

Table 1. Matrix correlations($\times 100$) between covariates

A high correlation can be observed for several features, particularly between X2 and X3, or among X9, X10 and X11. Surely, this is due to the fact that these variables can be very similar. For example, X2 and X3 represent gray level values for the cluster of microcalcifications and the ROI containing it, and both regions may nearly contain the same pixel values, this resulting in a high similarity between them. However, there are other features with a low correlation, for example the properties based on gray level values and the properties based on either distances or sizes.

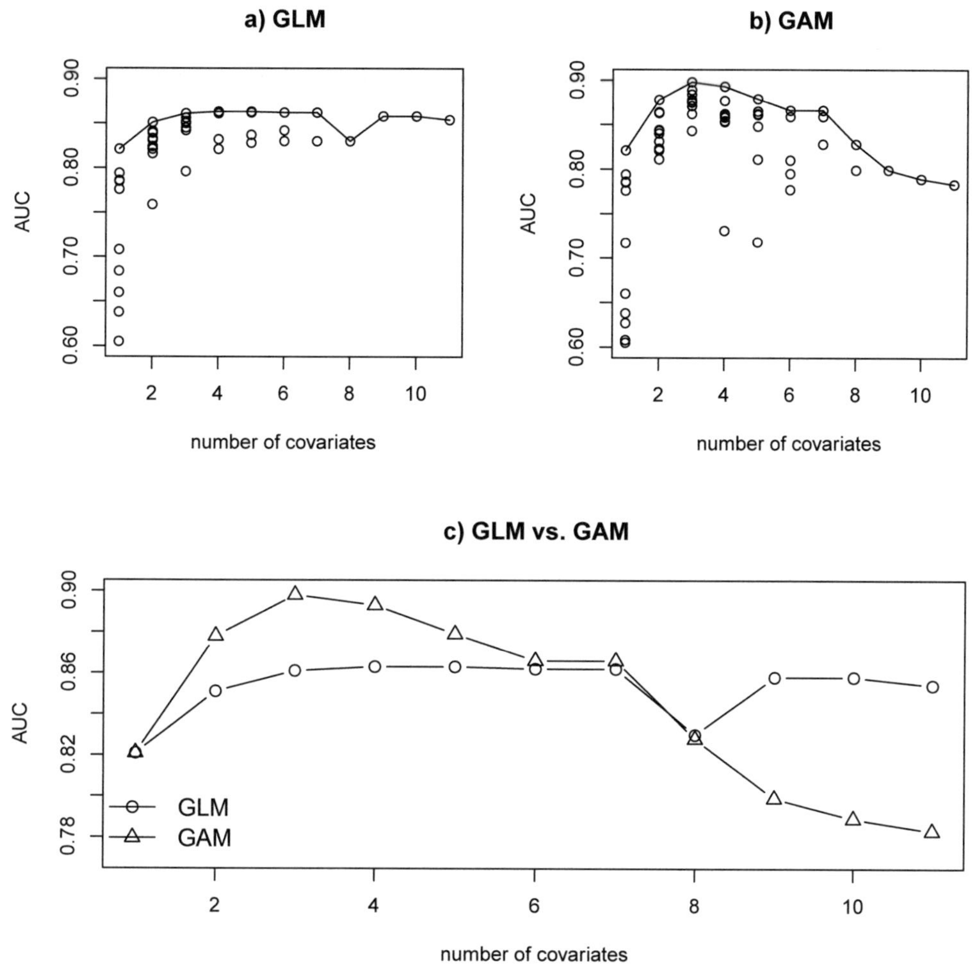

Fig. 3. Possible subset model. For each subset size, the AUC is shown for a) GLM, b) GAM and c) GLM vs. GAM.

When the correlations were calculated, the subset selection for the whole set of covariates was performed, and the corresponding AUCs were obtained for each model. Figure (3) presents the values for all the possible subset model combinations, employing GLMs and GAMs. This figure can be interpreted as follows: The x axis gives the number of covariates included in the statistical model, while the y axis represents the AUC obtained with the model employing the number of covariates indicated by the x value. For example, for a number of covariates equal to 1, a line of vertical points corresponding to different AUC values is represented, the first of them with a value close to 0.60 in both the GLM and the GAM. The last value obtained is greater than 0.80 in both models. All of them correspond to the AUC values obtained with one different covariate between X_1 and X_{11}. The intermediate values are the AUCs yielded by the models constructed employing the rest of covariates.

From Figure (3), it can be observed that, if only one covariate is considered, the best AUC obtained in the GLM is lower than in the rest of cases; however, the AUC is very similar when selecting 2 or more covariates.

When applying the GAM the situation is different, providing the best results for the AUC values when three covariates are considered. Finally, the comparison of the best models for both GLM and GAM indicates that GAM performs better when a number up to 8 covariates are considered. If this number increases, best results are provided by GLMs. Table (2) lists the AUC values obtained for both types of models with different number of covariates.

From Table (2), it can be observed that for both the linear and the additive models, if we only consider one variable in the model, best results were obtained for X10, that is, for the difference in gray level values between the average gray level value of the cluster avglcluster, and the average gray level value of the ROI, avglROI.

	GLM		GAM	
q	variables	AUC	variables	AUC
1	10	82.10	10	82.10
2	8	85.10	1	87.80
3	4	86.10	11	89.80
4	2	86.30	8	89.30
5	3	86.30	9	87.90
6	1	86.20	3	86.60
7	5	86.20	4	86.60
8	6	83.00	2	82.80
9	7	85.80	5	79.90
10	9	85.80	6	78.90
11	11	85.40	7	78.30

Table 2. AUC values for the different models and number of covariates in each subset.

As an increasing number of variables are included in the study, that is, as different covariates were considered in both models, greater values for AUCs were obtained; particularly, better results were achieved for GAMs when a number up to 8 covariates were included in the model, and better results were obtained for GLMs for 9 or more variables considered. In the previous models, no distinction was considered for the type of tissue, and a unique analysis was performed for both GLM and GAM. However, to study the effect of the previous models in the breast tissue, different analyses were performed for clusters of microcalcifica- tions embedded on both fatty and dense tissue. Different subset combinations were again obtained for both GLMs and GAMs, and the corresponding AUCs were calculated (Tables (3,4). From these tables, it can be observed that best AUCs are obtained for fatty tissue, while for dense parenchyma are always lower in the corresponding models. This is consistent with the fact that, for fatty tissue, the contrast value, that is, the difference between the microcalcification and the background surrounding it, is greater than for dense tissue. Thus, detection is

	fatty		dense	
q	variables	AUC	variables	AUC
1	10	79.20	8	73.60
2	3	86.40	7	74.50
3	11	86.70	1	74.90
4	4	87.00	2	74.90
5	2	86.40	3	74.90
6	5	86.40	4	74.90
7	6	85.80	11	72.30
8	7	85.70	5	72.10
9	8	85.70	6	69.90
10	1	85.60	9	73.60
11	9	85.60	10	74.90

Table 3. AUC values for the different GLMs and number of covariates in each subset, for both fatty and dense breast tissue

	fatty		dense	
q	variables	AUC	variables	AUC
1	10	79.20	1	79.00
2	3	86.10	11	84.40
3	5	86.90	5	85.10
4	11	85.30	6	86.80
5	1	81.80	7	86.60
6	9	87.90	3	87.00
7	2	81.20	9	87.70
8	4	80.10	10	87.00
9	6	69.10	2	66.70
10	7	87.00	4	64.10
11	8	62.60	8	70.50

Table 4. AUC values for the different GAMs and number of covariates in each subset, for both fatty and dense breast tissue

improved even for radiologists. The dense parenchyma always presents greater difficulties to peform a correct diagnosis.

Appart from this, we can also perceive that, when one covariate is included in the model, best results are obtained by X10 again; however, if more variables are present, selection is not the same in both GLM and GAMs, and it does not match the selection performed when the tissue type was not separately considered. Moreover, for fatty tissue GLM performs better, while, by contrary, for dense breasts the optimal results are obtained when employing GLMs to select covariates.

Figure (4) shows the AUC values for the best subset model combinations, employing GLMs and GAMs, for both fatty and dense tissue. Figure 5 represents the AUCs for the global analysis, and for both fatty and dense tissue, for the best GLM and GAM.

It can be observed that, for GLM, results obtained for fatty tissue are higher than those obtained for dense tissue. However, when employing the GAM, differences are lower, and a more reduced number of covariates have to be included in the study.

Sensitivity and false positive rates were also calculated for the best GLM and the best GAM. For linear models, results yielded a sensitivity of 88.31%, at a false positive rate of 3.7 FPs per image. For the same sensitivity, the false positive fraction achieved when reducing false

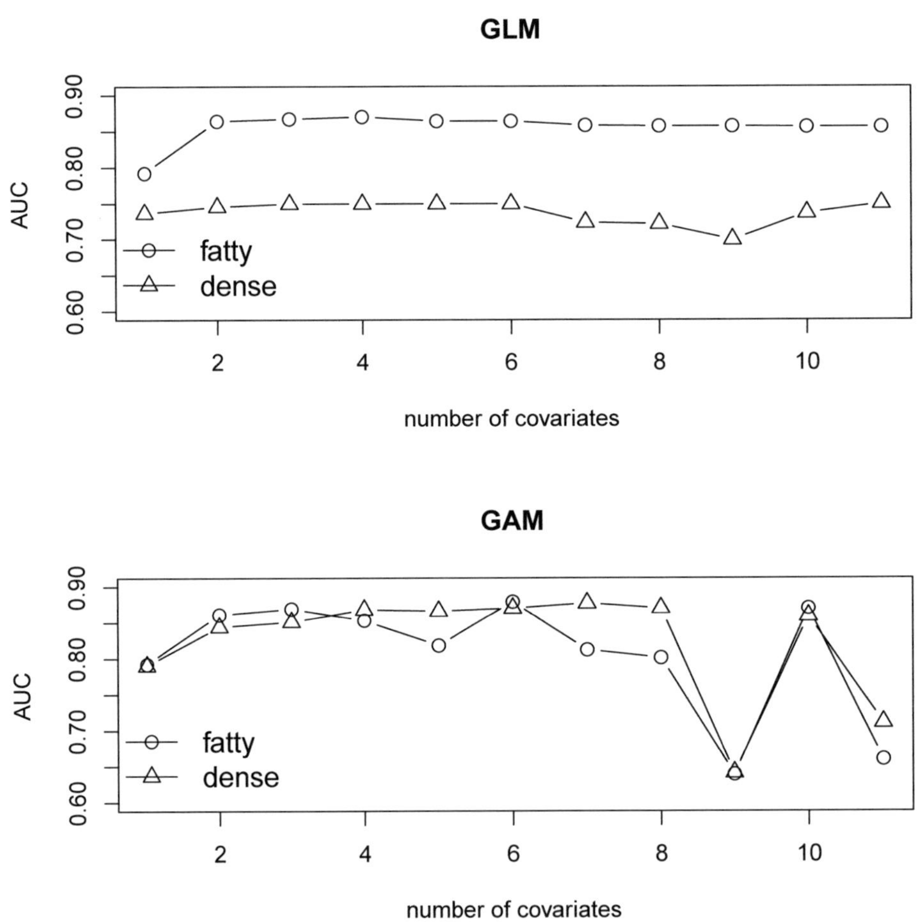

Fig. 4. "Optimal" models for both fatty and dense tissue. For each subset size, the AUC is shown for each model.

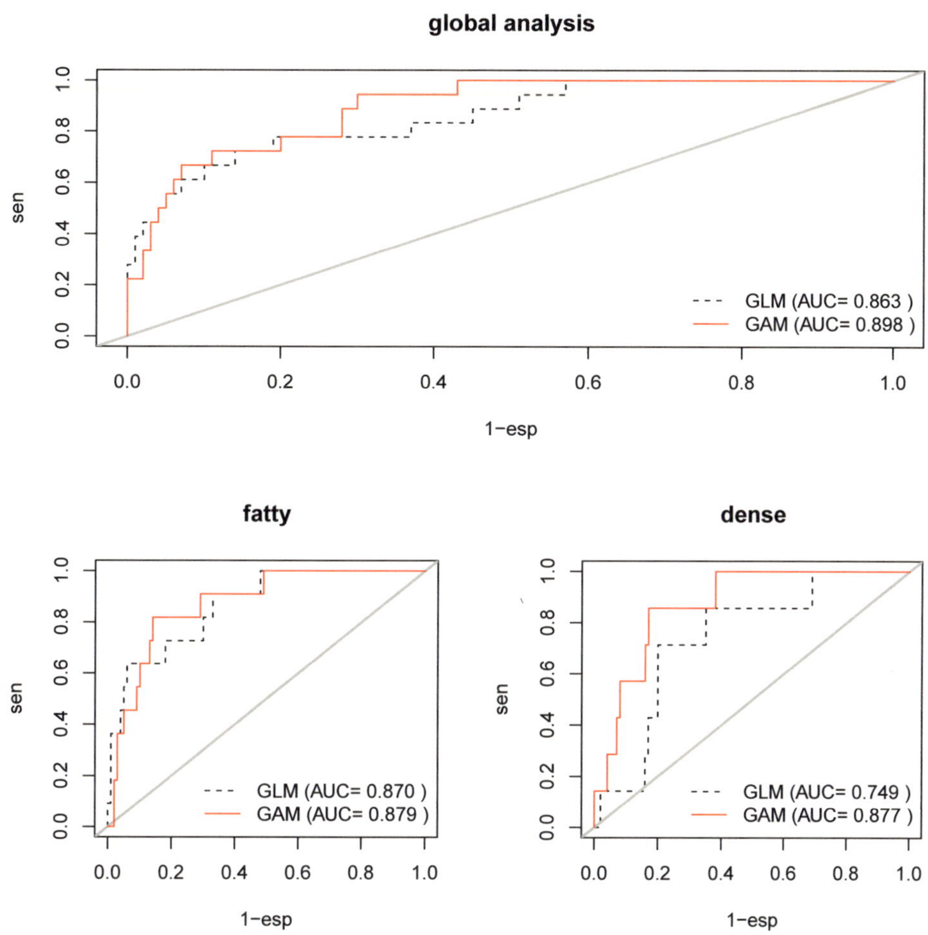

Fig. 5. ROC curves obtained for the GAM and GLM, for the global analysis, and for both types of breast tissue

positives with additive models was 2.7, this demonstrating the benefits of this type of models for discriminating tasks, employing factors and interactions.

6. Conclusion

In this work, GLMs and GAMs were applied to the reduction of false positives yielded by a CAD system devoted to the detection of clusters of microcalcifications. Results indicate that not all the features extracted from the detected clusters are useful for the discrimination between true and false detections: Moreover, there are features that are relevant when the different type of tissue is considered, and their influence is different depending on the breast parenchyma.

After the reduction of false positives, the system is capable of discriminating and detecting clustered microcalcifications from digital mammograms, this suggesting that this CAD scheme is competent to complement the radiologists' efforts in their daily clinical practice, to help them as second readers in the interpretation of mammograms, and also to improve their diagnostic performance.

Future work will address the issue of reducing the number of false positives, without decreasing the sensitivity, by applying different statistical models to our dataset. Another way to improve the results yielded by the CAD system would be to deal with a higher quality of the digital images, because subtle clusters can be more easily identified in the detection process if the image is digitized at a greater resolution. Thus, to further improve the sensitivity, high quality of the digitized images is required.

7. Acknowledgment

This work has been partially supported by Ministerio de Ciencia e Innovación, MTM2008-01603/MTM. Roca-Pardiñas' research was supported by grant MTM2008-03010 from the Spanish Ministry of Education & Science, and by grants PGIDIT07PXIB300191PR and PGIDIT10PXIB300068 PR from the Galician Regional Authority (Xunta de Galicia).

8. Appendix. Source code developed in R

The `R` code developed for calculating probability values for the GLMs and GAMs, as well as for obtaining the corresponding AUCs and plots is now given and explained. The starting point of this routines considers data covariates stored on the **X** covariates, while Y indicates if the data corresponds either to a true detection ($Y = 1$) or to a false positive cluster ($Y = 0$). The factor considered in the study is $F = 0$ for fatty tissue, and $F = 1$ for dense tissue.

The steps followed in the present work were the calculation of the correlation values, and the study of covariates, initially without taking into consideration the type of tissue, calculating in this situation the linear and additive models, employing the functions `stepGLM2` and `stepGAM2` respectively (described in this Appendix), and obtaining for both cases the corresponding areas uner the ROC curve, using the `empiricROC` function. Plots and tables were also obtained.

The same analysis was next calculated, but separating the data by the type of tissue where they were embedded in the breast. Graphs, tables and Auc were also obtained. The `R` code is listed below.

```
##################################################################
# Correlations calculation
cor(X)

##################################################################
# Selection of covariates employing the AUC criterion for the GLMs
# and GAMs

##################################################################
GLMresults=stepGAM(X,Y,"glm"); GAMresults=stepGAM(X,Y)

# Particular studies differentiating the type of tissue
ii<-F==0; X0=X[ii,];Y0=Y[ii]
```

```
ii<-F==1; X1=X[ii,];Y1=Y[ii]
GLM0results=stepGAM(X0,Y0,"glm")
GLM1results=stepGAM(X1,Y1,"glm")
GAM0results=stepGAM(X0,Y0)
GAM1results=stepGAM(X1,Y1)

####################################################################
# Output graphs and tables

# GLMs and GAMs comparison in global study
layout(matrix(c(1,2,3,3), 2, 2, byrow=TRUE))
plot(GLMresults$aucs,xlab="number of covariates",ylab="AUC",
main="GLM",ylim=c(0.6,0.9))
lines(GLMresults$aucopt)

plot(GAMresults$aucs,xlab="number of covariates",ylab="AUC",
main="GAM",ylim=c(0.6,0.9))
lines(GAMresults$aucopt)

plot(GLMresults$aucopt,xlab="number of covariates",ylab="AUC",
ylim=c(0.77,0.90),type='b',pch=1,main="GLM vs. GAM",cex=1.24)
lines(GAMresults$aucopt,type='b',pch=2,cex=1.25)
legend("bottomleft",c("GLM","GAM"),lty=1,pch=c(1,2),
box.lty=0,cex=1.25)

# GLMs and GAMs comparison considering the type of tissue
# GLMs results
par(mfcol=c(2,1))
plot(GLM0results$aucopt,xlab="number of covariates",ylab="AUC",
type='b',pch=1,ylim=c(0.6,0.90),cex=1.25,main="GLM")
lines(GLM1results$aucopt,type='b',pch=2,cex=1.25)
legend("bottomleft",c("fatty","dense"),lty=1,pch=c(2,1),
box.lty=0,cex=1.25)

plot(GAM0results$aucopt,xlab="number of covariates",ylab="AUC",
type='b',pch=1,ylim=c(0.6,0.90),cex=1.25,main="GAM")
lines(GAM1results$aucopt,type='b',pch=2,cex=1.25)
legend("bottomleft",c("fatty","dense"),lty=1,pch=c(2,1),
box.lty=0,cex=1.25)


####################################################################
# Calculation of the GAMs
stepGAM<-function(X,Y,option="gam") {
# X: Covariables matrix
# Y: Response vector
n=dim(X)[1]
nvar=dim(X)[2]
```

```
variables=1:nvar
auc0=NULL; formula0=NULL; inside=NULL
nvars=NULL;aucs=NULL;ROCs=NULL

test<-seq(1,n,4)
Wtraining=rep(1,n);Wtraining[test]=0
for (ivar in 1:nvar) {
 ii=! (variables %in% inside)
 variables=variables[ii]
 auc=NULL
 for (j in 1:length(variables)) {
  if (option=="gam") {formula=paste("+s(X[,",j,"])",sep="")}
else {formula=paste("+(X[,",j,"])",sep="")}
  formula=paste(formula0,formula,sep="")
  formula=paste("Y~",formula,sep="")
  if (option=="gam") {modelo=gam(as.formula(formula),
   family="binomial",weights=Wtraining)}
else {modelo=glm(as.formula(formula),family="binomial",
  weights=Wtraining)}
  muhat=predict(modelo,type="response")
  a=EmpiricalROC(Y[Wtraining==0],muhat[Wtraining==0])
  aux=a$auc
  nvars=c(nvars,ivar);aucs=c(aucs,aux);auc=c(auc,aux)
  jj=length(a$t)
  ROCs=rbind(ROCs,cbind(rep(ivar,jj),rep(aux,jj),a$t,a$ROC))}
  inside=c(inside,variables[which.max(auc)])
  auc0=c(auc0,max(auc))
  if (option=="gam")  {formula0=paste("s(X[,",inside,"])",
   sep="",collapse="+")}
  else { formula0=paste("(X[,",inside,"])",sep="",collapse="+")}}
return(list(aucs=cbind(nvars,aucs),
aucopt=cbind(1:nvar,auc0),models=inside,roc=ROCs))
}

###################################################################
# Calculation and plotting of the empiric AUCs
EmpiricalROC<-function (group,Y){
YE=Y[ group==1]; YS=Y[ group==0]
t=seq(0,1,0.01); F=quantile(YS,probs=(1-t),type=1)
ROC=1-sapply(F, function(x) mean( YE <= x ))
ROC=as.vector(ROC)

t=c(0,t,1); ROC=c(0,ROC,1)
m<-length(YS);n<-length(YE)
xmat<-matrix(rep(YS,n),nrow=n,byrow=T)
ymat<-matrix(rep(YE,m),nrow=n,byrow=F)
diffmat<-ymat-xmat
auc<-(length(diffmat[diffmat>0])+
```

```
0.5*length(diffmat[diffmat==0]))/(m*n)
auc=round(auc,digits=3)
plot(t,ROC,type='s',col='red',xlab="1-esp",ylab="sen")
abline(a=0,b=1,col='grey')

lines(t,ROC,col='blue',type='s')
text(0.9,0.1,paste("auc=",auc))
result=list(t=t,ROC=ROC,auc=auc)}
```

9. References

Banik, S.; Rangayyan, R.M. & Desautels J.E.L. (2011). Detection of architectural distortion in prior mammograms. *IEEE Transactions on Medical Imaging*, Vol.30, No.2, (February 2011), pp. 279-294, ISSN 0278-0062

Doi, K. (2007). Computer-aided diagnosis in medical imaging: Historical review, current status and future potential. *Computerized Medical Imaging and Graphics*, Vol.31, No.4, (June 2007), pp. 198-211 ISSN 0895-6111.

Duijm, L.E.M.; Groenewoud, J.H.; Fracheboud, J. & de Koning, H.J. (2007). Additional double reading of screening mammograms by radiologic technologists: impact on screening performance parameters. *Journal of the National Cancer Institute*, Vol.99, No.15 (August 2007), pp. 1162-1170, ISSN 1460-2105.

Hastie, T.J. & R. Tibshirani, J. (1990) *Generalized Additive Models*, Chapman & Hall, ISBN 0-412-34390-8, London.

Hosmer, D.W. & Lemeshow, S. (2000) *Applied logistic regression*, John Wiley and Sons, ISBN 0-471-35632-8, New York.

Hupse, R. & Karssemeijer, N. (2009). Use of normal tissue context in computer-aided detection of masses in mammograms. *IEEE Transactions on Medical Imaging*, Vol. 28, No.12, (December 2009), pp. 2033-2041, ISSN 0278-0062

Keogan, M.T.; Lo, J.Y.; Fred, K.S.; Raptopoulos, V.; Blake, S.; Kamel, I.R.; Weisinger, K.; Rosen, M.P. & and Nelson, C.R. (2002). Outcome analysis of patients with acute pancreatitis by using artificial neural network. *Academic Radiology*, Vol. 9, Mo.4, (April 2002), pp. 410-419, ISSN 1076-6332

Kopans, D.B. (1989). *Breast Imaging*, Lippincott, ISBN 9780397507610, Philadelphia.

Krupinski, E.A. & Nishikawa, R.M. (1997). Comparison of eye position versus computer identified microcalcification clusters on mammograms. *Medical Physics*, Vol.24, No.1, (January, 1997) pp. 17-23, ISSN 0094-2405

Lado, M.J.; Tahoces, P.G.; Méndez, A.J.; Souto, M. & Vidal J.J. (2001). Evaluation of an automated wavelet-based system dedicated to the detection of clustered microcalcifications in digital mammograms. *Medical Informatics and the Internet in Medicine*, Vol. 26, No.3, (July 2001), pp. 149-163, ISSN 1463-9238

Lado, M.J.; Cadarso-Suárez, C.; Roca-Pardiñas, J. & Tahoces, P.G. (2006). Using generalized additive models for construction of non-linear classifiers in computer-aided diagnosis systems. *IEEE Transactions on Information Technology in Biomedicine*, Vol.10, No.4, (April 2006), pp. 246-253, ISSN 1089-7771

Lado M.J.; Cadarso-Suárez, C.; Roca-Pardiñas, J. & Tahoces, P.G. (2008). Categorical variables, interactions and generalized additive models. Applications in computer-aided diagnosis systems. *Computer in Biology and Medicine*, Vol.38, No.4, (April 2008), pp. 475-483, ISSN 1879-0534

Li, F.; Arimura, H.; Suzuki, K.; Shiraishi, J.; Li, Q.; Abe, H.; Engelmann, R.; Sone, S.; MacMahon, H. & Doi, K. (2005). Computer-aided detection of peripheral lung cancers missed at CT: ROC analyses without and with localization. *Radiology*, Vol.237, No.11, (November 2005), pp. 684-690, ISSN 1527-1315

McCullagh, P. & Nelder, J.A. (1989) Generalized Linear Models, Chapman & Hall, ISBN 0-412-31760-5, London.

Mandelson, M.T.; Oestreicher, N.; Porter, P.L.; White, D.; Finder, C.A.; Tapli, S.H. & White, E. (2000). Breast density as a predictor of mammographic detection: comparison of interval- and screen-detected cancers. *Journal of the National Cancer Institute*, Vol.92, No.13 (July 2000), pp. 1081-1087, ISSN 1460-2105

Metz, C.E. (1986). ROC methodology in radiologic imaging. Investigative Radiology, Vol.21, No.9, September(1986), pp. 720-733, ISSN 0020-9996

Murphy, W.A. & DeSchryver-Kecskemeti, K. (1978). Isolated clustered microcalcifications in the breast: Radiologic-pathologic correlation. *Radiology*, Vol.127, No.5, (May 1978), pp. 335-341, ISSN 1527-1315

Obuchowski, N.A. (2005). ROC analysis. *American Journal of Roentgenology*, Vol. 184, No.2, (February 2005), pp. 364-372, ISSN 1546-3141

Park, S.C.; Chapman, B.E. & Zhen, B. (2011). A multistage approach to improve performance of computer-aided detection of pulmonary embolisms depicted on CT images: Preliminary investigation. *IEEE Transactions on Biomedical Engineering*, Vol.58, No.6, (June 2011), pp. 1519-1527, ISSN 0018-9294

Schousboe, J.T.; Kerlikowske, K.; Loh, A.; Cummings, S.R. (2011). Personalizing mammography by breast density and other risk factors for breast cancer: analysis of health benefits and cost-effectiveness. *Annals of Internal Medicine*, Vol.155, No.1, (July 2011), pp. 10-20, ISSN 1539-3704

Saveland, J.M. & Neuenschwander, L.F. (1990) A signal detection framework to evaluate models of tree mortality following fire damage. Forest Science, Vol.36, No.1, (January 1990), pp. 66–76, ISSN 1420-1143

Siegel, R.; Ward, E.; Brawley, O. & Jemal, A. (2011). Cancer statistics, 2011. The impact of eliminating socioeconomic and racial disparities on premature cancer deaths. *CA Cancer Journal for Clinicians*, Vol.61, No.4, (August 2011), pp. 212-236, ISSN 1542-4863

Tourassi, G.D.; Eltonsy, N.H.; Graham, J.H.; Floyd, C.E. & Elmaghraby, A.S. (2005). Feature and knowledge based analysis for reduction of false positives in the computerized detection of masses in screening mammography. *Proceedings of the 27th Annual Conference fo the IEEE EMB*, pp. 6524-6527, ISBN 0-7803-8741-4, Shanghai, China, September 1-4, 2005.

Van Dijck, J.A.; Verbeek, A.L.; Hendriks, J.H. and Holland, R. (1993). The current detectability of breast cancer in a mammographic screening program. A review of the previous mammograms of interval and screen-detected cancers. *Cancer*, Vol.72, No. 6, (June 1993) pp. 1933-1938, ISSN 1097-0142

Wood, S. (2006) *Generalized additive models: an introduction with R*, CRC Statistics, ISBN 9781584884743, United Kingdom.

Yoshida, H.; Masutani, Y.; MacEneaney, P.; Rubin, D.T. & Dachman, A.H. (2002). Computerized detection of colonic polyps at CT colonography on the basis of volumetric features: Pilot study. *Radiology*, Vol.222, No.2, (February 2002), pp. 327-336, ISSN 1527-1315